DIFFERENTIAL DIAGNOSIS IN PEDIATRIC RADIOLOGY

It is the
"wise and carefully considered differential diagnosis"
rather than the
"prodigious diagnostic stab"
which solves the problem most often.

DIFFERENTIAL DIAGNOSIS IN PEDIATRIC RADIOLOGY

Leonard E. Swischuk, M.D.

Professor of Radiology and Pediatrics
Director, Division of Pediatric Radiology
Child Health Center
The University of Texas Medical Branch
Galveston, Texas

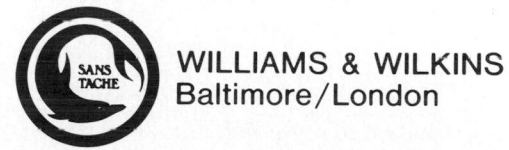

WILLIAMS & WILKINS
Baltimore/London

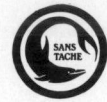

Editor: Toni M. Tracy
Copy Editor: Christopher Wienert
Design: Bert Smith
Illustration Planning: Lorraine Wrzosek
Production: Carol L. Eckhart

Made in the United States of America

Library of Congress Cataloging in Publication Data

Swischuk, Leonard E., 1937– .
   Differential diagnosis in pediatric radiology.

   1. Pediatric radiology. 2. Children—Diseases—Diagnosis. 3. Diagnosis, Differential. I. Title. RJ51.R3S89 1984   618.92′007572   83-21703 ISBN 0-683-08054-7

Composed and printed at the
Waverly Press, Inc.

To
My Family
My
Most Cherished
Possession

PREFACE

Most often the practice of radiology consists of arriving at a differential diagnosis for a radiologic finding or constellation of findings. Of course, there are situations where findings are so pathognomonic that only one diagnosis is possible, but these occasions are relatively rare. Therefore, after the radiologist finds the abnormality, his main job is to offer a weighted (if possible) differential diagnosis. It is to this end that this book is addressed and, to go beyond a simple gamut book, a reasonable amount of text and illustrative material accompanies the summarizing tables.

As usual, in producing a book such as this, many people are involved and without their support it would be very difficult to accomplish the project. I would, therefore, like to express my sincere appreciation to my secretary, Carmen Floeck, and our photographer, Mr. Milan Autengruber, for their mounds and mounds of work. In addition, I would like to express my appreciation to Melvyn Schreiber, M.D, our department chairman and Carlos Keith Hayden, Jr., M.D., my long time colleague and associate for their support in my daily work. To Charles J. Fagan go my thanks for his assistance and hard work in constructing Table 3.1A.

Leonard E. Swischuk, M.D.

CONTENTS

CHAPTER 2—FACE, SINUSES, MASTOIDS, AND NECK

CHAPTER 3—ABDOMEN

CHAPTER 4—BONES AND SOFT TISSUES

CHAPTER 5—HEAD

CHAPTER 6—THE SPINE

Chapter 1

CHEST

AERATION DISTURBANCES

Bilaterial Overaeration

Generally, bilateral overaeration of the lungs results from overly deep inspiratory efforts or expiratory obstruction (emphysema) of the lungs (Table 1.1). In terms of an overly deep inspiratory effort, the problem often simply is that of an overexuberant normal breath, accentuated by a voluntary Valsalva maneuver. What happens is that the technician tells the child to take a deep breath and "hold it," and in response, the patient performs a Valsalva maneuver. In infants, the same phenomenon occurs just before a cry. Fortunately, such artifactual overaeration usually is more pronounced on one view of the chest than the other, and in this way, one can determine that overaeration is not fixed. This is important because, if overaeration is fixed, further evaluation of the problem is required.

Another cause of bilateral, nonobstructive overinflation of the lungs is air hunger, a phenomenon present in patients who are oxygen deficient. In such patients, as long as pulmonary compliance is relatively normal, overbreathing to better oxygenate the blood leads to overdistended lungs. This most commonly occurs in patients with cyanotic heart disease (10). Another form of "air hunger" occurs in the acidotic infant, and actually, this is a much more common situation than hypoxemia. Acidotic patients, in an attempt to blow off excessive carbon dioxide, "overbreathe" and overinflate their lungs (Fig. 1.1). The finding, of course, is nonspecific and can occur with any number of metabolic disturbances leading to acidosis, but in the pediatric patient (especially the infant), it most commonly is due to severe diarrhea and dehydration (6). These patients also tend to demonstrate transient microcardia and decreased pulmonary blood flow due to the low blood volume induced by the severe degree of fluid loss. Such decreased blood flow causes the pulmonary blood vessels to become smaller than normal, the lungs to be oligemic, and hyperlucency to be even more pronounced (8).

When airway obstruction is the cause of overaeration, increased lung size and radiolucency are more fixed, and the obstruction can be central (trachea or upper airway) or peripheral (bronchial). Central obstruction is far less common, and in most cases, the obstruction usually is located from somewhere just below the glottis to the carina. Obstructions above this level tend to cause underaeration more than

overaeration (i.e., inspiratory obstruction predominates). With peripheral obstruction, air trapping is diffuse and the lungs become large and radiolucent. Clinically, these patients often demonstrate expiratory wheezing and stridor.

Lesions causing central obstructions usually are extratracheal compressive lesions, for endotracheal lesions such as inflammatory granulomas, tumors, foreign bodies, tracheal stenoses (congenital or acquired), and ectopic endotracheal thyroid tissue are

Table 1.1 Bilateral Overaeration

A. Nonobstructive overaeration	
Overexuberant inspiration Air hunger—dehydration—acidosis	Commonest
Air hunger—cyanotic heart disease	Moderately common
B. Obstructive emphysema (peripheral)	
Viral lower respiratory tract infection (bronchitis, bronchiolitis)	Commonest
Asthma	Common
Cystic fibrosis	Moderately common
Immunologic deficiency Thermal bronchiolitis	Relatively rare
Cutix laxa Antitrypsin deficiency Multiple peripheral F.B.	Rare
C. Obstructive emphysema (central)	
Vascular ring	Moderately common
Mediastinal mass or cyst Enlarged lymph nodes Laryngotracheal foreign body	Relatively rare
Endotracheal mass	Very rare

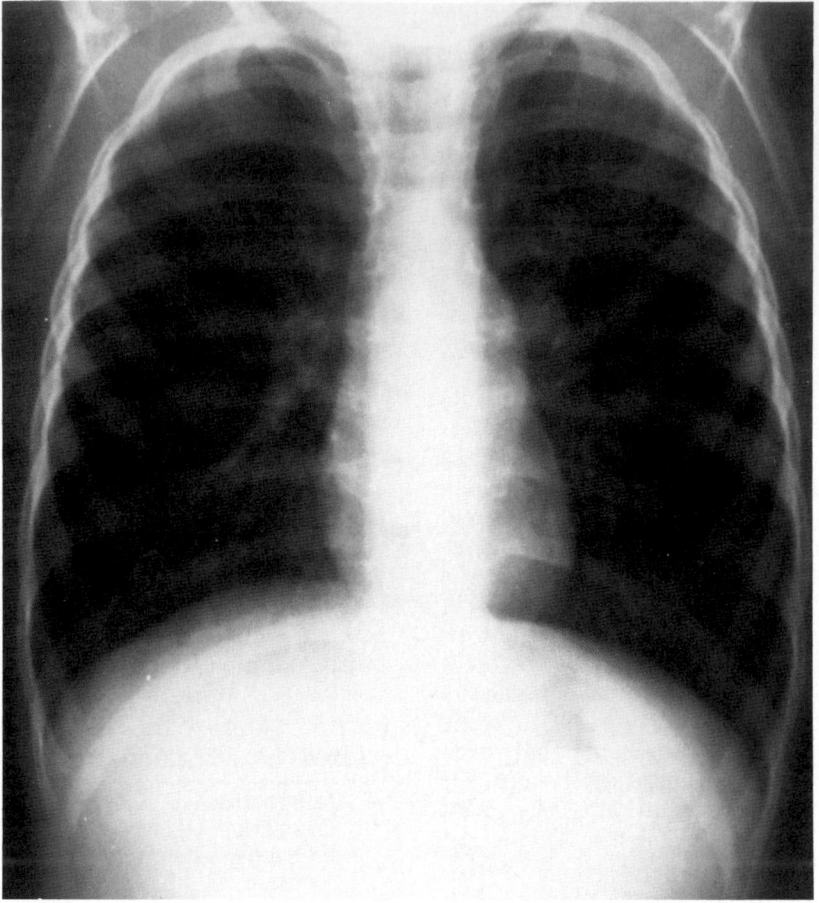

Fig. 1.1. Overaeration due to dehydration. Note the overdistended but clear lungs. Also note that the heart is smaller than normal (dehydration causes microcardia).

relatively rare. Extratracheal lesions causing airway compression include entities such as abnormal blood vessels, mediastinal cysts or tumors (primary and secondary), and enlarged lymph nodes (inflammatory or tumorous).

In terms of vascular abnormalities, congenital anomalies, rather than acquired aneurysms or other dilations are the usual problem. In this regard, often one is dealing with a true vascular ring and the main roentgenographic clue to its presence is a right side aortic arch (Fig. 1.2). The reason for this is that in the two most common vascular rings (double aortic arch and right side aorta with aberrant left subclavian artery and ligamentum arteriosus or ductus arteriosus), a right aortic arch is present (10). With double aortic arch, the two arches encircle the trachea and esophagus, while with aberrant left subclavian artery, the right aortic arch, aberrant left subclavian artery traveling behind the esophagus, and the ligamentum arteriosum or ductus arteriosus extending from the left subclavian artery to the pulmonary artery comprise the ring (Fig. 1.3). Both of these rings have a right side aortic arch, and thus, if the aortic arch is on the left, a vascular ring causing airway obstruction is a very remote possibility.

A right side aortic arch produces one or more of the following findings: deviation of the trachea to the left, ipsilateral indentation and compression of the trachea, and a right paratracheal mass or lump. This latter finding, of course, represents the aortic knob which usually is somewhat higher in position than it would be if it were normal and on the left (Fig. 1.2). In addition, there is absence of the aortic knob on the left, and on lateral view, when a vascular ring exists, anterior tracheal deviation frequently also occurs.

After these observations are made, confirmation of the presence of a vascular ring is best accomplished with a barium esophagram, where the vessels comprising the ring produce opposing indentations on the esophagus. Occasionally, these indentations lie directly across from one another, but more often, they are offset so as to produce a reverse-S configuration (Fig. 1.2). Of course, posterior indentation of the esophagus also is present, but since such indentation can be seen with other asymptomatic arterial anomalies, it is the reverse-S configuration which is most important to note. After this, just which of the two vascular rings exist is best demonstrated with aortography.

Less commonly, compression of the trachea is due

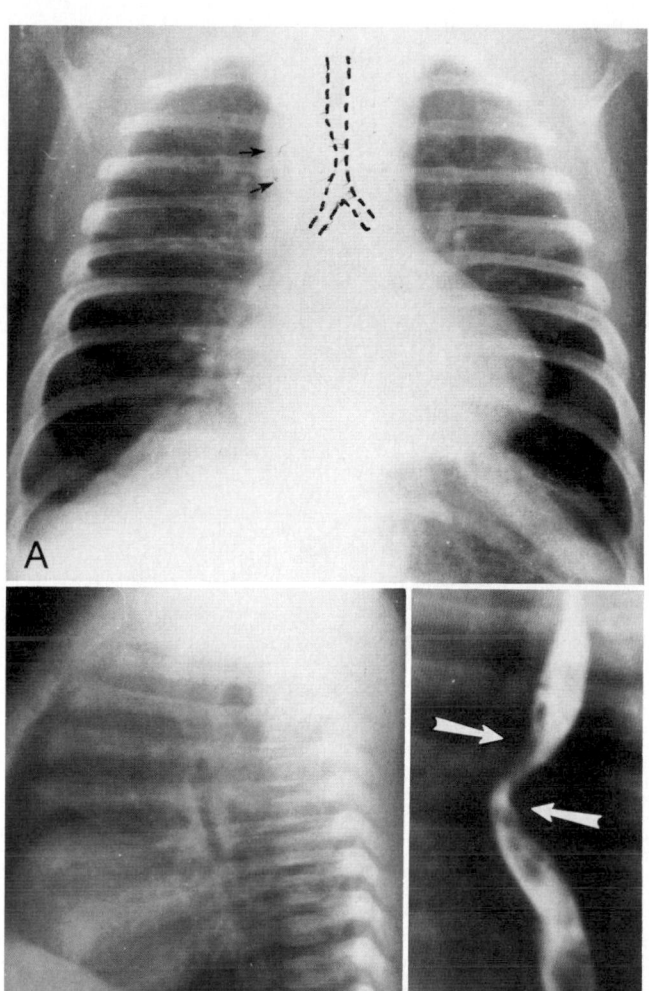

Fig. 1.2. Overaeration with vascular ring. A. Frontal view demonstrating marked overaeration of both lungs. Note subtle evidence of a right side aortic arch (arrows). In infants, this finding usually is subtle; but, in older children, the findings are more distinct and consist of an aortic knob on the right and associated indentation and deviation of the trachea to the left (see Fig. 1.36A). B. Lateral view demonstrates marked overaeration and flattening of the diaphragmatic leaflets. This patient had chronic wheezing and expiratory stridor. C. Barium swallow demonstrating characteristic reverse-S indentation of the esophagus (arrows). In other cases, the indentations lie directly across from each other.

to an anomalous innominate or left common carotid artery (Fig. 1.4). The former is much more common, but even in these cases, the indentation produced by the anomalous vessel usually is associated with no symptoms (9). Occasionally, severe obstruction of the airway results (1), but most often the finding should be treated with caution and significance attached only

if other causes of airway obstruction have been excluded. Tracheal compression with these anomalies is anterior, and the indentation is demonstrable on lateral chest films only (Fig. 1.4). The tracheal deformity is the same for both anomalous innominate or left common carotid artery, and results from the fact that the origin of these vessels from the aortic arch either is too far to the left (innominate artery), or too far to the right (left common carotid artery). In either case, as the vessel crosses the mediastinum, it becomes "stretched" and, as such, causes compression of the anterior surface of the trachea. Although bronchoscopy and bronchography have been used to demonstrate the presence of these vessels, if one requires complete documentation of the anomaly, one should turn to aortography. However, this seldom is required because the indentation is rather characteristic and, except for the severe cases, surgery is not performed. If it is, it takes the form of tacking the artery to the posterior surface of the sternum. However, it is best to let these infants grow out of their problem, for by the age of 4 or 5, or even sooner, anatomical rearrangements in the growing mediastinum are such that compression disappears (1, 8). Consequently, such tracheal indentation is not seen in older children.

Mediastinal cysts, tumors, or enlarged lymph nodes causing compression of the airway usually are identified by the unilateral or bilateral mediastinal widening which they produce. In addition, compression and deformity of the tracheal air column are seen, but overall, the plain film findings are nonspecific. Barium esophagrams also usually are nonspecific, and eventually one must employ procedures such as CT scanning, aortography, venography, or ^{131}I isotope studies (thyroid masses) for final delineation. Indeed, most times CT scanning will be performed before any of the more invasive procedures are contemplated. If the compressing mass is large enough, and touches the chest wall, ultrasonography also is useful. One problem with ultrasonography, however, is that if the mass does not touch the chest wall, the air space between the wall and the lesion interferes with proper imaging. Bronchography seldom is necessary in the investigation of these lesions.

Obstructive emphysema secondary to widespread peripheral bronchial or bronchiolar obstruction most classically occurs in viral lower respiratory tract infection (including infantile bronchiolitis), asthma, and cystic fibrosis (2–4) (Fig. 1.5). With viral lower respiratory tract infection, one of the main problems is bronchial infection with bronchospasm. Bronchial inflammation leads to mucosal edema, hypersensitive bronchi with exaggerated constriction during expiration, air-trapping, and obstructive emphysema. The entire problem is seen in its worst form in acute infantile bronchiolitis. Indeed, in the most severe cases, the lungs hardly change in size between inspiration and expiration; the thoracic cage is grossly overdistended and the diaphragmatic leaflets flattened or even slightly inverted. Interestingly enough, most

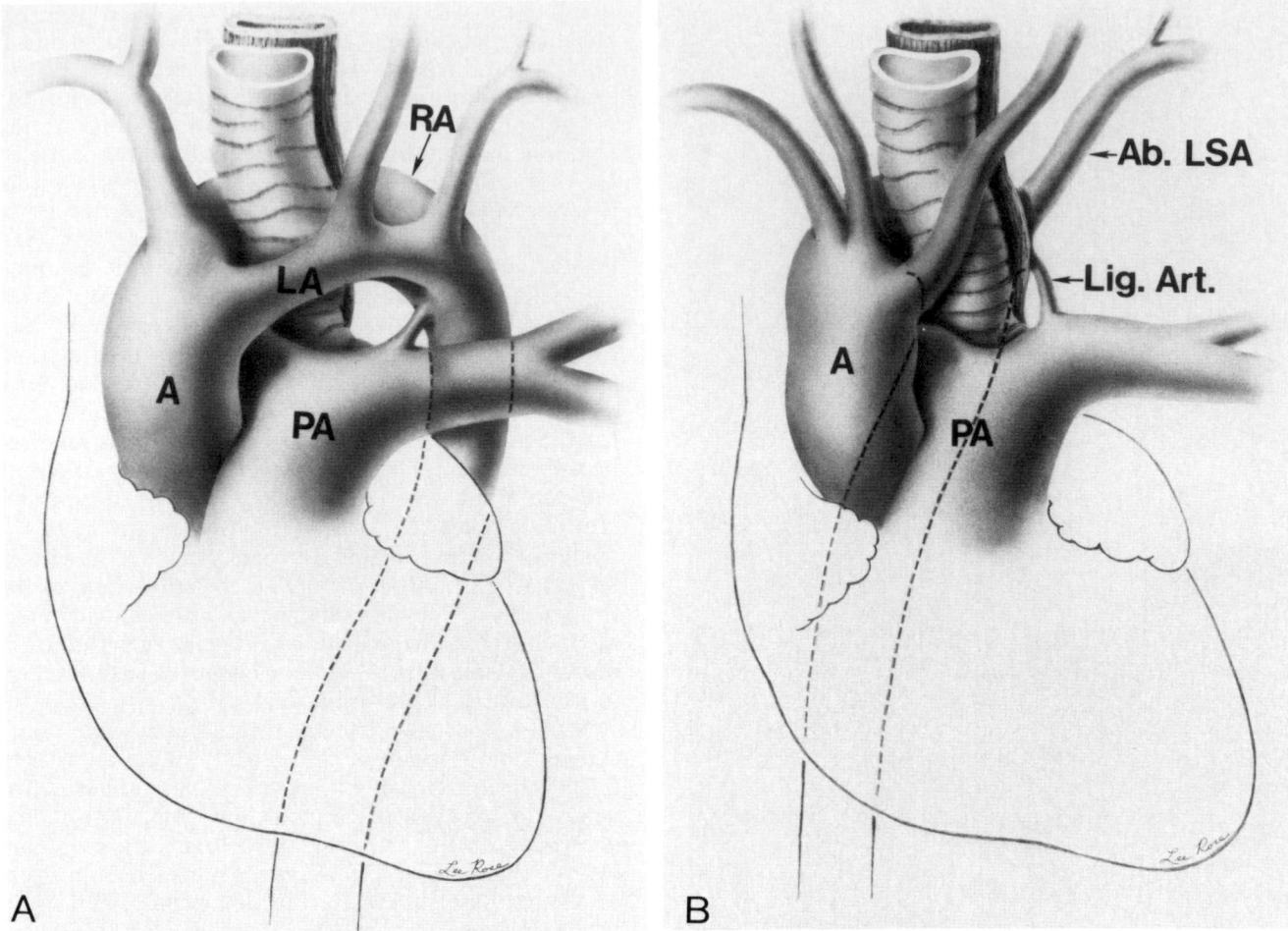

Fig.1.3. The two most common vascular rings. A. **Double aortic arch.** Note the two arches of the aorta; the right (RA) usually is larger and higher than the left (LA). Both unite behind the esophagus and the resultant encircling ring is obvious. Aorta (A), Pulmonary artery (PA). B. **Right aortic arch with aberrant left subclavian artery and ligamentum arteriosum or ductus arteriosus.** The ring in this anomaly is completed by the ligamentum arteriosum (Lig. Art.) or patent ductus arteriosus which connects the aberrant left subclavian (Ab. LSA) artery (passing behind the esophagus) with the left pulmonary artery (passing in front of the trachea). Aorta (A), Pulmonary artery (PA).

of these infants do not demonstrate parenchymal infiltrates, although a good many show parahilar-peribronchial infiltrates (bronchial inflammation) leading to shaggy hilar regions. To a lesser extent, similar peripheral bronchial obstruction occurs with viral lower respiratory tract infections throughout childhood, but it is the infant with bronchiolitis (0 to 2 years of age with peak incidence around 6 months) who demonstrates overaeration most profoundly.

Findings similar to those seen with viral bronchiolitis also can be seen in infants with cystic fibrosis, and actually, it is not uncommon for these infants to present with a bronchiolitis-like picture on a number of occasions before the proper diagnosis is established. However, infants with cystic fibrosis tend to demonstrate more in the way of parahilar-peribronchial infiltrates and areas of atelectasis from the onset. Nonetheless, it is not uncommon at all for the first one or

two episodes in an infant with cystic fibrosis to be interpreted as being due to repeated bouts of viral bronchiolitis.

In the older child with viral lower respiratory tract infection, parahilar-peribronchial infiltration is the rule, and many times, patchy parenchymal infiltrates (usually areas of atelectasis), commonly are present. The same holds true for asthma, cystic fibrosis, and certain immunologic deficiency states. In addition, similar findings can be produced with chronic esophageal reflux or swallowing abnormalities leading to pulmonary disease. However, most common will be viral lower respiratory tract infection, with or without underlying asthma.

Generalized overaeration due to bronchial or bronchiolar constriction, generally unassociated with pulmonary infiltrates, also can be seen with Alpha$_1$ antitrypsin deficiency (1), congenital cutis laxa (5), and

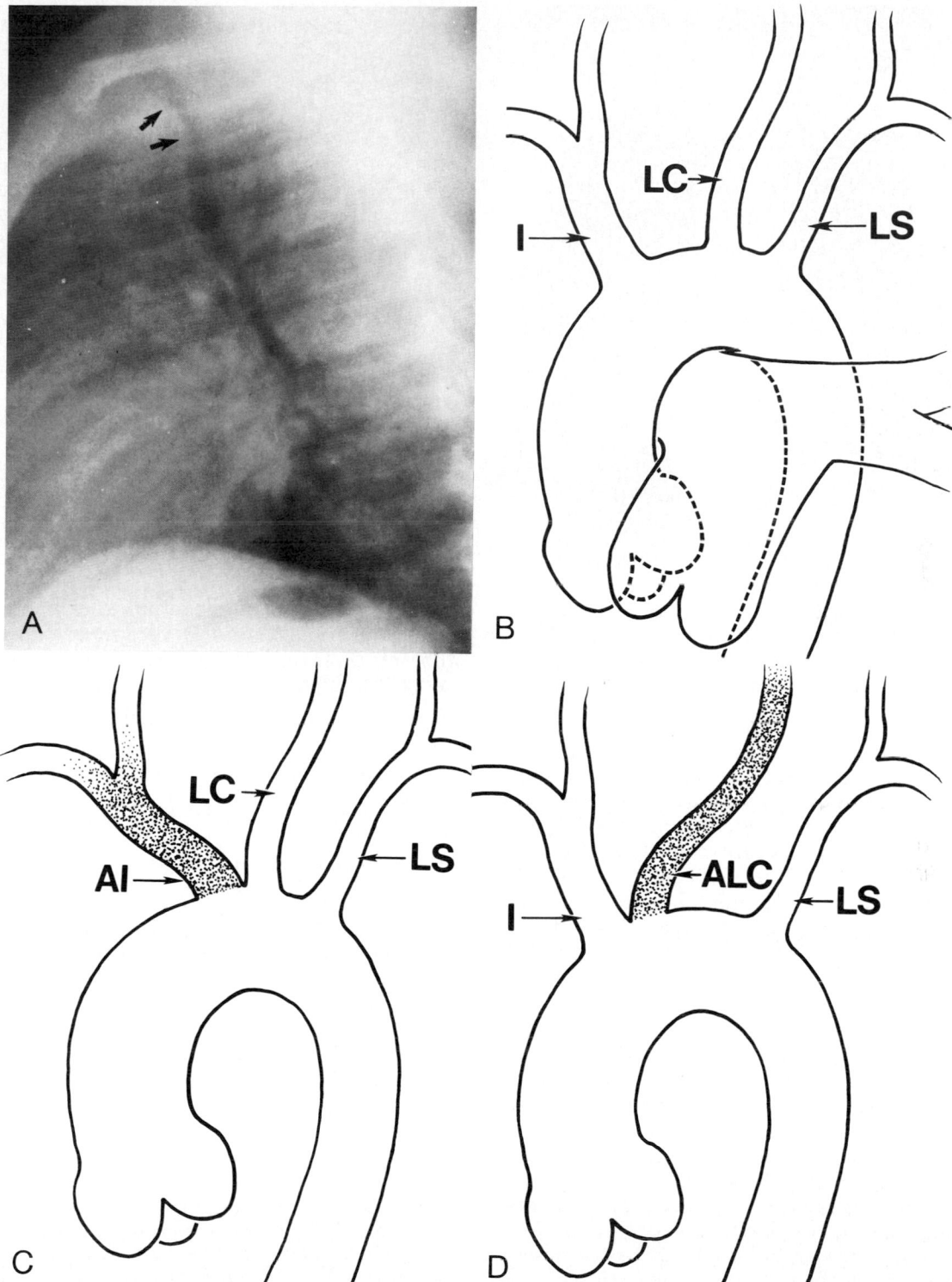

Fig. 1.4. Anomalous innominate or left common carotid artery. A. Note the characteristic indentation and posterior displacement of the trachea (arrows) which can be produced by either one of these anomalies. The anomalous innominate artery, however, is much more common. Even then, though, the indentation most often is asymptomatic. B. **Normal arrangement of vessels.** Note normal separation of the three great arteries; the innominate (I), left common carotid (LC), and left subclavian (LS) arteries. C. **Anomalous innominate (AI) artery.** The innominate artery arises too far to the left. D. **Anomalous left common carotid (ALC) artery.** The left carotid artery arises too far to the right.

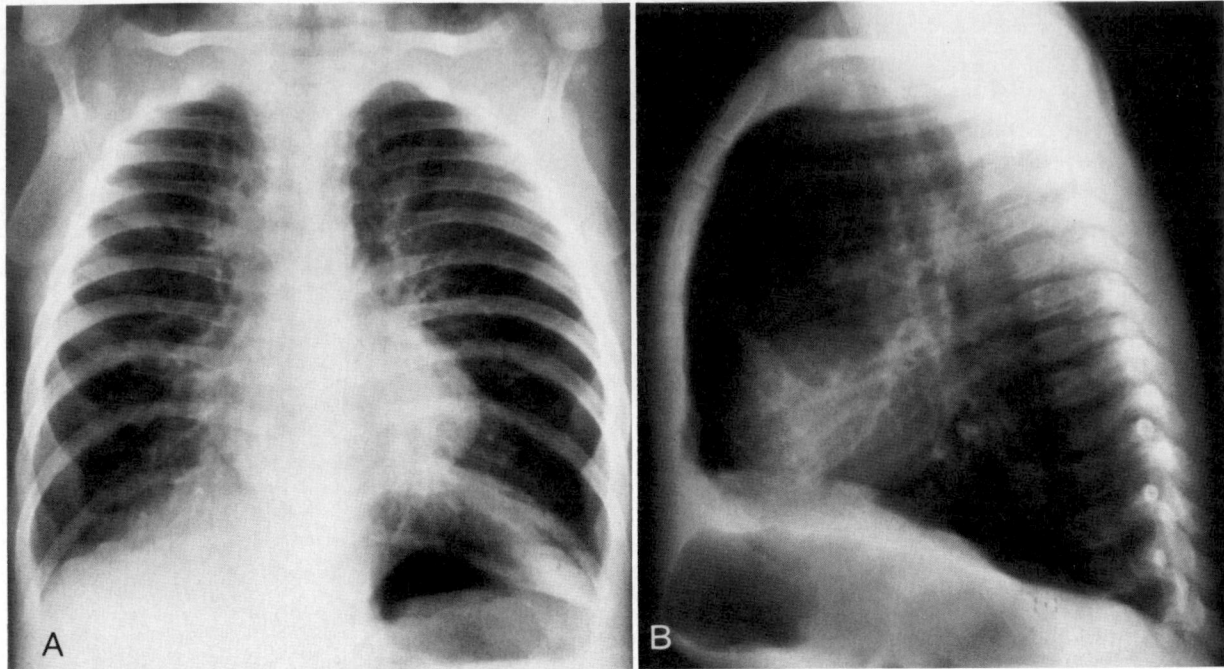

Fig. 1.5. Overaeration in diffuse bronchial disease. A. Frontal view demonstrating marked overaeration of the lungs and extensive parahilar-peribronchial infiltrates in this infant with cystic fibrosis. B. Lateral view demonstrating the same findings. Similar findings can be seen in patients with viral lower respiratory tract infection and asthma. In bronchiolitis, often there is less in the way of parahilar-peribronchial infiltration.

thermal bronchiolar damage secondary to smoke or hot air inhalation. However, all of these conditions are rather rare. Similarly, so are multiple foreign body fragments scattered in numerous bronchi, bilaterally.

Finally, a word regarding **intercostal bulging and cervical herniation of the lungs,** as seen with obstructive emphysema, is in order. It is true that such bulging of the lungs through the various soft tissue spaces of the thoracic cage occurs with obstructive emphysema, but it also can be seen in a normal infant performing a Valsalva maneuver, just before starting to cry. In addition, although **flattening of the diaphragmatic leaflets is a common feature of obstructive emphysema, to a degree, it also can be seen in nonobstructive overaeration. Most often, this also occurs in the normal patient performing a voluntary Valsalva maneuver.** I have seen this on numerous occasions and the finding also has been noted by Riggs (7). Consequently, before one accepts flattening of the diaphragmatic leaflets as a definite finding, one should be sure that it is present on both views. Only then can one be certain that it is due to fixed airway obstruction.

References

1. Berdon WD, Baker DH, Bordiuk J, Mellins R: Innominate artery compression of trachea in infants with stridor and apnea. *Radiology* 92:272–278, 1969.

2. Eggleston PA, Ward BH, Pierson WE, Bierman CW: Radiographic abnormalities in acute asthma in children. *Pediatrics* 54:442–449, 1974.

3. Kirkpatrick JA, Wagner ML: Roentgen manifestations of bronchiolitic inflammatory disease. *Pediatr Clin North Am* 10:633–642, 1963.

4. Koch DA: Roentgenologic considerations of capillary bronchiolitis. *Am J Roentgenol* 82:433–436, 1959.

5. Merton DF, Rooney R: Progressive pulmonary emphysema associated with congenital generalized elastolysis (cutis laxa). *Radiology* 113:691–692, 1974.

6. Nathan MH: Diagnosis of dehydration, acidosis, and gastroenteritis in infants from chest radiography. *Radiology* 83:297–305, 1964.

7. Riggs WW Jr: *Pediatric Chest Roentgenology—Recognizing the Abnormal.* St. Louis, Warren H. Green, 1979, p 198–203.

8. Swischuk LE: Microcardia: an uncommon diagnostic problem. *Am J Roentgenol Radium Ther Nucl Med* 103:115–118, 1968.

9. Swischuk LE: Anterior tracheal indentation in infancy and early childhood: normal or abnormal? *Am J Roentgenol Radium Ther Nucl Med* 112:12–17, 1971.

10. Swischuk LE: *Plain Film Interpretation in Congenital Heart Disease,* ed 2. Baltimore, Williams & Wilkins, 1979, pp 210–226.

11. Talamo RC, Levison H, Lynch MJ, Hercz A, Hyslop NE Jr, Bain HW: Symptomatic pulmonary emphysema in childhood associated with hereditary A_1 antitrypsin and elastase inhibitor deficiency. *J Pediatr* 79:20–26, 1971.

Bilateral Underaeration

The most common cause of bilateral underaeration is a poor inspiratory effort, and while many times this occurs because the infant is too sick, weak, or depressed to initiate good respiratory activity, more often than not, it is due to faulty radiographic technique (Table 1.2). However, underaeration also can be due to diaphragmatic elevation secondary to large abdominal masses or fluid collections, diaphragmatic paralysis, and central obstruction of the airway (1, 2). Airway obstruction leading to bilateral underaeration can be caused by foreign bodies (either central in the trachea or bilateral in the bronchi), intraluminal tumors or granulomas, extrinsic masses or cysts, and compressing vascular anomalies or aneurysms. These lesions, in themselves, of course, are not rare, but usually they produce overaeration, and the circumstance of their causing bilateral underaeration is rather uncommon, and frequently missed. Other causes of chronically shallow inspirations include muscular or neurogenic disease.

In those cases where impaired air entry is the cause of underaeration, paradoxical inspiratory phase widening of the superior mediastinum and cardiac silhouette occurs (2). Under normal circumstances, of course, during inspiration, both the superior mediastinum and cardiac silhouette become smaller, but with inspiratory obstruction, negative intrathoracic pressures increase and paradoxical enlargement of the heart and mediastinum occurs. It is not always easy to appreciate these changes, however, and to avoid missing them, one must keep the phenomenon in mind and be certain that the film is, in fact, an inspiratory film.

Table 1.2 Bilateral Underaeration

Poor inspiration	}	Commonest
Abdominal distention (mass, fluid, etc.)	}	Common
Primary muscle disease Neurogenic disease Diaphragmatic paralysis	}	Moderately common
Inspiratory airway obstruction	}	Relatively rare

References

1. Blazer S, Naveh Y, Friedman A: Foreign body in the airway: a review of 200 cases. *Am J Dis Child* 134:68–71, 1980.
2. Capitanio MA, Kirkpatrick JA: Obstructions of the upper airway in children as reflected on the chest radiograph. *Radiology* 107:159–161, 1973.

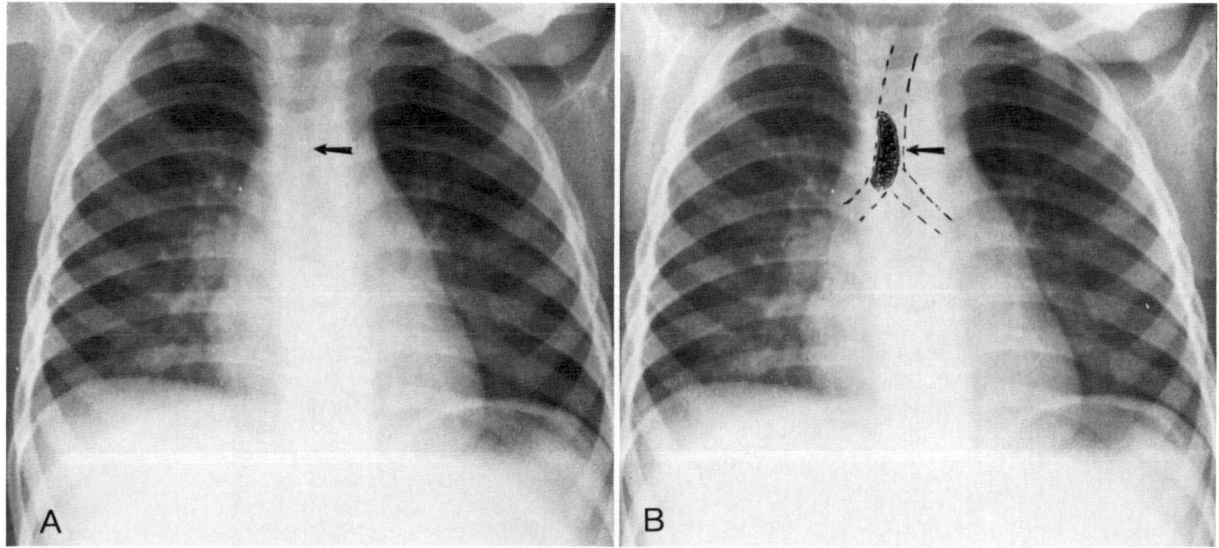

Fig. 1.6. Underaeration with tracheal foreign body. A. This is an inspiratory film (note distended trachea), but the lungs are underaerated. The reason is that there is a peanut, just vaguely visible (arrow) in the trachea. B. Peanut and trachea outlined. Courtesy of C. J. Fagan, M.D.

Unequal Lung Aeration, Size, and Vascularity (Which Side Is Abnormal?)

To one degree or another, lung size, aeration, and vascularity (pulmonary blood flow) are interrelated, but the relationships are not always the same. In other words, in some cases, a lung may be enlarged, hyperlucent, and undervascularized, while in others, it may be large, hyperlucent, but normally vascularized. Each set of circumstances represents a different pathophysiologic disturbance, and knowledge as to just which is present usually is available from plain chest films. A problem arises, however, when one is uncertain as to which side is abnormal. This is a frequent dilemma, but if one applies three or four simple rules to one's analysis of the initial inspiratory film, and the subsequent inspiratory-expiratory film sequence, one almost always will be able to decide which lung is abnormal (Table 1.3).

Customarily, the decision as to which lung is abnormal has been accomplished by noting mediastinal shift. In some cases, this can be done with relative ease, but in others, it is more difficult (i.e., is the mediastinum pushed or pulled to one side?). If one cannot make this decision, then one cannot decide which side is abnormal, and because of this, I have come to rely on other findings. However, before embarking on their discussion, it might be emphasized

Table 1.3 Unequal Lung Size, Aeration, and Blood Flow (Which Side is Abnormal?)

Inspiratory film
1. Side with normal or ↑ vascularity usually is normal
2. Side with ↓ vascularity usually is abnormal
3. Small, *completely* opaque side is abnormal

Inspiratory-expiratory films
1. Side which changes size less, or not at all, is abnormal

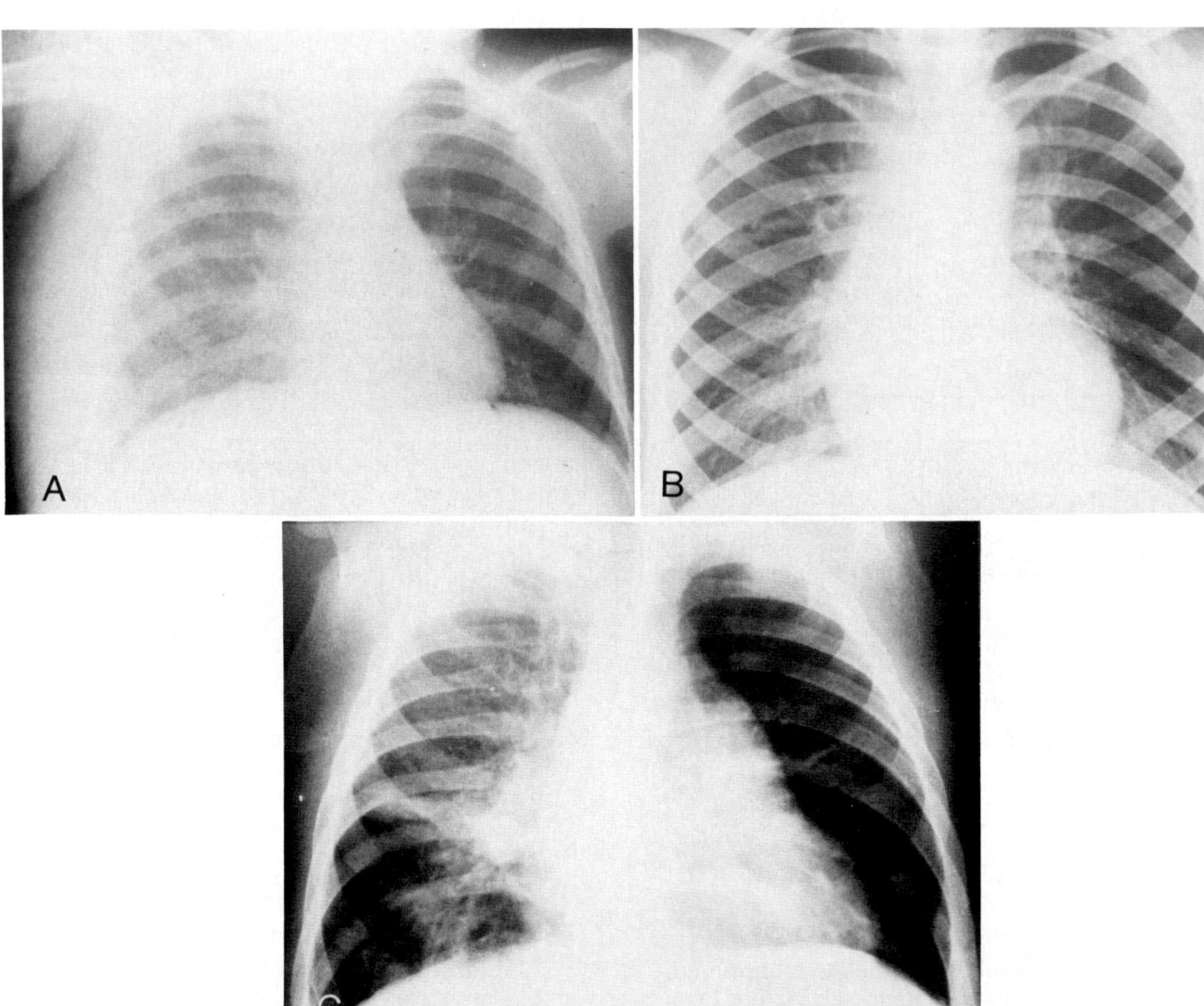

Fig. 1.7. "Apparent" unequal aeration. A. The left lung appears more radiolucent than the right, but the vascularity is equal. Density over right lung is due to edmatous soft tissues secondary to a burn. B. The left lung is slightly more radiolucent than the right. This is due to absence of the left pectoralis muscle. Note associated underdevelopment of the upper four ribs on the left. C. Rotation to the left causes the left lung to appear more radiolucent. The mediastinal edge also appears sharper. This patient had a viral lower respiratory tract infection with parahilar-peribronchial infiltrates and some linear atelectasis on the right. Actually, lung aeration is equal, but appears unequal because of rotation.

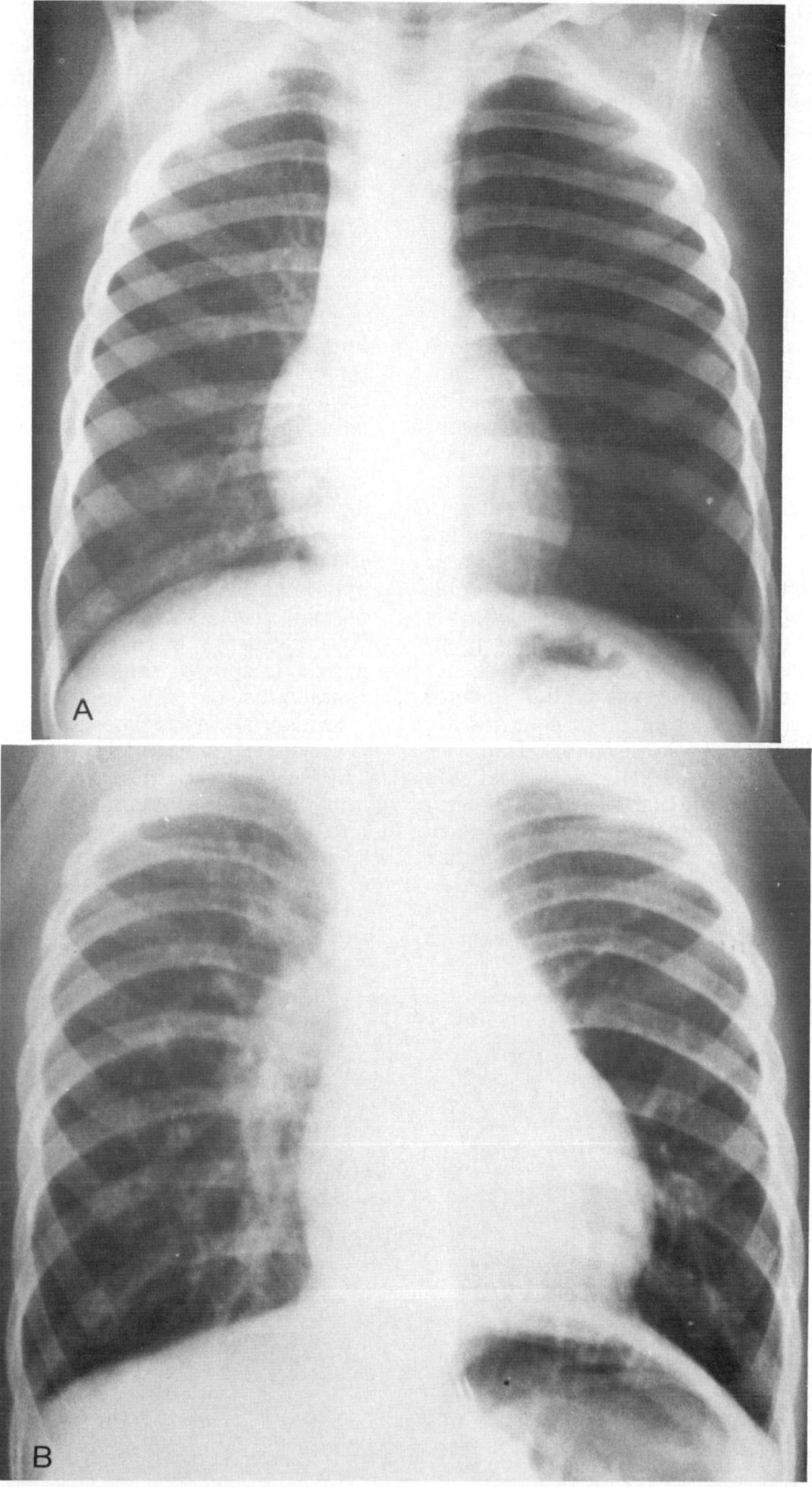

Fig. 1.8. Hyperlucent lung with decreased vascularity. A. The left lung is hyperlucent, slightly larger than the right, and shows diminished vascularity. The problem is obstructive emphysema due to a foreign body in the left bronchus. B. This patient also demonstrates decreased vascularity on the left, but in addition, the left lung is small and radiolucent. The problem is left lung hypoplasia. In both cases, decreased vascularity is the clue to the radiolucent lung being the abnormal one.

that certain artifactual physical factors such as thick, overlying soft tissues, absence of soft tissue, poor tube centering, grid cut-offs, patient rotation, etc., be entirely eliminated as causes of "apparently" unequal aeration (Fig. 1.7). This seems straightforward, but it is important.

RULE 1: IF VASCULARITY IS DECREASED, THE LUNG IS ABNORMAL

This rule holds whether the lung is large or small. Decreased pulmonary blood flow in such lungs can be due to pulmonary artery obstruction, hypoplasia, absence, or spasm (Fig. 1.8). Spasm usually is a reflex phenomenon (secondary to hypoxia and subsequent acidosis) which occurs when a lung ceases to ventilate normally (i.e., infection, obstruction). It is as if the pulmonary artery knew that there was little use in sending blood to the nonventilating lung, and although the phenomenon is nonspecific, it can occur rather quickly after ventilation is interfered with. With pulmonary artery hypoplasia or absence (agenesis), it is not difficult to see why pulmonary blood flow is diminished and similarly, with pulmonary artery obstruction, the problem often also is straightforward (i.e., intravascular embolus or extrinsic compression by an adjacent mediastinal cyst or tumor). However, obstruction more often is more generalized and it is due to widespread peripheral compression of the vessels by obstructed emphysematous lungs. In such cases, compression probably acts in concert with reflex arterial spasm (i.e., nonventilating lung), and together these factors can reduce blood flow to near zero. With this degree of abnormality, there is no problem in

convincing one's self that pulmonary blood flow is decreased, and that the lung should be abnormal. In less striking cases, however, uncertainty may prevail, and then one best go on to inspiratory-expiratory films.

RULE 2: IF PULMONARY VASCULARITY IS NORMAL OR INCREASED, THE LUNG PROBABLY IS NORMAL

This is the corollary of rule 1. In other words, if a lung demonstrating decreased pulmonary vascularity is abnormal, then one demonstrating normal or increased blood flow should be normal. This may seem an almost foolishly simplistic rule, but one will come to see its usefulness when one is dealing with a large, radiolucent, or hyperlucent lung on one side and a small, radiolucent lung on the other (Fig. 1.9). If the large lung, in such cases, is compensatorily overinflated, even though one's first temptation is to call it abnormal (because it is so large) one will reverse one's opinion once its pulmonary vasculature is assessed. The vascularity in these cases will be normal or engorged, in spite of the fact that the lung is large and overaerated.

Evidence of such bloodflow shift may be more obvious in certain cases that others for usually it takes a little time for the shift to develop. As a consequence, it might be less pronounced in acute problems such as foreign bodies, and very florid in chronic problems such as unilateral pulmonary artery and lung agenesis or hypoplasia. Nonetheless, one often is surprised to see how rapidly such blood shift can occur with an acute problem.

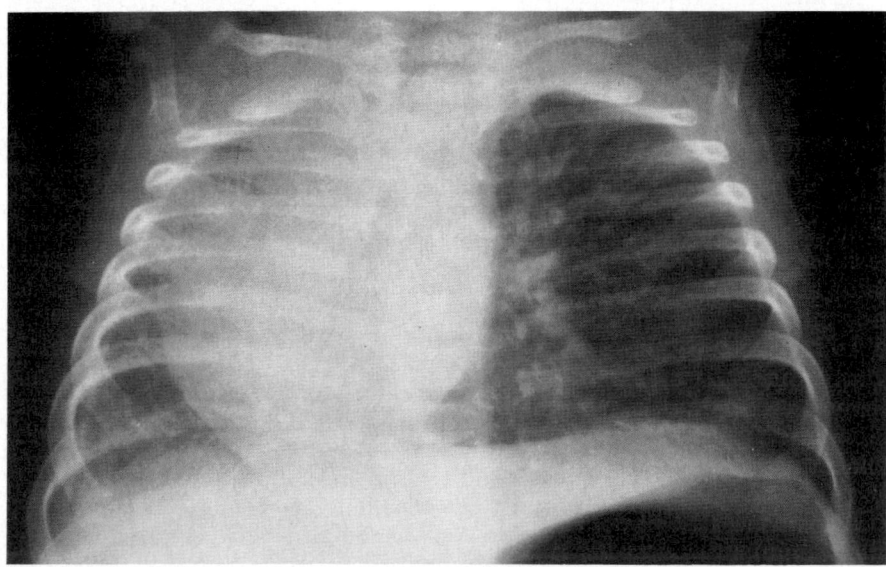

Fig. 1.9. Hyperlucent lung with normal or increased vascularity. At first one might pick the more radiolucent and larger left lung as the abnormal one (i.e., obstructive emphysema). However, note that its vascularity is normal, and in fact, increased. For this reason, it could not be abnormal and the real problem is partial agenesis (upper lobe) of the right lung with compensatory overaeration of the left lung. More than normal volumes of blood are flowing through the left lung because the right lung cannot accept a normal flow of blood.

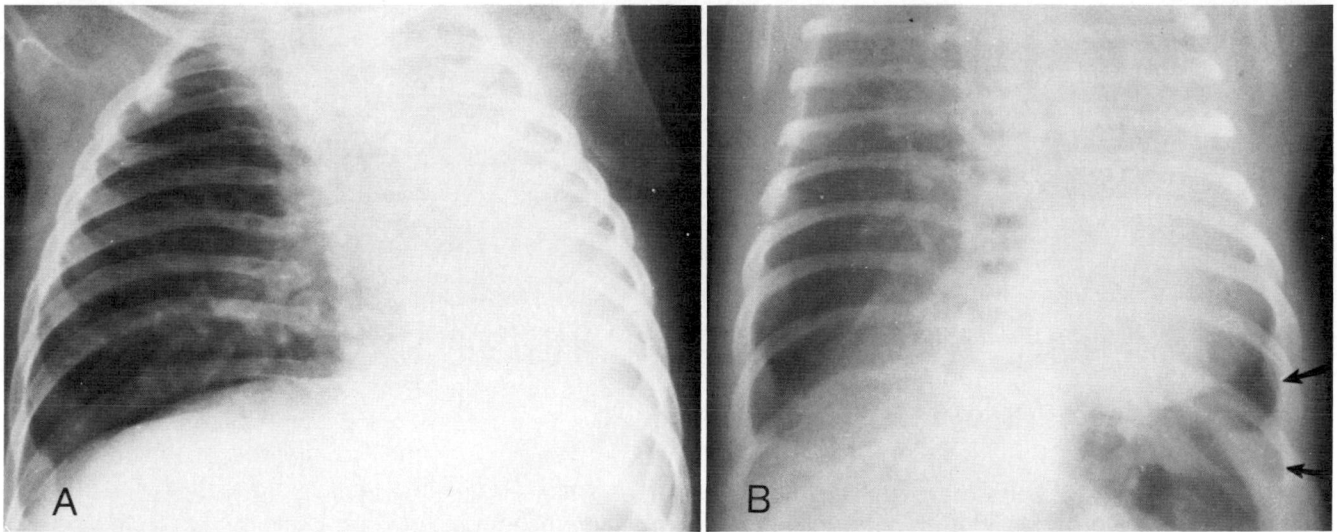

Fig. 1.10.   Small, totally opaque hemithorax versus almost totally opaque hemithorax. A. Note the small, totally opaque left hemithorax in this young infant. No air at all is present in the left lung. The problem was left lung agenesis. The right lung shows compensatory emphysema, and as might be expected, slightly engorged pulmonary vascularity. B. This patient presents with an almost similar picture except that there is a triangle of aerated lung (arrow) in the left costophrenic angle. Even though the left hemithorax is nearly totally opaque, this triangle of aerated lung should cause one to look at the other side more critically. In actual fact, it is this other side (right lung) which is abnormal. It is emphysematously overdistended because of congenital lobar emphysema, and is causing compression of the left lung. However, even though the right lung is markedly enlarged, it cannot completely compress the left lung and some aeration (triangular radiolucency) remains.

RULE 3: A SMALL, COMPLETELY OPAQUE HEMITHORAX IS THE ABNORMAL HEMITHORAX

The **key word** to the proper interpretation of cases demonstrating this finding is "**complete.**" In other words, the involved hemithorax must be completely opaque, and the best way to evaluate this is to inspect the costophrenic angle. If the angle is opaque, then the hemithorax is totally opaque, and if it is not, then the hemithorax is not completely opaque. This is an important distinction because, if a small hemithorax is deemed totally opaque, it is the abnormal one and the problem should be either total atelectasis or agenesis (Fig. 1.10A). Atelectasis in such cases can be presumed resorptive (i.e., secondary to obstruction), and not compressive (i.e., compression by an overdistended contralateral lung), for no matter how large a pathologically obstructed, overdistended lung becomes, it does not compress the other lung to the point of total opacification (Fig. 1.10B). This rule, however, holds for the inspiratory film only, for if the film is made during expiration, the normal lung can be totally compressed. This phenomenon is difficult, if not impossible, to accomplish during inspiration. As a sidepoint, the same pathophysiology exists with large, opaque masses in the chest, for no matter how large they become, they seldom cause total compression and opacification of the other lung during inspiration.

RULE 4: WITH INSPIRATION-EXPIRATION, THE LUNG CHANGING SIZE LEAST, OR NOT AT ALL, IS THE ABNORMAL LUNG

The preceding three rules are applied to the inspiratory chest film, and thereafter the inspiratory-expiratory film sequence should be obtained. It will either confirm one's inspiratory film impressions or solve the problem in those cases where uncertainty persists. Once the inspiratory-expiratory film sequence is obtained, no matter what one's initial inspiratory film impression is, one can be assured that the lung which changes size least, or not at all, is the abnormal lung. This is true of a lung which is hypoplastic, emphysematous because of obstruction, atelectatic, or agenetic. The reason for this is that all one is doing is documenting the fact that either air movement or parenchymal distensibility are abnormal. The degree of abnormality, of course, decrees the degree of change, but virtually always, discrepancy between the two sides exists (Figs. 1.11 and 1.12). The only exception occurs with mild unilateral, congenital hypoplasia of a lung, where the mildly hypoplastic lung functions in near normal or completely normal fashion.

In the vast majority of cases, with the four rules applied, seldom does one need fluoroscopy for the assessment of unequal aeration. This, of course, is not to denounce the procedure, but merely to indicate that

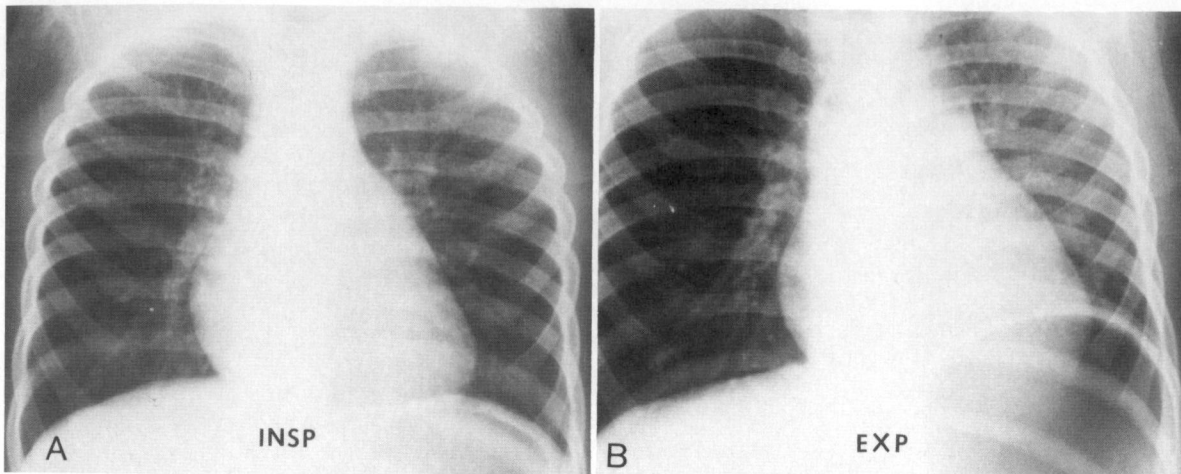

Fig. 1.11. Value of inspiratory-expiratory film sequence. A. On this inspiratory view, one would have considerable difficulty determining that an obstructing foreign body is present on the right. Clinically, however, this was the prime consideration. B. Expiratory view clearly demonstrates air trapping in the right lung, consistent with a foreign body in the right main bronchus.

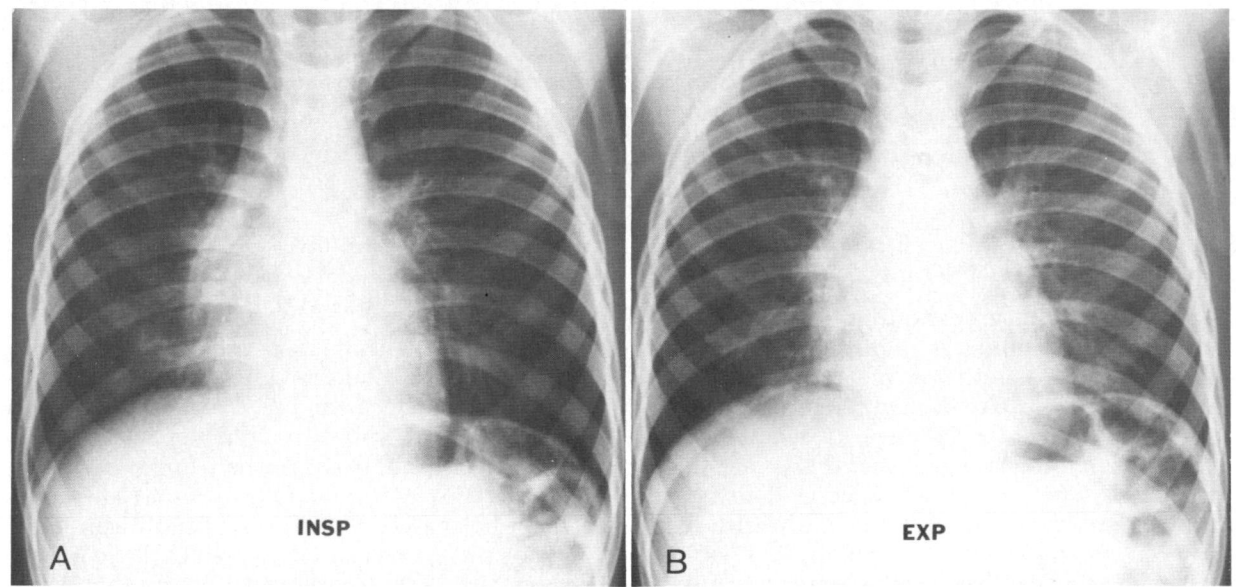

Fig. 1.12. Inspiratory-expiratory sequence—lung which changes size least is the abnormal lung. A. On this **inspiratory view,** note that the left lung is much larger than the right. However, vascularity is about the same on both sides and it might be difficult to determine which lung is abnormal. B. **Expiratory film** clearly shows that the left lung is the one which changes volume most markedly. The right lung, in fact, has not changed size at all, and on expiration, is the larger lung. This clearly indicates obstructive emphysema on the right, which in this patient with asthma, was due to an obstructing mucous plug.

plain films usually suffice. However, if fluoroscopy is performed, one will note characteristic mediastinal shifts and ipsilateral diaphragmatic immobilization. After assessment of the inspiration-expiratory film sequence, one's next decision usually will be whether to use isotope scans (either ventilation or perfusion), bronchoscopy, bronchography, angiography, or tomography to obtain further information. To some extent, this will depend on the presenting history; i.e., acute problems usually go on to bronchoscopy, while chronic problems may require a number of these other studies before the problem is finally resolved.

Large Opaque Hemithorax

A large opaque hemithorax is due most often to large accumulations of fluid in the pleural space, and in the pediatric age group, pus (empyema) is the most common fluid (Table 1.4). Other types of fluid include serous, bloody, or chylous effusions, but after the newborn period, chyle accumulations are uncommon. For the most part, they occur after thoracic surgery or chest trauma, and are due to thoracic duct injuries. Bloody effusions usually occur in association with chest trauma, but occasionally, such bleeding can occur with rupture of a congenital aneurysm of the ductus arteriosus (usually an infant) or a blood dyscrasia. However, all of these situations are relatively uncommon, and consequently, in the pediatric age group, **pleural fluid is pus until proven otherwise.**

Roentgenographically, it is impossible to differentiate one type of fluid from another, and even though chyle contains fat, it does not appear significantly more radiolucent than other types of fluid. Perhaps with CT scanning, utilizing attenuation factors, it would be possible to determine that chyle is present, but on plain films, it is a difficult task. Overall, then, the findings with any type of fluid depend primarily on the volume of fluid, and in advanced cases, contralateral shift of the mediastinum is seen. In addition,

inversion of the ipsilateral diaphragmatic leaflet often occurs (especially on the left), and of course, the lung on the same side is so compressed that neither parenchymal aeration nor an air bronchogram is seen (Fig. 1.13). In less advanced cases, however, the lung is less compressed, the opaque hemithorax near normal or normal in size, and the findings confusing. The reason for this is that residual aeration of the lung is present and to the uninitiated suggests that consolidation, rather than fluid in the pleural space, is the problem (see Fig. 1.19).

Empyemas can be seen with any number of bacterial infections, but most commonly occur with staphylococcal, hemophilus, and pneumococcal pneumonias. Staphylococcal pneumonia has a wide age range, while hemophilus pneumonia tends to occur in infants and young children (under the age of 2 yr). Pneumococcal pneumonias have an age range comparable to staphylococcal infections, except that they are a little less

Table 1.4 Large Opaque Hemithorax

1. Fluid (massive accumulation)	}	Commonest
Pus (empyema)	}	Commonest
Effusion with Lymphoma (abdomen or chest) Neuroblastoma (abdomen or chest) Metastases Renal disease Subdiaphragmatic infection	}	Common
Effusion with Tuberculosis Fungus Primary chest tumor Pancreatitis Liver tumor Other abdominal tumors	}	Relatively rare
Blood Chyle	}	Relatively rare
2. Large mass or cyst	}	Relatively rare
3. Diaphragmatic hernia	}	Neonatal problems
4. Fluid-filled lung (bronchial atresia CLE)		

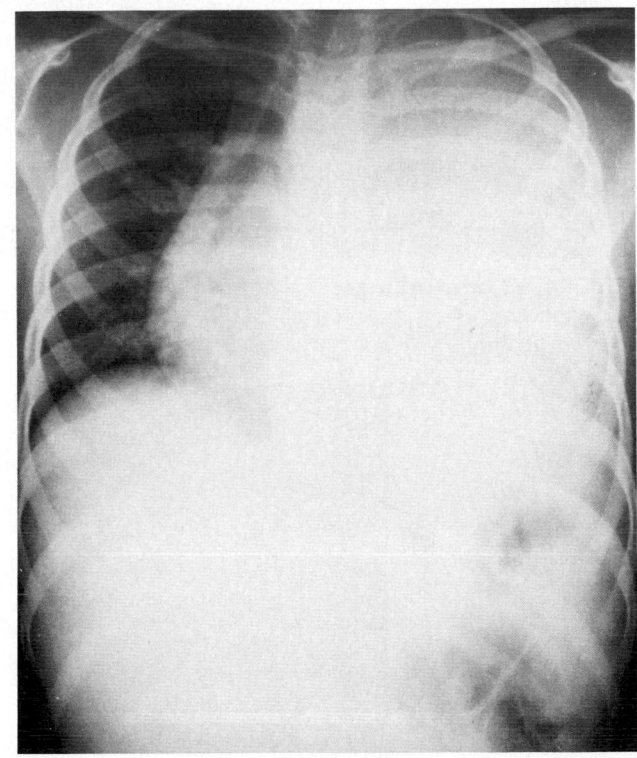

Fig. 1.13. Large opaque hemithorax—empyema. There is no problem in deciding that the abnormality is on the left. The entire left hemithorax is opacified, the mediastinum shifted to the right, and the left diaphragmatic leaflet and stomach depressed. In addition, there is no air in the peripheral bronchi of the left lung. This patient had a pneumococcal empyema which was completely compressing the left lung. For lesser degrees of this problem, where a confusing air bronchogram in a partially compressed lung may be seen, see Figure 1.19.

common in the young infant. With massive serous pleural effusions, a number of underlying diseases can be present, but most commonly one will be dealing with kidney disease such as the nephrotic syndrome or an intrathoracic or abdominal tumor such as lymphoma or neuroblastoma. Other intrathoracic tumors (i.e., teratoma, mesothelioma, etc.) presenting as a massive pleural effusion are less common, but occasionally the situation does arise (Fig. 1.14). Quite rarely, massive pleural effusions can be seen with primary pulmonary tuberculosis, fungal disease, and viral infections (1, 4). Pleural effusions with the col-

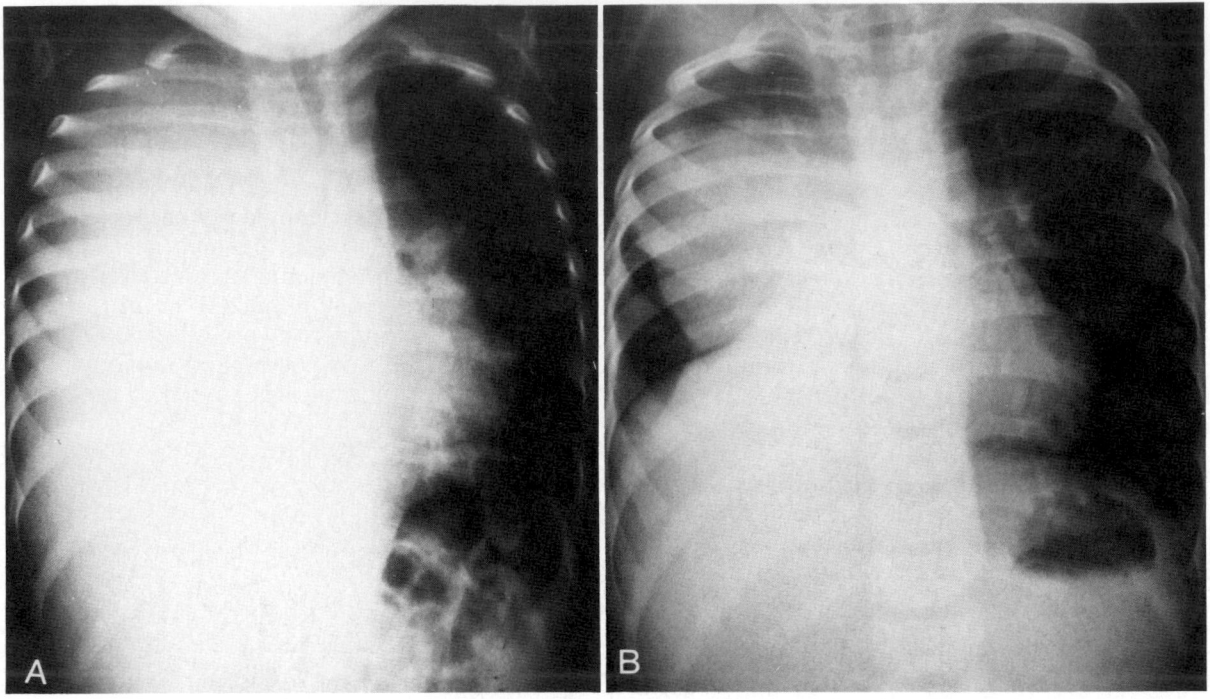

Fig. 1.14. Large opaque hemithorax—large pleural effusion with underlying tumor. A. The findings are nonspecific and suggest a large fluid accumulation on the right. B. After thoracentesis, a large mass remains. This was a teratoma.

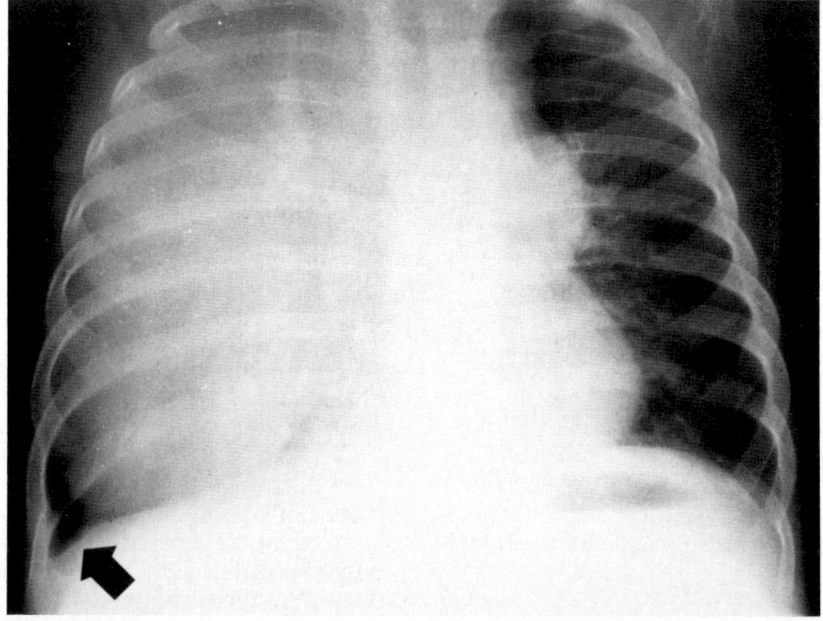

Fig. 1.15. Large opaque hemithorax—large mass. A large lymphoma infiltrated thymus gland is producing the opaque right hemithorax in this patient. The clue to the fact that the problem is a large mass rather than a large collection of pleural fluid is that there is a triangle of aerated lung in the right costophrenic angle (arrow).

lagen vascular diseases and acute glomerulonephritis, are common, but to have the effusion so massive that total unilateral chest opacification results is rare. On the right, massive unilateral pleural effusions can occur with subphrenic or hepatic tumors or abscesses, and on the left with subphrenic abscesses or pancreatic infections. Pancreatitis, less frequently, produces the same findings on the right.

Other causes of a totally opaque hemithorax are unlikely to occur beyond the neonatal period, for they include the fluid-filled lung of congenital lobar emphysema or bronchial atresia (2, 3), the solid right lung syndrome (5), and the airless diaphragmatic hernia. Occasionally, one can encounter a patient with a large cyst or intrathoracic mass which causes near total opacification of a hemithorax, but in most of these cases, residual aeration of the ipsilateral lung, seen as a triangular radiolucency in the costophrenic angle, occurs (Fig. 1.15). It is most important to make this latter observation, for when the radiolucent tri-

angle is seen, massive accumulation of fluid in the hemithorax cannot be the cause of opacification. For this reason, one would not want to perform a thoracentesis, a procedure which is mandatory when fluid is the cause of opacification.

References

1. Cho CT, Hiatt WO, Behbehani AM: Pneumonia and massive pleural effusion associated with adenovirus type 7. *Am J Dis Child* 126:92–94, 1973.
2. Fagan CJ, Swischuk LE: The opaque lung in lobar emphysema. *Am J Roentgenol Radium Ther Nucl Med* 114:300–304, 1972.
3. Griscom NT, Harris GBC, Wohl MEB, Vawter GF, Eraklis AJ: Fluid-filled lung due to airway obstruction in the newborn. *Pediatrics* 43:383–390, 1969.
4. Pinckney L, Parker BR: Primary coccidioidomycosis in children presenting with massive pleural effusion. *Am J Roentgenol* 130:247–249, 1978.
5. Swischuk LE, Hayden CK Jr, Richardson J: Neonatal opaque right lung. *Radiology* 141:671–673, 1981.

Small Opaque (Hazy) Hemithorax

For the most part, a distinctly small, hazy, or opaque hemithorax indicates a volume loss problem, and almost always one is dealing with atelectasis or pulmonary agenesis (Table 1.5). Of course, whether the lung is hazy or totally opaque depends on the degree of abnormality present. With partial agenesis (one or two lobes only) or incomplete atelectasis, the hemithorax is hazy, while with complete atelectasis and

total unilateral pulmonary agenesis, it is opaque (Fig. 1.16 and also see Fig. 1.9C). Atelectasis, of course, is much more common and leading the list of causes are conditions such as improper endotracheal tube positioning, mucous plugs (most often secondary to viral lower respiratory tract infection and/or asthma), and foreign bodies. Then come endobronchial granulomas and tumors, but they are far less common than mucous

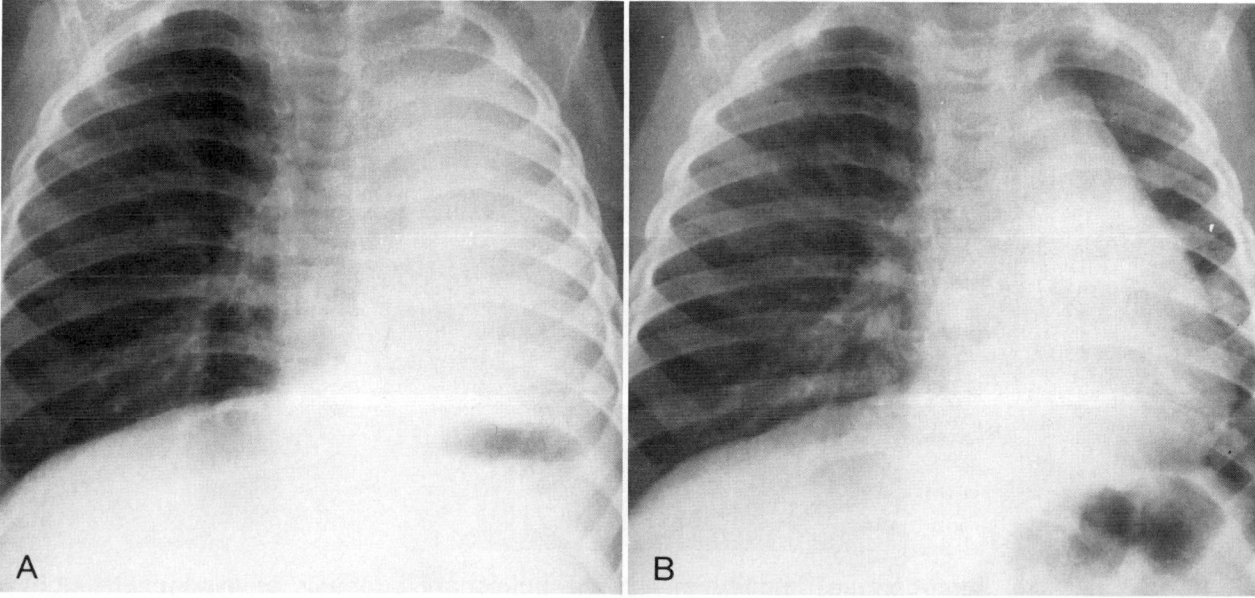

Fig. 1.16. Small opaque hemithorax—total atelectasis. A. The left hemithorax is small and totally opaque. There is no triangular radiolucency in the left costophrenic angle. This should suggest that the problem is on the left. In addition, the pulmonary artery branches in the large right lung are far too prominent for the right lung to be the abnormal one. A foreign body was present on the left, and the right lung was compensatorily overinflated. B. Twenty-four hr earlier, same patient, only partial collapse of the left lung is present. Because of this, the lung, although small, is not opaque.

plugs and foreign bodies. Similarly, so are extrinsic, compressive lesions such as strategically located mediastinal cysts, masses, or abnormal vessels.

As regards abnormal vessels, the one most commonly encountered (although still quite rate) is the aberrant left pulmonary artery, or so-called pulmonary sling (1, 3–6). In this condition, the left pulmonary artery, as it arises anomalously from the right pulmonary artery, swings around the right side of the carina and compresses the right bronchus (see Fig. 1.36C). Most often, there is variable atelectasis of the right lung, but occasionally, obstructive emphysema can result (1). This condition is discussed more fully later (p 34), but at the moment, it might be noted that the aberrant left pulmonary artery, and indeed, all

vascular abnormalities, eventually are best identified with pulmonary angiography or aortography.

As noted earlier, when atelectasis or agenesis are partial, the involved hemithorax is small and hazy rather than small and opaque (Fig. 1.17). Partial agenesis, for the most part, is a problem of the right lung, and usually the upper and middle lobes are the ones which are agenetic. The anomaly commonly is associated with abnormalities such as accessory diaphragm, abnormal veins (scimitar syndrome), sequestration, and A-V fistula. It also has been termed the hypogenetic right lung syndrome (2). Overall, the condition is rather innocuous, but to the uninitiated, the x-rays in these children almost always are misinterpreted for a pulmonary infection or massive atelectasis

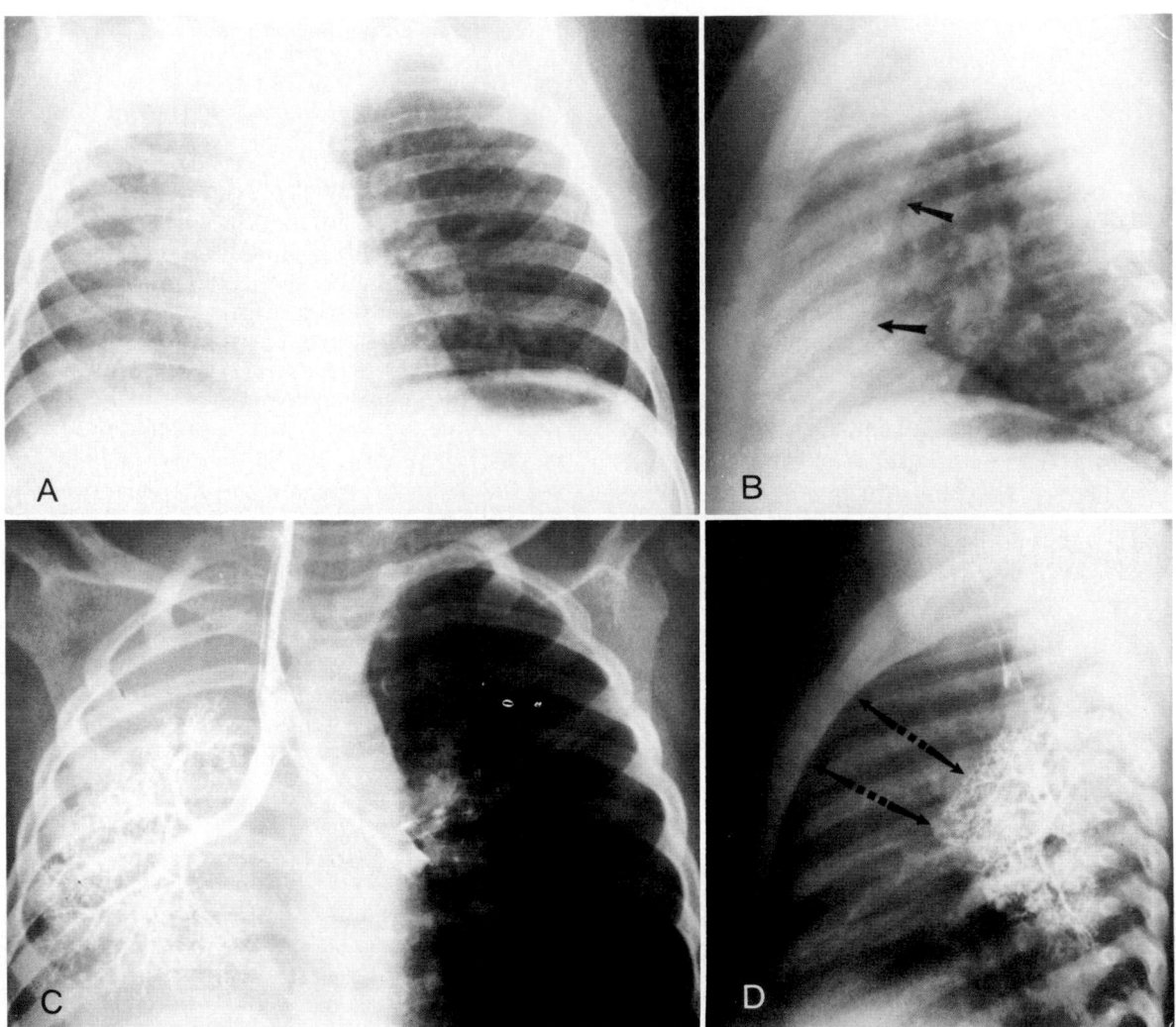

Fig. 1.17. Small hazy (semi-opaque) hemithorax—partial pulmonary agenesis or hypogenetic right lung syndrome. A. Note that the right hemithorax is smaller than the left. It also is hazy and there is ipsilateral shift of the mediastinum. B. Lateral view demonstrating the typical retrosternal density seen with agenesis of the right, upper, and middle lobes (arrows). This is due to the aerated lower lobe abutting areolar soft tissue replacing the absent middle and upper lobes. C. Bronchogram demonstrating absence of the right upper and middle lobe bronchi. Only the lower lobe bronchus and its branches are present. D. Lateral view showing absence of any lung tissue in the anterior compartment (where the right middle and upper lobes should be).

(Fig. 1.18). Indeed, many of these patients are subject to procedures such as bronchoscopy, bronchography, pulmonary angiography, and isotope perfusion or ventilation studies, and while all of these studies can clearly define where the problem lies, if one is familiar with the condition, investigation beyond the chest film can be avoided.

Table 1.5 Small or Normal Size Opaque Hemithorax

A. Small opaque or hazy hemithorax		
Atelectasis	}	Commonest
Pulmonary agenesis	}	Relatively rare
B. Normal size opaque or hazy hemithorax		
Pleural fluid on supine film	}	Commonest
Developing empyema or other fluid	}	Moderately common
Total lobe consolidation (all lobes on one side)	}	Very rare

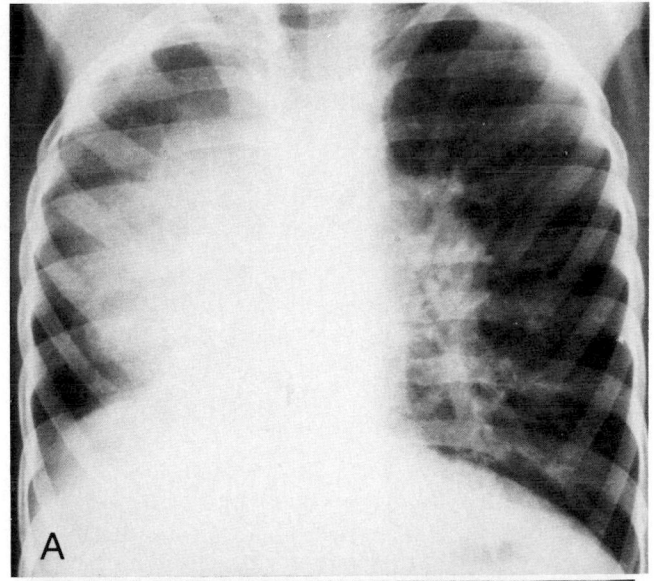

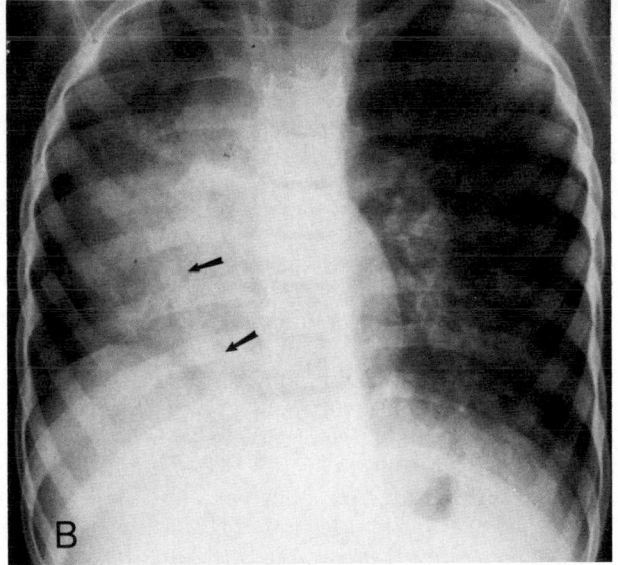

Fig. 1.18 A and B.

Fig. 1.18. Small hazy (semi-opaque) hemithorax mimicking pneumonia. A. A pneumonia might erroneously be suggested on the right. However, one should ask, "Why is there so much volume loss on the right?" and "Why is the pulmonary artery and its branches so prominent on the left?" These are unusual findings for an acute pneumonia, and overall, should suggest that the problem is on the right, chronic, and due either to atelectasis or agenesis. B. Another view (overpenetrated) in the same patient 3 yr earlier demonstrates a characteristic abnormal vein (scimitar syndrome). This is in keeping with the diagnosis of a hypogenetic right lung with middle and upper lobe agenesis. The abnormal vein is less clearly visualized in Figure A.

Normal Size Opaque or Hazy Hemithorax

There are a few instances where a hemithorax is opaque or hazy and yet relatively normal in size (Table 1.5). Most often, this occurs when fluid layers along the posterior chest wall in a patient who is examined in the supine position. With the aerated lung located above the fluid, the end result is a hazy but relatively normal sized hemithorax. A similar problem can occur with pus loculated along the posterior or anterior chest wall. Another time, when a hemithorax is opaque or hazy, and yet of relatively normal size, is during the development of an empyema. Although a similar problem can arise with other fluid accumulations, most often it occurs with empyema. In such cases, the volume of fluid is not large enough to completely compress the lung, but yet large enough to cause considerable opacification of the hemithorax (Fig. 1.19). In such cases, because the lung is incompletely compressed, some parenchymal aeration, and certainly an air bronchogram, remain, and because of this, one often is led to believe that consolidation is the problem. However, one should realize that total consolidation of an entire lung (all lobes) is very uncommon. Although consolidating pneumonias can occur in two different lobes of the two lungs, involvement of two adjacent lobes is rather uncommon, and the involvement of all three lobes would be most unusual. Consequently, when one encounters a film such as the one seen in the patient demonstrated in Fig. 1.19, thoracentesis should be the next step, for fluid in the pleural space is the problem. It is impor-

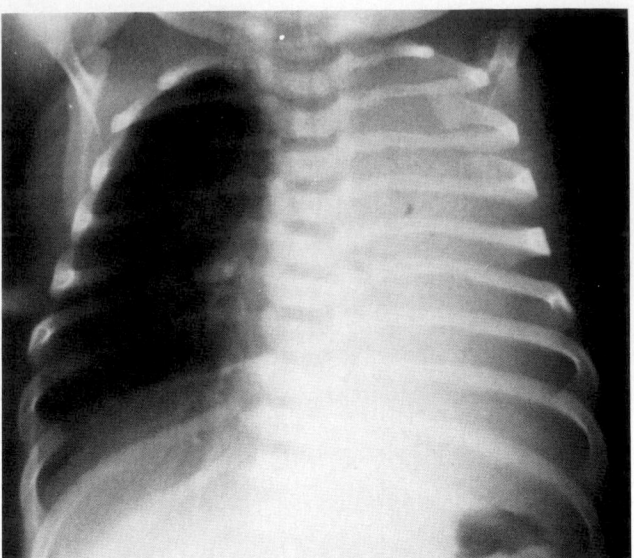

Fig. 1.19. Small or normal size, opaque hemi-thorax—developing empyema. The left hemithorax in this patient is opaque, but normal size. However, fluid is present in the pleural space, and an empyema is developing. One can determine this by noting that the air bronchogram ends about 3 cm from the chest wall. The space between the most peripheral portion of the air bronchogram and chest wall is full of pus. The

tant to be aware of this concept of the developing empyema, for since its configurations are so varied, this is the one way in which one can get on the right track early. Ultrasound is an excellent modality with which to demonstrate the fluid in these patients.

References

1. Capitanio MA, Ramos R, Kirkpatrick JA: Pulmonary sling: roentgen observations. *Am J Roentgenol Radium Ther Nucl Med* 112:28–34, 1971.
2. Felson B: Pulmonary agenesis and related anomalies. *Sem Roentgenol* 7:17–30, 1972.
3. Jue KL, Raghib G, Amplatz K, Adams P Jr, Edwards JE: Anomalous origin of the left pulmonary artery from the right pulmonary artery. *Am J Roentgenol* 95:598–610, 1965.
4. Philip T, Sumerling MD, Fleming J, Grainger RG: Aberrant left pulmonary artery. *Clin Radiol* 23:153–159, 1972.
5. Taybi H: Congenital malformations of the larynx, trachea, bronchi and lungs. In Kaufman HJ (ed): *Progress in Pediatric Radiology.* Chicago, Year Book Medical Publishers, 1967, p 237.
6. Tesler UF, Balsara RH, Niguidula F: Aberrant left pulmonary artery (vascular sling): report of five cases. *Chest* 66:402–407, 1974.

combination of findings should not be misinterpreted for a consolidating pneumonia of the entire left lung, for this would be a very unusual situation.

Large Radiolucent (Hyperlucent) Hemithorax

Most often, when one encounters a large, hyperlucent hemithorax, one is dealing with obstructive or compensatory emphysema of an entire lung (Table 1.6), and when emphysema is compensatory, almost always it is secondary to complete atelectasis or agenesis of the contralateral lung. Occasionally, it is due to contralateral pneumonectomy, but in childhood, this is a rare situation. In any of these cases, the large, hyperlucent lung is easy to identify, and with its normal or increased vascularity, should be chosen as the normal lung (Fig. 1.20; also see Figs. 1.10A and 1.16). Of course, once again, it does take time for such blood flow shift to occur, and generally, the compensatorily overinflated lung develops a greater degree of hypervascularity with a chronic problem such as pulmonary agenesis than with acute atelectasis. However, even with acute atelectasis, contralateral blood flow can appear increased at surprisingly early stages (Fig. 1.20).

If all cases of a compensatorily overinflated lung were secondary to total atelectasis or agenesis on the other side, very little problem in interpretation would arise. However, in some cases, partial agenesis (a lobe or two) or near static endobronchial obstruction of the other lung occurs, and the lung is neither totally collapsed nor grossly overinflated (Figs. 1.17 and 1.21). As a result, one has a situation where the lungs may be unequal in size (often not by much) but yet both

radiolucent. In such cases, the chance of erroneous diagnosis is great, and only the astute observer will note that the vascularity in the smaller lung is slightly decreased. This observation, however, is critical because it then designates the smaller lung as abnormal. Once having made this observation, the inspiratory-expiratory film sequence can be utilized to confirm one's findings. During inspiration and expiration, the smaller, abnormal lung changes its size very little or not at all (Fig. 1.21). In these cases, the abnormality of air flow to and from the lung is such that, during inspiration, enough air gets into the lung to prevent the development of atelectasis, and during expiration, not enough is trapped to allow the lung to become

Table 1.6 Large Hyperlucent (Radiolucent) Hemithorax

Obstructive emphysema	}	Commonest
Compensatory emphysema[a]		
Ordinary pneumothorax	}	moderately common
Anterior pneumothorax		
Cystic disease of the lung		
Large pneumatocele	}	Relatively rare
Diaphragmatic hernia (stomach)		

[a] Changes size on inspiration-expiration.

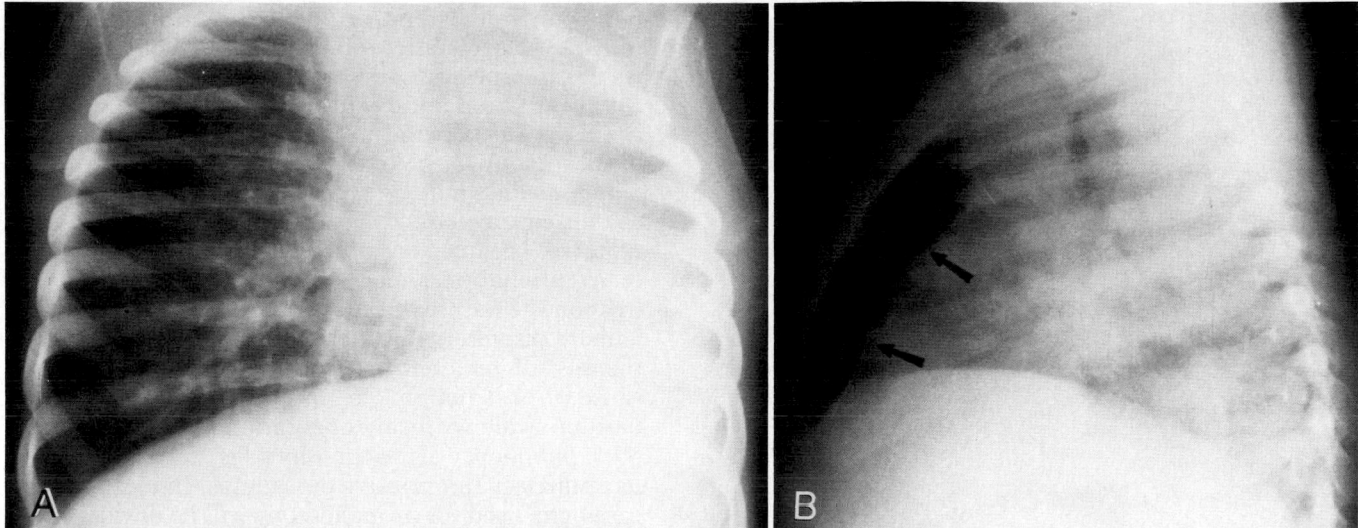

Fig. 1.20. Large hyperlucent lung; compensatory emphysema. A. Note the large, hyperlucent right lung. However, also note that the pulmonary vascularity is engorged. This lung, therefore, must be the normal lung. The other lung is collapsed secondary to mucous plugging from a viral lower respiratory tract infection. B. Lateral view demonstrating anterior mediastinal herniation (arrows) of the compensatorily overinflated right lung, a common phenomenon with an overdistended lung.

progressively enlarged. The end result is a "balanced-obstructed" lung.

When classic obstructive emphysema (i.e., progressive enlargement of a lung) is the cause of a large, hyperlucent lung, the emphysematous lung is fixed in overdistention, and its vascularity usually is diminished (Fig. 1.22). The degree of diminution of the vascularity depends on the degree and duration of overdistention, and thus, in early or mild cases, vascularity still may appear relatively normal (see Fig. 1.11). Eventually, however, it becomes decreased, but in a few cases, residual prominence of the pulmonary vascularity can erroneously suggest that vascularity, overall, still is normal (Fig. 1.23).

Most commonly, obstructive emphysema is caused by an endobronchial foreign body, but next most common is a mucous plug. Such a plug usually is seen with viral lower respiratory tract infections and/or asthma. Endobronchial lesions such as inflammatory granulomas (i.e., tuberculosis), endobronchial tumors, etc., are much less common causes of obstructive emphysema and so are extrinsic, compressive lesions such as mediastinal cysts, tumors, and abnormally dilated or located blood vessels.

Congenital lobar emphysema is another common cause of hyperlucency of one side of the chest, but usually the condition presents in infancy. On the other hand, there are those cases where the patient grows into later childhood with little or no respiratory difficulty. In any case, it is the left upper, and then the right upper lobe which are involved most often, and if emphysema is pronounced, the entire lung may falsely appear emphysematous (Fig. 1.24A). If one is fortunate enough to also see the triangular, compressed

lower lobe, just against the spine, the diagnosis of upper lobe obstructive emphysema is almost assured. Thereafter, bronchoscopic confirmation of the diagnosis and subsequent surgery are in order. However, if the patient is asymptomatic, the enlarged lobe may be left alone.

Further investigation, after obstructive emphysema is determined to be present, depends on whether the problem is acute or chronic. If it is acute and present in a patient with asthma or a viral lower respiratory tract infection, a mucous plug is most likely and little else needs to be done. The patient should be encouraged to cough, but regardless, the plug usually eventually dislodges on its own. If, however, by clinical history, the presumptive diagnosis is a foreign body, bronchoscopy is the next step. Seldom is there need for other roentgenographic studies, but if uncertainty prevails, one can obtain decubitus views (2) which can substantiate that the questionably obstructed lung is really obstructed (see Fig. 1.22). These views also are useful when fluoroscopy is unavailable, and the reason they work is that if the dependent lung (the lower one in the decubitus position) is the obstructed lung, it acts as an air cushion and does not deflate. Normally, the dependent lung deflates because of compression of that side of the chest, and the phenomenon can be enhanced by asking the patient to exhale at the same time the film is being obtained. Seldom is it necessary to fluoroscope a patient for suspected foreign body, but if fluoroscopy is performed, one will note lack of motion of the depressed, ipsilateral diaphragmatic leaflet and contralateral shift of the mediastinum on expiration.

If the problem is chronic, isotope ventilation and

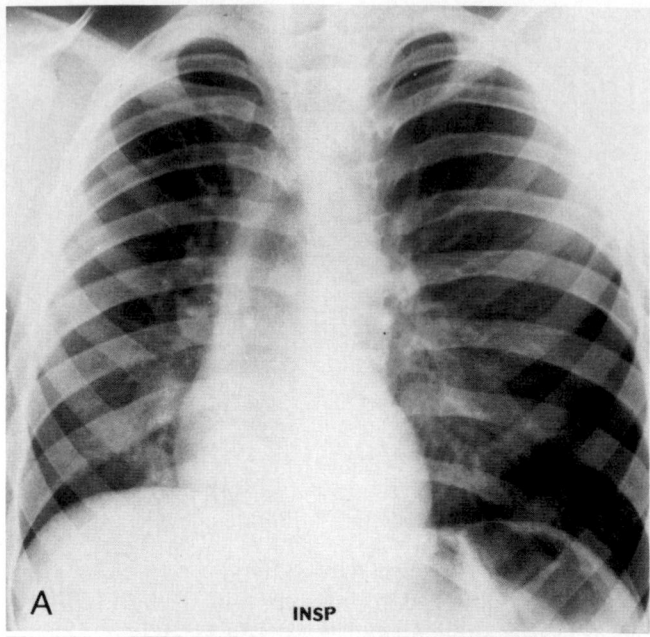

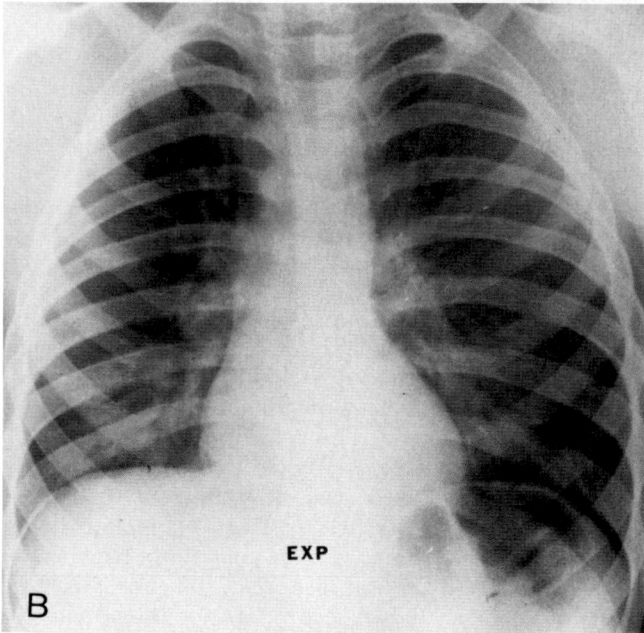

Fig. 1.21. Large hyperlucent lung; compensatory emphysema with inspiratory-expiratory films. A. On this inspiratory view, the large, overdistended left lung might be picked as the abnormal lung. This is especially likely to occur since the vascularity in the left lung is not engorged, and in fact, is not that different from the vascularity in the right lung. However, this observation is important because, if a lung as large as the left lung were enlarged because of obstructive emphysema, the vascularity almost surely would be unequivocally decreased. Since it is not, one must now suspect that compensatory, rather than obstructive, emphysema is the problem on the left. This being the case, the left lung should be the normal one. B. Expiratory film con-

perfusion studies and/or pulmonary arteriograms often are performed. However, the results of these studies are nonspecific, for they show nothing more than that ventilation and perfusion are decreased. Because of this, eventually most of these patients also come to bronchoscopy.

If a mediastinal cyst, mass, or abnormal vessel is visualized on plain films, bronchoscopy may not be required because barium swallow and tomography (conventional or computed) can shed enough further light on the nature of the lesion (certainly the location is more discretely outlined) to allow for its definitive therapy. If an abnormal vessel is suspected as the cause of obstruction (i.e., esophageal indentation on barium swallow, focal indentation on the bronchus, etc.), pulmonary arteriography or aortography are the most directly informative procedures. In most of these cases, the need for bronchoscopy will be obviated, and by the same token, bronchography seldom is required.

Conditions producing findings similar to obstructive emphysema of one or the other of the lungs include cystic diseases of the lung, large postinflammatory pneumatoceles, left side diaphragmatic hernias with an air-filled stomach in the chest (1, 3, 4), and pneumothorax (6, 7). As far as cystic disease of the lungs is concerned, occasionally, a large solitary cyst or postinflammatory pneumatocele can occupy a hemithorax, but more often the problem is multiple cysts in congenital adenomatoid malformation (5). Although initially the cysts in this lesion are very small and fluid-filled (in the neonatal period), as the patient grows older, there is progressive replacement of the fluid with air (via the ducts of Lambert and pores of Kohn by the air-drift phenomenon) and improved visualization of the cysts. At first they appear small and bubbly, then larger and more thin-walled, and eventually, so large that they coalesce and virtually obliterate the septae between them. It is in these latter two stages that the findings are difficult to differentiate from those of an emphysematous lung or a large pneumothorax (Fig. 1.24B).

Diaphragmatic hernias, on the left side, containing an air-filled stomach are a rather uncommon cause of a large, unilateral hyperlucent hemithorax, but the findings can be puzzling (Fig. 1.24C). Such hernias can be secondary to blunt abdominal trauma (either acute or on a delayed basis), but most are delayed

firms this impression in that it clearly demonstrates that the left lung changes size most. The right lung has changed size very little and now has become the more radiolucent and larger of the two lungs. This suggests that a certain degree of obstructive emphysema is present on the right, and indeed, an obstructing mucous plug in this patient with asthma was the problem.

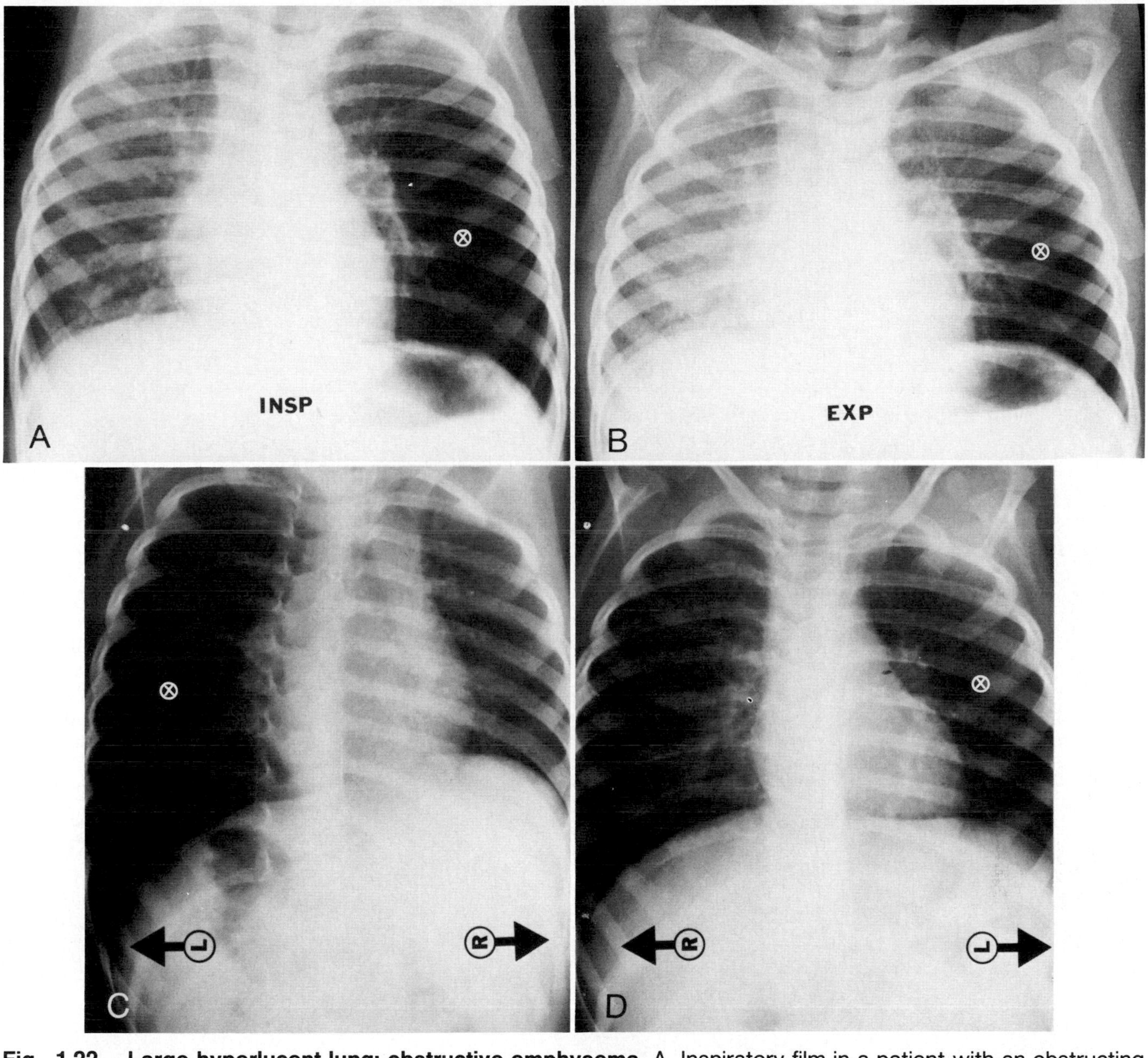

Fig. 1.22. Large hyperlucent lung; obstructive emphysema. A. Inspiratory film in a patient with an obstructing foreign body on the left. The left lung, especially the left lower lobe, is large, hyperlucent, and undervascularized. B. Expiratory film confirms air trapping in the left lung, especially in the left lower lobe. C. Decubitus film with the right side down demonstrates the right lung to collapse (become smaller and hazy). The left lung is radiolucent and remains overdistended. D. Decubitus film with left side down. Note that the left lung has remained radiolucent (air cushion effect due to obstructive emphysema). The right lung is normal. The findings confirm obstructive emphysema of the left lung ⊗.

congenital herniations through the foramen of Bochdalek. Finally, massive pneumothoraces also can produce a large, hyperlucent hemithorax, but the findings usually are very straightforward (Fig. 1.24D). Anterior pneumothoraces, on the other hand, occurring in patients lying in the supine position can pose a more perplexing problem. Such pneumothoraces most commonly occur in the neonate (7), but also occur in older children (6). In such cases, radiolucency of the hemithorax is due to air accumulating over the anterior surface of the lung, and also to compression of the lung by the pleural air. Together, these factors cause pulmonary blood flow to be diminished and the lung to become hyperlucent. The degree of increased radiolucency depends on the volume of free air present.

Another clue to the presence of an anterior pneu-

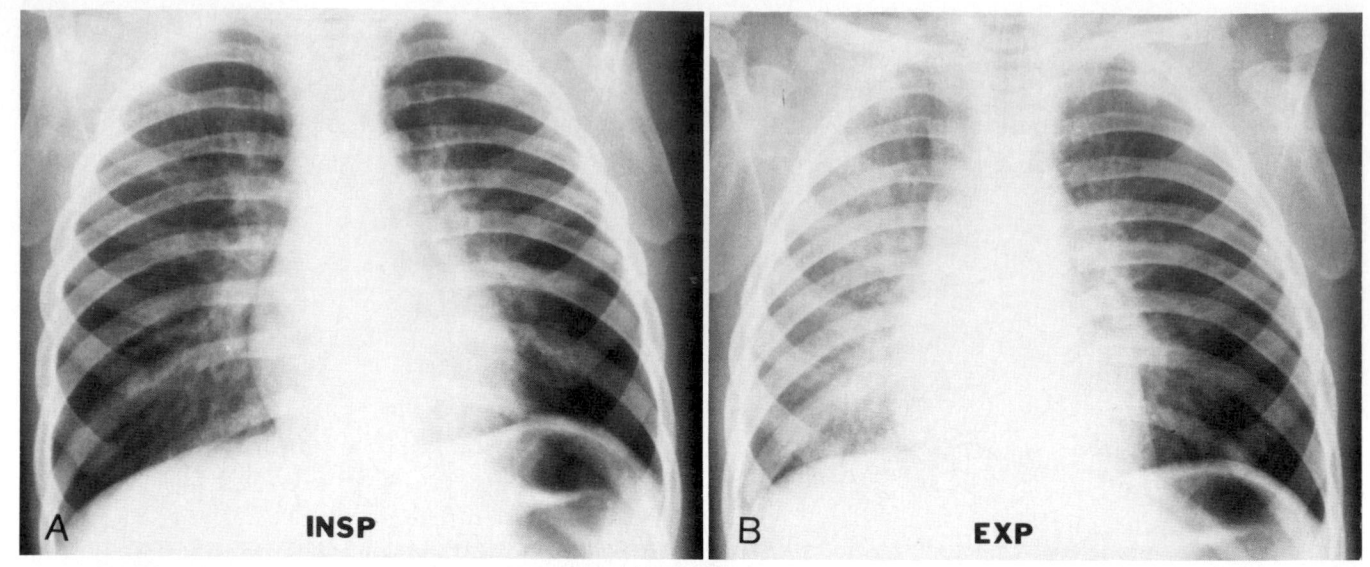

A   **INSP**   B   **EXP**

Fig. 1.23.

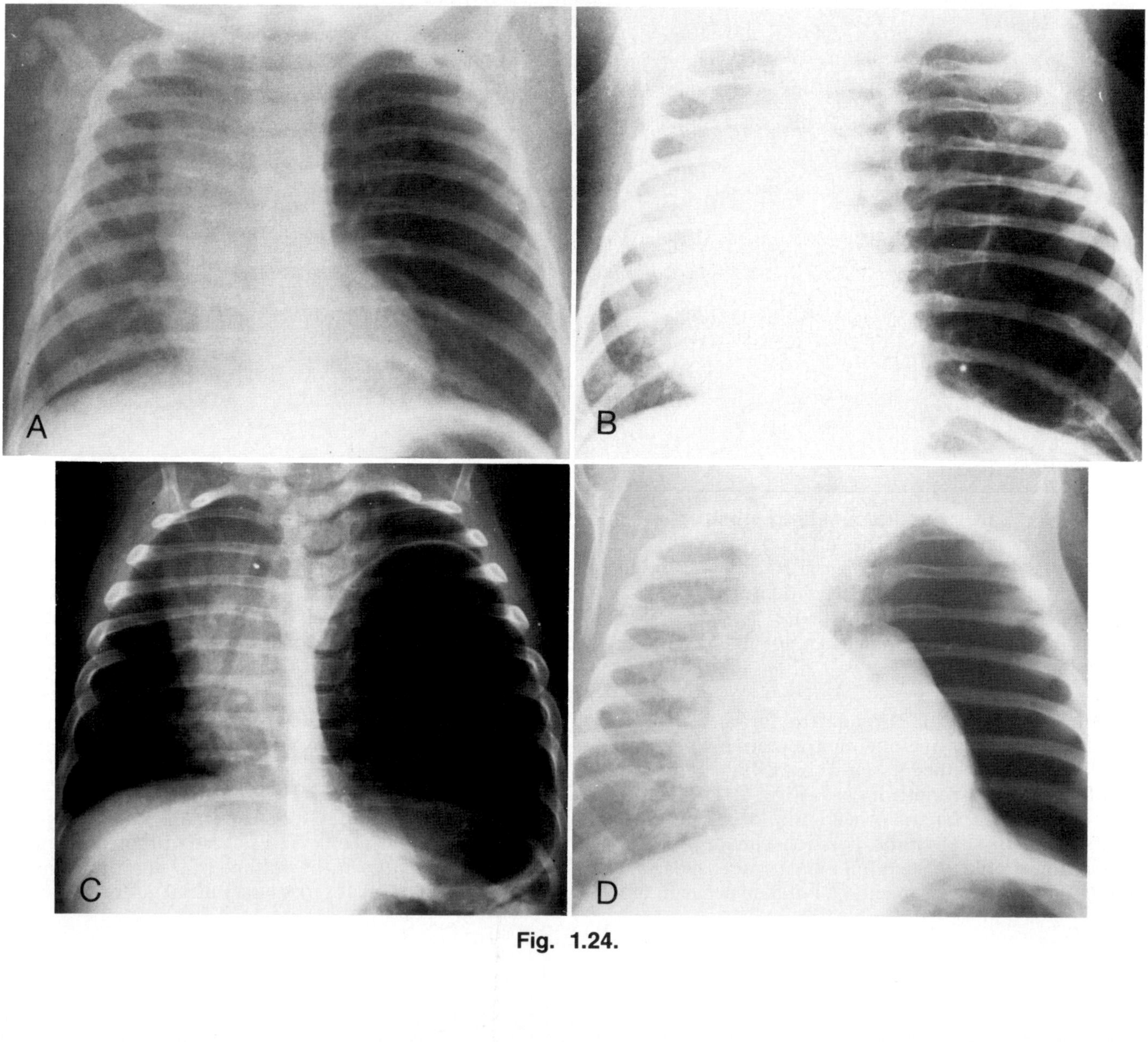

Fig. 1.24.

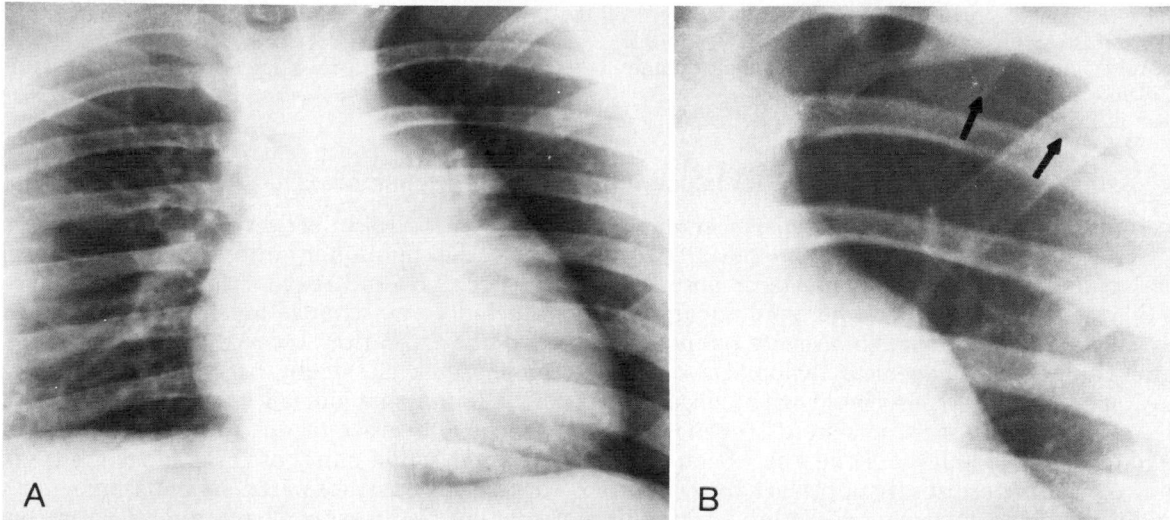

Fig. 1.25. Anterior pneumothorax causing hyperlucent hemithorax. A. Note that the left lung appears more radiolucent than the right and that the ipsilateral mediastinal edge is sharper than that on the right. This is due to an anterior accumulation of air; i.e., anterior pneumothorax. B. Film obtained a few moments later, on expiration, demonstrates typical findings of a pneumothorax (arrows).

mothorax is that the ipsilateral mediastinal edge usually appears sharper than its mate on the other side (Fig. 1.25). This is not an absolutely pathognomonic finding, for similar sharpness can be seen with an emphysematously overdistended lung (see Fig. 1.22) or a hypoplastic, underperfused lung (see Fig. 1.26). However, it still is a very useful sign of anterior pneumothorax.

The reason the ipsilateral mediastinal edge is sharper with anterior pneumothorax is that free air, rather than normal lung tissue abuts the mediastinal edge. In the other entities, the ratio of air to blood in the lungs is altered in favor of air. In other words, since with obstructive emphysema, the blood vessels are compressed and constricted, and with congenital hypoplasia, they are absent or small, less blood than normal is carried through the lungs. The lungs then become hyperlucent and at the same time, the presence of fewer, smaller, and less filled blood vessels

causes less blurring (increased sharpness) of the ipsilateral mediastinal edge. With anterior pneumothorax, of course, no blood vessels at all are present along side the heart, and because of this, the mediastinal edge is sharpest in this condition.

References

1. Brill PW, Gershwind ME, Krasna IH: Massive gastric enlargement with delayed presentation of congenital diaphragmatic hernia: report of three cases and review of the literature. *J Pediatr Surg* 12:667–674, 1977.
2. Capitanio MA, Kirkpatrick JA: The lateral decubitus film, an aid in determining air-trapping in children. *Radiology* 103:460–462, 1972.
3. Glasson MJ, Barter W, Cohen DH, Bowdler JD: Congenital left posteriolateral diaphragmatic hernia with previously normal chest x-ray. *Pediatr Radiol* 3:201–205, 1975.
4. Hurdiss LW, Taybi H, Johnson LM: Delayed appearance of left-sided diaphragmatic hernia with infancy. *J*

Fig. 1.23. Large hyperlucent lung; obstructive emphysema with deceptive pulmonary vascularity. A. The left lung is small and, at first, one might interpret the vascularity to be normal. However, on closer inspection, one should note that in the left lower lobe, the vascularity is diminished. B. Expiratory film clearly confirms that the left lung is obstructed in that it changes size very little, if at all, during expiration. Note, however, that the right lung is deflated. In A, it was overaerated due to compensatory emphysema. An obstructing foreign body was present on the left.

Fig. 1.24. Large hyperlucent hemithorax; other causes. A. **Congenital lobar emphysema.** Note the overdistended left lung. Vascularity is diminished, but the often present, secondarily compressed lower lobe is not visualized in this patient. For a good example of such compression, on the right side, see the case illustrated in Figure 1.10A. B. **Congenital adenomatoid malformation.** At this stage of the disease, the cysts become very large and the septae quite thin. The lung is hyperlucent and devascularized. C. **Delayed diaphragmatic hernia with gastric herniation.** Note the distended stomach in the left hemithorax. Courtesy of Virgil Graves, M.D., Great Falls, Montana. D. **Large tension pneumothorax on the left.** The pneumothorax was secondary to air trapping as part of a viral lower respiratory tract infection. The findings are straightforward.

Pediatr 88:990–992, 1976.

5. Madewell JE, Stocker JT, Korsower JM: Cystic adenomatoid malformation of the lung: morphologic analysis. *Am J Roentgenol* 124:436–448, 1975.
6. Swischuk LE: *Emergency Radiology of the Acutely Ill or Injured Child.* Baltimore, Williams & Wilkins, 1979, pp 107–108.
7. Swischuk LE: Two lesser known but useful signs of neonatal pneumothorax. *Am J Roentgenol* 127:623–627, 1976.

Small, Radiolucent (Hyperlucent) Hemithorax

The commonest causes of a small, hyperlucent hemithorax are congenital pulmonary hypoplasia (with ipsilateral pulmonary artery hypoplasia or absence), and the Swyer-James syndrome where pulmonary hypoplasia is acquired secondary to a severe pulmonary infection (Table 1.7). Congenital hypoplasia of the lung may or may not be associated with congenital heart disease, but when it is, persistent truncus arteriosus and tetralogy of Fallot are one's best bets. With persistent truncus arteriosus, hypoplasia can occur on either side, but with tetralogy of Fallot, it usually occurs on the left. In the absence of congenital heart disease, left side hypoplasia also is favored, for if underdevelopment of the right lung occurs, usually it takes the form of right upper and/or middle lobe agenesis. The lower lobe is normal, but in combination with agenesis of the other lobes, a small, hazy, and not a small, radiolucent hemithorax results (see Fig. 1.17).

With congenital hypoplasia of the lung, little or no symptoms usually exist, and in my experience, these lungs are not particularly prone to repeated pulmonary infections. Indeed, most of the time their discovery is totally incidental. Increased radiolucency of these lungs results from decreased pulmonary blood flow (i.e., hypoplastic or absent pulmonary artery), and in some cases, the findings are quite striking (Fig. 1.26). An important feature of these lungs is that they change size on inspiration-expiration, and even though the degree of change may not be as great as in a totally normal lung, significant change does occur (Fig. 1.26). It is this feature, more than any other, which serves to distinguish the congenitally hypoplastic lung from the one acquired in the Swyer-James or MacLeod syndromes (1–4, 6).

Classically, the Swyer-James lung results from a severe inflammatory episode which produces an obliterative bronchiolitis. This is especially prone to occur with viral infections (1, 3), but also can be seen with other pulmonary infections, chronic foreign bodies, etc. The end result is a small, hyperlucent lung which does not change much in size between inspiration and expiration. Indeed, on expiration, obstructive emphysema classically becomes evident. However, I have found that not all such lungs demonstrate recognizable degrees of obstructive emphysema, and in addition, while many of these lungs are totally clear, others demonstrate parenchymal scarring or reticulation. For this reason, I have, at least in my own mind, expanded the classic definition of the Swyer-James lung to include such variations. From the purist's standpoint, however, the lung should be free of infiltrates, small, hyperlucent, and demonstrative of obstructive emphysema. Obstructive emphysema in these lungs results from the obliterative bronchiolitis but air first enters the lung parenchyma by the air-drift phenomenon. In other words, air from adjacent normal lung tissue passes through the pores of Kohn and ducts of Lambert into the parenchyma of the involved lung, and then, because the bronchioles are obstructed, accumulates under tension.

When a small, hyperlucent lung is demonstrated to be congenital in origin, there is little reason to perform any other roentgenographic studies, for no specific therapy usually is indicated. Of course, isotope perfusion scans will be abnormal, and pulmonary arteriograms will show ipsilateral pulmonary artery hypoplasia or absence, but these findings are expected and no different from those seen in the Swyer-James lung (Fig. 1.27). If, on the other hand, a patient is decreed to have a Swyer-James lung, then it must be determined whether the lung is a problem to the patient. This can take the form of repeated pulmonary infections or cyanosis resulting from arterial desaturation due to intrapulmonary shunting. The latter complication is best assessed with cardiac catheterization, blood gas studies, and pulmonary angiography. Bronchial disease is best assessed with bronchograms which may show one of two abnormal patterns. The first is that seen in the classic Swyer-James lung where the obliterative bronchiolitis leads to nonfilling of the peripheral bronchioles and a normal bronchial tree proximal to this level. In other cases, however, widespread bronchiectatic changes in the more proximal bronchi can occur (Fig. 1.27).

After congenital or acquired pulmonary hypoplasia, the next most common cause of a small hyperlucent hemithorax is bronchial obstruction. At first, this may appear to be a strange statement, for most often one

Table 1.7 Small Hyperlucent Hemithorax

Pulmonary artery and lung hypoplasia[a] Swyer-James lung[b]	Commonest
Bronchial obstruction	Moderately common
Postradiation lung[b] Pulmonary vein atresia or stenosis[b] Pulmonary embolus[a]	Rare

[a] Changes size on inspiration-expiration.
[b] May show scarring, reticulation, etc.

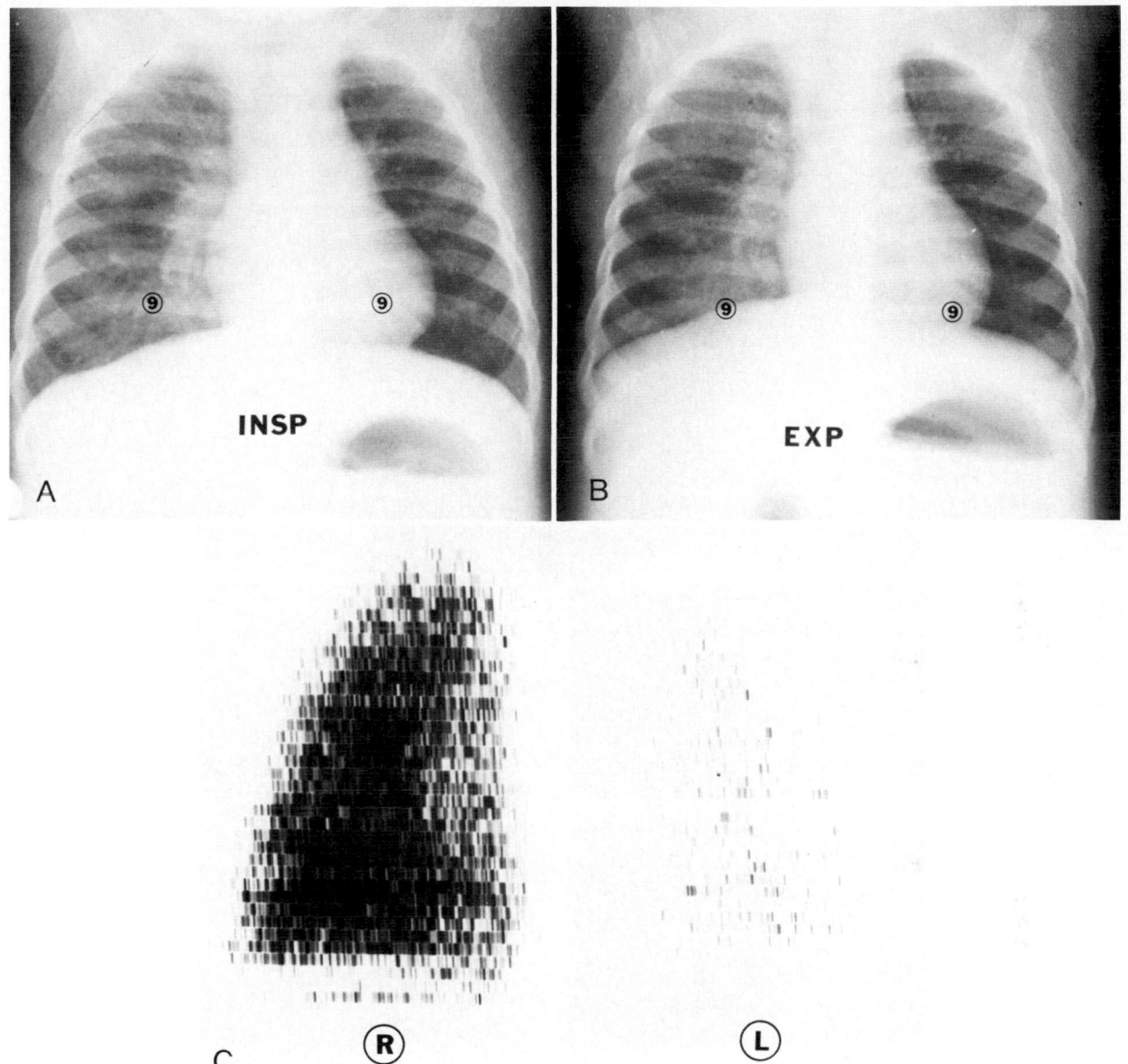

Fig. 1.26. Small hyperlucent hemithorax; pulmonary hypoplasia. A. On this inspiratory view, note that the left lung is smaller, but more radiolucent (undervascularized) than the right lung. This also is causing increased sharpness of the left mediastinal edge. The ninth ribs ⑨ are marked. B. Expiratory film in the same infant demonstrates that both lungs change size during expiration, but the left does so a little less than the right. The ninth ribs ⑨ are marked again. C. Isotope perfusion study demonstrates markedly decreased perfusion of the left lung.

thinks of atelectasis or obstructive emphysema as the two findings associated with this problem. However, at a certain stage of bronchial obstruction, the involved lung may appear smaller and more radiolucent than normal. Most often, this occurs with mucous plugs in patients with asthma or viral lower respiratory tract infection, and unless one is aware of this problem, the finding can be overlooked. In most cases, it is the inspiratory-expiratory film sequence which finally clarifies the situation (Fig. 1.28).

Other rather rare causes of a unilateral, small hy-

perlucent hemithorax include the postirradiation lung, pulmonary embolus (very rare in children), and pulmonary vein atresia or stenosis (5). A final variation of the small, hyperlucent lung is one which demonstrates some degree of reticularity. For the most part, if one encounters such a lung, the best possibilities are unilateral pulmonary vein atresia or stenosis, acquired hypoplasia with parenchyma scarring, and occasionally, the postirradiation lung. Cases of unilateral pulmonary vein atresia may be difficult to differentiate from the Swyer-James lung until pulmonary

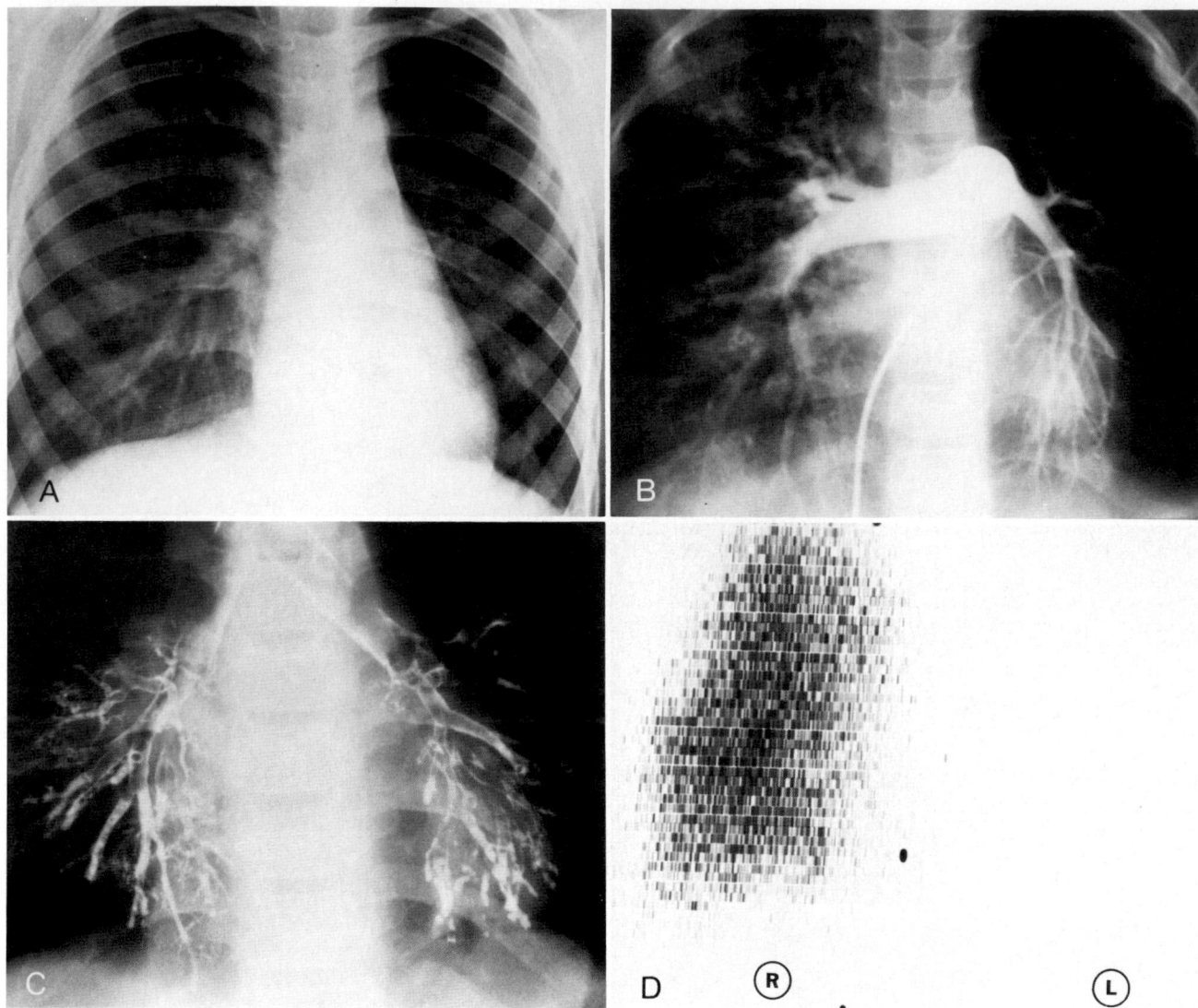

Fig. 1.27. Small hyperlucent hemithorax; acquired hypoplasia (Swyer-James lung). A. Note the small, hyperlucent, and undervascularized left lung. The right lung shows slight compensatory overaeration and increased pulmonary blood flow. This patient, when an infant, had a normal chest film, and then acquired a severe infection on the left. B. Pulmonary arteriogram demonstrates characteristic decreased flow to the left lung and small, constricted pulmonary arteries. Those in the left lower lobe are crowded because of a degree of left lower lobe atelectasis. On the chest film in A, note that some infiltrate is present behind the left side of the heart. C. Bronchogram demonstrating moderate bronchiectatic changes on the left, especially on the left lower lobe, and less filling of the small peripheral bronchioles than on the normal right side. Also note that both the right and left major bronchi are about equal in size. If congenital hypoplasia were the problem, the left bronchus would be significantly smaller than the right (recall, however, that the normal left bronchus often is a little smaller than the right). Also note that the bronchi of the left lower lobe are crowded, confirming the presence of atelectasis. D. Perfusion isotope scan demonstrates virtually no isotope activity in the left lung.

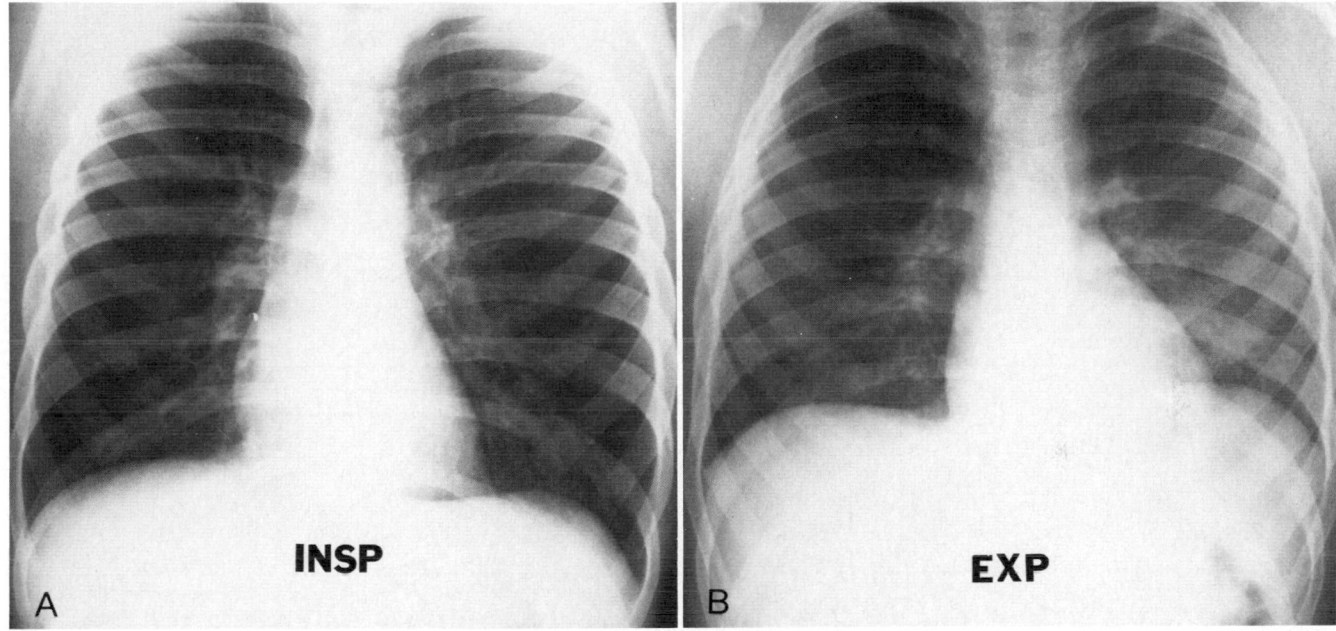

Fig. 1.28. Small hyperlucent hemithorax; endobronchial obstruction. A. On this inspiratory view, note that the right lung is more radiolucent than the left. In addition, it is a little smaller than the left lung. Also note that some compensatory anterior mediastinal herniation of the left lung has occurred. One might be confused as to which lung is abnormal, but since pulmonary blood flow is less on the right, the right lung should be the abnormal one. B. Expiratory film demonstrates that the left lung changes volume markedly, while the right lung has remained about the same in size. In fact, now it is the larger, more radiolucent lung. The problem was an obstructing mucous plug on the right, secondary to asthma. In these patients, the endobronchial obstruction is of such a degree and/or duration that neither total atelectasis or gross obstructive emphysema occur. Obviously, both the intake and exit of air are altered, but the ratio of these airflow abnormalities are such that a small obstructed lung results (i.e., less than normal volumes of air enter the lung and cause it to be small, but at the same time, during expiration, enough air is trapped to keep the lung from collapsing.

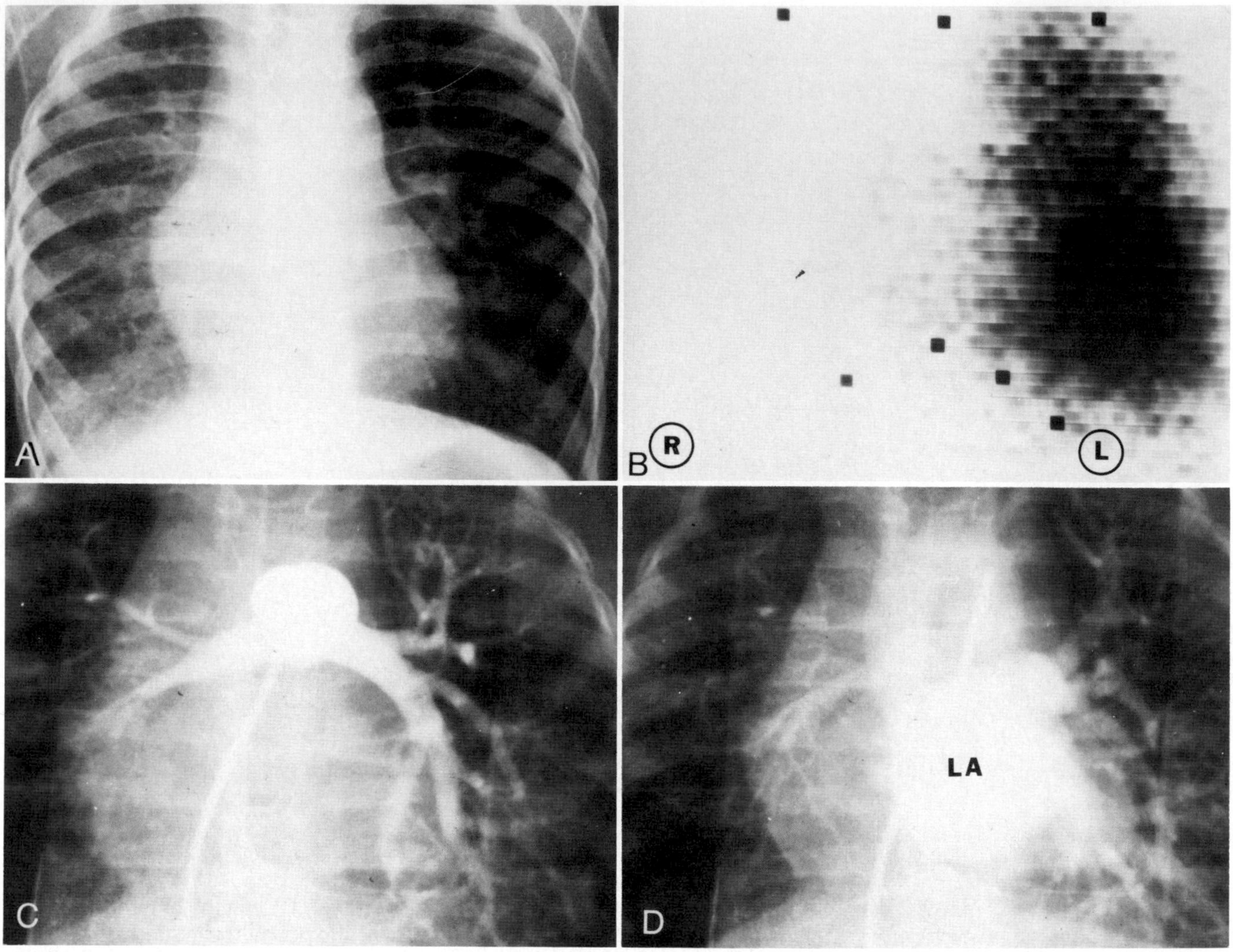

Fig. 1.29. Small reticular lung. A. Note that the right lung is smaller than the left, but also note that it possesses a diffuse reticularity, especially in its lower half. For the most part, such reticulation should suggest unilateral pulmonary vein atresia or a variation of the Swyer-James lung. However, pulmonary vein atresia will be less common. B. Isotope perfusion study demonstrates no isotope uptake in the right lung. C. Pulmonary arteriogram, early phase. Note markedly diminished blood flow to the right lung and characteristically small, constricted, and tapered pulmonary artery branches. D. Pulmonary arteriogram, later phase. The small vessels on the right are the pulmonary artery branches visualized in C. They demonstrate extreme stasis of contrast material, and hence markedly impaired pulmonary blood flow. Also note that there are no draining pulmonary veins on the right. On the left, veins are present, and in fact, are a little larger than normal. Left atrium (LA). A bronchogram in this patient was normal. Final diagnosis was pulmonary vein atresia.

arteriograms are performed. In pulmonary vein atresia, draining pulmonary veins will not be visualized (Fig. 1.29). The reticulations present in these patients are due to chronic interstitial pulmonary edema and fibrosis, and probably also to compensatorily dilated lymphatics. In the Swyer-James lung, reticularity is due to pulmonary fibrosis, and similarly, if it is seen in the postirradiation lung, fibrosis is the cause.

References

1. Cumming GR, MacPherson RI, Chernick V: Unilateral hyperlucent lung syndrome in children. *J Pediatr* 78:250–260, 1971.
2. Kogutt MS, Swischuk LE, Goldblum R: Swyer-James syndrome (unilateral hyperlucent lung) in children. *Am J Dis Child* 125:614–618, 1973.
3. MacLeod WM: Abnormal transradiancy of one lung. *Thorax* 17:230–239, 1962.
4. MacPherson RI, Cumming GR, Chernick V: Unilateral hyperlucent lung: a complication of viral pneumonia. *J Can Assoc Radiol* 20:225–231, 1969.
5. Swischuk LE, L'Heureux, P: Unilateral pulmonary vein atresia or stenosis (diagnostic roentgenographic and clinical features). *Am J Roentgenol* 135:667–672, 1980.
6. Swyer P, James C: Case of unilateral pulmonary emphysema. *Thorax* 8:133–136, 1953.

FOCAL AERATION DISTURBANCES

Focal aeration disturbances, either atelectatic or emphysematous, can result from any of the problems leading to similar aeration disturbances involving the entire lung. These conditions have been discussed in previous sections and do not require reiteration, except to note that the commonest cause of focal atelectasis is mucous plugging due to viral lower respiratory tract infection or asthma. The commonest cause of obstructive emphysema is a foreign body (1, 5). In addition, it might be noted that mixed aeration disturbances frequently are present in some patients. For the most part, this occurs with endobronchial lesions such as granulomas, tumors, or multiple foreign bodies, but unless one is aware of the phenomenon, the findings can be puzzling. This is especially true when the right middle lobe is involved (Fig. 1.30).

An unusual condition resulting in a focal aeration disturbance consisting of localized overinflation of a portion of the lung (usually a lobe) is the bronchial atresia-mucocele syndrome (2–4, 6). In the newborn,

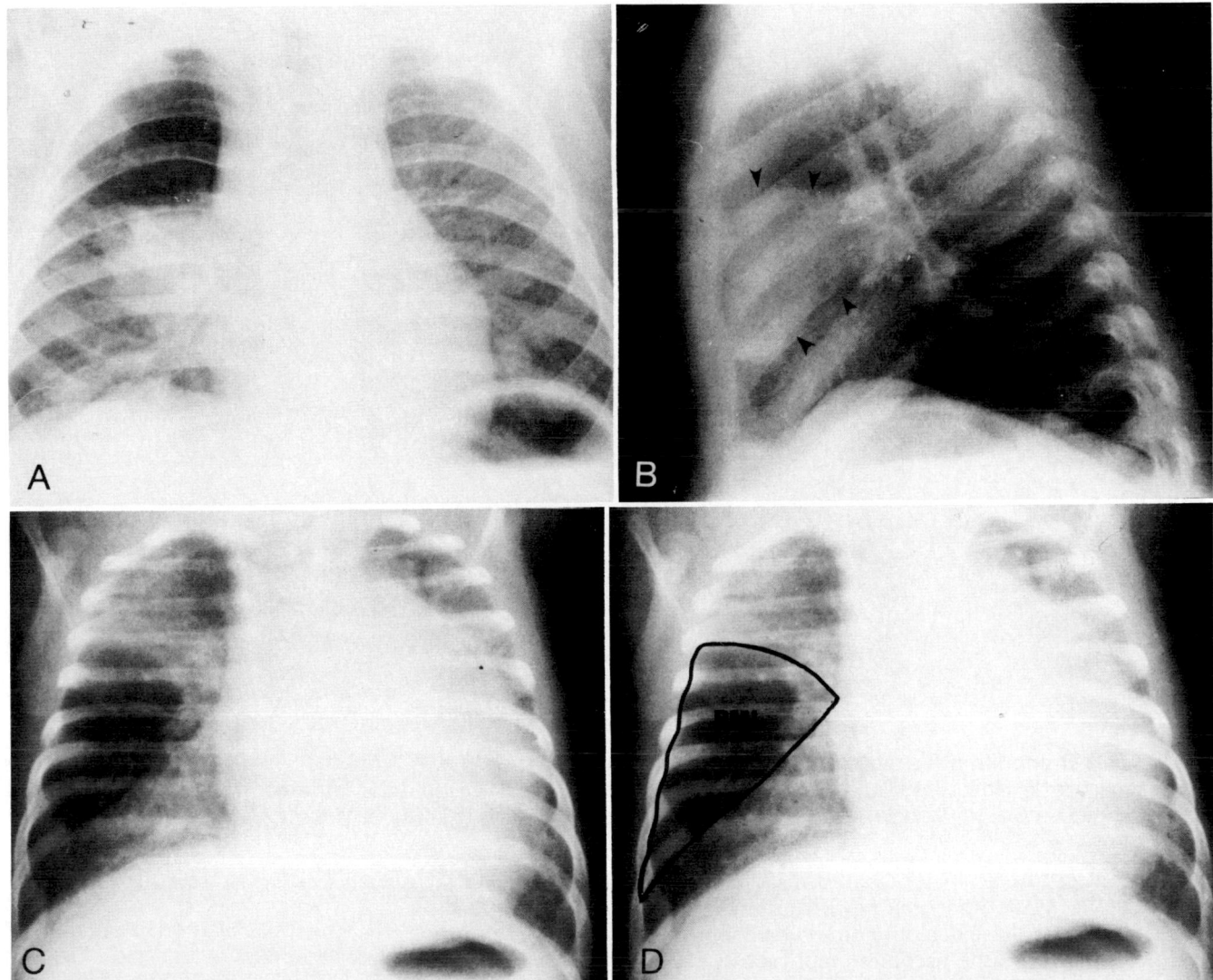

Fig. 1.30. Focal aeration disturbances. A. Right middle lobe atelectasis and right upper lobe emphysema. Note what at first appears to be a large, dense, right hilum (arrows). Also note that the right upper lobe is more radiolucent than the remaining lung. There is moderate obstructive emphysema present. B. Lateral view demonstrates the density seen on frontal view to be a partially collapsed right middle lobe (arrows). These findings were secondary to a large endobronchial granuloma due to atypical tuberculous infection. C. **Middle lobe emphysema.** Note the triangular radiolucency in the right midlung field. This is characteristic of an overdistended right middle lobe, and the densities above and below are the partially collapsed right upper and lower lobes. D. Diagrammatic outlining of the emphysematous right middle lobe (RML). This patient had congenital right middle lobe emphysema and also had a large ventricular septal defect (note cardiomegaly and vascular engorgement).

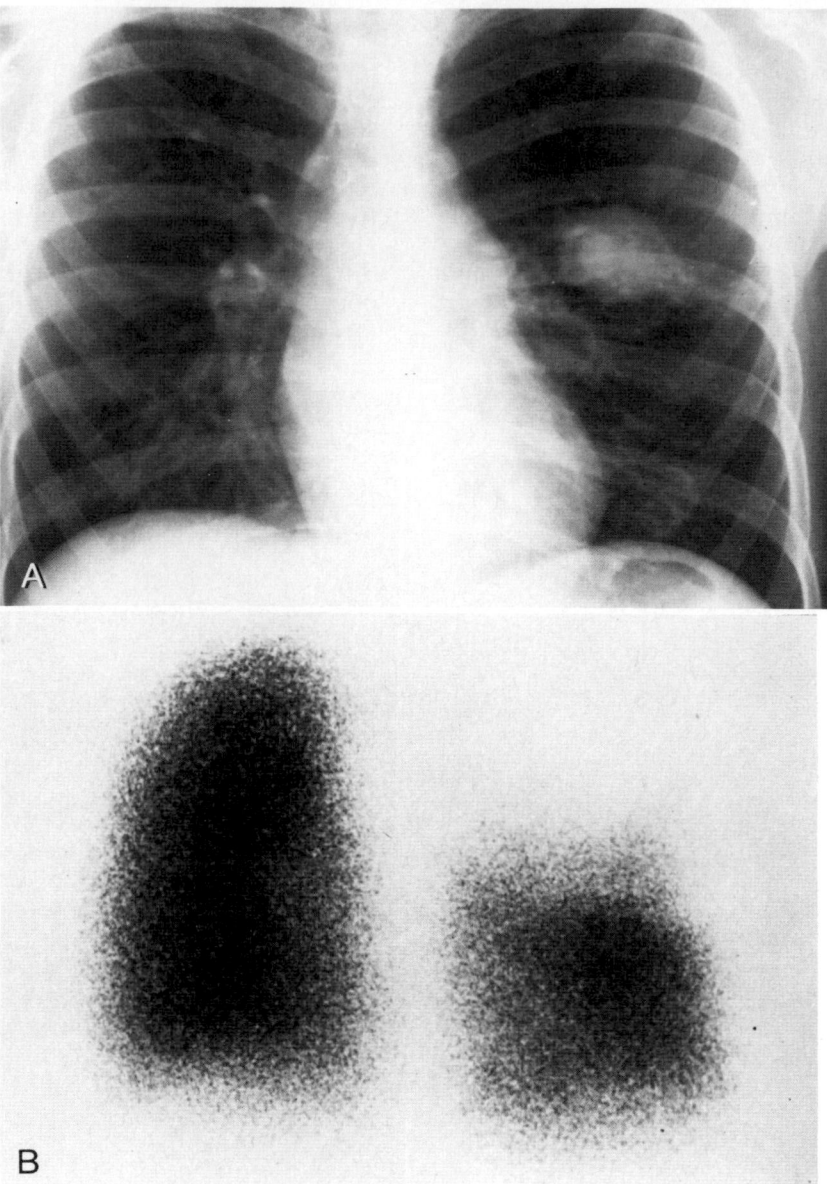

Fig. 1.31.   Bronchial atresia with mucocele-hyperinflation syndrome. A. Note the hyperinflated left upper lobe. The vascularity is diminished, and the lobe is larger than normal. Also note the large central nodule representing impacted mucus (i.e., mucocele). B. Isotope scan showing no uptake in left upper lobe.

this lesion can present with a solid, fluid-filled lobe distal to the atretic portion of the bronchus. The findings then are those of a pulmonary mass, but later, as fluid clears, the lung becomes emphysematous (by way of the air-drift phenomenon through the pores of Kohn). Mucous impactions, just distal to the site of bronchial atresia, present as a nodule or small mass on the chest film, and in combination, the findings are pathognomonic (Fig. 1.31).

References

1. Eggleston PA, Ward BH, Pierson WE, Bierman CW: Radiographic abnormalities in acute asthma in children. *Pediatrics* 54:442–449, 1974.
2. Genereux GP: Bronchial atresia: a rare cause of unilateral lung hypertranslucency. *J Can Assoc Radiol* 22:71–82, 1971.
3. Oh KS, Dorst JP, White JJ, Haller JA Jr, Johnson BA, Byrne WD: Syndrome of bronchial atresia or stenosis with mucocele and focal hyperinflation of the lung. *John Hopkins Med J* 138:48–53, 1976.
4. Schuster SR, Harris GBC, Williams A, Kirkpatick J, Reid L: Bronchial atresia: a recognizable entity in the pediatric age group. *J Pediatr Surg* 13:682–689, 1978.
5. Shopfner CE: Aeration disturbances secondary to pulmonary infection. *Am J Roentgenol Radium Ther Nucl Med* 120:261–273, 1974.
6. Talner LB, Gmelich JT, Liebow AA, Greenspan RH: The syndrome of bronchial mucocele and regional hyperinflation of the lung. *Am J Roentgenol Radium Ther Nucl Med* 110:675–686, 1970.

TRACHEOBRONCHIAL AIR SHADOW ABNORMALITIES

The tracheal air shadow almost always is visible in infants and children, but in the young infant, since the trachea is mobile, the air column may become very tortuous during expiration (Fig. 1.32). Characteristically, during inspiration, it deviates to the right (4), and in some cases, produces an almost right angle configuration at the level of the thoracic inlet (Fig. 1.32). This should not be misinterpreted for deviation due to a mass, for when a mass or vascular ring deviate the trachea, acute bends are not present; rather, focal curving defects occur (Fig. 1.33).

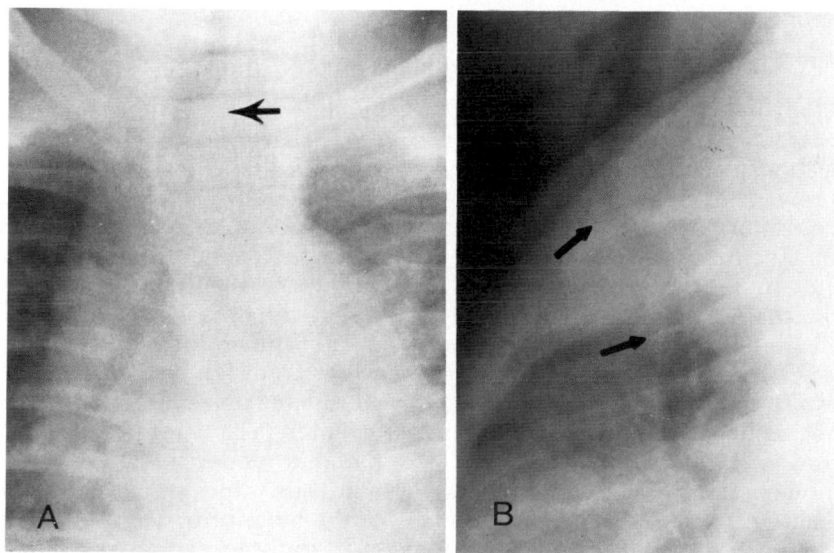

Fig. 1.32. Normal tracheal buckling. A. Frontal view showing characteristic deviation of the trachea to the right on expiration. Note the almost right angle bend (arrow) at the level of the thoracic inlet. B. Lateral view demonstrating extreme tortuosity of the entire airway causing a "pseudomass" configuration to develop behind the pharynx and upper trachea.

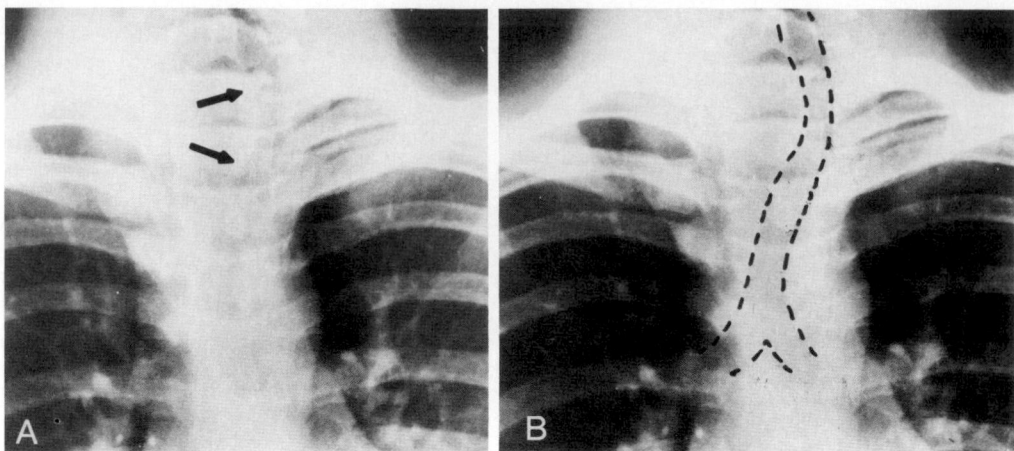

Fig. 1.33. Pathologic tracheal deviation. A. Note minimal compression and marked deviation of the trachea to the left (arrows) by a thyroid adenoma. The superior mediastinum also is wider than normal. B. Diagrammatic representation of tracheal deviation seen in A.

Generalized Tracheal Diameter Changes

It has been stated that in infants, if during inspiration the trachea is less than 3 mm in diameter, it should be considered abnormal (6). This is probably true, but the whole problem is rather rare, for there are very few, if any, causes of narrowing of the entire trachea on inspiration. Even cases of congenital trachea stenosis usually are more focal than generalized. On expiration, however, the problem is more common, for there are certain situations where the trachea narrows to a diameter of less than 3 mm during the expiratory phase of respiration. In some of these cases, the trachea simply appears hypercollapsible, and even though it is quite narrow during expiration, no particular symptoms arise, and obstructive emphysema does not appear to be present. On the other hand, the same phenomenon can occur in infants with bronchiolitis and/or those who might develop asthma (Fig. 1.34, A and B). This phenomenon often is explained on the basis of generalized tracheomalacia (2, 11), but there is considerable question as to whether such a condition

actually exists. If it does, it is rare, and it is more likely that most of these infants have so called hyperreactive airway disease.

A generalized increase in the diameter of the trachea and major bronchi is an uncommon problem, but does occur in the condition known as tracheobronchomegaly (1, 9, 13, 19). In these cases, elastic tissue deficiency allows the trachea and bronchi to distend to greater than normal diameters during inspiration (Fig. 1.34, C and D), and although the condition has been considered congenital, most likely it is the result of an acquired peripheral necrotizing bronchiolitis. In these patients, air does not enter the obliterated bronchioles, and thus, during inspiration, there is overdistention of the more proximal bronchi and trachea (13). However, the trachea may not dilate as much as the bronchi (i.e., Fig. 1.34C). Apart from this condition, generalized increase in diameter of the trachea is rather uncommon.

Focal Tracheobronchial Narrowings

Focal, often eccentric, tracheobronchial narrowings can result from the compressive effects of abnormally located or dilated blood vessels and paratracheal cysts, masses, or inflammations (Fig. 1.34). They also can result from encroachment upon the airway by endotracheal or endobronchial lesions. Circumferential narrowings are less common, and usually due to congenital or acquired stenoses, or focal areas of tracheomalacia. None of these lesions are particularly common, but with the widespread use of endotracheal tubes in the neonate, acquired tracheal stenosis is becoming more common. Usually these narrowings are located within 1 inch of the vocal cords.

Focal tracheomalacia occurs with any lesion which

causes compression of the trachea in utero. Consequently, it can be seen with compressing vascular anomalies or rings, paratracheal cysts or masses, or even the dilated proximal esophageal pouch of esophageal atresia. In these cases, there is inhibition of normal cartilage development and focal softening of the trachea. In the older infant and child, focal tracheomalacia usually is the result of damage to the trachea by the placement of endotracheal tubes or severe local infections such as croup. In many of these cases, actual fixed fibrotic stenosis eventually develops.

Congenital stenosis of the trachea and bronchi is rather uncommon (8, 17), but does occur (Fig. 1.35).

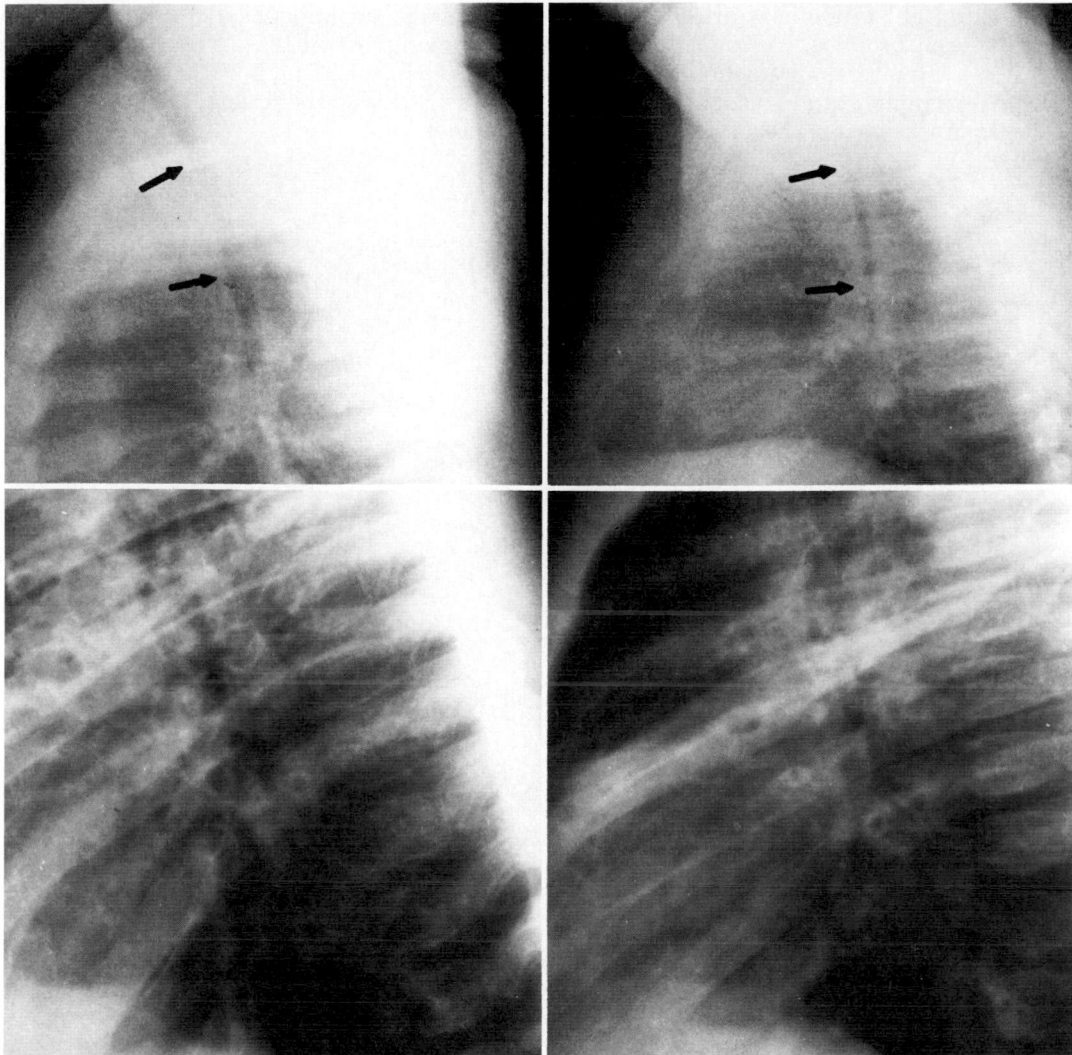

Fig. 1.34. Hypercollapsible trachea. A. Inspiratory view demonstrating a normal tracheal diameter (arrows). B. Expiratory view demonstrates marked diminution of tracheal diameter (arrows). This patient had wheezing which cleared with epinephrine. Eventually, the infant developed asthma. C. **Tracheobronchomegaly.** Inspiratory view demonstrating large cystic structures scattered throughout the lung. These are overly dilated bronchi. D. Expiratory film. Characteristically, the bronchi collapse, (i.e., note how much smaller the cystic areas appear).

These narrowings, of course, can occur anywhere along the tracheobronchial tree and thus differ from narrowings produced by certain masses or vascular anomalies which often have a favorite location. Certainly this is true of the vascular abnormalities causing tracheal compression, and the three most characteristic are the: (*a*) right aortic arch (with or without a vascular ring); (*b*) anomalous innominate or left common carotid arteries; and (*c*) anomalous left pulmonary artery or so-called pulmonary sling (7, 10, 12, 14, 16, 18). Right aortic arch abnormalities produce a characteristic right side tracheal indentation and contralateral shift of the trachea. The indentation is located just above the level of where it would occur if a normal left-side aortic knob were present (Fig.

1.36A). A similar indentation occurs on the barium-filled esophagus, and if the right aortic arch is part of a vascular ring, the barium swallow will demonstrate a characteristic double, opposing, or reverse "S" indentation of the esophagus (see Fig. 1.2).

The indentations produced by the anomalous innominate and left common carotid arteries are identical and located just at the level of the manubrium (Fig. 1.36B). The anomalous innominate artery, however, is far more common, and while a few infants with this indentation may be symptomatic, even to the point of apneic spells (3), the vast majority are asymptomatic (15). These lesions are discussed in more detail on p 2.

With the pulmonary sling, the left pulmonary artery, arising from the right pulmonary artery, swings around the trachea, and produces an indentation on the right (Fig. 1.36C). On lateral view, since the artery travels between the esophagus and trachea, a characteristic posterior indentation on the trachea is produced (Fig. 1.36D).

Finally, an unusual, but not uncommon, tracheal narrowing can occur with impacted esophageal foreign bodies (Fig. 1.35 C, D). Paraesophageal edema is the cause here, and the problem resolves after foreign body removal.

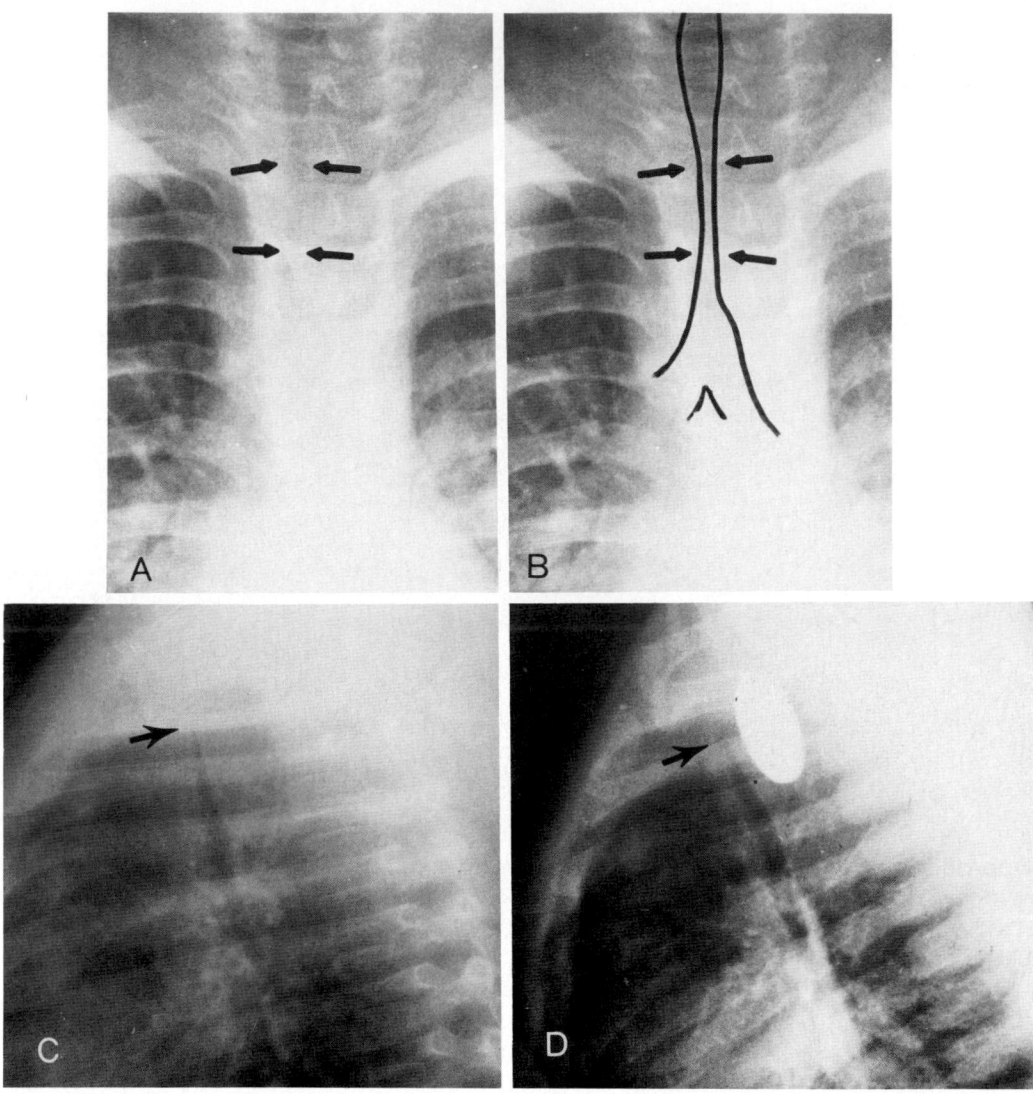

Fig. 1.35. Focal tracheal narrowing. A. Congenital stenosis. Note loss of tracheal air column and tracheal narrowing (arrows). B. Diagrammatic representation of the stenotic portion of the trachea. C. Esophageal foreign body (coin) causing paraesophageal inflammation and compression of the trachea (arrow). D. Same patient. Narrowing (arrow) persists after the coin has been removed. Such narrowing can develop within 2 or 3 days after the foreign body becomes lodged, and characteristically remains for a few days after its removal.

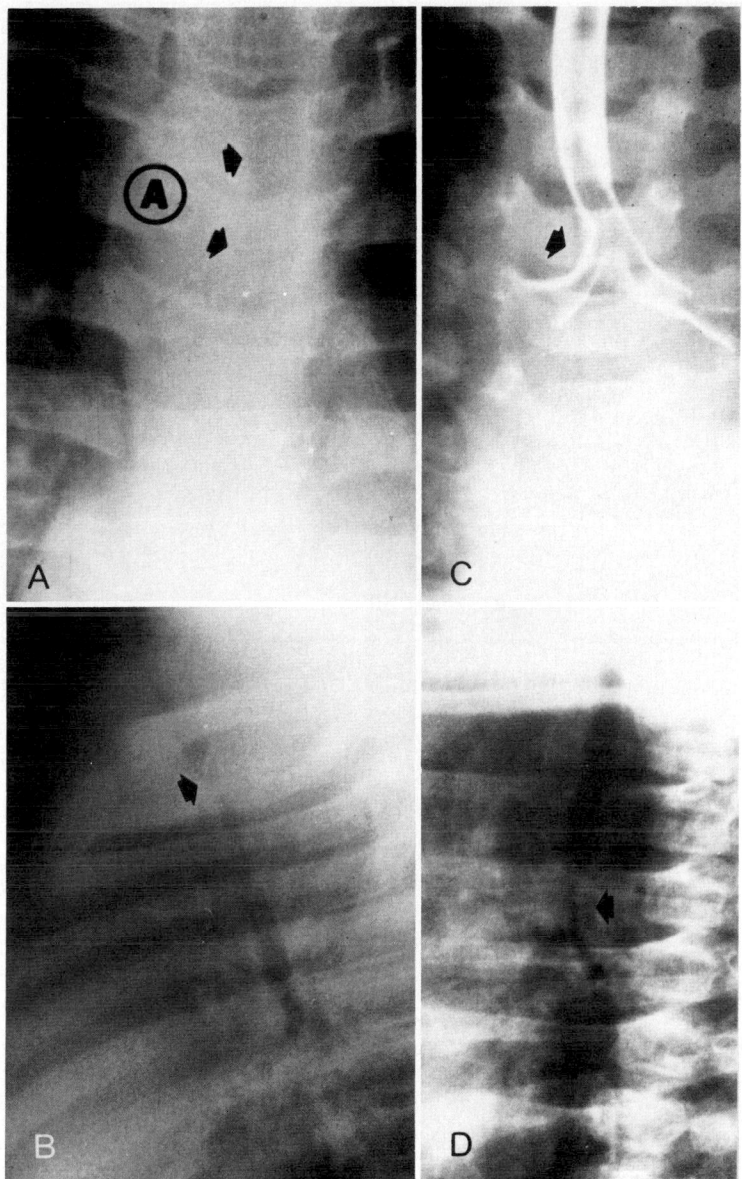

Fig. 1.36. Tracheal deviations due to vascular anomalies. A. Right aortic arch. Note the aorta (A) on the right producing deviation and indentation of the trachea (arrows). The aorta descends on the right (note the slanted paraspinal stripe just below the aortic knob). The soft tissue stripe lateral to the aorta is the superior vena cava. **B. Anomalous innominate artery.** Note characteristic anterior tracheal indentation (arrow) produced by an anomalous innominate artery. **C. Pulmonary sling.** Characteristic indentation, on the right, just at the level of the carina (arrow). D. Lateral view, same patient, demonstrating characteristic posterior indentation and compression of the trachea (arrow). C and D are courtesy of Joe Jackson, M.D., Corpus Christi, Texas.

Air Bronchogram

When air is seen in the bronchi, the term "air bronchogram" is used, and while such a phenomenon occurs in the trachea and major bronchi in normal individuals, when it is seen beyond the second branching of the bronchial tree, it becomes pathologic. In such cases, the pulmonary parenchyma for one reason or another, loses its normal aeration and becomes hazy or opaque. As a result, the air in the small bronchi becomes visible as an air bronchogram, and basically, lung opacification is due either to atelectasis or the accumulation of some type of fluid in the alveoli (i.e., exudate, edema, or blood). Exudate (pus) is seen with consolidating pneumonias, edema fluid from any number of cardiac or noncardiac causes, and blood from

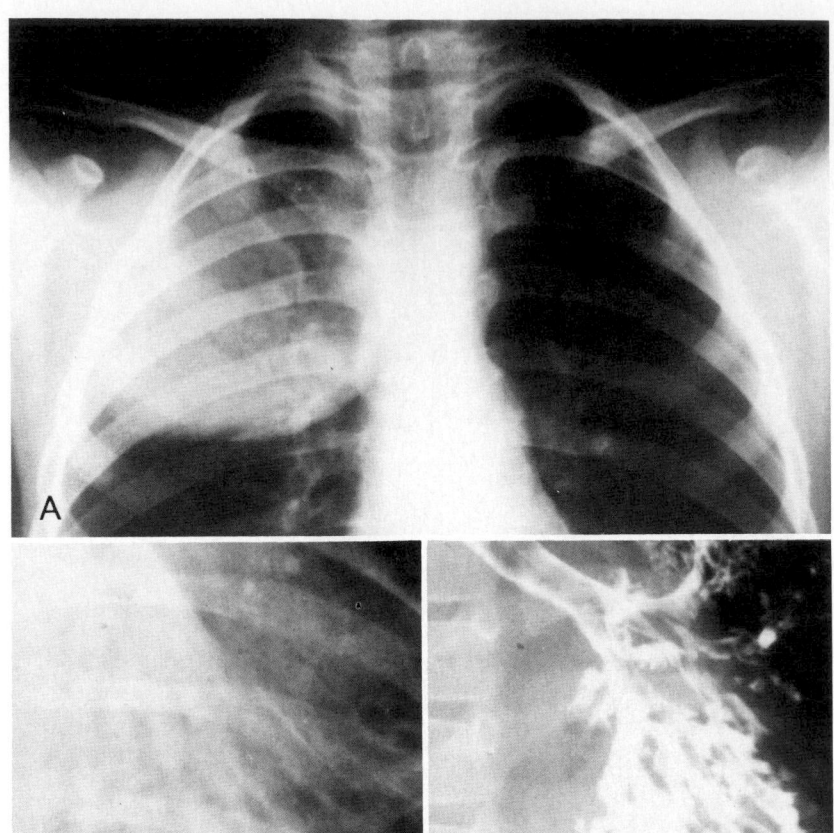

Fig. 1.37. Air bronchogram. A. Consolidating pneumonia. Note the air bronchogram in the consolidated right upper lobe. *Klebsiella* pneumonia. B. Air bronchogram with atelectasis and bronchiectasis. Note the dilated, tortuous air-filled bronchi in the left lower lobe. They are crowded together because of atelectasis and dilated because of bronchiectasis. C. Bronchogram demonstrating the left lower lobe bronchiectatic changes.

contusions, venous infarctions, or intrapulmonary bleeding. In any of these cases, the findings are about the same (Fig. 1.37A), but with compressive atelectasis, the air-filled bronchi in the collapsed lobe are clustered close together. If bronchiectasis also is present, the bronchi become nodular and dilated (Fig. 1.37, B and C).

Rarely, air bronchograms can be seen with extensive interstitial disease (i.e., see Fig. 1.69B), and in such cases, although the alveoli are relatively free of disease, the interstitium is so thickened by infiltrate, edema, or fibrosis that the alveoli are compressed to a near airless state. Alveolar disease, then, is erroneously suggested because the roentgenogram cannot differentiate between alveoli which are packed full of fluid and those squeezed shut by extensive interstitial infiltrate (i.e., both are airless).

References

1. Bateson EM, Woo-Ming M: Tracheobronchomegaly. *Clin Radiol* 24:354–358, 1973.
2. Baxter JD, Dunbar JS: Tracheomalacia. *Ann Otol Rhinol Laryngol* 72:1013–1023, 1963.
3. Berdon WD, Baker DH, Bordiuk J, Mellins R: Innominate artery compression of trachea in infants with stridor and apnea. *Radiology* 92:272–278, 1969.
4. Chang L, Lee F, Gwinn J: Normal lateral deviation of the trachea in infants and children. *Am J Roentgenol Radium Ther Nucl Med* 109:247–251, 1970.
5. Cook RCM, Bush GH: Tracheal compression as a cause of respiratory symptoms after repair of oesophageal atresia. *Arch Dis Child* 53:246–248, 1978.
6. Donaldson SW, Thompsett AC Jr: Tracheal diameter in the normal newborn infant. *Am J Roentgenol Radium Ther Nucl Med* 67:785–787, 1952.
7. Ericsson NO, Soderlund S: Compression of trachea by anomalous innominate artery. *J Pediatr Surg* 4:424–431, 1969.
8. Holinger PH: Congenital anomalies of the tracheobronchial tree. *Postgrad Med* 36:454–462, 1964.
9. Hunter TB, Kuhns LR, Roloff MA, Holt JF: Tracheobronchiomegaly in an eighteen month old child. *Am J Roentgenol* 123:687–690, 1975.
10. Jue KL, Raghib G, Amplatz K, Adams P Jr, Edwards

JE: Anomalous origin of the left pulmonary artery from the right pulmonary artery. *Am J Roentgenol* 95:598–610, 1965.

11. Levin SJ, Adler P, Scherer RA: Collapsible trachea (tracheomalacia): a non-allergic cause of wheezing in infancy. *Ann Allergy* 22:20–25, 1964.

12. Maurseth K: Tracheal stenosis caused by compression from innominate artery. *Ann Radiol* 9:287–294, 1966.

13. Mitchell RE, Burgy RG: Congenital bronchiectasis due to deficiency of bronchial cartilage (Williams-Campbell syndrome). *J Pediatr* 87:230–232, 1975.

14. Möes CAF, Izukawa T, Trusler GA: Innominate artery compression of the trachea. *Arch Otolaryngol* 101:733–738, 1975.

15. Swischuk LE: Anterior tracheal indentation in infancy and early childhood: normal or abnormal? *Am J Roentgenol Radium Ther Nucl Med* 112:12–17, 1971.

16. Swischuk LE: *Plain Film Interpretation in Congenital Heart Disease*, ed 2. Williams & Wilkins, Baltimore, 1979, pp 205–226.

17. Taybi II: Congenital malformations of the larynx, trachea, bronchi and lungs. In Kaufman HJ (ed): *Progress in Pediatric Radiology*, Chicago, Year Book Medical Publishers, 1967, pp 231–255.

18. Tesler UF, Balsara RH, Niguidula F: Aberrant left pulmonary artery (vascular sling): report of five cases. *Chest* 66:402–407, 1974.

19. Williams HE, Landau LI, Phelan PD: Generalized bronchiectasis due to extensive deficiency of bronchial cartilage. *Arch Dis Child* 47:423–428, 1972.

FREE AND LOCULATED AIR

Free air can accumulate in the pleural space (pneumothorax), mediastinum (pneumomediastinum), pericardial cavity (pneumopericardium), and in the heart itself (pneumocardium). The most common of these, of course, is pneumothorax.

Pneumothorax

Pneumothorax, beyond the neonatal period, is not extremely common in children, and spontaneous pneumothorax, as opposed to adults, is quite rare (10). However, recently a familial form has been noted (16), but generally, when pneumothorax is present in a child, some underlying problem such as chest trauma, asthma (1, 5), ruptured pneumatocele, etc., is the cause (Table 1.8). Chest trauma, however, probably is most common.

With pneumothorax, air can outline the lung circumferentially, or can accumulate along any of its surfaces. This is important to appreciate, for one can encounter subpulmonic, medial, and anterior air accumulations, and when any of these occur alone, they may be missed or misinterpreted. Classically, however, free air tends to produce a band of hyperlucency (vascular marking free) between the chest wall and the underlying lung (Fig. 1.38A).

Medial pneumothoraces, that is, collections of air between the mediastinum and the inner lung edge, most commonly occur in the neonate (11, 14), but can be seen in older children. They must be differentiated from the normal radiolucent halo around the heart, occasionally produced by juxtapositioning of the left cardiac border and the lower lobe pulmonary artery, and from pneumopericardium. When a medial pneumothorax is suspected, decubitus views should be obtained as the air will shift (rise) to a more familiar location, that is, against the lateral chest wall.

Anterior pneumothoraces, that is, free air layered over the anterior surface of the lungs in patients examined in the supine position, also pose considerable diagnostic problems. Although first described in the neonate (14), they also can occur in older children. When present, they produce hyperlucency of the involved hemithorax (due to increased air in the pleural space and compression of the lung below it), and exaggerated sharpness of the ipsilateral mediastinal edge (see Fig. 1.25). This latter finding is due to air abutting the mediastinum and is important to note because often, no other findings of pneumothorax are present.

Table 1.8 Free and Loculated Air

1. Pneumothorax		
Chest trauma	}	Commonest
Ruptured cyst or pneumatocele		
Asthma		Relatively uncommon
Foreign body		
Other obstructive emphysema		
Esophageal perforation		Rare
Spontaneous pneumothorax		
2. Mediastinal air		
A. Pneumomediastinum		
Asthma	}	Commonest
Chest trauma	}	Moderately common
Foreign body		
Paroxysmal coughing		Relatively rare
Esophageal perforation		
B. Air in mediastinal viscera (hiatus hernia, obst esophagus)		Relatively uncommon
3. Pneumopericardium		
Trauma	}	Commonest
Other causes	}	Relatively rare
4. Pneumocardium		
Penetrating trauma	}	Commonest
Other causes	}	Relatively rare

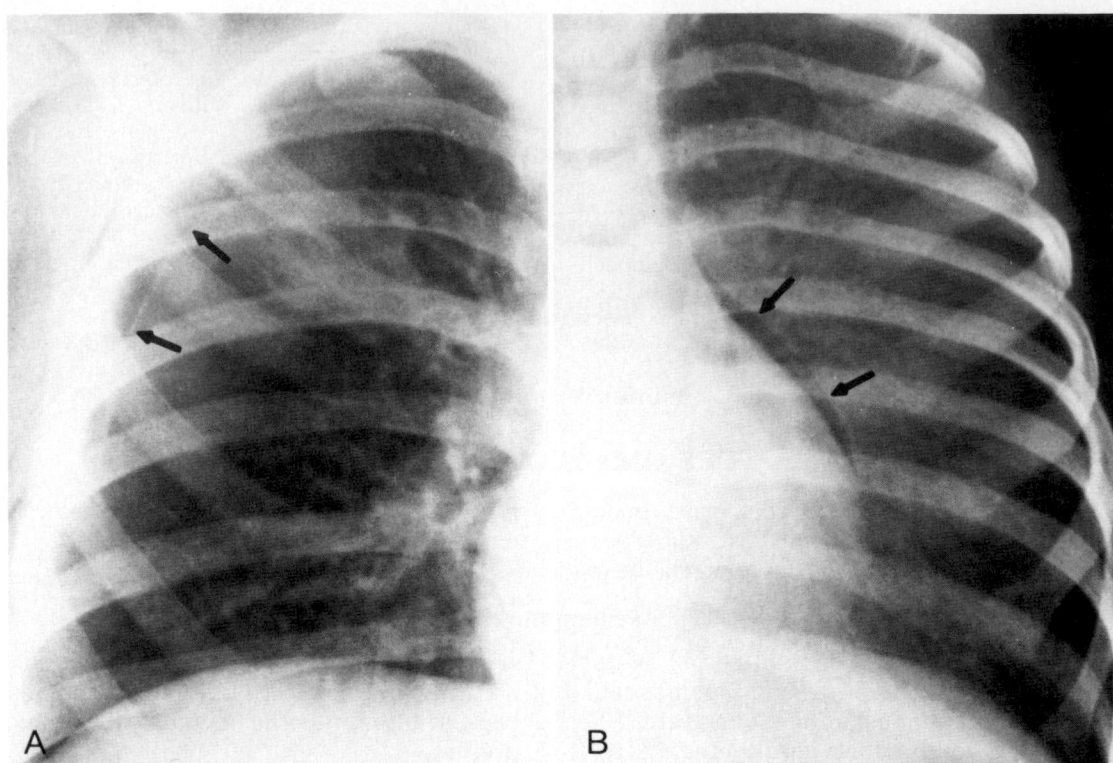

Fig. 1.38. A. **Typical pneumothorax.** Note the free edge of the right lung (arrow). Some air also is present outside the chest wall because of penetrating chest trauma. B. **Medial pneumothorax.** Note the medial pneumothorax (arrows) in this patient whose lung was biopsied for verification of *Pneumocystis carinii* pneumonia (i.e., hazy lungs).

Pneumomediastinum

The commonest cause of pneumomediastinum in the pediatric age group is airway obstruction as seen in asthma (1, 5, 6, 9, 10), and although pneumomediastinum also can occur with obstructing foreign bodies, other focal or generalized airway obstructions, all of these situations are rather uncommon (Table 1.8). Next most commonly after asthma, pneumomediastinum can be seen with chest trauma, and iatrogenically after endoscopy or positive pressure ventilation. Paroxysms of coughing also occasionally can lead to pneumomediastinum (i.e., pertussis pneumonia), but the situation does not arise very often. Pneumomediastinum secondary to spontaneous esophageal perforation also is rare.

Air in the mediastinum produces irregular gas collections within the soft tissues of the superior mediastinum, and often extends into the soft tissues of the neck or chest wall. This is termed subcutaneous interstitial emphysema (Fig. 1.39) and indeed, there may be more air in the extrathoracic soft tissues than in the mediastinum itself. Air in the mediastinum often is visualized better on lateral, than on frontal views, and occasionally can track downward and produce similar irregular collections of air in the lower mediastinum. In other cases, air can pass into the abdominal cavity producing pneumoperitoneum. On rare occasions (except in the neonate), pneumomediastinal

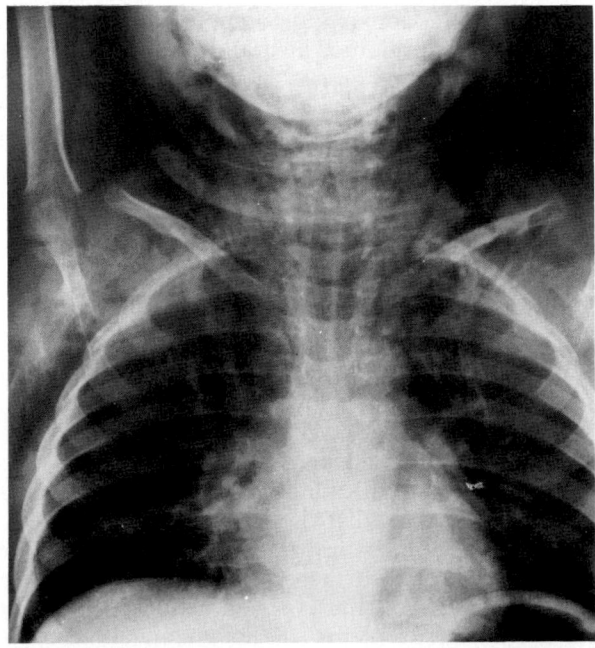

Fig. 1.39. Pneumomediastinum. Note characteristic irregular air collections throughout the superior mediastinum, extending into the neck. This patient had a punctured trachea.

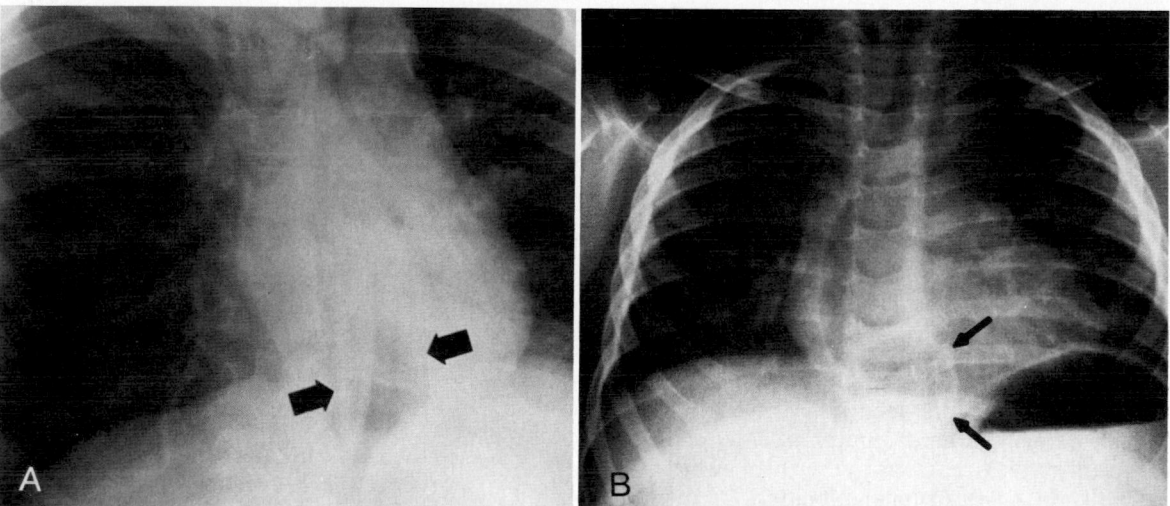

Fig. 1.40. Central mediastinal air collections. A. Air in inferior pulmonary ligament. Note typical appearance of such air (arrows) in this location. This patient also had left lower lobe atelectasis, right upper lobe atelectasis, and air in the superior mediastinum. All of these changes resulted from massive aspiration of foreign material. B. **Hiatus hernia.** Note the typical appearance of air in the hiatus hernia (arrows). Air also is present in the remainder of the esophagus, which also is wider than normal. This is termed mega-aeroesophagus, and is a reliable plain film sign of gastroesophageal reflux.

air may accumulate along the diaphragmatic leaflets (between the diaphragm and the parietal pleura), and mimic a subpulmonic pneumothorax. If such air crosses the superior surface of the diaphragm, it will outline the diaphragm in its entirety (7). Finally, it might be noted that pneumomediastinal air also can accumulate in the inferior pulmonary ligaments, and as such, produce a characteristic oblong or oval air collection behind the heart (Fig. 1.40A). Such air

collections commonly occur with blunt chest trauma (2–4, 13) and with positive pressure assisted ventilation. They must be differentiated from the circular to oval collection of air in a hiatus hernia (Fig. 1.40B). Air in a dilated esophagus (1 cm in diameter or more) also can be seen with esophageal reflux (Fig. 1.40B). This finding, termed mega-aeroesophagus, is most common in the perinatal period and in children with cerebral palsy or mental retardation (15).

Pneumopericardium

Pneumopericardium generally is uncommon in the pediatric age group, but can be seen with chest trauma and positive pressure assisted ventilation. Of course, the latter mechanism accounts for a good many pericardial air collections in the neonate, but in older children, the problem is much less common. With small volume air collections within the pericardial cavity, air may not surround the entire heart, but most often enough air is present to allow visualization of the pericardial sac (thin white stripe) itself (Fig. 1.41).

Fig. 1.41. Pneumopericardium. A. Note air within the pericardial sac, outlining the sac itself (arrows). Air also is present around the great vessels, and associated pneumomediastinum has outlined the thymus gland. B. All of these latter structures are identified; aorta (A), pulmonary artery (P), and thymus (T).

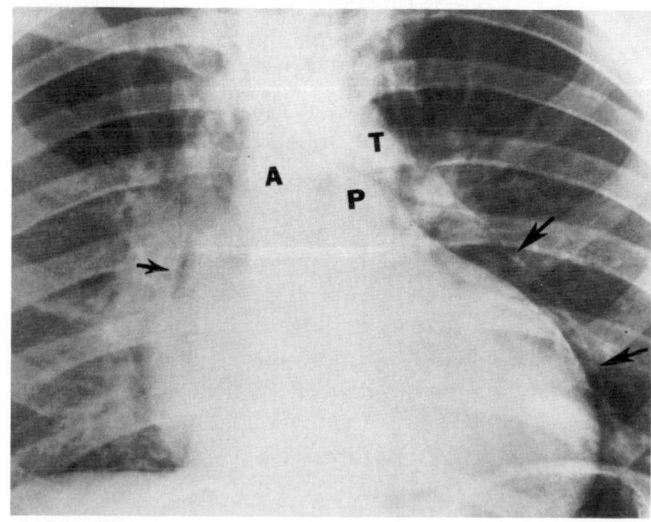

Fig. 1.41.

Pneumocardium

Air within the heart is quite rare and almost always is secondary to penetrating trauma of the chest, or trauma to the large peripheral blood vessels resulting in air embolus of the heart. However, it also can be seen on an iatrogenic basis, secondary to positive pressure ventilation (usually neonate), and after having been accidentally introduced into the vascular system during intravenous injections.

Free Air and Fluid

Air, when combined with fluid, in any of the foregoing compartments results in air-fluid levels on upright or decubitus views. In the pleural space, such air-fluid levels can be seen with pyo- or hemopneumothorax. Air-fluid levels in the pleural space also occur with esophageal perforation, and air-fluid levels in the mediastinum can be seen with hiatus hernia, inferior pulmonary ligament pneumatocele, esophageal obstruction, and occasionally, with pneumopericardium. Multiple air-fluid levels, located behind the sternum, and often just off midline on frontal view, are characteristic of colon interpositions. These patients usually have had either a lye stricture or esophageal atresia requiring the replacement of the esophagus by a portion of their own colon. Tunneling the stomach into the chest also occasionally is utilized to accomplish the same end. In either case, the air-filled segment of transposed intestinal tract can be seen behind the sternum (Fig. 1.42).

mediastinal air cyst. A case report. *Pediatr Radiol* 4:120–121, 1976.

4. Hyde I: Traumatic paramediastinal air cysts. *Br J Radiol* 44:380–383, 1971.
5. Jorgensen J, Falliers C, Bukantz S: Pneumothorax and mediastinal and subcutaneous emphysema in children with bronchial asthma. *Pediatrics* 31:824–832, 1963.
6. Kirsh M, Orvald T: Mediastinal and subcutaneous emphysema complicating acute bronchial asthma. *Chest* 57:580–581, 1970.
7. Levin B: Continuous diaphragm sign: newly recognized sign of pneumomediastinum. *Clin Radiol* 24:337–338, 1973.
8. Lillard RL, Allen RP: The extrapleural air sign in pneumomediastinum. *Radiology* 85:1093–1098, 1965.
9. McGovern J, Roett K, Haywood TJ, Hensel AE Jr: Mediastinal and subcutaneous emphysema complicating atopic asthma in infants and children. *Pediatrics* 27:951–960, 1961.
10. McSweeney WJ, Stempel DA: Non-iatrogenic pneumo-

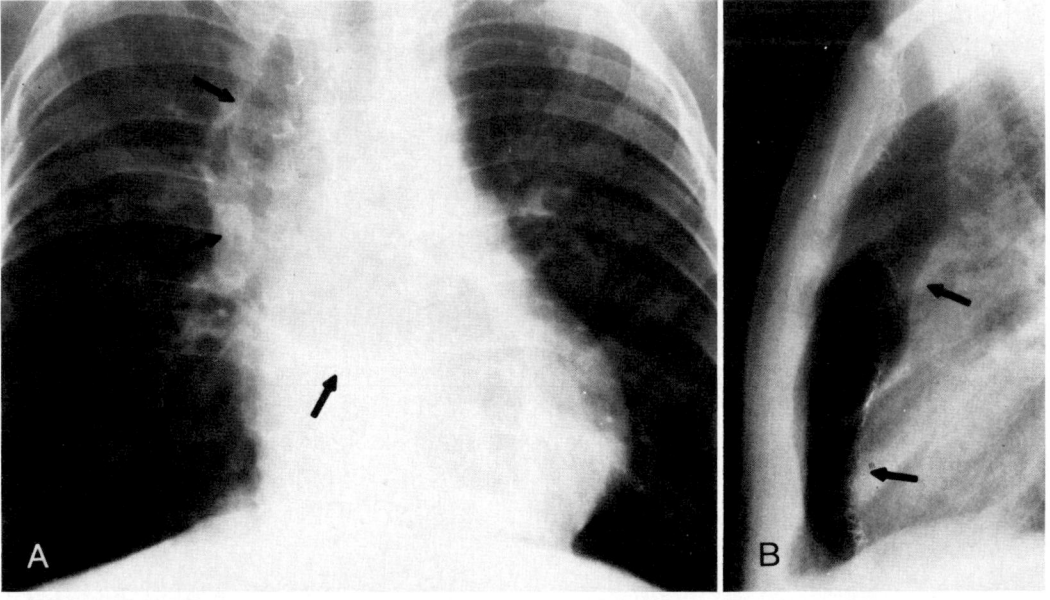

Fig. 1.42. Retrosternal stomach tunnel. A. Note air outlining the retrosternally transfered stomach (arrows). B. Lateral view demonstrating similar findings (arrows).

References

1. Bierman CW: Pneumomediastinum and pneumothorax complicating asthma in children. *Am J Dis Child* 114:42–50, 1967.
2. Fagan AH, Rogers BM, Talbert JL: Traumatic mediastinal pneumatoceles. *Radiology* 120:11–18, 1976.
3. Felman AH, Rogers BM, Talbert JL: Traumatic para-

mediastinum in infancy and childhood. *Pediatr Radiol* 1:139–144, 1973.
11. Moskowitz PS, Griscom NT: the medial pneumothorax. *Radiology* 120:143–147, 1976.
12. Ozonoff M: Pneumomediastinum associated with asthma and pneumonia in children. *Am J Roentgenol* 95:112–117, 1965.
13. Ravin C, Smith GW, Lester PD, McLoud TC, Putman

CE: Post-traumatic pneumatocele in the inferior pulmonary ligament. *Radiology* 121:39–41, 1976.

14. Swischuk LE: Two lesser known but useful signs of neonatal pneumothorax. *Am J Roentgenol* 127:623–627, 1976.

15. Swischuk LE, Hayden CK Jr, van Caillie B: Megaaeroesophagus in childhood: a sign of esophageal sphincter dysfunction. *Radiology* 141:73–76, 1981.

16. Wilson WG, Aylsworth AS: Familial spontaneous pneumothorax. *Pediatrics* 64:172–175, 1979.

PLEURAL SPACE AND FISSURE THICKENING

Thickening of the Pleural Space

Thickening of the pleural space can be generalized or localized and when generalized, most often is due to some type of fluid collection. Thickening of the pleura (fibrosis) is less common in children, and as far as fluid is concerned, any type of fluid can accumulate in the pleural space. However, pus (i.e., empyema) and serous effusions are the commonest (Table 1.9). Empyema can accompany any number of bacterial pneumonias, but most commonly is seen with staphylococcal, Hemophilus influenzae, and diplococcus (streptococcus) pneumoniae infections (3, 5). Pleural fluid accumulations with viral and mycoplasma pneumoniae respiratory tract infections are rare (2).

Serous pleural effusions commonly occur with renal diseases such as acute glomerulonephritis, nephrotic syndrome, chronic renal failure, and with tumors such as lymphoma and neuroblastoma in the abdomen or chest. Serous effusions also occur with other tumors in the chest, iatrogenic fluid overload, and congestive heart failure due to a number of causes. Blood in the pleural space most commonly occurs with chest trauma, occasionally with bleeding disorders, catheter erosions, or aortic rupture, and least frequently with rupture of a ductus arteriosus aneurysm. With aortic rupture, fluid often accumulates over the left apex, as the point of rupture is in that portion of the transverse arch which lies in communication with the left pleural space. Blood leaks over the top of the lung to produce the so-called apical cap (4), a finding which when seen with a widened mediastinum should suggest aortic rupture. Apical caps, however, can occur for other reasons and one due to an underlying rib fracture is seen in Figure 1.44. If chyle accumulates in the chest of patients beyond the neonatal period, chest trauma or thoracic surgery are the usual causes and the chylothorax results from thoracic duct injury.

The most typical appearance of fluid in the pleural space is that which results when fluid accumulates over the lateral and apical portions of the lung (Fig. 1.43). Similar fluid accumulations can be seen on lateral view, occurring either along the anterior or posterior chest walls. Posteriorly, a costophrenic angle meniscus can be a clue to the presence of such fluid. If fluid accumulates over the diaphragmatic leaflets, a subpulmonic effusion results and an abnormality of diaphragmatic contour is seen (see Fig. 1.92). Over the apex, pleural fluid accumulation must be differentiated from normal soft tissues which, to the uninitiated, may have an appearance virtually indistinguishable from fluid (Fig. 1.44). This finding is common in children as well as adults and is due to normal subpleural fat and muscle (6).

Thickening of the pleural space due to fibrosis, is less common in children, but frequently must be differentiated from pleural fluid. For the most part, this is accomplished with decubitus views which show that fibrous thickening does not change its configuration while fluid does. However, one must remember

Table 1.9 Pleural Space and Fissure Thickening

1. **Pleural space thickening**

A. Fluid	}	Commonest
Empyema Serous effusion	}	Commonest
Blood	}	Moderately common
Chyle	}	Rare
B. Pleural fibrosis	}	Moderately common
C. Underlying rib lesions	}	Relatively rare
D. Pleural tumor	}	Very rare

2. **Pleural fissure thickening**

A. Fluid		
Serous effusion	}	Commonest

Purulent effusion
    Blood
    Adjacent pulmonary
      edema
	}	Moderately common

Chyle	}	Relatively rare

3. **Localized subpleural thickening**

A. Underlying rib lesions	}	Commonest

Fracture with hematoma
    Osteomyelitis with pus
    Metatases to rib[a]
    Leukemia-Lymphoma[a]
	}	Moderately common

Primary bone tumor	}	Very rare
B. Pleural tumor	}	Very rare

[a] May be diffuse and cause widespread thickening.

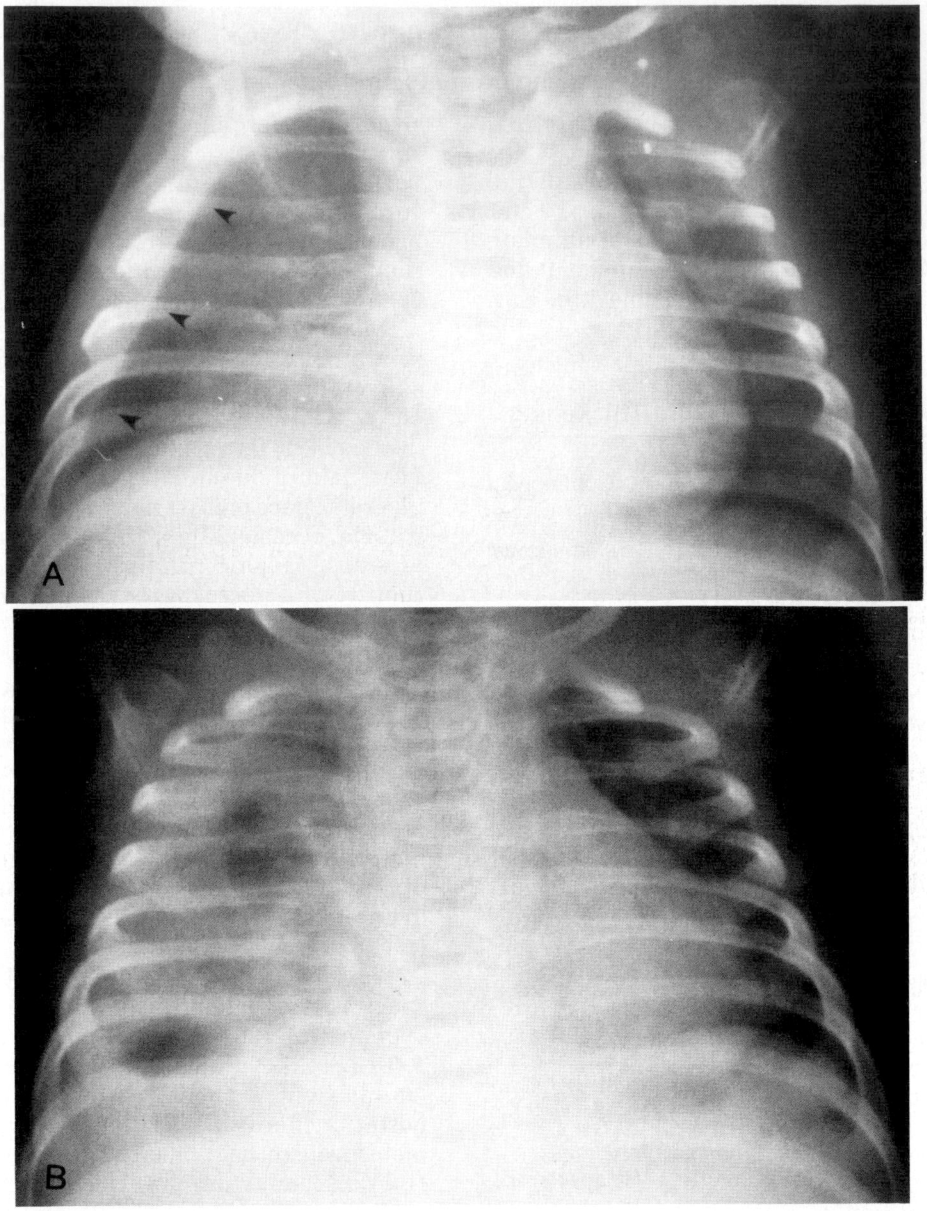

Fig. 1.43. Pleural fluid. A. Note characteristic appearance of pleural fluid accumulating laterally (arrows). One should recall that this fluid actually surrounds the lung and this is why the whole lung itself appears a little hazy. B. Later on, typical pneumatoceles have developed in this patient with staphylococcal empyema and pneumonia.

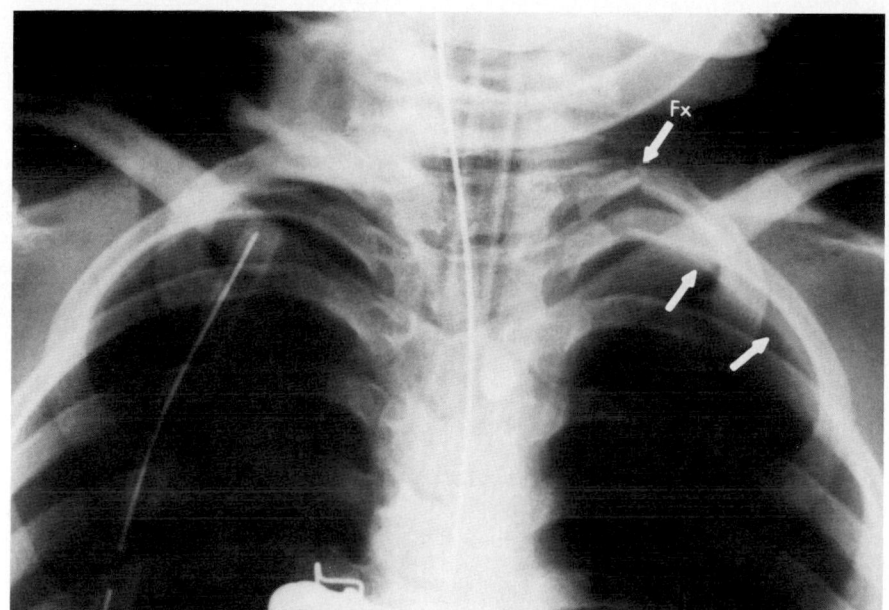

Fig. 1.44. Pleural fluid over apex of lung. Note characteristic appearance of fluid over the apex of the left lung (left arrow). Also note the fracture of the first rib (Fx). A tube is in place for a pneumothorax on the right. The "apparent" fluid collection over the right apex is not fluid at all, but normal soft tissue commonly seen in this area in children.

that in some cases of empyema, or clotted blood, the fluid is so thick or so loculated, that it does not shift. Nonetheless, decubitus views are still worthwhile for differentiating pleural thickening due to fibrosis from pleural thickening due to the accumulation of fluid.

Localized Thickenings of the Pleura

Localized thickenings of the pleura almost always are due to some underlying lesion of the rib, or old infection, trauma, or surgery (Table 1.9). These include hematoma with fracture, osteomyelitis with pus, and metastases to the ribs (Fig. 1.45). When extensive, the latter may be more diffuse than localized. Primary bone tumors and primary pleural tumors are quite rare. **Pleural fissure thickening**, when minimal, can be due to accumulation of fluid in the fissure, or the accumulation of fluid in the immediate subpleural space (Fig. 1.46, A, B, C). Actually, in the early stages of interstitial pulmonary edema, the latter probably is more common and results from the distention of subpleural lymphatics. When the finding is due to actual pleural fluid, the fluid most often is serous (Table 1.9), and the degree of thickening depends on the degree of fluid present. In more severe cases, actual loculations of fluid can be seen (Fig. 1.46D). Thickening of the pleural fissures secondary to fibrosis is uncommon in the pediatric age group, but occasionally can occur after infection or trauma.

Localized **thickening over the apex** of the lungs most often is due to normal soft tissues. Thereafter one should consider some type of fluid collection, and lastly an underlying rib lesion, or pleural fibrosis. As far as fluid collections are concerned the causes are the same as for generalized fluid accumulations. However, over the apex one should be aware of the propensity for blood to accumulate here with aortic rupture (4).

References

1. Bean WJ, Jordan RB, Gentry H, Nice CM: Fissure lines in the pediatric roentgenogram. *Am J Roentgenol Radium Ther Nucl Med* 106:109–113, 1969.
2. Fine NL, Smith LR, Sheedy PF: Frequency of pleural effusions in mycoplasma and viral pneumonias. *N Engl J Med* 283:791–793, 1970.
3. Highman JH: Staphylococcal pneumonia and empyema in childhood. *Am J Roentgenol* 106:103–108, 1969.
4. Simeone JF, Minagi H, Putman CE: Traumatic disruption of the thoracic aorta: significance of the left apical extrapleural cap. *Radiology* 117:265–268, 1975.
5. Smith PL, Gerald B: Empyema in childhood followed roentgenographically: decortication seldom needed. *Am J Roentgenol* 106:114–117, 1969.
6. Vix V: Extrapleural costal fat. *Radiology* 112:563–565, 1974.

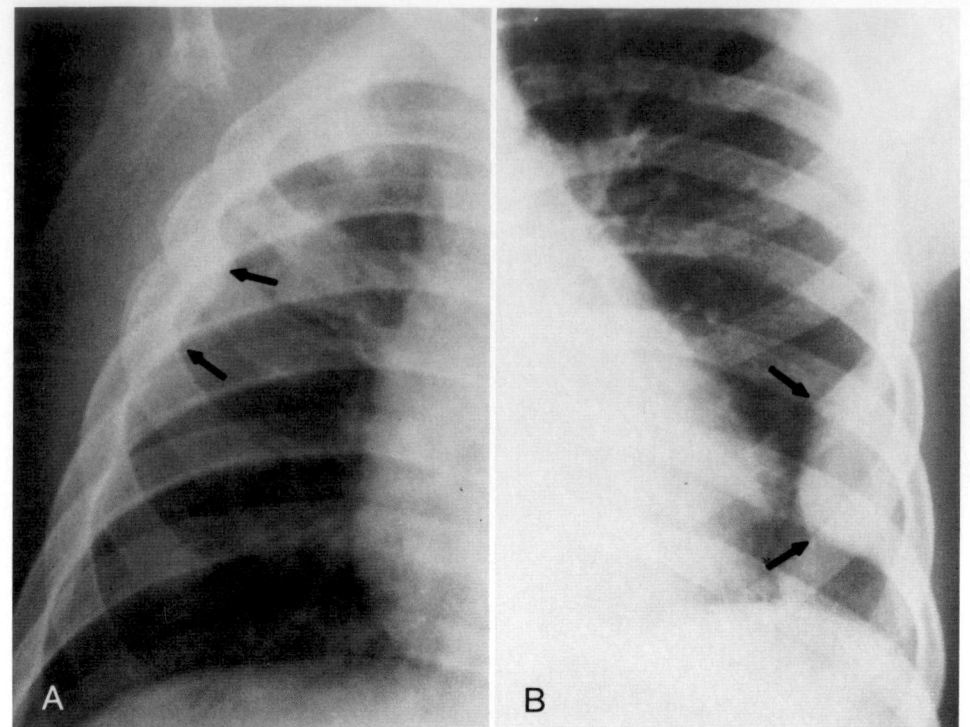

Fig. 1.45.

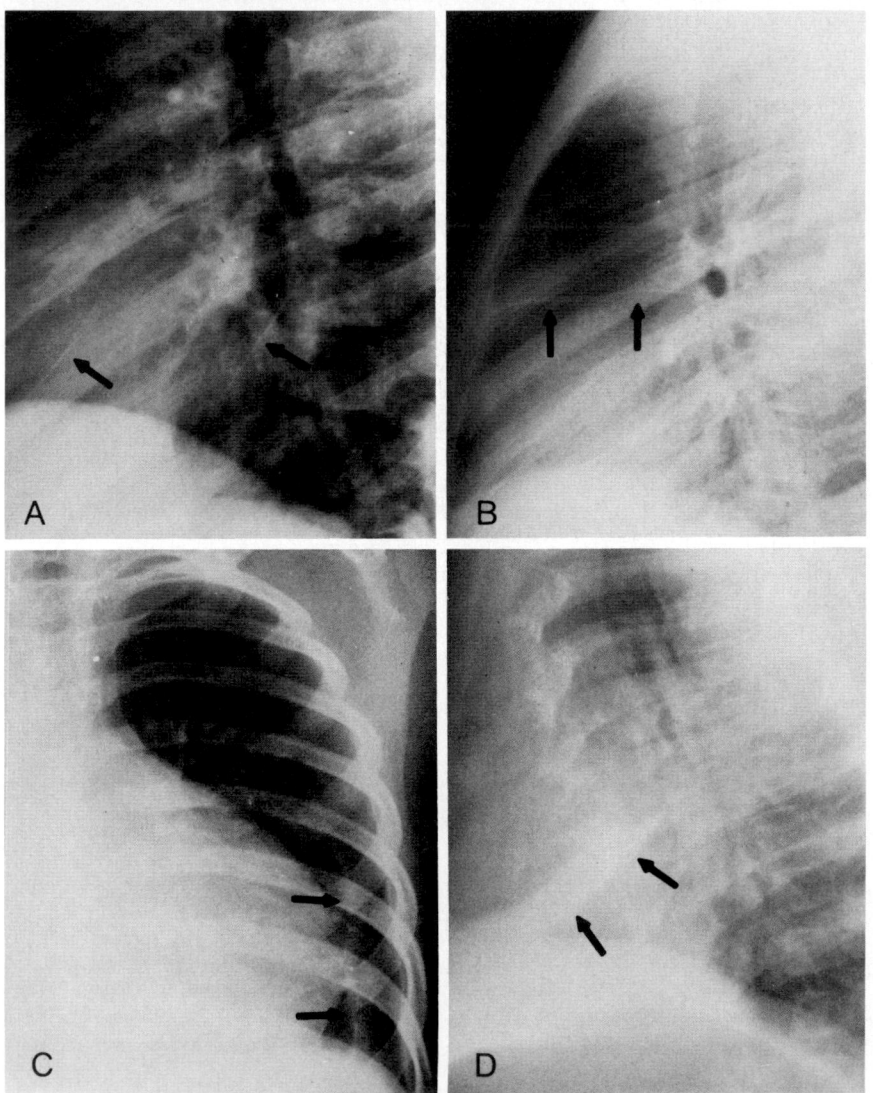

Fig. 1.46.

CALCIFICATIONS IN THE CHEST

A number of different calcifications can occur in the chest of a child, but almost always, when calcification is seen, the disease process is chronic or healed. Such calcifications, for the most part, are flocculent, irregular, curvilinear, or punctate, (Table 1.10).

Table 1.10 Calcifications in the Chest

1. Flocculent or irregular
   - Healed, peripheral granulomas (nodules)
   - Old inflamed lymph nodes } Most common

   - Old thrombi in IVC or SVC } Moderately common

   - Necrotic or treated tumor
   - Calcific pericarditis
   - Pleural calcifications
   - Teratoma
   - Old pulmonary hematoma
   - Old pneumonia
   - Hamartoma
   - Cardiac valve
   - Myocardial infarction } Rare
2. Linear and curvilinear
   - Pleura
   - Pericardium
   - Vascular } Relatively uncommon

   - Calcification in wall of cyst } Rare
3. Punctate calcifications
   - Old healed granulomatous disease } Most common

   - Calcification ligamentum arteriosum
   - Osteogenic sarcoma metastases } Relatively uncommon

   - Chickenpox pneumonia
   - Pulmonary microlithiasis
   - Hypercalcemia states
   - Sarcoidosis } Very rare

Flocculent and Irregular Calcifications

This type of calcification commonly is seen in granulomatous pulmonary nodules or lymph nodes (Fig. 1.47, A and B). Most commonly, the underlying infection is tuberculosis or fungal disease, but every so often, similar calcifications can be seen in tumors undergoing necrosis, either spontaneously or after therapy (Fig. 1.47C). Flocculent calcification, within a pulmonary nodule, is most characteristic of a ha-

Fig. 1.45. Local pleural thickenings. A. Note typical localized pleural thickening (arrows). Also note periosteal new bone deposition on the adjacent ribs. This was the site of former tube placement for drainage of fluid. B. Another case with a typical area of localized subpleural fluid collection (arrows). This was pus due to osteomyelitis of the rib which became roentgenographically visible later on.
Fig. 1.46. Pleural fissure thickening. A. **Normal.** Note the normal, thin pleural fissures (arrows). B. **Early fluid.** Note that the minor fissure (arrows) in this patient with glomerulonephritis and pulmonary edema is thicker than the fissures in A. C. So-called vertical fissure (arrows). This is the major fissure visualized in displaced, oblique position; a phenomenon which usually occurs when cardiomegaly is present. D. Loculated pleural effusion in the major fissure causes marked thickening of the fissure (arrows).

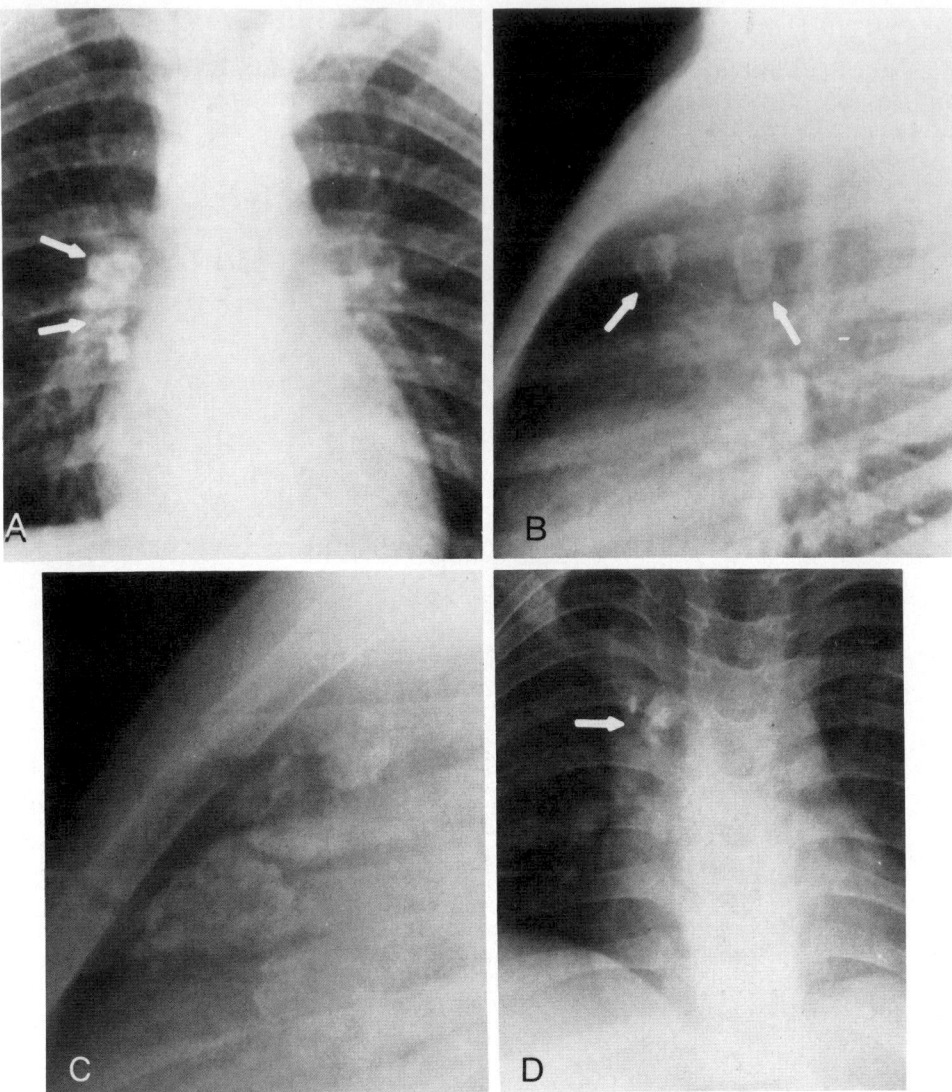

Fig. 1.47. Irregular calcifications. A. Note typical irregular calcification of lymph nodes in the right hilar region (arrows) in this patient with old healed tuberculosis. B. Lateral view showing the calcified, shell-like periphery of the paratracheal and anterior mediastinal lymph nodes (arrows). C. Old calcified posttreatment lymphoma lymph nodes in the mediastinum. D. Note the typically irregularly calcified thrombus in the superior vena cava (arrow). Also note the tip of the adjacent shunt tube in this patient shunted for hydrocephalus.

martoma (see Fig. 1.56B). These lesions, of course, are rare, but the flocculent calcification belies the presence of cartilage, and as such, is a significant diagnostic feature of the lesion.

Irregular calcifications, of various sizes, also occur in old thrombi in the superior and inferior vena cavae (2, 5, 9), and while many are idiopathic (probably the result of dehydration, sepsis, or infection in infancy), others are the result of indwelling catheters or shunt tubes for hydrocephalus. The characteristic location

of these calcifications is what identifies them as such (Fig. 1.47D). In addition, however, some are bullet-shaped. Other less common causes of irregular or fluocculent calcification include calcific pericarditis, pleural calcification secondary to old infections, calcification in an old pulmonary hematoma, calcification in an old pneumonia, calcification in a cartilaginous rib tumor, and rarely calcification of the myocardium after infarction in the neonatal period (3), or calcification of diseased cardiac valves (7).

Linear and Curvilinear Calcifications

These calcifications occur within the walls of blood vessels or cysts, or in serous membranes such as the pericardium and pleura. With these latter structures,

calcification almost always is secondary to old inflammatory disease or trauma, and poses no real difficulty in identification. Vascular calcifications are relatively

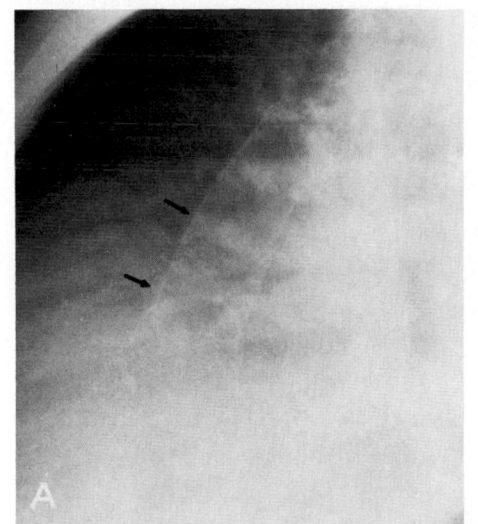

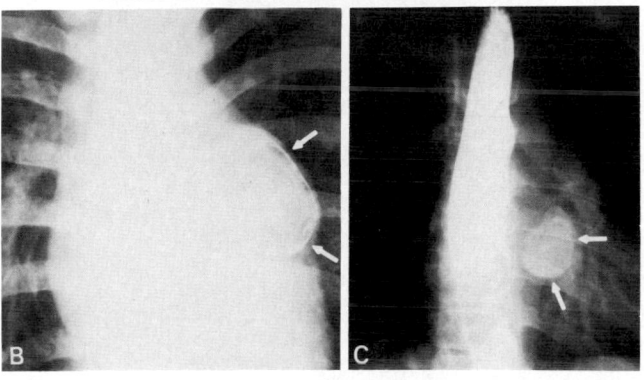

Fig. 1.48. Curvilinear calcifications. A. Linear calcification in aorta in patient with possible Singleton-Mertin syndrome. B. Typical calcification (arrow) in the dilated patch used for correction of tetralogy of Fallot. C. Unusual calcification in bronchogenic cyst (arrows). Nature of cyst presumed on the basis of location. Skin test negative, patient not from endemic Echinococcal area and the cyst was found as an incidental lesion.

uncommon in the pediatric age group, but idiopathic calcification of the great vessels can occur in the young infant (8), and within the aorta of older children with the Singleton-Merten syndrome (4) (Fig. 1.48A). Calcifications in great vessel aneurysms, mycotic or otherwise, are uncommon (10), and so is calcification of the patch used for correction of infundibular stenosis in tetralogy of Fallot. In these cases, aneurysmal dilation of the repaired infundibular region precedes the appearance of calcification, but when calcification occurs, it is rather characteristic (Fig. 1.48B). Calcification within the walls of bronchogenic cysts is rare

(Fig. 1.48C), but calcification of acquired cysts, such as echinococcal cysts, is considerably more common. Overall, however, the frequency of this latter cyst being encountered depends on the geographic location of one's practice. In our area, it is extremely uncommon.

Curvilinear lymph node calcifications resulting in so-called eggshell calcifications are rare in children. However, some calcified lymph nodes, either tuberculous or fungal, occasionally can calcify in such a fashion (see Fig. 1.47B).

Punctate Calcifications

Punctate, parenchymal calcifications can be single or multiple, and most often result from tuberculous or histoplasmic infections (Fig. 1.49A). Of course, they also can be seen with other fungal diseases, and their main differential diagnosis, especially when multiple, is that of normal blood vessels seen on end. Other causes of multiple punctate calcifications in the parenchyma include chickenpox, pneumonia (usually immunologically suppressed patients), and pulmonary microlithiasis. Both problems, however, are extremely rare in children. Calcification due to bone formation within metastatic nodules from osteogenic sarcoma

can be punctate, but such nodules seldom are discovered before the presence of the primary tumor is known.

A peculiar, small, often punctate, calcification is that which occurs in the ligamentum arteriosum (1). This calcification is located just between the aorta and pulmonary artery, and although often punctate, it also can be comma or flame-shaped (Fig. 1.49B). The location of this calcification is what suggests its origin most strongly because, characteristically, it lies between the pulmonary artery and aorta.

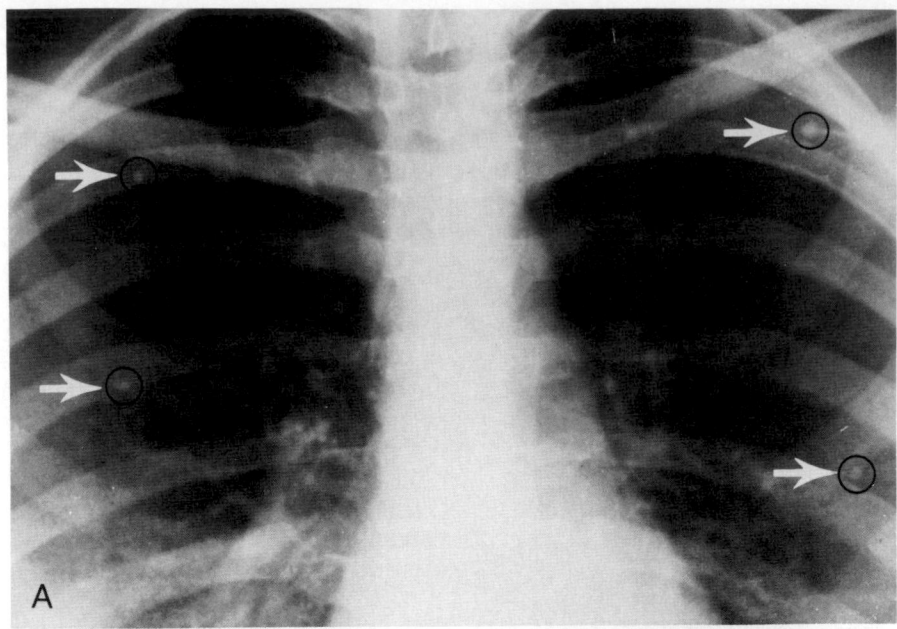

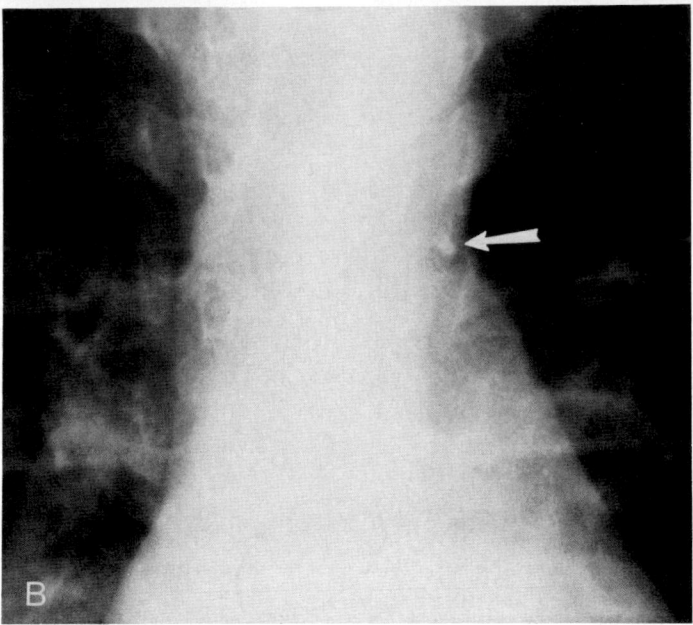

Fig. 1.49. Punctate calcifications. A. Note numerous small punctate calcifications in this patient with healed histoplasmosis (arrows). These densities are located too far out in the periphery to be blood vessels seen on end. When central, however, they can be difficult to differentiate from blood vessels seen on end. Also, note calcifications in right hilar nodes. B. Small punctate calcification (arrow) in typical location of ligamentum arteriosum.

Miscellaneous Calcifications

Diffuse calcification of the lungs is very uncommon, but can be seen with chronic hypercalcemic states such as end stage chronic renal failure (6). In such cases, calcium is deposited in the interstitium of the lungs, much the same as in other soft tissues of the body. Formed calcifications representing bony structures, or even teeth, are characteristic of teratomas, but these tumors also can present with nonspecific irregular calcifications.

References

1. Currarino G, Jackson JH Jr: Calcifications of ductus arteriosus and ligamentum Botalli. *Radiology* 94:139–142, 1970.
2. Kassner EG, Baumstark A, Kinkhabwala MN, Ablow RC, Haller JO: Calcified thrombus in the inferior vena cava in infants and children. *Pediatr Radiol* 4:167–171, 1976.
3. Kogutt M: Personal communication.

4. Singleton EB, Merten DF: An unusual syndrome of widened medullary cavities of the metacarpals and phalanges, aortic calcification and abnormal dentition. *Pediatr Radiol* 1:2–7, 1973.
5. Singleton EB, Rosenberg HS: Intraluminal calcification of the inferior vena cava. *Am J Roentgenol* 86:556–560, 1961.
6. Slovis TL, Chand N, Shanovos TO, Fleischmann LE, Brough AJ: Pulmonary calcifications in a child with renal failure. *Pediatr Radiol* 6:112–115, 1977.
7. Swischuk LE: *Plain Film Interpretation of Congenital Heart Disease,* ed 2. Williams & Wilkins, Baltimore, 1979, p 41.
8. Swischuk LE: *Radiology of the Newborn and Young Infant,* ed 2. Williams & Wilkins, Baltimore, 1980.
9. Tseng CH, Chang GKJ, Lora F: Congenital calcified thrombosis of inferior vena cava, bilateral renal veins and left spermatic vein. *Pediatr Radiol* 6:176–177, 1977.
10. Viat P, Cattelain C, Gallez A: Acquired pulmonary artery aneurysm in an infant. *Pediatrics* 65:89–93, 1980.

PULMONARY CAVITIES

This section deals with large pulmonary cavities for small pulmonary nodules which cavitate have been dealt with in the section on pulmonary nodules (see p 55). Larger cavities most often are the result of pneumatoceles or pulmonary abscesses (Table 1.11), and an abscess usually is a complication of a bacterial pneumonia. However, abscesses also can be seen with infections secondary to chronic foreign bodies in the tracheobronchial tree (14). Air-fluid levels frequently are present in the abscess and the wall is variably thickened and hazy around its periphery (Fig. 1.50A). Haziness is due to surrounding inflammation, and in most cases, serves to distinguish the abscess from a pneumatocele, or rarely, a congenital pulmonary cyst (Fig. 1.50B). The reason for this is that, unless these latter lesions become infected, their walls remain thin and discrete. An abscess has this appearance only after being treated.

The commonest cause of a pneumatocele is infection, and most commonly, the infection is staphylococcal pneumonia (4). However, pneumatoceles also can be seen with other acute bacterial pneumonias (1, 11), and even tuberculosis (15). In any given case, the pneumatoceles can be single or multiple (Fig. 1.50, C–E), and in some cases, can become so large that a tension phenomenon is induced (Fig. 1.50D). Occa-

sionally, pneumatoceles can rupture and produce a pneumothorax, but most often, they slowly resolve and disappear; indeed, even without a trace that ever they were present. Other causes of pneumatoceles include hydrocarbon pneumonitis (2, 3, 5, 9) and histiocytosis-X (8). In all of these cases, pneumatoceles result from bronchial obstruction (i.e., by inflammatory exudate, endobronchial granulomas, extrensic pressure from lymph nodes or peribronchial infiltrates), causing air trapping and alveolar rupture distal to the point of obstruction.

Another form of lung pneumatocele is that which occurs with blunt, compressive chest trauma (6, 7, 16). Although it is not known exactly how such a pneumatocele develops, it is believed that compressive forces cause temporary occlusion of a bronchus, buildup of pressures beyond the point of occlusion, and then rupture of the temporarily overdistended alveoli. These pneumatoceles, usually quite innocuous, may be single or multiple (Fig. 1.50C), and similar air collections can occur in the inferior pulmonary ligament (see Fig. 1.40A).

Cavitary primary tuberculosis is very rare in children (16), and actually, most reported cases probably are cases of pneumatocele formation rather than cases of necrotic cavity development. Other rare cavitary lesions include cavitating posttraumatic pulmonary hematomas, cavitating infarcts, and echinococcal cysts (12, 18). These latter cysts, of course, may be more common in certain geographic areas than others. Multiple large, thin-walled, cystic cavities also can be seen with congenital adenomatoid malformation of the lung. This lesion, initially solid and fluid-filled in the neonate, gradually has the fluid in the cystic areas replaced with air, and as air accumulates, the cysts become quite large (13). Indeed, they can fill the entire hemithorax, even to the point of mimicking a pneumothorax (see Fig. 1.24B).

Table 1.11 Pulmonary Cavities

Pneumatocele—inflammatory[a] Pulmonary abscess[a]	Commonest
Pneumatocele—traumatic[a] Pneumatocele—hydrocarbon pneumonia[b] Echinococcal cyst[c]	Moderately common
Solitary cyst Adenomatoid malformation (multiple) Pneumatocele histiocytosis Pneumatocele—tuberculosis Cavitary tuberculosis Cavitating pneumonia Cavitating hematoma Cavitating infarct	Relatively rare

[a] Frequently multiple.
[b] May be multiple.
[c] In endemic areas; rare elsewhere.

References

1. Asmar BI, Thirumoorthi MC, and Dajani AS: Pneumococcal pneumonia with pneumatocele formation. *Am J Dis Child* 132:1091–1093, 1978.
2. Baghassarian OM, Weiner S: Pneumatocele formation complicating hydrocarbon pneumonitis. *Am J Roentgenol* 95:104–111, 1965.
3. Bergeson PS, Hales SW, Lustgarten MD, Lipow HW: Pneumatoceles following hydrocarbon ingestion. *Am J*

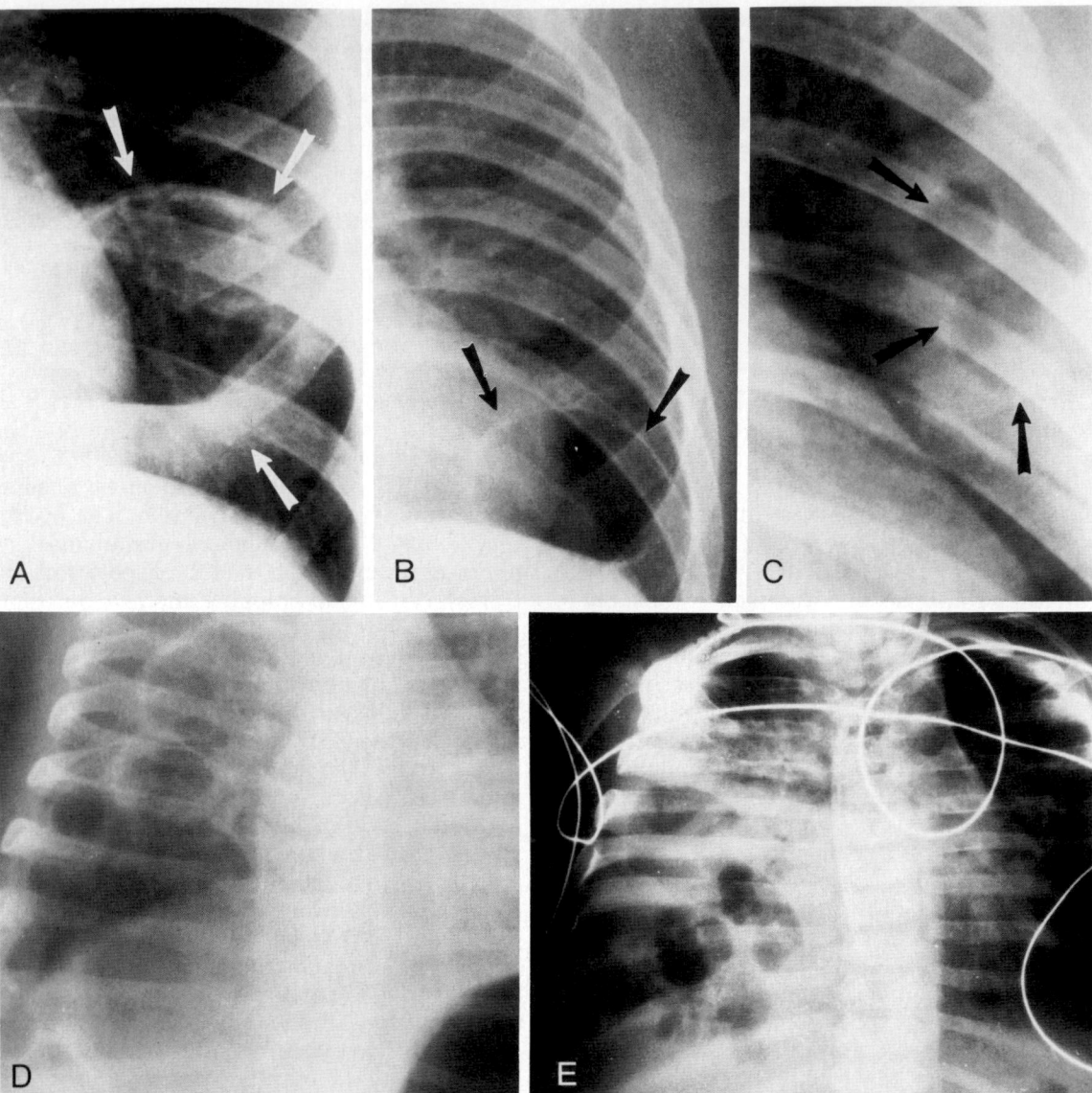

Fig. 1.50. Cavities in the lung. A. **Abscess.** Note the rather thick, fuzzy wall and an air-fluid level (arrows). B. **Congenital lung cyst** with a thin wall (arrows) in the left lower lobe. A solitary pneumatocele would look the same. C. **Posttraumatic pneumatoceles** (arrows) with surrounding evidence of pulmonary contusion. D. **Multiple pneumatoceles** in the right lung secondary to staphylococcal pneumonia. E. **Pneumatoceles in tuberculosis.** These are uncommon, and ordinarily, this film would be more representative of staphylococcal infection. However, this patient had tuberculosis.

Dis Child 129:49–54, 1975.

4. Boisset GF: Subpleural emphysema complicating staphylococcal and other pneumonias. *J Pediatr* 81:259–266, 1972.
5. Campbell JB: Pneumatocele formation following hydrocarbon ingestion. *Am Rev Respir Dis* 101:414–418, 1970.
6. Fagan CJ, Swischuk LE: Traumatic lung and paramediastinal pneumatoceles. *Radiology* 120:11–18, 1976.
7. Felman AH, Rodgers BM, Talbert JL: Traumatic paramediastinal air cyst. *Pediatr Radiol* 4:120–121, 1976.
8. Godwin JD, Webb WR, Savoca CJ, Gamsu G, Goodman PC: Multiple thin-walled cystic lesions of the lung. *Am*

J Roentgenol 135:593–604, 1980.

9. Harris VJ, Brown R: Pneumatoceles as a complication of chemical pneumonia after hydrocarbon ingestion. *Am J Roentgenol* 125:513–537, 1975.
10. Hyde I: Traumatic parmediastinal air cysts. *Br J Radiol* 44:380–383, 1971.
11. Johnson F: Cavitating lesions in a cold agglutinin positive pneumonia. *Pediatr Radiol* 6:181–182, 1977.
12. Katz R, Murphy S, Kosloske A: Pulmonary echinococcosis: a pediatric disease of the southwestern United States. *Pediatrics* 65:1003–1006, 1980.
13. Madewell JE, Stocker JT, Korsower JM: Cystic ade-

nomatoid malformation of the lung: morphologic analysis. *Am J Roentgenol* 124:436–448, 1975.

14. Marks PH, Turner JAP: Lung abscesses in childhood. *Thorax* 23:216, 1968.
15. Matsaniotis N, Kattamis CH, Economov-Mavrou, C, Kyriaakou M: Bullous emphysema in childhood tuberculosis. *J Pediatr* 71:703, 1967.

16. Ravin C, Smith GW, Lester PD, McLoud TC, Putman CE: Post-traumatic pneumatocele in the inferior pulmonary ligament. *Radiology* 121:39–41, 1976.
17. Solomon A, Rabinowitz L: Primary cavitating tuberculosis in childhood. *Clin Radiol* 23:483–485, 1972.
18. Thumler J, Munoz A: Pulmonary and hepatic echinococcosis in children. *Pediatr Radiol* 7:164–171, 1978.

BUBBLY LUNGS

Bubbly lungs most commonly are seen in the neonate, and beyond this age, are rather uncommon. On a unilateral basis, they can be seen with cystic adenomatoid malformation (1), and bilaterally or unilaterally, with bronchiectasis (Fig. 1.51). Bronchiectasis, of course, is much more common, and focally, most often is seen with chronic foreign bodies or severe pulmonary infections which destroy bronchial walls. On a diffuse basis, bubbly lungs are seen most often in cystic fibrosis, and then, certain immunologic deficiency states. Bubbly lungs also can result from pulmonary interstitial emphysema (2) in children requiring ventilatory assistance (i.e., positive pressure assisted ventilation).

References

1. Madewell JE, Stocker JT, Korsower JM: Cystic adenomatoid malformation of the lung: morphologic analysis. *Am J Roentgenol* 124:436–448, 1975.
2. Westcott JL, Cole SR: Interstitial pulmonary emphysema in children and adults: roentgenographic features. *Radiology* 111:367–378, 1974.

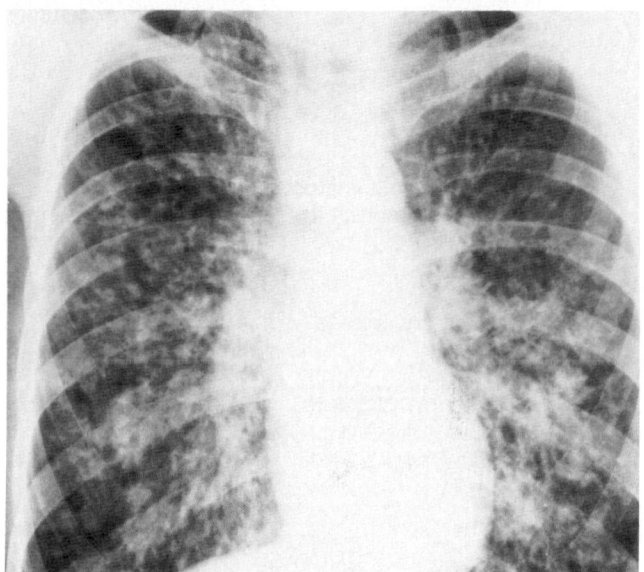

Fig. 1.51. Bubbly lungs. Note the fine architecture of the bronchiectatic spaces (i.e., bubbles) in this patient with bronchiectasis from cystic fibrosis.

LARGE OR PROMINENT HILAR REGIONS

Hilar prominence or enlargement can be bilateral or unilateral (Table 1.12), and overall, the commonest cause is lymph node enlargement. The second most common cause is pulmonary artery dilation. In some cases of hilar lymph node enlargement, the nodes are discretely outlined, while in others, adjacent inflammatory changes cause the edges of the nodes to be fuzzy (Fig. 1.52A). For the most part, this pattern is due to associated interstitial, peribronchial infiltrate and classically occurs with viral lower respiratory tract infections (2, 4, 7). However, it also can be seen with asthma (chronic bronchitis or superimposed viral infection), cystic fibrosis, aspiration pneumonia (3), and *Mycoplasma pneumoniae* infection. Generally this pattern is not seen with the common bacterial pneumonias. When bilateral adenopathy is discrete, one's first consideration still should be viral lower respiratory tract infection, but in addition, one should give serious consideration to fungal infections, metastatic disease, the reticuloendothelioses, and the leukemia-lymphoma group of diseases. Much less commonly (mostly because the diseases are rare), one also can encounter bilateral adenopathy with sarcoidosis (3) and Wegener's granulomatosis.

When bilateral hilar prominence is due to enlargement of the pulmonary arteries, the most common underlying problem is pulmonary hypertension, and its cause usually is an underlying left-to-right shunt or a cardiac admixture lesion (Fig. 1.52B). In either case, excessive volumes of blood flowing through the lungs, in time, induce muscular hypertrophy of the peripheral pulmonary arterioles, elevated pulmonary artery pressures, and then, pulmonary hypertension. Pulmonary hypertension secondary to left side obstructing lesions such as aortic stenosis, coarctation of the aorta, mitral stenosis, and myocardial disease, is less common, especially in young infants. In the older pediatric patient, however, enough time goes by so that the left side lesion can cause chronic pulmonary arteriolar changes and pulmonary hypertension. In addition, acquired rheumatic valvular disease is more prevalent in the older child. Idiopathic pulmonary hypertension is rare in the pediatric age group and so is hypertension due to pulmonary artery emboli.

A very rare cause of bilateral pulmonary artery enlargement leading to prominent hilar regions is congenital absence of the pulmonary valve (1, 5, 6).

Table 1.12 Large or Prominent Hilar Regions

Bilateral		
1. Adenopathy	}	Commonest
Viral infection	}	Commonest
Cystic fibrosis Fungus infections *Mycoplasma pneumoniae* infections Reticuloendothelioses Metastases Leukemia-lymphoma Chronic aspiration	}	Moderately common
Sarcoidosis Wegener's granulomatosis Bacterial pneumonias (bi- lateral) Tuberculosis	}	Relatively rare
2. Pulmonary artery enlarge- ment	}	Moderately common
Pulmonary hypertension	}	Commonest
Absent pulmonary valve	}	Very rare
Unilateral		
1. Adenopathy	}	Commonest
Tuberculosis	}	Commonest

Fungus infections
Mycoplasma pneumoniae
  infection
Bacterial pneumonia
Superior segment, lower
  lobe pneumonia artefact
	}	Common

Metastases Viral infection Lingular or right mid lobe atelectasis artefact Leukemia-lymphoma	}	Relatively uncommon
2. Pulmonary artery enlarge- ment	}	Relatively uncommon
Absent pul valve w/unil ab- sent pul art	}	Relatively rare
Pulmonary stenosis w/left PA enlarged	}	Rare

These cases, often associated with tetralogy of Fallot, demonstrate gross insufficiency of the absent pulmonary valve, and characteristically, show massive enlargement of the main, right, and left pulmonary artery branches (Fig. 1.52C). The peripheral pulmonary vascularity in these patients is very thin, and the zone of demarcation between the dilated proximal pulmonary artery and its peripheral branches often is so abrupt that hilar masses are suggested. In addition, in many of the cases associated with tetralogy of Fallot, the left pulmonary artery is absent, and then, enlargement of the right hilar region only occurs.

The commonest cause of **unilateral hilar enlargement** in the pediatric age group is inflammatory disease (Fig. 1.53), and most commonly, it will be primary tuberculosis (8). In some of these cases, adenopathy may be discrete but in others it may be obscured by frequently present atelectasis, or even obstructive emphysema (Fig. 1.54). Bilateral adenopathy in primary pulmonary tuberculosis is rather uncommon.

Other causes of unilateral hilar lymph node enlargement include fungal disease, *Mycoplasma pneumoniae* and bacterial pneumonias, and very occasionally, viral lower respiratory tract infection. With most viral lower respiratory tract infections, bilateral adenopathy is the rule. Unilateral hilar enlargement also can occur with metastatic disease, the leukemia-lymphoma group of diseases, and absence of the pulmonary valve with concomitant absence of the left pulmonary artery (i.e., right hilar enlargement is present). Indeed, anytime one pulmonary artery is absent, the other tends to enlarge and produce a unilaterally prominent hilar region. Another cause of unilateral hilar prominence due to an enlarged pulmonary artery is pulmonary stenosis. Although this finding is not particularly common in childhood, it can be seen, and is due to poststenotic dilation of the main pulmonary artery and the left branch. The jet of blood passing through the stenotic valve is so directed that it causes dilation of these two structures.

Finally, and before leaving the topic of unilateral hilar enlargement, one should make note of the artefactually prominent hilar region produced by a superior segment lower lobe pneumonia. On lateral view, of course, the hilar region is not enlarged, and the pneumonia is clearly identified to lie posterior to the hilar region. However, on frontal view, since it is superimposed on the hilar region, it makes it appear as though the hilar region itself were enlarged (Fig.

Fig. 1.52. Bilateral hilar prominence. A. Adenopathy. Characteristic bilateral hilar adenopathy in a patient with viral lower respiratory tract infection. B. **Large pulmonary arteries** causing prominent bilateral hilar regions (the left is partially obscured by the heart) in a patient with a large VSD and pulmonary hypertension. C. **Large pulmonary arteries** causing large bilateral hilar regions in a patient with dilation secondary to absence of the pulmonary valve.
Fig. 1.53. Unilateral hilar prominence. A. Right hilar adenopathy in a patient with histoplasmosis. B. Note the prominent left hilar region produced by a large pulmonary artery. The problem was pulmonary stenosis with poststenotic dilation of the main pulmonary artery and its left branch (arrows).

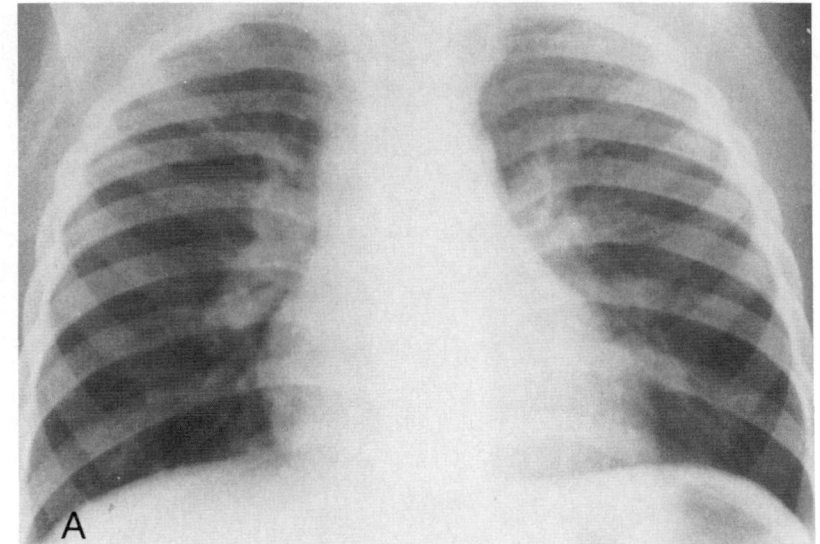

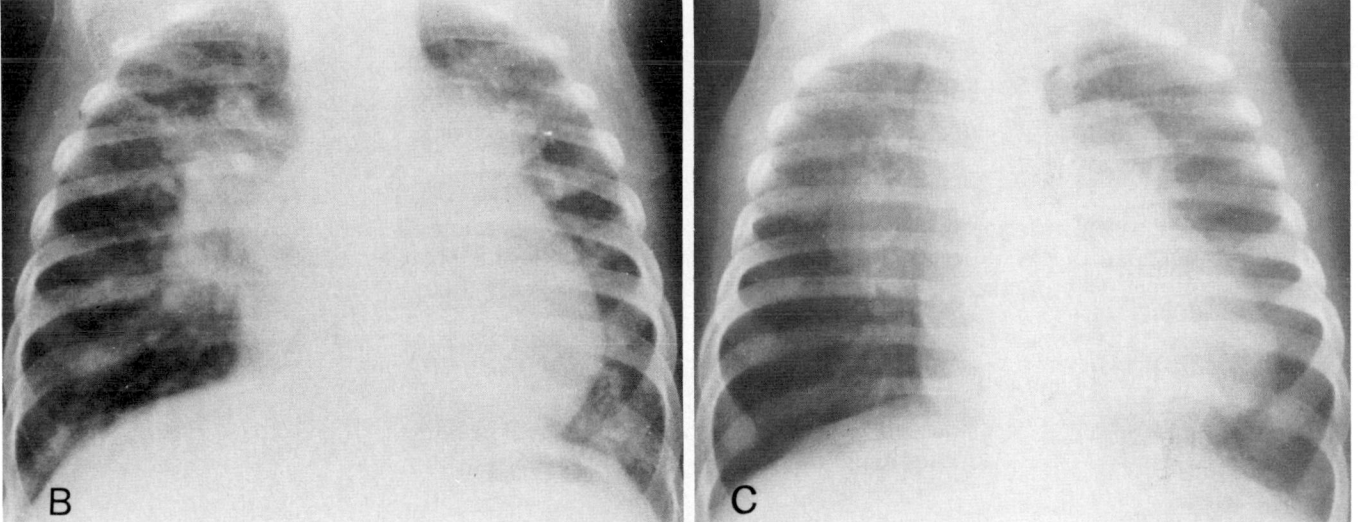

Fig. 1.52.

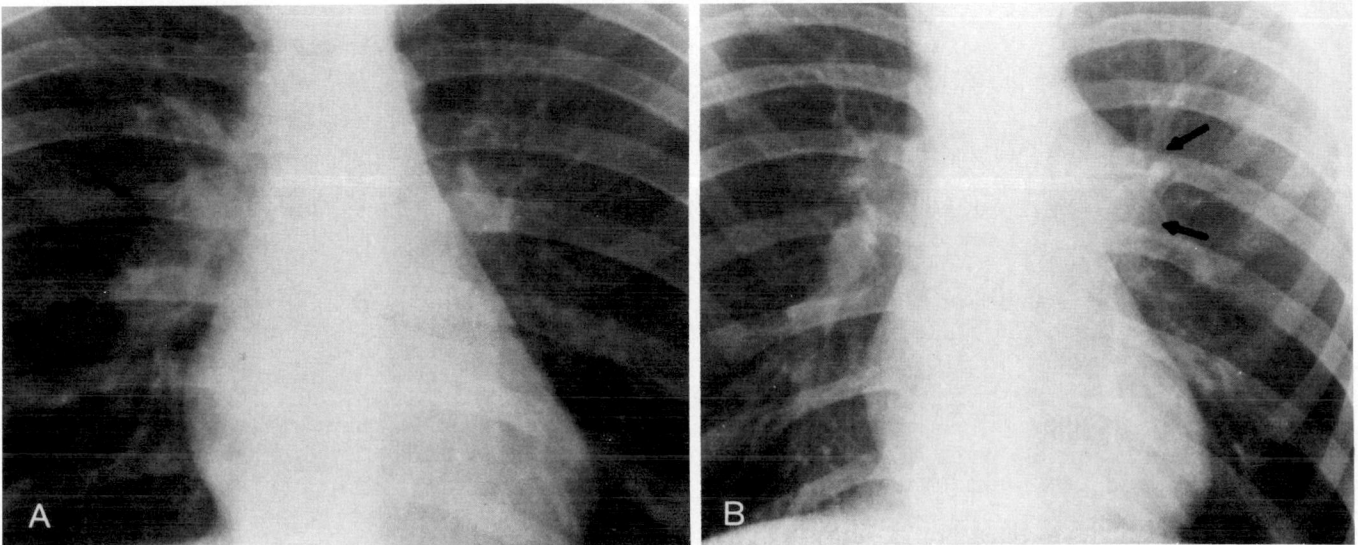

Fig. 1.53.

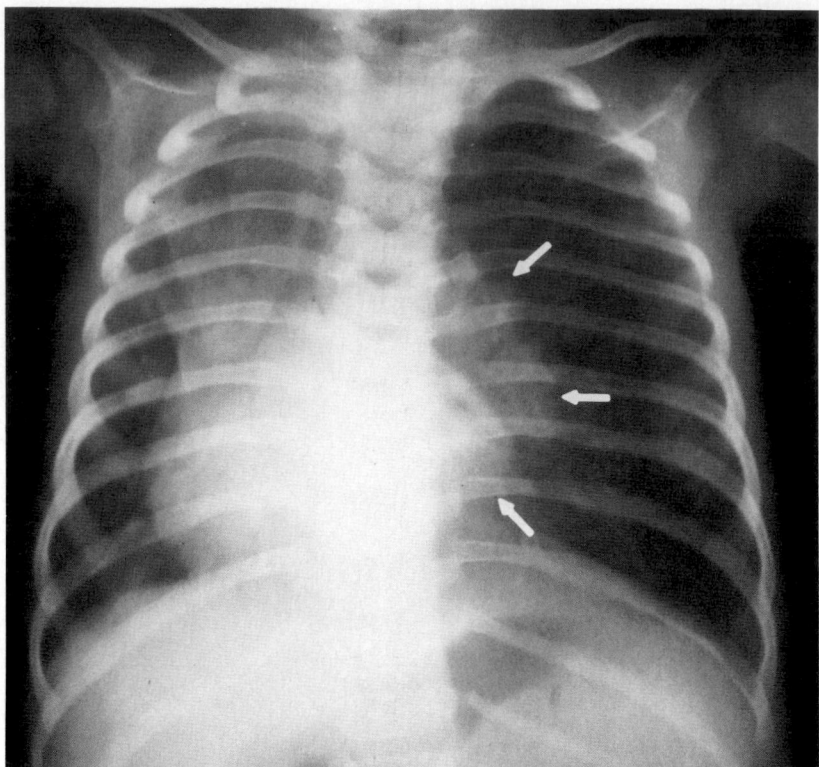

Fig. 1.54. Unilateral adenopathy and obstructive emphysema. The left hilar adenopathy (arrows) could be overlooked because of the large, obstructed left lung and associated mediastinal shift to the right. The problem was tuberculosis with bronchial obstruction.

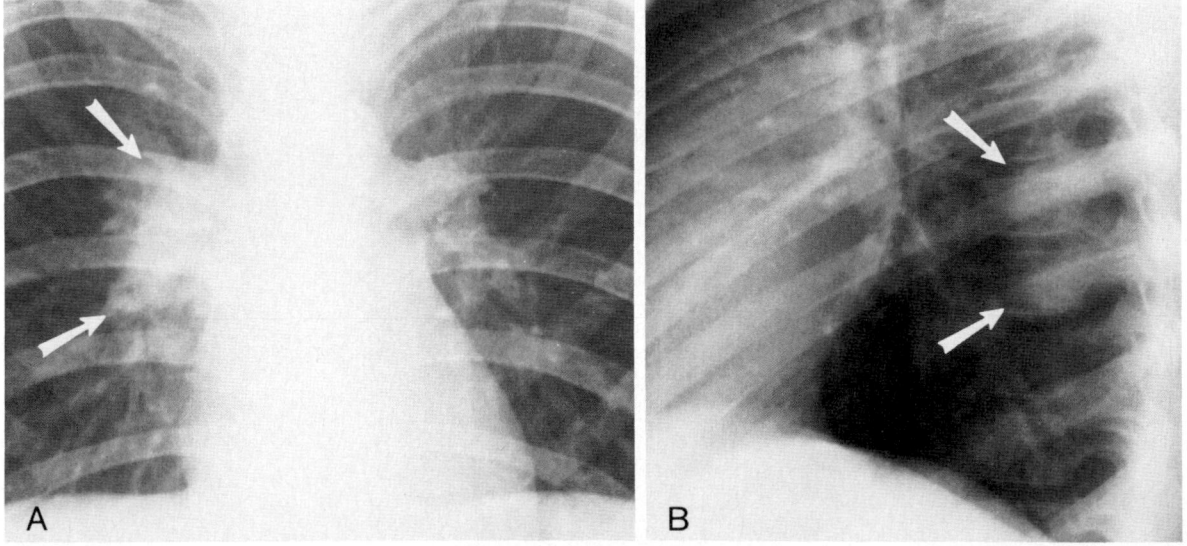

Fig. 1.55. Superior segment pneumonia mimicking unilateral adenopathy. A. Note the dense, prominent hilar region on the right (arrows). B. Lateral view shows that it is due to superimposition of a superior segment, lower lobe pneumonia (arrows).

1.55, A and B). A similar problem occasionally can arise with anterior segment, right upper lobe atelectasis or consolidation.

References

1. Bove E, Shaher RM, Alley R, McKneally M: Tetralogy of Fallot with absent pulmonary valve and aneurysm of the pulmonary artery: report of two cases presenting as obstructive lung disease. *J Pediatr* 81:339–343, 1972.
2. Conte P, Heitzman ER, Markarian B: Viral pneumonia roentgen-pathological correlations. *Radiology* 95:267–272, 1970.
3. Merten DF, Kirks DR, Grossman H: Pulmonary sar-

coidosis in childhood. *Am J Roentgenol* 135:673–679, 1980.
4. Osborne, D: Radiologic appearance of viral disease of the lower respiratory tract in infants and children. *Am J Roentgenol* 13:29–33, 1978.
5. Osman MZ, Meng CCL, Girdany BR: Congenital absence of the pulmonary valve: report of eight cases with review of the literature. *Am J Roentgenol Radium Ther Nucl Med* 106:58–69, 1969.
6. Pernot C Hoeffel JC, Henry M, Stehlin H, Worms AM,

Louis JP: Congenital absence of the pulmonary valve: radiological findings in infants. *Ann Radiol* 15:217–222, 1972.
7. Scanlon GA, Unger JD: The radiology of bacterial and viral pneumonias. *Radiol Clin North Am* 11:317–338, 1973.
8. Weber AL, Bird KT, Janower ML: Primary tuberculosis in childhood with particular emphasis on changes affecting the tracheobronchial tree. *Am J Roentgenol* 103:123–132, 1968.

PULMONARY NODULES

Pulmonary nodules can be solitary or multiple, calcified or uncalcified, and cavitary or solid (Table 1.13). The commonest cause of a solitary nodule in a child is infection, and in this regard, the commonest is healed tuberculosis. Tuberculous nodules may or may not contain calcification, and are much more common than similar nodules caused by fungal infections (Fig. 1.56A). Residual nodules (healed granulomas) from other pulmonary infections are quite rare, including those seen with acute or healed atypical measles pneumonia (7, 8, 16, 17).

A relatively common cause of an apparent lung nodule is acute, consolidating pneumonia (Fig. 1.57B), and most frequently, the problem is pneumococcal infection. The fact that the consolidation presents as a pulmonary nodule is strictly fortuitous for it just happens that at this early stage of consolidation, the pneumonia can appear nodular or spherical (12). A few hours later, its configuration changes and it becomes more diffuse and typical. As a side point, it might be noted that these pneumonias need not always appear as a nodule, for many appear as a pulmonary or mediastinal mass. In all of these cases, the clue to proper diagnosis is the clinical history, for these children invariably have findings such as tachypnea, cough, high fever (103°F or over) or chest pain, clearly suggesting that a pulmonary infection is the problem.

All other causes of a solitary pulmonary nodule are rare, and one of the rarest is a pulmonary tumor. For the most part, one cannot tell one tumor from another except in those cases where typical flocculent cartilage calcifications are present, and then, a hamartoma should be the diagnosis (Fig. 1.56B). Solitary pulmonary metastases can occur, but usually more than one nodule is present by the time these patients present to the clinician. Occasionally, a small bronchogenic cyst can present in the periphery of the lung and suggest a pulmonary nodule, but more often they are located in juxtaposition to the tracheobronchial tree (Fig. 1.57A). Uncommonly, these cysts can calcify (see Fig. 1.48B).

When a nodule is associated with trailing vascular feeders and drainers, one can suggest the diagnosis of pulmonary varix or AV malformation, and conventional or computerized tomography, along with zeroradiography, can delineate these vessels to better advantage. If a pulmonry nodule is associated with hyperinflation and hyperlucency of the lung around, and

Table 1.13 Pulmonary Nodules

1. Solitary nodule	
Granuloma—tuberculous[a] }	Commonest
Granuloma—fungus[a] Consolidating pneumonia Metastases[d]	Moderately common
Hamartoma[a] Small abscess[d] Small cyst Nipple shadow Other primary neoplasia Sarcoidosis[b,d] Pulmonary varix or AVM Cutaneous nodules Mucous plugs (asthma) Mucocele (bronchial atresia) Healed (posttraumatic) hematoma[b,d] Postinfarct[b,d] Collagen vascular disease[d] Atypical measles[b] Old pneumonia[b] Primary tumor	Relatively rare
2. Multiple nodules	
Granulomas[a] (TB, fungus) }	Commonest
Metastases[d] }	Moderately common
Laryngeal papillomatosis[d] Multiple abscess[c] Multiple emboli[d]	Relatively rare
Wegener's granulomatosis[c] Sarcoidosis[b,d] Mucous plugs Cutaneous nodules (artefact) Collagen vascular disease[d] Lymphoma Multiple hamartomas[b?] Other primary tumors	Rare

[a] Commonly calcify.
[b] May calcify.
[c] Commonly cavitate.
[d] May cavitate.

distal to it, bronchial atresia with a mucocele should be the diagnosis (4, 10, 13). In these cases, bronchial atresia exists from birth, but as time goes by, mucous accumulates distal to the area of atresia and forms a

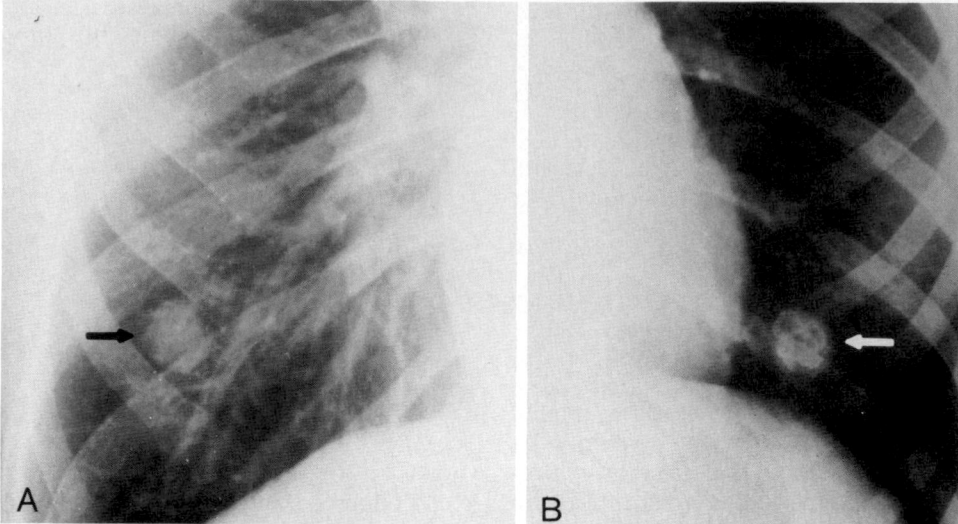

Fig. 1.56. Solitary pulmonary nodules. A. Typical nodule, uncalcified, in the left lower lobe (arrow). Most often this turns out to be a granuloma, and in this patient, the histoplasmosis skin test was positive. These nodules also frequently show central calcification. B. Hamartoma with typical flocculent calcification of cartilage (arrow).

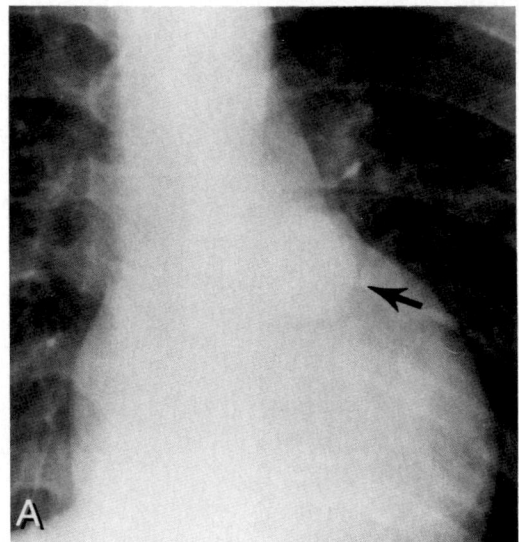

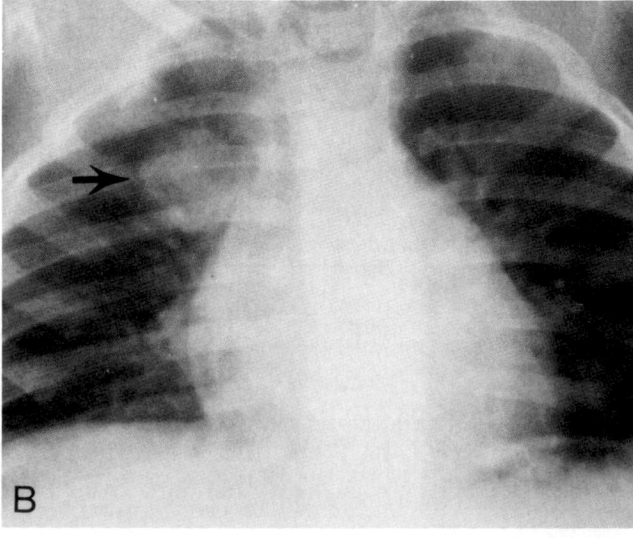

mucocele (see Fig. 1.31). The lung distal to the obstruction receives air by the air-drift phenomenon (i.e., air from the adjacent normal lung passes to the abnormal lung through the pores of Kohn and ducts of Lambert), and then becomes distended. This leads to hyperlucency and oligemia of the involved lobe, and the plain film findings are virtually diagnostic. Similar nodular accumulations of mucous can occur on a transient basis in asthmatics, but they are not associated with regional hyperinflation (15).

Lesions on the skin which might project through the lungs as a pulmonary nodule, or nipple shadows producing the same phenomenon, generally are uncommon in the pediatric age group. Of course, the simplest way to determine whether such a pseudonodule is present is: (a) to be aware of the typical location of a nipple shadow (i.e., lower third of the lung fields), and (b) to know whether the patient has any cutaneous lesions (i.e., neurofibromatosis). Unfortunately, this latter piece of information is not always available, and then, if one does not judge the nodule to be within the pulmonary parenchyma on both frontal and lateral views, one has to suspect it as being a skin lesion. Oblique views also often can be utilized to demonstrate that such a nodule is not in the chest. Other causes of a solitary pulmonary nodule include a small abscess, sarcoidosis, healed (post-trau-

Fig. 1.57. Solitary pulmonary nodules. A. Small nodule due to a bronchogenic cyst (arrow). The typical location suggests the diagnosis. B. Nodular consolidating pneumonia (arrows). The finding, at first, would suggest a pulmonary nodule, but the patient had a high fever and clinical findings typical of pneumonia. Such nodular pneumonias are not uncommon in childhood, and usually are due to pneumococcal infections.

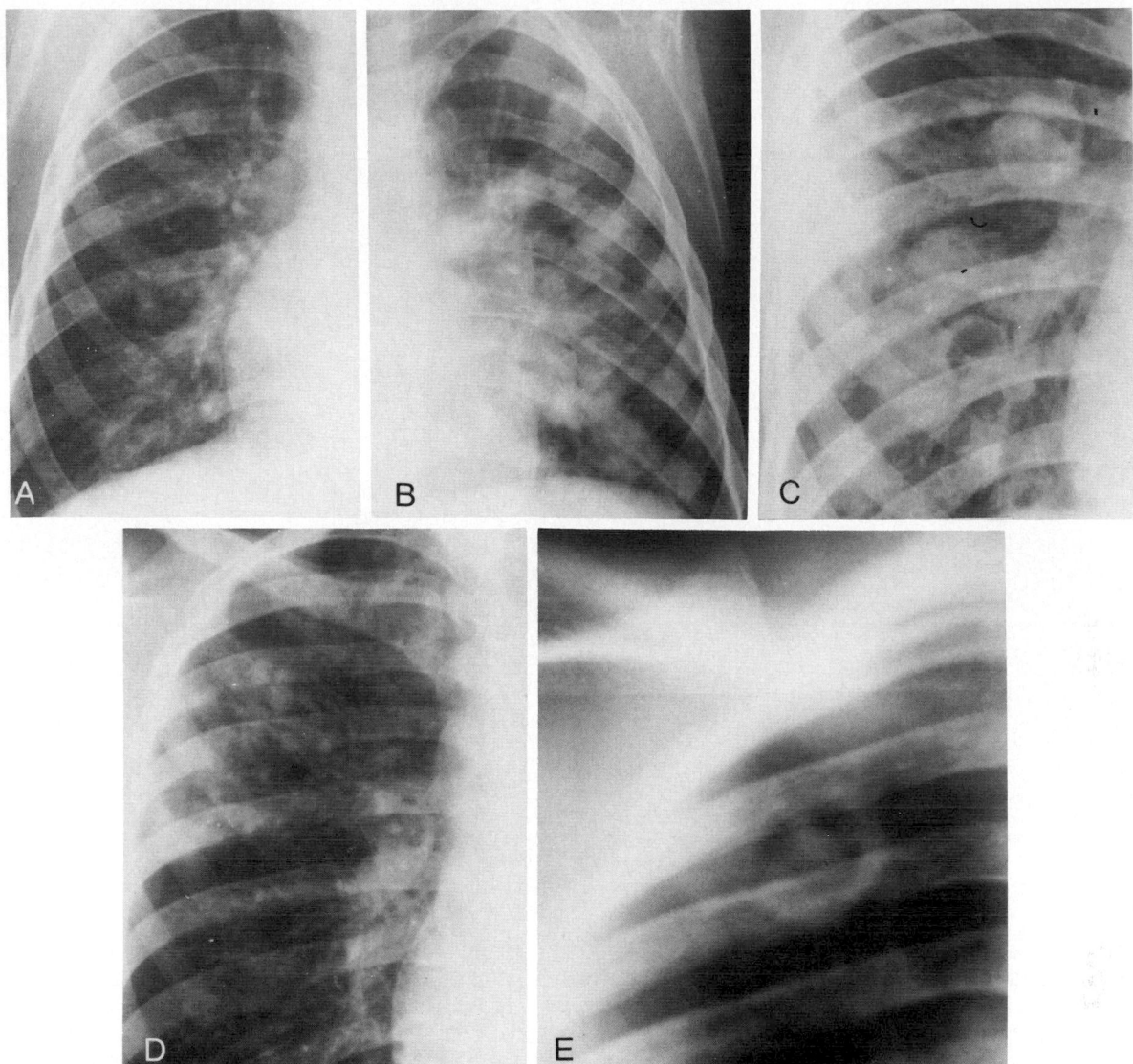

Fig. 1.58. Multiple pulmonary nodules. A. Multiple, but somewhat indistinct, pulmonary nodules in juvenile papillomatosis. The development of such nodules is common after surgical intervention. B. Numerous, ill-defined nodules due to granulomas in actinomycosis. C. Typical appearance of metastatic nodules, some which have cavitated. They are smooth-edged and of variable size. D. Mucous plugs in cystic fibrosis. Note numerous mucous plugs presenting as nodules in the lung. They are especially prominent in the right upper lobe. E. Small cavitary nodule with central nidus. Typical of aspergillosis. The small nidus often is termed the fungus ball. This patient had immunologic deficiency.

matic) hematoma, healed pulmonary infarct, collagen vascular disease, and old healed pneumonia (Table 1.13).

The two most common causes of **multiple nodules** in the chest are granulomas and pulmonary metastases (Table 1.13). Granulomas, however, are more common and, for the most part, include tuberculous and fungal infection (Fig. 1.58B). Fungal infections are a more common cause, and the nodules usually are quite uniform in size and may show punctate calcifications (see Fig. 1.49A). Metastatic nodules often show greater variation in size (Fig. 1.58C), and in

addition, often are sharper and cleaner-looking than granulomas.

Metastatic pulmonary nodules, as a rule, do not calcify, but those due to osteogenic sarcoma may show ossification within their substance. Such ossification cannot be distinguished from calcification, but on a practical basis, the fact that a primary osteogenic sarcoma is present usually is well known before metastatic nodules develop. Consequently, there usually is no differential diagnosis. Another interesting cause of multiple pulmonary nodules is juvenile laryngeal papillomatosis (14). These patients first present with

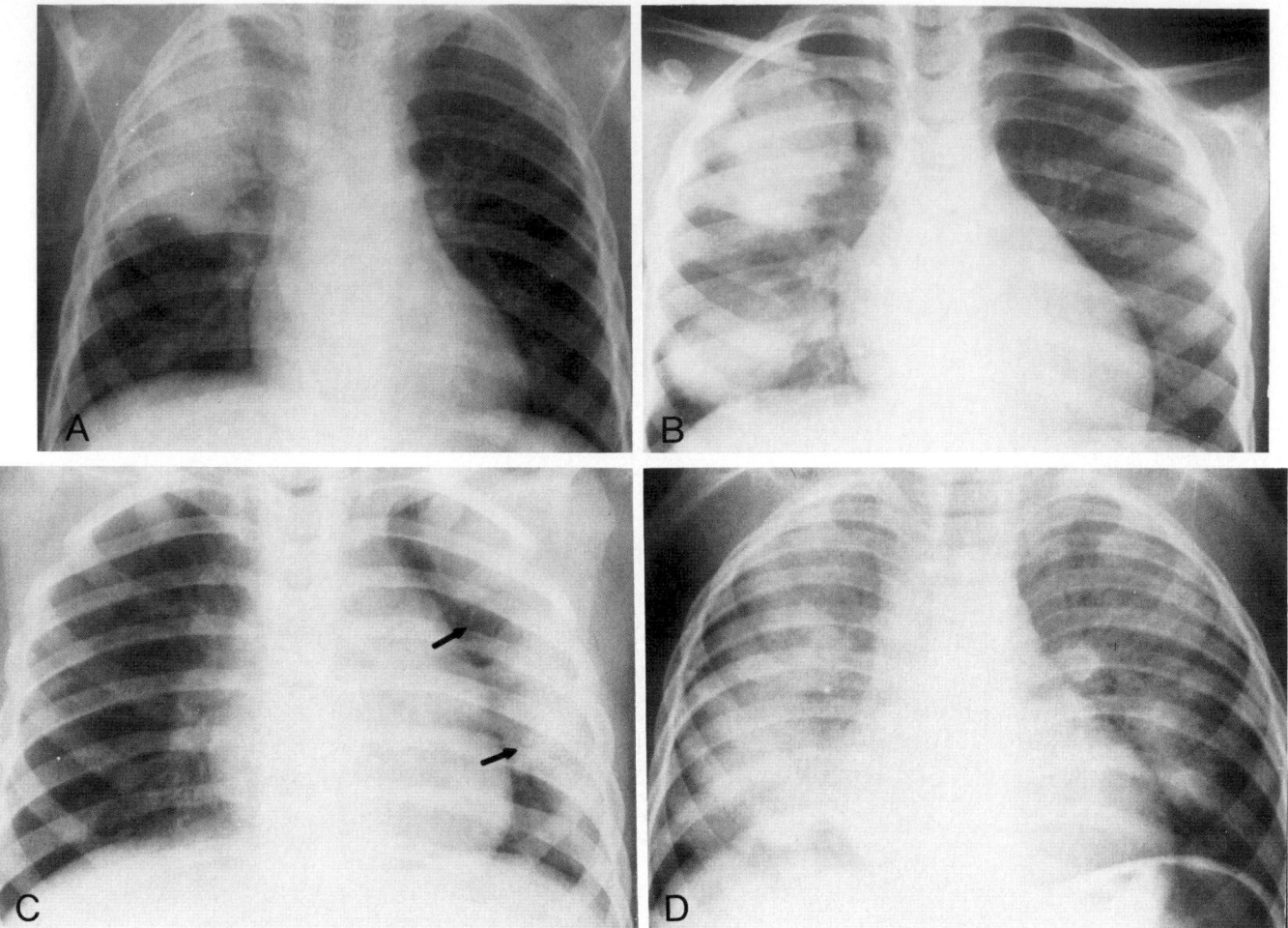

Fig. 1.59. Consolidations. A. Typical, well-developed consolidation of the right upper lobe. Note the central air bronchogram and the relatively normal position of the minor fissure. This indicates very little volume loss. B. Two more consolidations, this time located more centrally within the lobes of the right lung. Note that there is a little volume loss in the right upper lobe (minor fissure is elevated). C. Peripheral consolidation on the left due to pulmonary contusion (arrows). D. Bilateral central consolidations due to bleeding into the lung in idiopathic pulmonary hemosiderosis.

hoarseness due to a papilloma growing in or around the vocal cords. Once surgical intervention or tracheostomy is accomplished, seeding of the papilloma into the distal bronchial tree occurs, and then pulmonary nodules develop (Fig. 1.58A). Some of these nodules may cavitate. Other causes of multiple pulmonary nodules include: multiple pulmonary abscesses (2), multiple emboli, Wegener's granulomatosis (11), multiple hemangiomas of the lung (1), multiple hamartomas (3, 6), sarcoidosis, collagen vascular diseases, lymphoma, and mucous plugs in cystic fibrosis (Fig. 1.59D) or asthma (15).

Calcifications within pulmonary nodules have, to some extent, been dealt with earlier, but, in addition to granulomas and the rare pulmonary hamartoma, they can be seen with healed hematomas, old infarcts, and old healed pneumonias. Calcification within a nodule usually can be verified with conventional or computerized tomography, but the latter modality is more sensitive (9). Tomography also is useful in demonstrating cavities within nodules, and in this regard, cavitation occurs most commonly with multiple pulmonary abscesses, septic emboli, Wegener's granulomatosis, and laryngeal papillomatosis (5). However, it also can be seen with metastatic disease (Fig. 1.58C), sarcoidosis, the collagen vascular diseases, and aspergillosis (5). In this latter condition, a small, free-rolling, nodule may be seen within the cavity, the so-called fungus ball (Fig. 1.58E).

References

1. Brill PW, Symchych P, Winchester P: Capillary hemangioma of the lung. *Radiology* 124:184, 1977.
2. Felman AH, Shulman ST: Staphylococcal osteomyelitis, sepsis and pulmonary disease. *Radiology* 117:649–655, 1975.
3. Futrell JW, McKillop DB, Izant RJ Jr: Angiomatous

lymphoid hamartoma in an infant. *Am J Dis Child* 128:96–99, 1974.

4. Genereux GP: Bronchial atresia: a rare cause of unilateral lung hypertranslucency. *J Can Assoc Radiol* 22:71–82, 1971.

5. Godwin JD, Webb WR, Savoca CJ, Gamsu G, Goodman PC: Multiple thin-walled cystic lesions of the lung. *Am J Roentgenol* 135:593–604, 1980.

6. Hull MT, Gonzalez-Crussi F, Grosfeld JL: Multiple pulmonary fibroleiomyomatous hamartomata in childhood. *J Pediatr Surg* 14:428–431, 1979.

7. Margolin FR, Gandy TK: Pneumonia of atypical measles. *Radiology* 131:653–655, 1979.

8. Mitnick, J, Becker, MH, Rothberg, M, Genieser, NB: Nodular residua of atypical measles pneumonia. *Am J Roentgenol* 134:257–260, 1980.

9. Muhm JR, Brown LR, Crowe JK, Sheedy PF II, Hattery RR, Stephens DH: Comparison of whole lung tomography and computed tomography for detecting pulmonary nodules. *Am J Roentgenol* 131:981–984, 1978.

10. Oh KS, Dorst JP, White JJ, Haller JA Jr, Johnson BA, Byrne WD: Syndrome of bronchial atresia or stenosis with mucocele and focal hyperinflation of the lung. *Johns Hopkins Med J* 138:48–53, 1976.

11. Orlowski JP, Clough JD, Dyment PG: Wegener's granulomatosis in the pediatric age group. *Pediatrics* 61:83–90, 1978.

12. Rose RW, Ward BH: Spherical pneumonias in children simulating pulmonary and mediastinal masses. *Radiology* 106:179–182, 1973.

13. Schuster SR, Harris GBC, Williams A, Kirkpatrick J, Reid L: Bronchial atresia: a recognizable entity in the pediatric age group. *J Pediatr Surg* 13:682–689, 1978.

14. Smith L, Gooding CA: Pulmonary involvement in laryngeal papillomatosis. *Pediatr Radiol* 2:161–166, 1974.

15. Swischuk LE: *Emergency Radiology of the Acutely Ill or Injured Child.* Williams & Wilkins, Baltimore, 1979, pp 90.

16. Wood BP, Bernstein RM: Pulmonary nodular "pneumonia" during the acute atypical measles illness. *Ann Radiol* 21:193–198, 1978.

17. Young LW, Smith DI, Glasgow LA: Pneumonia of atypical measles, residual nodular lesions. *Am J Roentgenol Radium Ther Nucl Med* 110:439–448, 1970.

INFILTRATES

Basically, pulmonary infiltrative patterns can be categorized as follows: (a) lobar consolidation, (b) fluffy or patchy parenchymal infiltrates, (c) streaky or wedgeshaped infiltrates, (d) parahilar-peribronchial infiltrates, (e) reticular or reticulonodular infiltrates, (f) hazy to opaque lungs, and (g) miliary infiltrates. In addition, some infiltrates tend to cluster around the hilar regions while others are more basal in distribution. Each pattern has its own list of differential diagnostic possibilities, and even though considerable overlap often occurs, it is of value to know which entities are most likely to produce the different patterns. Not only does this aid in directing immediate therapy, but it also assists in unraveling difficult problems.

Lobar Consolidation

Lobar consolidation results when the alveoli become full of fluid, and most commonly the fluid is a purulent exudate secondary to a bacterial infection (Fig. 1.59, A and B). Overall, the commonest infection is pneumococcal pneumonia, but in children under 2 to 3 years of age, *Hemophilus influenzae* pneumonia is more common. Staphylococcal and *Mycoplasma pneumoniae* infections (4, 14, 27) are next most common as causes of lobar consolidations. Fungal infections generally do not produce isolated lobar consolidations, except perhaps for actinomycosis, and viral consolidations, if they exist, are very rare. Other bacterial infections which can produce consolidating pneumonias include *Klebsiella pneumoniae, Aerobacter aerogenes,* and *Streptococcus,* but these organisms are not nearly as commonly encountered as those mentioned earlier. Similarly, although Gram-negative infections can produce consolidation, they are not particularly common in children.

Roentgenographically, in any given case, the entire lobe eventually becomes consolidated, but initially, the infiltrate tends to begin in the periphery. With mature consolidations, air in the bronchi stands out as the air bronchogram. Pleural effusions commonly are associated, and indeed, many times develop into frank empyemas. Most lobar consolidations are associated with only slight volume loss or gain of the involved lobe. The rather uncommon *Klebsiella pneumoniae* can produce considerable expansion of the lobe, and bulging of the adjacent fissures (see Fig. 1.37), but overall, slight volume loss is more common with consolidations. When volume loss is more pronounced, a problem arises in differentiating the findings from simple atelectasis (Fig. 1.60, A and B). Generally, when consolidation occurs, since the alveoli are full of exudate, volume loss is minimal, but with a partially healed pneumonia, considerable atelectasis can be present. In the end, one may have to make the differentiation clinically, but meanwhile it might be noted that when atelectasis is the only, or predominant problem, volume loss usually is marked (Fig. 1.60, C and D). In this regard, it becomes essential to appreciate the characteristic fashion in which the various lobes collapse (Fig. 1.61), and that in any given case, the findings will be more difficult to evaluate on one or the other of the two standard views of the chest.

The problem of differentiating consolidation from atelectasis is not academic. Indeed, in the assessment of respiratory infections, it is the commonest problem encountered. The reason for this is that atelectasis

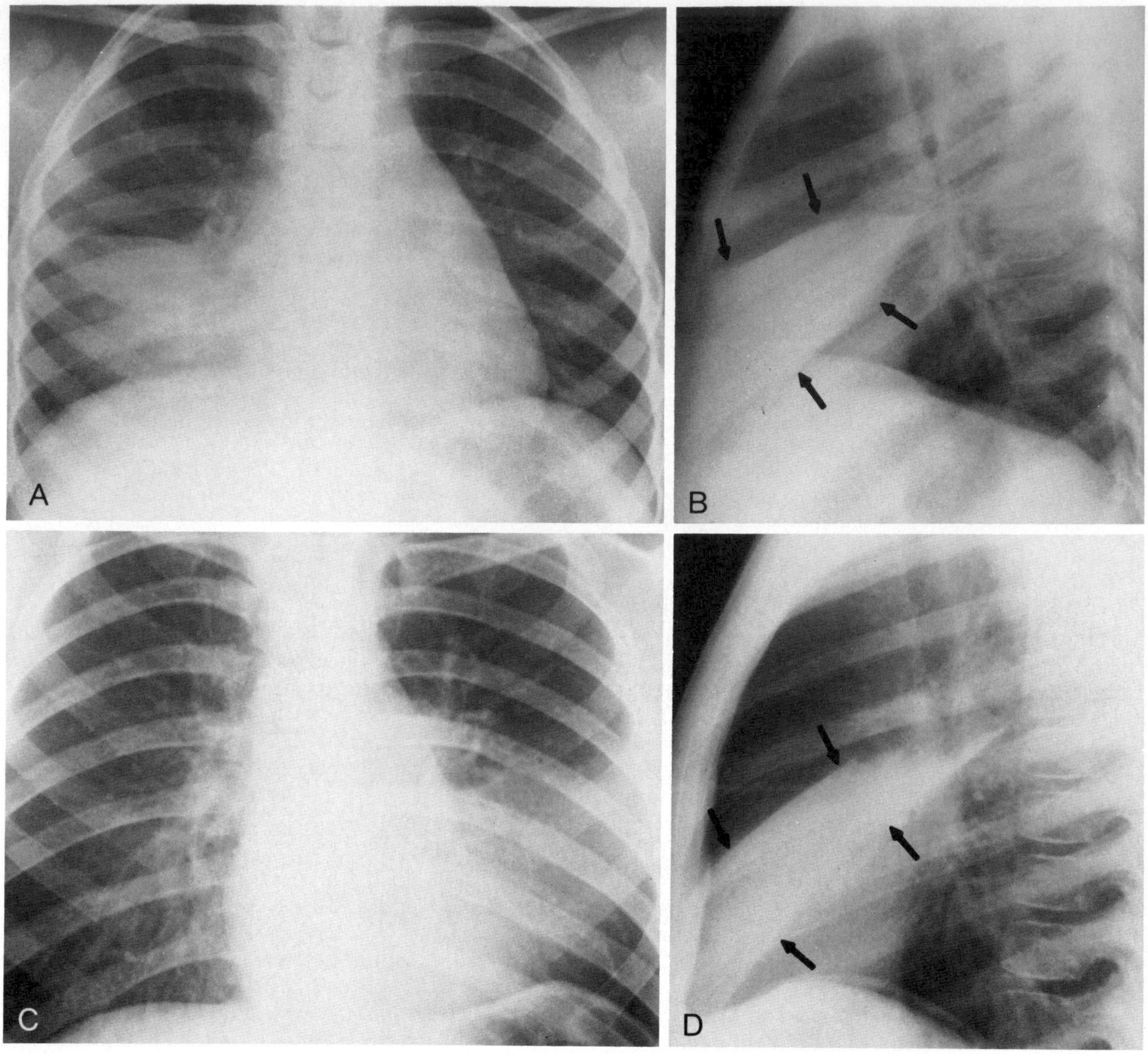

Fig. 1.60. Consolidation: infiltrate or atelectasis? A. **Consolidating pneumonia with volume loss.** Note typical right middle lobe consolidation. Little volume loss is suggested. B. On later view, however, more than usual collapse of the right middle lobe is present (arrows). Clinical correlation is most important here. The patient had a fever 104°F and abrupt onset of cough and chest pain. This does not occur with atelectasis. C. **Atelectasis mimicking pneumonia.** Note the homogenous density on the left. D. Lateral view shows characteristic collapse of the lingula (arrows). Such a profound degree of collapse usually does not occur with lobar pneumonias. Patient had asthma and was afebrile.

secondary to mucous plugging of a bronchus is very common in viral lower respiratory tract infections (5, 24), and these infections are the most common in children. Because of this, if one encounters a peripheral infiltrate in such a patient, even though it might resemble a consolidation, statistically, the best bet is atelectasis. As a side point, the same holds true for patients with asthma, and the reason for this is that both asthma and viral disease are bronchial problems. In the end, however, some cases of "atelectasis versus

consolidation" cannot be resolved with roentgenology alone, and then, clinical correlation is essential. In this regard, patients with consolidation due to pneumonia usually present with high fevers and abrupt onset of toxic symptoms, while patients with atelectasis frequently aren't even aware that they have a collapsed lobe.

Other conditions which might present with consolidation of a lobe include pulmonary contusion (Fig. 1.59C), pulmonary infarction, bleeding into the lung

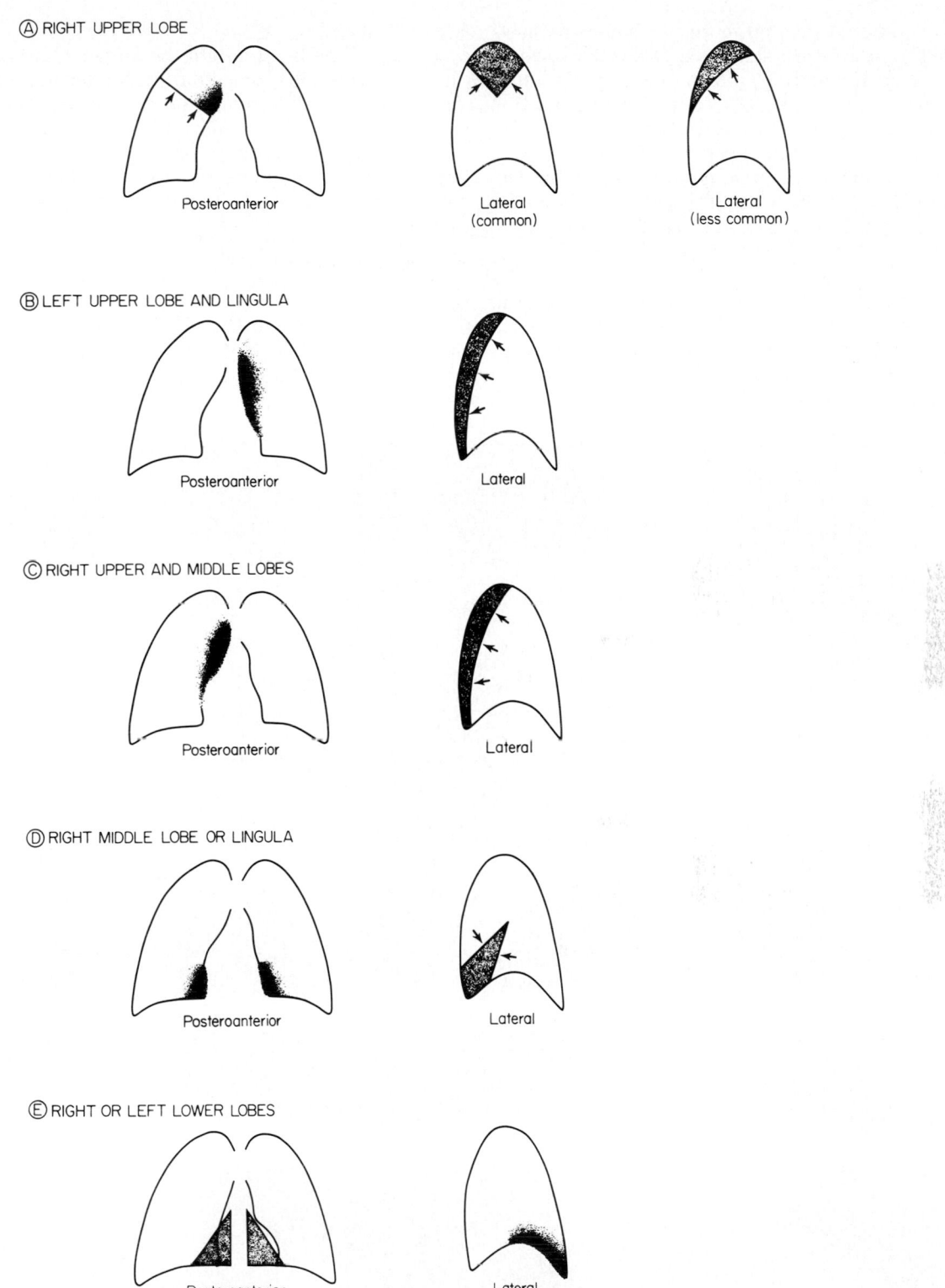

Ⓐ RIGHT UPPER LOBE

Posteroanterior

Lateral
(common)

Lateral
(less common)

Ⓑ LEFT UPPER LOBE AND LINGULA

Posteroanterior

Lateral

Ⓒ RIGHT UPPER AND MIDDLE LOBES

Posteroanterior

Lateral

Ⓓ RIGHT MIDDLE LOBE OR LINGULA

Posteroanterior

Lateral

Ⓔ RIGHT OR LEFT LOWER LOBES

Posteroanterior

Lateral

Fig. 1.61. Atelectasis: varying configurations. A. Right upper lobe atelectasis. B. Left upper lobe and lingular atelectasis. C. Right upper lobe and right middle lobe atelectasis. D. Right middle lobe or lingular atelectasis. E. Right lower lobe or left lower lobe atelectasis. Arrows indicate direction of collapse and displacement of the involved major fissures. From Swischuk LE: Emergency Radiology of the Acutely Ill or Injured Child. Baltimore, Williams & Wilkins, 1979.

from idiopathic pulmonary hemosiderosis (Fig. 1.59D), or a lesion such as a gastroenterogenous cyst or AV malformation, and pulmonary vein atresia localized to one lobe (34). In the latter condition, consolidation results from pulmonary edema, either secondary to back pressures on the lung from the obstructed vein, or from pulmonary infarction. However, all of these conditions, with the exception of pulmonary contusion, either are rare to begin with, or rare in childhood.

Finally, it might be noted that in infancy, right upper lobe consolidation can be mimicked by a normal, large right thymic lobe when the infant is turned to the right. A similar problem can occur on the left, but most often it does so on the right. In some cases, there is complete opacification of what would appear to be the right upper lung, and the unwary should avoid this pitfall.

Fluffy or Patchy Infiltrates

These infiltrates can be scattered diffusely throughout both lung fields or localized to one lobe. In either case, they are rather nonspecific (Figs. 1.62 and 1.63). Basically, these infiltrates have ill-defined margins, and, for the most part, they reflect alveolar disease, where the alveoli are full of exudate, edema fluid, or blood. When these infiltrates occur bilaterally, most commonly they are due to infection; i.e., most often staphylococcal pneumonia, but also *Hemophilus influenzae, Mycoplasma pneumoniae,* and streptococcal in-

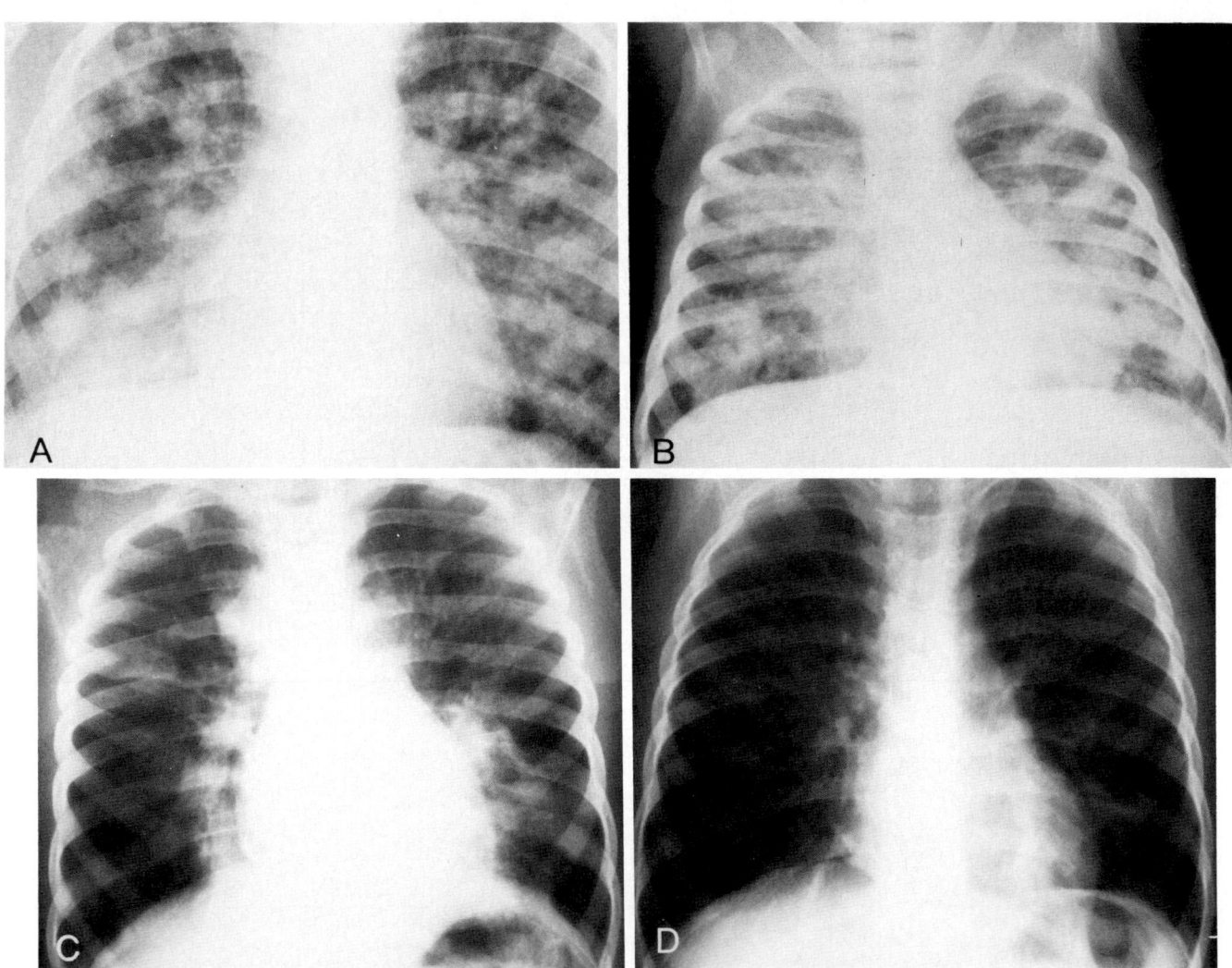

Fig. 1.62. Patchy or fluffy infiltrates. A. Note widespread patchy infiltrates in this patient with idiopathic pulmonary hemosiderosis (acute episode with pulmonary hemorrhage and edema). B. Another infant with similar infiltrates due to staphylococcal pneumonia. C. **Patchy atelectasis mimicking pneumonia.** Note widespread patchy infiltrates in both lungs. However, they are clustered toward the hilar regions of the lung, and this should favor segmental atelectasis over bacterial pneumonitis. D. Less than 24 hr later, almost all of the apparent infiltrates have disappeared. Only a few vertical streaks of atelectasis remain in the lung bases. C and D from Swischuk LE: Emergency Radiology of the Acutely Ill or Injured Child. Baltimore, Williams & Wilkins, 1979.

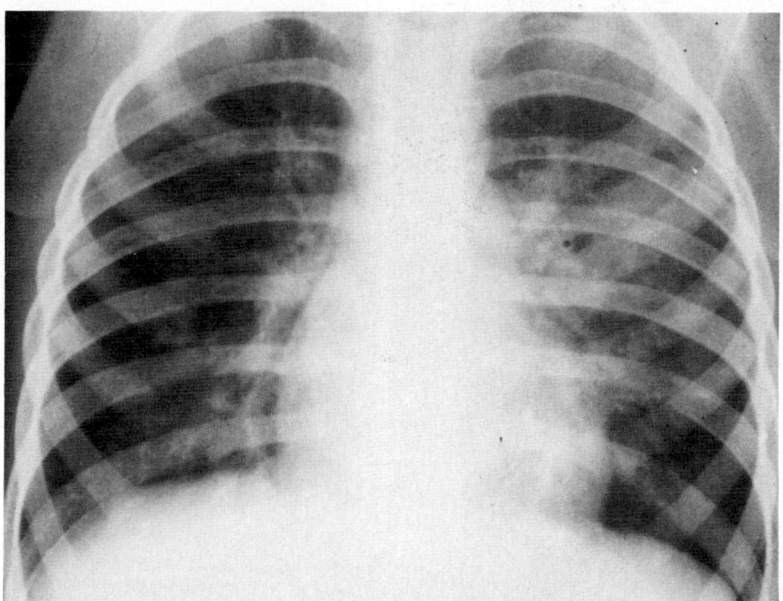

Fig. 1.63. Patchy infiltrates in one lobe. Note the patchy, somewhat hazy, infiltrate in the left upper lobe and lingula. On this view, it would be impossible to determine whether this is due to bacterial pneumonia or atelectasis. On lateral view, however, there was no evidence of volume loss. Under these circumstances, atelectasis is unlikely and a pneumonia should be considered. More often than not, it will be bacterial or Mycoplasmic in origin.

fections. As a rule, however, they do not occur with pneumococcal infections.

Other, less common, conditions producing patchy alveolar infiltrates include aspiration pneumonia, immunologic disease, fungal infections, sarcoidosis, milk allergy (3, 7, 12), visceral larva migrans (36), idiopathic pulmonary hemosiderosis (in its active, bleeding stage) (20, 29) (Fig. 1.62A), uremic lung with edema or bleeding, allergic lung (inhalants or ingested materials) (18, 35), hydrocarbon pneumonitis, near drowning, Loeffler's allergic pneumonia, and lung hemorrhage.

Patchy, indeed, fluffy appearing infiltrates also can be seen with segmental atelectasis, and while this is not common with bacterial infections, it is very common with viral or *Mycoplasma pneumoniae* infections. The reason for this is that these infections involve the bronchi and peribronchial interstitium more than the alveoli (especially the viruses). This being the case, these infections are attendant with considerable bronchospasm and mucous secretion, and together, these factors lead to bronchial obstruction and atelectasis. Such atelectasis, when patchy is almost impossible to differentiate from patchy pneumonia. However, one clue to the fact that atelectasis is the problem is the clustering of the infiltrates around the hilar regions

(Fig. 1.62C). The peripheral lung fields remain relatively clear, a distribution quite different from the more generalized one seen with bacterial infiltrates (Fig. 1.62B). Nonetheless, in many cases, it is not until repeat films are obtained that one is convinced that atelectasis only is the problem (Fig. 1.62D). In addition, it should be reiterated that clinical correlation is of the utmost importance in such cases, for often the roentgenograms in these children appear a lot worse than the child's clinical condition actually is. A similar problem can arise in the early stages of pertusis infection, for initially, this is a bronchial problem (2). It is later on only, with superimposed infection, that alveolar involvement occurs.

Patchy infiltrates localized to one lobe usually are the result of bacterial or *Mycoplasma pneumoniae* infections. When such infiltrates are seen with viral infection, they usually are due to incomplete atelectasis of a lobe. Of course, this does not mean that they are easy to differentiate from true consolidations, but only to indicate that most such infiltrates in viral disease are due to atelectasis. Roentgenographically, in these cases, one again must look for evidence of lobe collapse on one or the other of the views of the chest (see Fig. 1.60).

Streaks and Wedges

Thin streaks and wedges commonly occur with fluid accumulations in the pleural fissures, and as Kerley A and B lines in interstitial pulmonary edema (Fig. 1.64C). When the streaks are more wedge-like, or triangular in shape, segmental atelectasis should be the problem (Fig. 1.64, A and B). Occasionally, how-

ever, extensive fluid accumulations in the pleural fissures can be somewhat wedge-shaped, but once again their fissural location should be a clue to correct diagnosis. Fibrotic streaking in the lungs generally is uncommon in children, except as seen with healed tuberculosis, and in these cases, often a calcified cen-

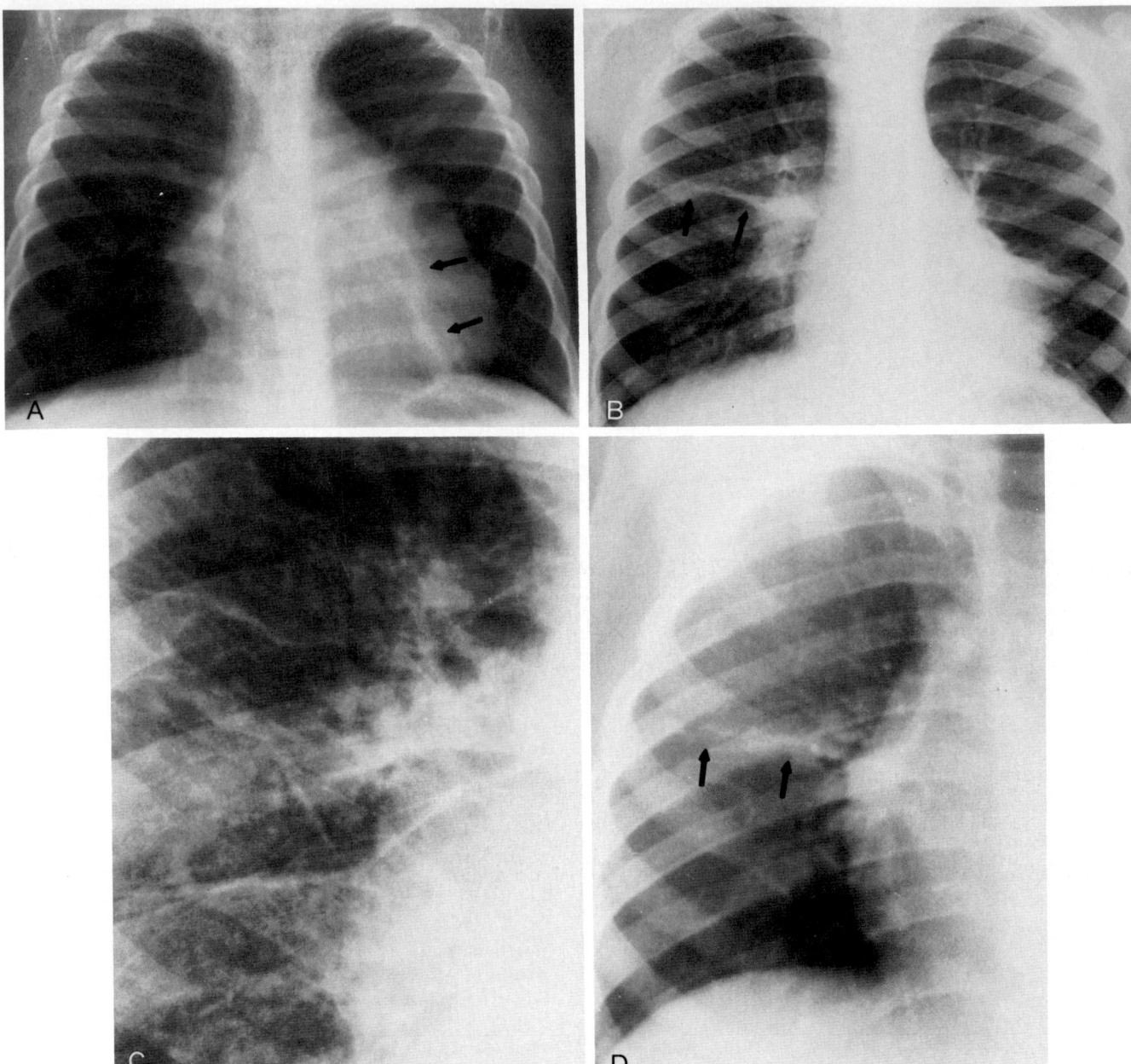

Fig. 1.64. Streaks and wedges. A. Note typical vertical streak of discoid atelectasis (arrows) behind the left side of the heart. This infant had a viral lower respiratory tract infection. B. Another patient with early atelectasis of the right upper lobe (arrows). This patient had asthma (i.e., note extensive parahilar-peribronchial infiltrates). A somewhat similar configuration can be seen with pleural effusions, along the interlobar fissures. For more streaks and wedges due to atelectasis, see Figure 1.62D. C. Numerous streaks secondary to interstitial pulmonary edema. These represent distended lymphatics and edema along interlobular septa, and the longer lines are referred to as Kerley A lines, while the shorter ones as Kerley B lines. D. Fibrotic streak (arrows) of healed tuberculosis. Note residual density in the right hilum, probably old scarred lymph nodes.

tral lymph node or peripheral Ghon lesion accompany the fibrotic streak (Fig. 1.64D). Fibrotic streaks re-

sulting from other pulmonary infections, except aspiration pneumonia, generally are uncommon.

Parahilar-Peribronchial Infiltrates

The term parahilar-peribronchial infiltrate infers that a bronchial infection (i.e., bronchitis and peri-

bronchitis) exists, and in some cases, actual thickening of the bronchial wall (i.e., seen on end as a circle or in length as parallel tram lines) is seen. Unfortunately, however, some patients with normal chests may show such ring-like configurations of the bronchus, and thus, unless multiple, the finding is a little difficult to assess. As a consequence, one's best diagnostic criterium for the diagnosis of a parahilar-peribronchial infiltrative pattern is "ragged" or "dirty" appearing parahilar regions (Fig. 1.65). Most commonly, parahilar-peribronchial infiltrates are seen with viral lower respiratory tract infection (5, 24, 32), and in many cases, are associated with bilateral hilar adenopathy (Fig. 1.65). The outward radiating pattern of the infiltrates attests to their peribronchial distribution, but at the same time, mimics the radiating pattern of passive vascular congestion. This should not be so surprising, for the peribronchial space is interstitial, and when passive vascular congestion occurs, it first occurs in this same interstitial compartment.

Mycoplasma pneumoniae infections also commonly produce this pattern of infiltration (4, 14, 27), but seldom is the pattern produced by the standard bacterial infections of childhood. Indeed, when bacterial infection is the cause of this type of infiltrate, it usually occurs as a mixed infection, often in a patient with cystic fibrosis, underlying immunologic disease, or iatrogenically suppressed immunity. In a perfectly normal child, it is highly unlikely that an acute bacterial infection would produce a parahilar-peribronchial infiltrate, and thus, when seen, viral lower respiratory tract infection (i.e., bronchitis more than pneumonitis) should first come to mind. Of course, if the viral infection lingers, secondary bacterial growth, both pathogen and nonpathogen, can develop, but even then, the parahilar-peribronchial pattern exists because of the primary viral infection.

Other conditions where parahilar-peribronchial infiltrates are seen include chronic asthma (especially with superimposed viral lower respiratory tract infection), interstitial pulmonary edema, and the early stages of pertussis infection (Fig. 1.65C). With pertussis, bronchial infection occurs first, and it is later only,

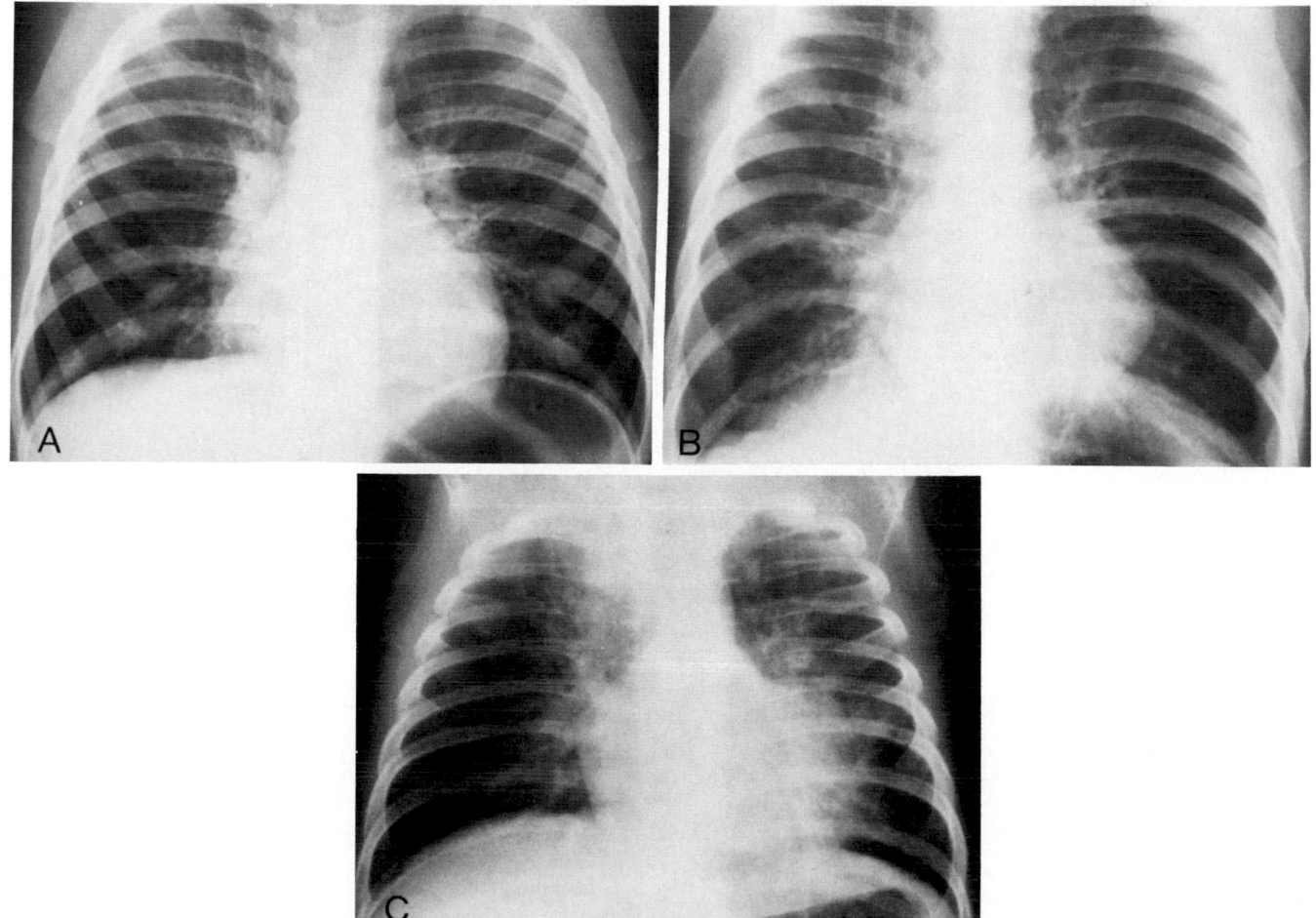

Fig. 1.65. Parahilar-peribronchial infiltrates. A. Typical appearance of radiating parahilar-peribronchial infiltrates, associated with hilar adenopathy in viral lower respiratory tract infection. B. Extensive parahilar-peribronchial infiltrates, associated with marked overaeration in an infant with cystic fibrosis. C. Parahilar-peribronchial infiltrates, with a more ragged interstitial pattern in an infant with pertussis.

that parenchymal infiltrates develop secondary to superimposed bacterial infection (2). Indeed, the parahilar-peribronchial pattern of early pertussis infection has led to the descriptive term "shaggy heart" but it should be noted that the commonest cause of this configuration is viral lower respiratory tract infection.

Reticular, Reticulonodular, and Honeycombed Infiltrates

These patterns intertwine, but basically reflect interstitial pulmonary disease (Figs. 1.66 and 1.67). Just which pattern predominates depends on how thick the lung interstitium becomes. When minimally thickened, delicate, even honeycombed, reticulations are seen, but when thicker, nodularity is superimposed. In addition, it is quite likely that when a number of reticulations overlap, nodular-like densities are seen at the point of overlapping. In still other cases, the nodules themselves become so large that they begin to coalesce and erroneously suggest the presence of alveolar (acinar) infiltrates (Fig. 1.68B). Of course, some alveolar disease probably coexists at this stage, for the thickened interstitium may so occlude the small peripheral airways that subsegmental atelectasis and secondary pneumonia develop. In addition, in certain inflammatory conditions, and certainly with pulmonary edema, when the interstitium becomes profoundly involved, the disease process extends into the alveoli (i.e., edema fluid seeps into the alveoli or some inflammatory cells extrude into the alveoli), but even then, it is important to appreciate that the disease process still basically is interstitial (Fig. 1.68C).

The commonest cause of reticular or reticulonodular infiltrates in children is viral pulmonary infection. Close behind is *Mycoplasma pneumoniae* infection, but it is quite uncommon to see this pattern of infiltration with the ordinary bacterial infections of childhood. It

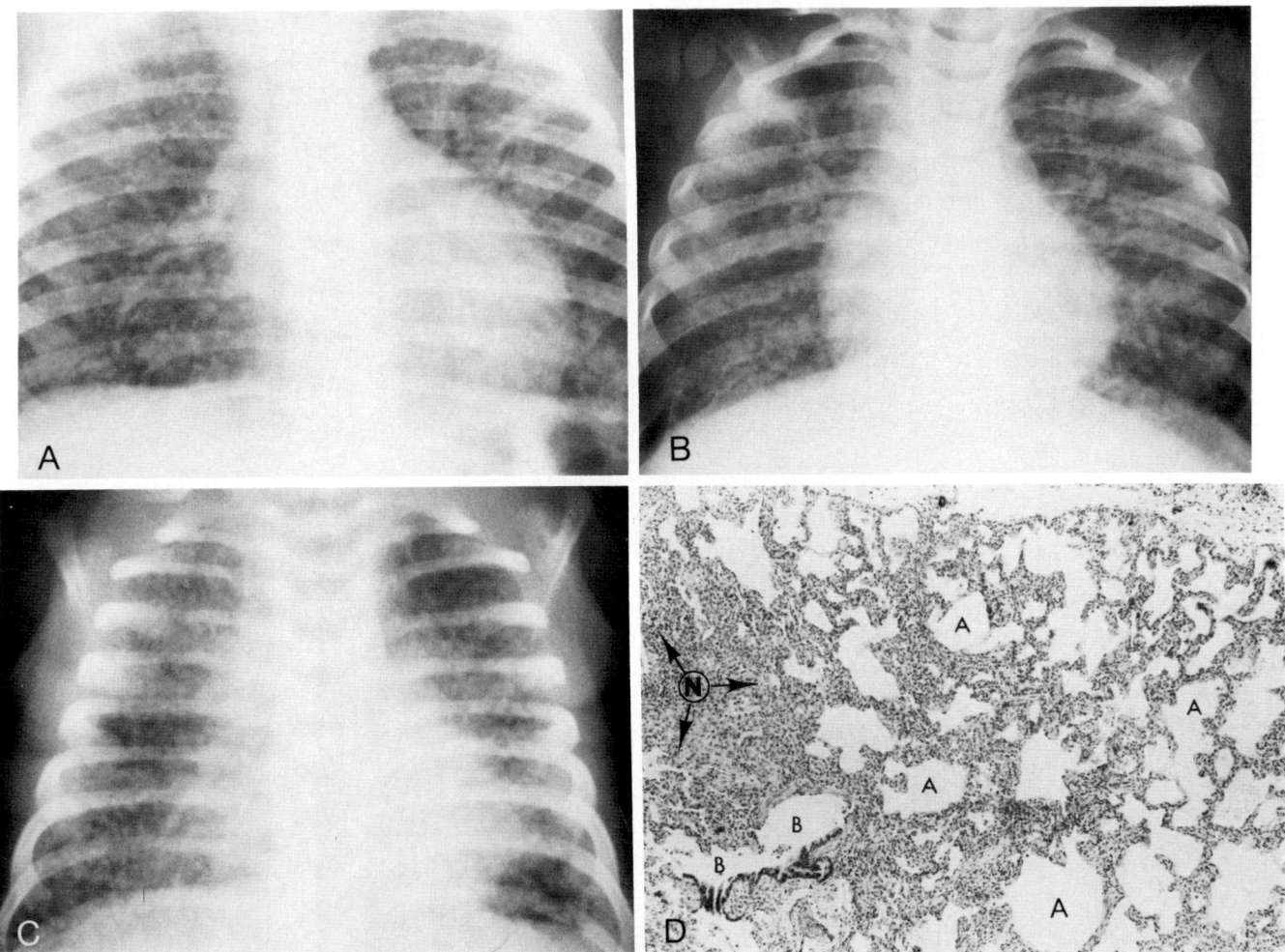

Fig. 1.66. Reticulonodular infiltrates. A. Typical reticulonodular infiltrates in patient with T-cell deficiency and cytomegalic inclusion virus pneumonitis. B. Reticulonodular infiltrates in histiocytosis-X. C. Nodular infiltrates in infant with viral interstitial pneumonia. D. Histologic material from infant in C. Note the clear alveoli (A), but also note the markedly thickened interstitium due to massive inflammatory cell infiltration. These areas show up as reticulations and the more pronounced area of infiltration, as nodules (N). Peripheral bronchiole (B).

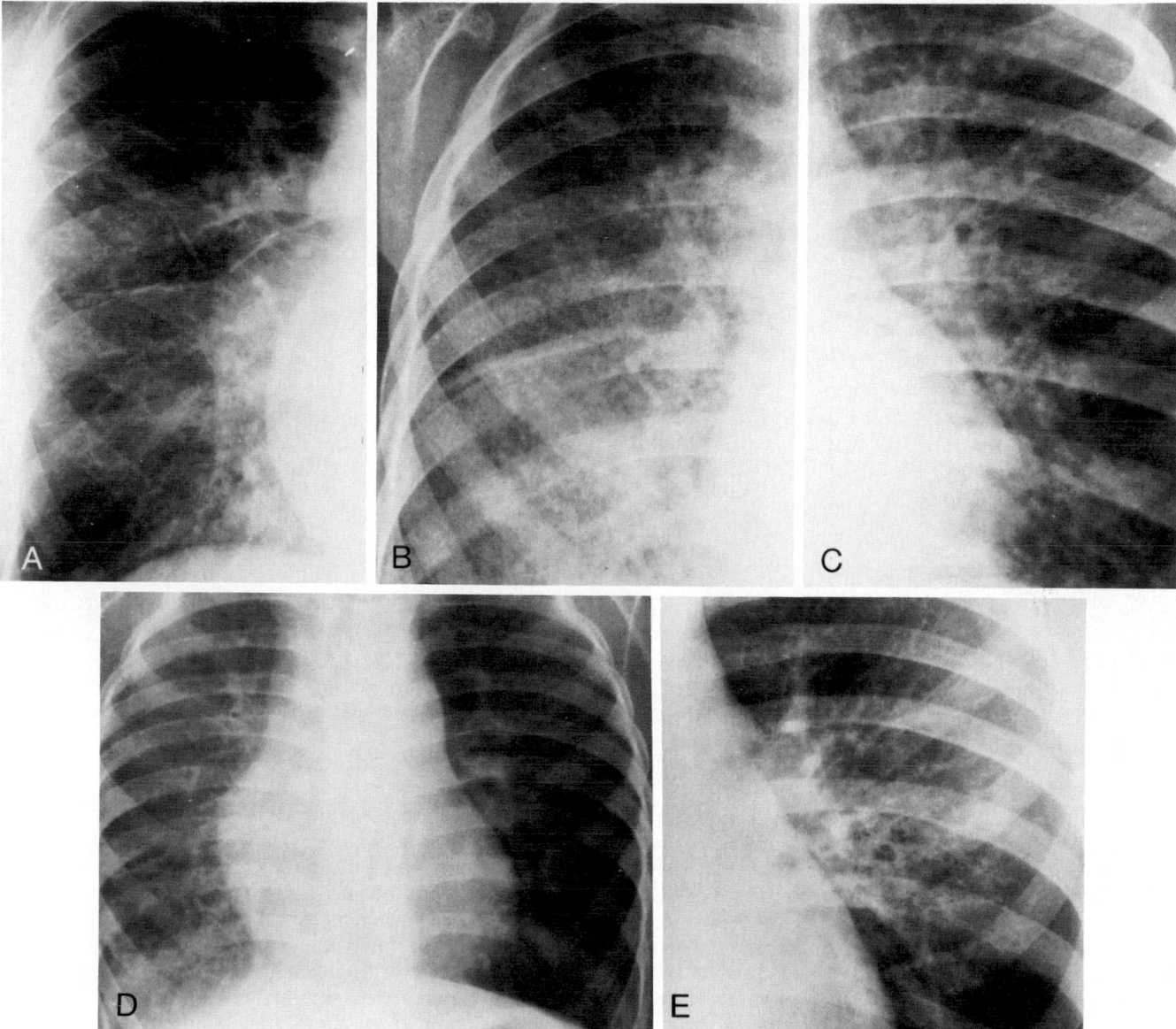

Fig. 1.67. Reticular infiltrates. A. Reticularity, bordering on honeycombing in a patient with interstitial pulmonary edema secondary to profound heart failure from thyrotoxicosis. The small transverse lines are Kerley B lines, while the long, oblique lines are Kerley A lines. B. Fine reticularity, bordering on honeycombing in patient with Niemann-Pick disease. C. Reticular infiltrates in patient with immunologic disease. D. Unilateral reticularity, especially well seen in the right lower lobe, in a generally small right lung. These findings are quite typical of unilateral pulmonary vein atresia. E. Reticular infiltrate in left upper lobe secondary to *Mycoplasma pneumoniae* infection.

is, however, seen with fungal infections, especially histoplasmosis, and with pulmonary edema. Pulmonary edema can be cardiac or noncardiac in origin, and in children, probably more often is noncardiac. For example, it can be seen with acute glomerulonephritis (17, 19), where the problem is fluid and electrolyte retention, or with the collagen vascular diseases where a vasculitis is the problem. For causes of pulmonary edema in childhood, see Table 1.16.

Other conditions causing reticular or reticulonodular infiltrates include pulmonary lymphangiectasia or hemangiomatosis (31), pulmonary vein atresia, idiopathic pulmonary hemosiderosis (chronic stage), the various causes of pulmonary fibrosis, the reticuloendotheliosis, lymphoma, sarcoidosis (21), leukemia, metastatic disease (lymphangiectatic spread), tuberous sclerosis, chronic aspiration, immunologic disease, cystic fibrosis, and occasionally, even *Pneumocystis carinii* pneumonia. In most of these conditions, the infiltrative pattern extends throughout both lung fields, but when it is localized to one lobe, *Mycoplasma pneumoniae* infection should be one's choice (Fig.

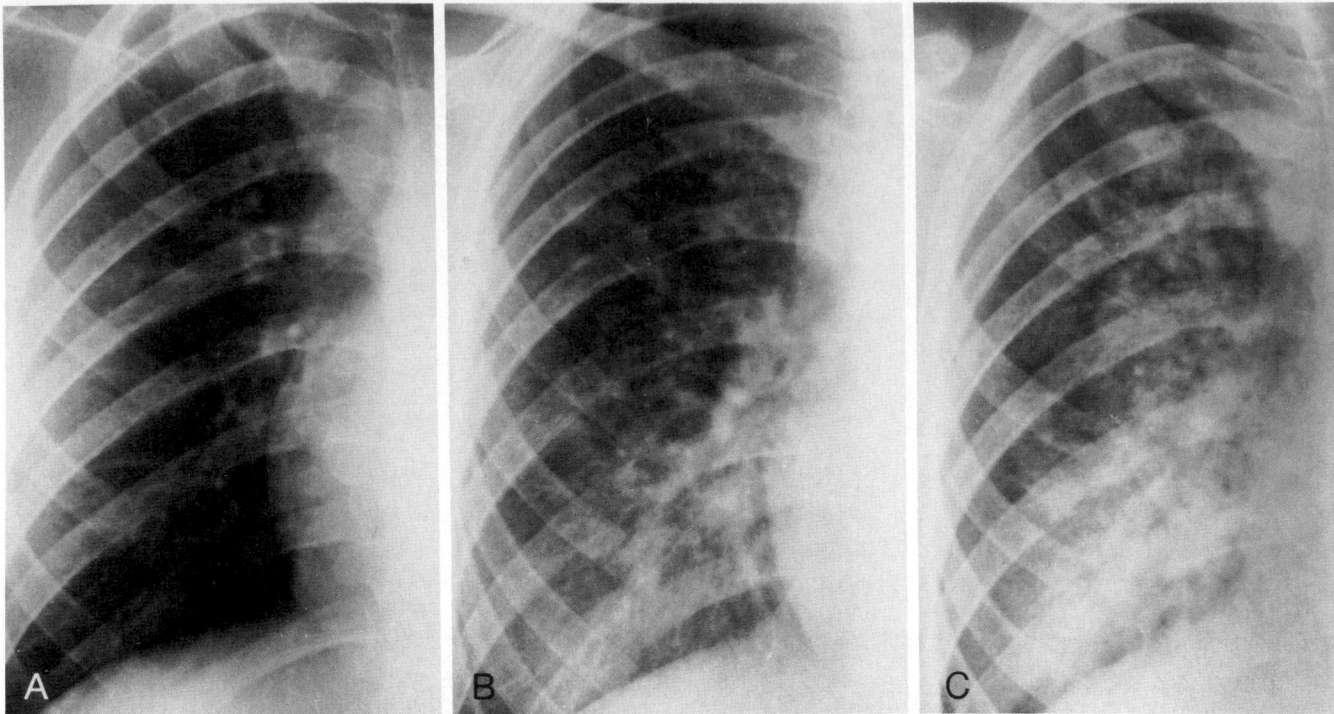

Fig. 1.68. Reticulonodular infiltrates: progressing to alveolar pattern. A. Normal chest in patient with renal failure. B. Early reticular infiltrates secondary to uremic pneumonitis. C. Advanced reticulonodular infiltrates seen the next day. This represents even more extensive interstitial involvement and thickening and, probably, some alveolar spillover.

1.67E). Such focal reticulation seldom, if ever, is seen with bacterial infection. Finally, it might be added that the so-called Kerley B and A lines of congestive heart failure (13) are in fact examples of reticular infiltrates. They result from dilated septal lymphatics and interstitial edema, and most commonly, are seen with lesions of the left cardiac valves or myocardium leading to congestive heart failure. However, they also can be seen with any cause of pulmonary edema.

Honeycombing, as mentioned earlier, represents a very delicate reticular infiltrate, and is most characteristic of pulmonary fibrosis. In the pediatric age group, idiopathic pulmonary fibrosis is rare, and more often, fibrosis occurs secondary to viral interstitial pneumonia, idiopathic pulmonary hemosiderosis (20, 29), chemotherapeutic agent and other drug toxicity (1, 26), neurofibromatosis, scleroderma, tuberous sclerosis, storage diseases, chronic pulmonary infection, chronic aspiration, immunologic deficiency states, and oxygen toxicity (10).

Hazy to Opaque Infiltrates

This pattern of infiltration also reflects interstitial disease, and is characterized by a diffuse, homogeneous haziness of the lungs. In more profound cases, haziness may be so dense that the lungs are nearly opaque. Most commonly, this pattern of infiltration is seen with pulmonary edema (cardiac or noncardiac) (9, 17, 19), viral interstitial pneumonitis, and *Pneumocystis carinii* pneumonia (6) (Fig. 1.69). In more advanced cases, an air bronchogram is clearly visible, and probably results from the fact that the interstitium is so thickened that it compresses the alveoli. In so doing, aerated lung is reduced to the point where alveolar disease is mimicked. Of course, in some of these cases, the disease process may extend into the alveoli (i.e., edema fluid spills into the alveoli or inflammatory cells are extruded into the alveoli), but it is important to remember that interstitial disease still is the predominant problem (Fig. 1.69, C and D).

Hazy lungs also can be seen with pulmonary fibrosis, idiopathic pulmonary hemosiderosis (fibrotic stage), lipoid pneumonia, shocked lung, pulmonary hemorrhage (including Goodpasteur's syndrome), near drowning, the hemolytic uremic syndrome, and the collagen vascular diseases (i.e., vasculitis with pulmonary edema or end stage fibrosis).

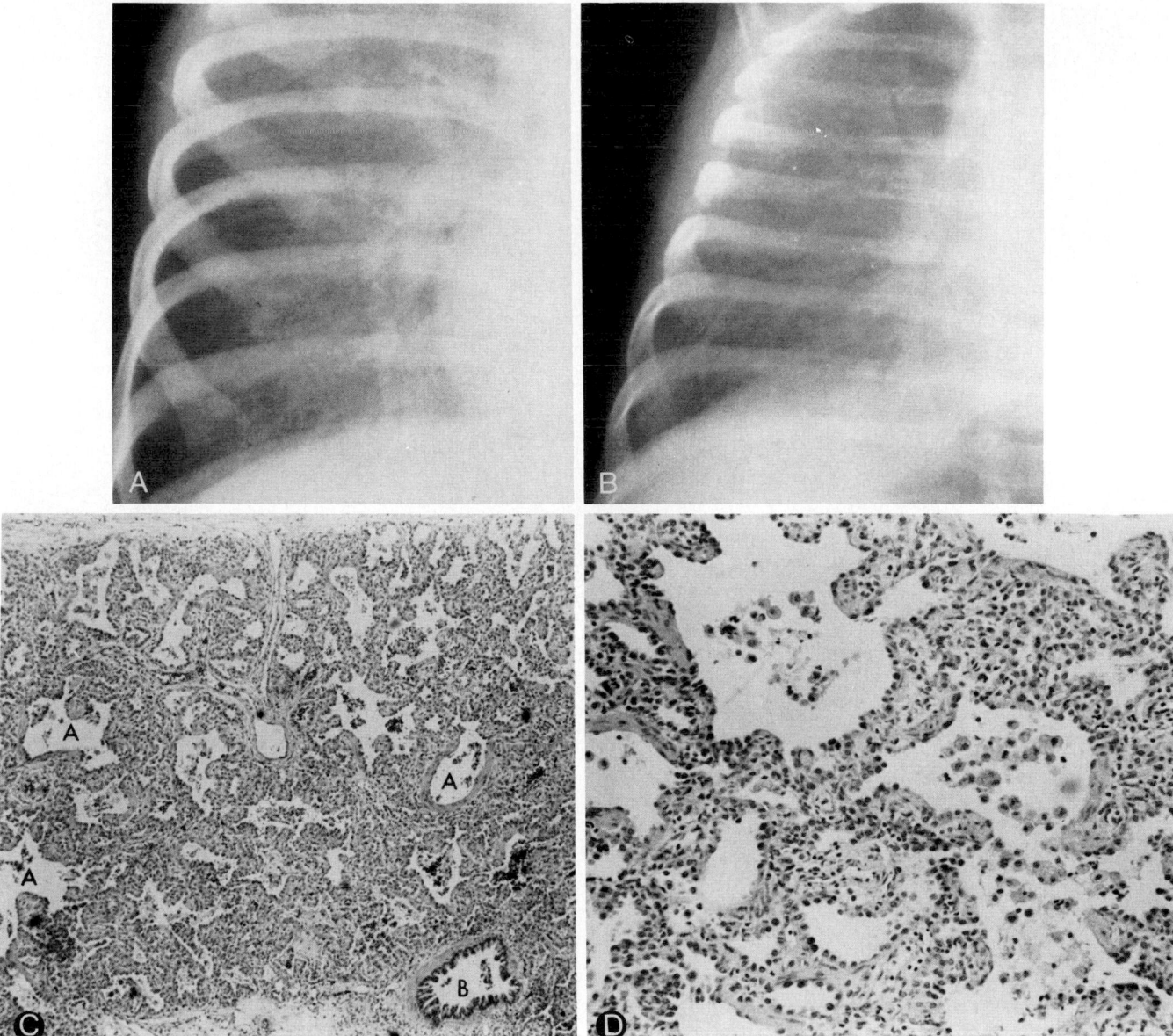

Fig. 1.69.   Hazy infiltrates. A. Typical diffuse hazy infiltrates of *Pneumocystis carinii* pneumonia. B. Another infant with biopsy proven viral interstitial pneumonitis producing diffuse haziness of both lungs. C. Histologic material from infant seen in B. Note the very thickened interstitium secondary to diffuse inflammatory cell infiltrate. Note that in some areas, the alveoli (A) still are open, but in others, they are completely compressed by the impinging interstitial thickening. Bronchiole (B). D. Higher power demonstrating that the alveoli contained only a few inflammatory cells, but that the interstitium is packed with inflammatory cells. On trichrome stain, early interstitial fibrosis also was present.

Miliary Infiltrates

Miliary infiltrates are interstitial infiltrates, and the small dots visualized result from the summation of numerous fine reticulations crossing one over the other. They are most characteristic of miliary tuberculosis (Fig. 1.70A). (28), but also can be seen with viral lower respiratory tract infection (viral pneumonitis), idiopathic pulmonary hemosiderosis (Fig. 1.70C), metastatic disease to the lungs, lymphoma, leukemia, aspirated foreign matter (16), and sarcoidosis. When miliary infiltrates become larger, a more reticulonodular pattern of infiltration results (Fig. 1.70B).

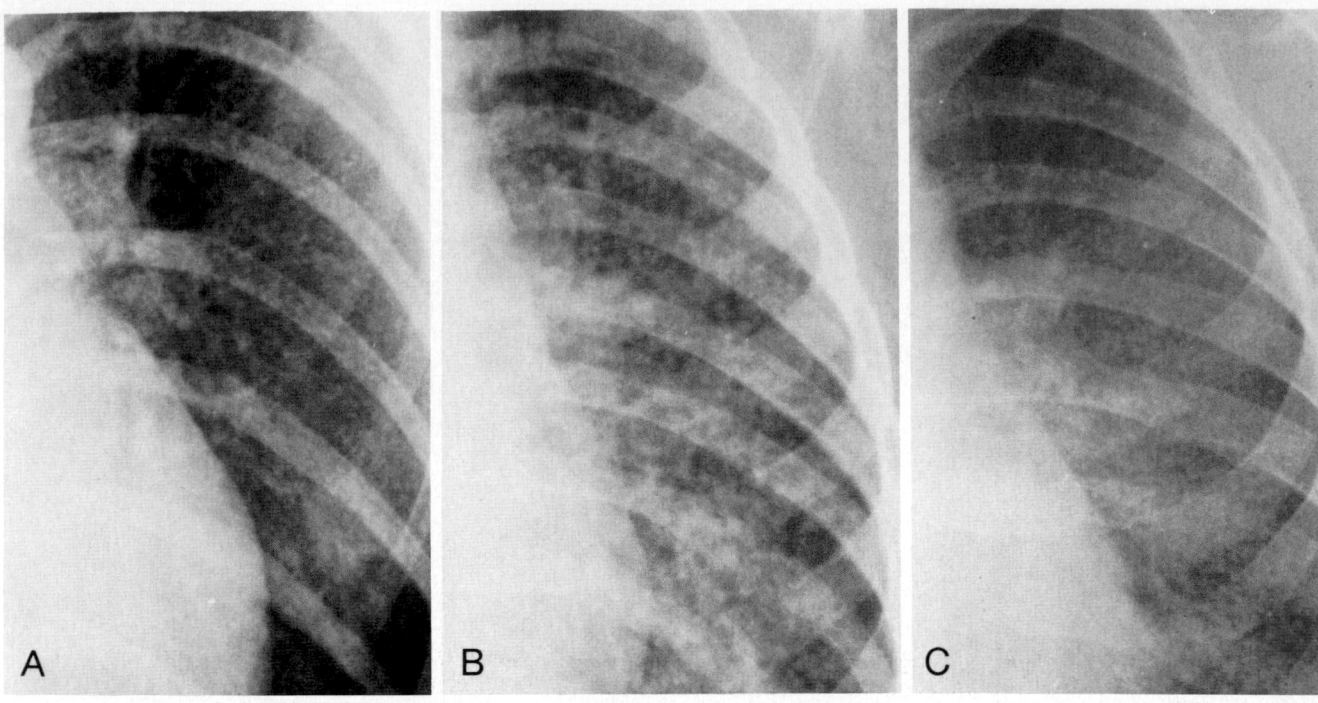

Fig. 1.70. **Miliary infiltrates.** A. Typical fine miliary infiltrates of tuberculosis. B. Slightly larger nodules in another infant with miliary tuberculosis. C. Fine miliary infiltrates in idiopathic pulmonary hemosiderosis (chronic phase with interstitial fibrosis).

Basal Infiltrates

Basically, basal infiltrates either are homogenous and hazy, or blotchy and patchy (Fig. 1.71). This latter pattern most commonly occurs with aspiration pneumonia, either hydrocarbon or regular aspiration (23). The basal and medial distribution of these infiltrates attests to the fact that aspiration occurred in the upright position. Diffuse, hazy infiltrates (Fig. 1.71A) reflect interstitial disease and most commonly occur with viral pulmonary infections such as desquamative interstitial pneumonia or lipoid interstitial pneumonia. However, a similar basal distribution also commonly is seen with cardiac and noncardiac pulmonary edema, and the vasculitis of collagen vascular disease (Fig. 1.71A). Just why these infiltrates so predominate in the lung bases is not known, but one reason may be that since the lungs are larger in their lower portions, any infiltrate present appears more pronounced in these areas. On the other hand, the degree of discrepancy between the relatively clear upper lobes and the hazy lower lobes is so great that it would suggest that some other etiologic factor is at play. In this regard, it may be that since most of these diseases lead to increased capillary permeability (i.e., severe damage to the interstitium and its vessels), gravity tends to favor the accumulation of the transudate (i.e., edema fluid) in the lower lobes. This may be enhanced by the normally greater flow of blood to the lower lobes.

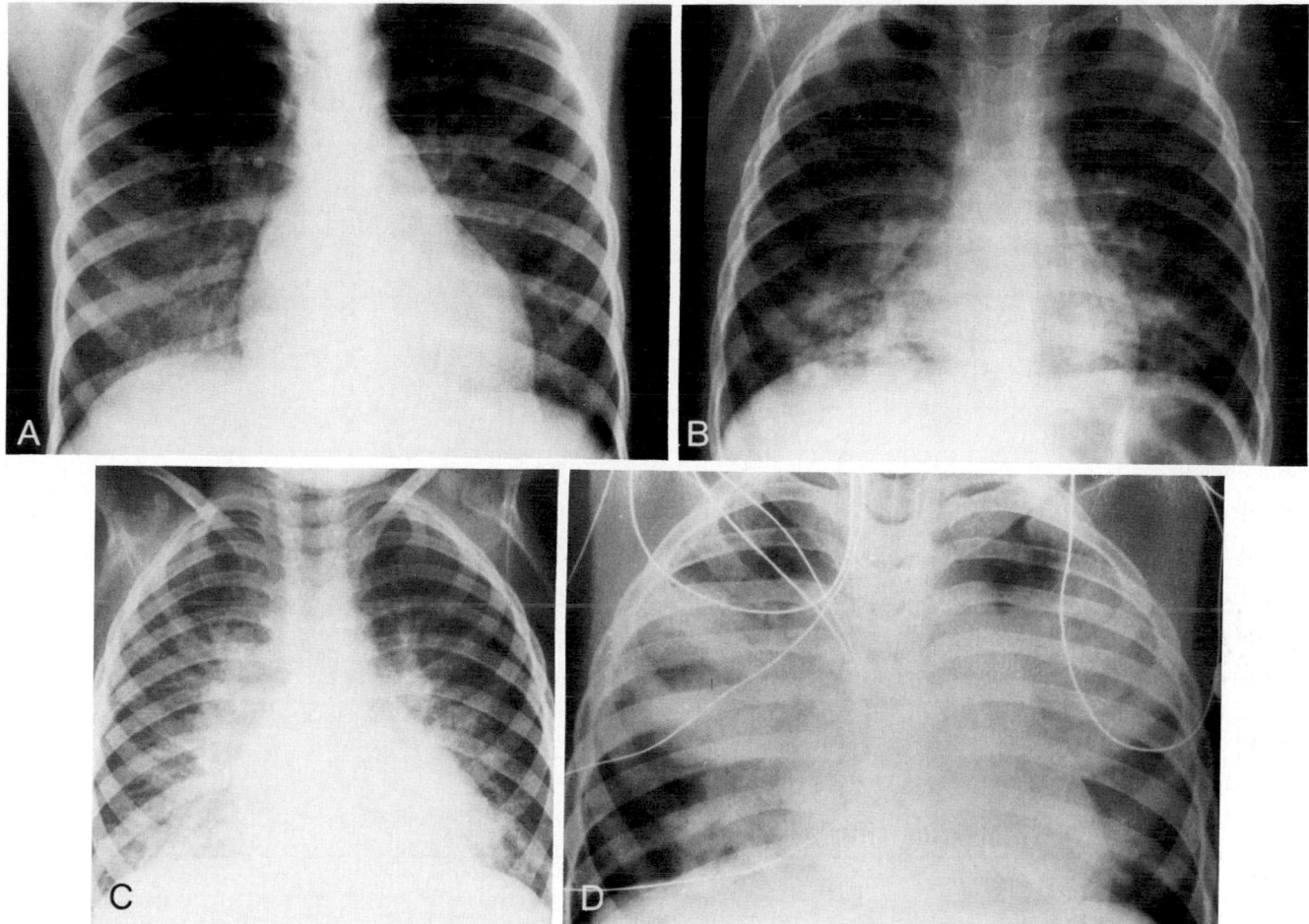

Fig. 1.71. Basal infiltrates. A. Note diffuse, basal haziness due to interstitial bleeding and edema in a patient with periarteritis nodosa. B. Typical fluffy and ragged, medial basal infiltrates due to hydrocarbon aspiration. C. **Basal and central infiltrates.** Typical distribution of reticular infiltrates in patient with pulmonary edema secondary to glomerulonephritis. The infiltrates are both central and basal. D. Dense **central infiltrates** due to iatrogenic fluid overload and pulmonary edema. Edema, at this stage, is alveolar. Note sparing of the apices and basal portions of the lungs. For central, interstitial infiltrates, see Figure 1.65.

Dense Central Infiltrates

Some of the conditions producing basal infiltrates also produce dense central infiltrates, and such infiltrates can be streaky or more homogeneous. Streaky, reticular infiltrates infer interstitial disease and have been dealt with in the section on parahilar-peribronchial disease (see Fig. 1.65). Dense, homogeneous infiltrates usually signify alveolar disease but can be seen with interstitial disease. Pulmonary edema is the most common cause of such infiltration (Fig. 1.71D), but it also can be seen with the hemolytic uremic syndrome, the active stage of pulmonary hemosiderosis (see Fig. 1.59D), pulmonary alveolar proteinosis, lipoid pneumonia, and rheumatic pneumonia (33).

In conclusion, it can be seen that although many infiltrative patterns are nonspecific, with an organized approach, one still can present the referring physician with a reasonable list of diagnostic possibilities for each pattern encountered. The more common conditions producing these patterns are summarized in Tables 1.14 and 1.15, and in addition, since pulmonary

Table 1.14 Pulmonary Infiltrate Patterns—Infections[a]

	Type of Infiltrate									
	Pneumo-coccus	Staphylo-coccus	Hemophi-lus	Strepto-coccus	Pertussis (Early)	Myco-plasma	Virus	Tuberculo-sis	Fungus	Pneumo-cystis car-inii
Consolidation	1	2	1	3	4	1	5	5	3[c]	4
Atelectasis (lobar)	5	5	5	5	3	1	1	1	3	5
Patchy, fluffy (bilateral, diffuse)	5	1	3	3	3[b]	2[b]	2[b]	5	1	3
Patchy, fluffy (lobar)	4	1	3	2	5	2	5	5	3	3
Patchy, fluffy (basal, bilateral)	5	5	5	5	5	5	4[b]	5	5	5
Parahilar-peribronchial	5	5	5	5	1	1	1	5	5	5
Reticulonodular	5	5	5	5	3	1[e]	1	3[d]	2	2
Honeycombed	5	5	5	5	5	5	5	5	5	5
Hazy to opaque	5	5	5	5	5	4	3	5	5	1
Hazy (basal)	5	5	5	5	5	3	2	5	5	3
Miliary	5	5	5	5	5	4	3	1	3	5
Diffuse steaks and wedges[b]	5	5	5	5	3	1	1	5	5	5

[a] Legend: 1, commonly seen in the condition; 2, moderately common in the condition; 3, occasionally seen in the condition; 4, rarely seen in the condition; 5, never, or nearly never, seen in the condition.
[b] Atelectasis usually.   [d] Usually nodular.
[c] Especially actinomycosis.   [e] Often one lobe only.

Table 1.15 Pulmonary Infiltrate Patterns—Noninfections[a]

	Pulmo-nary Edema	Pulmo-nary He-moside-rosis	Allergic Lung	Sarcoid-osis	Aspiration Pneumo-nia	Pulmo-nary Fi-brosis	Pulmo-nary Con-tusion	Pulmo-nary He-mor-rhage[g]	Reticulo-endothe-liosis	Leukemia-Lym-phoma	Asthma	Cystic Fi-brosis	Lymphan-giectasia-Heman-giomato-sis
Consolidate	3	5	5	5	2	5	1	3	5	5	3[d]	3[d]	5
Atelectasis (lobe)	5	5	5	5	1	5	5	5	5	5	1	1	5
Patchy, (bilat)	3	1	1	3	1	5	5	1	1	5	4[c,e]	2	5
Patchy, (lobe)	5	5	4	5	1	5	5	1	5	5	1[e]	2[e]	5
Patchy, (basal)	5	5	5	5	1	5	5	5	5	5	5	5	5
Parahilar peribron-chial	2	5	5	3	1	5	5	5	3	5	1	1	5
Reticulonod	2	1	3	2	3	1	5	5	2	2	4[c]	2	1
Honeycomb	5	3	5	3	5	1	5	5	1	5	5	2[f]	3
Hazy-opaque	1	2	5	4	3	1	5	2[b]	5	5	5	5	5
Hazy (basal)	2	3	5	5	5	4	5	5	5	5	5	5	5
Miliary	5	2	5	3	5	5	5	5	5	3	5	5	5
Streaks-wedge[e]	5	5	5	5	2	5	5	5	5	5	1[e]	1[e]	5

[a] Legend: 1, commonly seen in the condition; 2, moderately common in the condition; 3, occasionally seen in the condition; 4, rarely seen in the condition; 5, never, or nearly never, seen in the condition.
[b] Usually opaque.   [e] Atelectasis usually.
[c] With superimposed virus inf.   [f] Large honeycomb due to cystic change.
[d] With superimposed bacterial inf. only. [g] Including Goodpasteur's.

Table 1.16 Pulmonary Edema

Cardiac causes		
Left side cardiac failure		
Myocardial disease	}	Commonest
Valvular disease (obstruction, insufficiency)	}	Moderately common
Vascular obstructive disease (coarctation, etc.)	}	Relatively rare
Hyperkinetic cardiac failure		
Left-to-right shunt, admixture lesions	}	Moderately common
Anemia AV fistula	}	Relatively rare
Thyrotoxicosis	}	Very rare
Noncardiac causes		
Kidney disease		
Acute glomerulonephritis	}	Commonest
Chronic renal failure		
Iatrogenic fluid overload		
Near drowning		
Neurogenic (increased intracranial pressure)	}	Moderately common
Lung toxicity		
Rheumatic pneumonitis		
Allergic lung		
Toxic inhalants	}	Relatively rare
Vasculitis		
Collagen vascular diseases		
Idiopathic hemosiderosis		
Miscellaneous		
Pulmonary vein atresia		
Pulmonary vein obstruction acquired	}	Very rare

edema so commonly enters into the differential diagnosis of most of these patterns, it is worth being familiar with its various causes (Table 1.16).

References

1. Alvarado CS, Boat TF, Newman AJ: Late onset pulmonary fibrosis and chest deformity in two children treated with cyclophosphamide. *J Pediatr* 92:443–445, 1978.
2. Barnhard HJ, Kniker WT: Roentgenologic findings in pertussis. With particular emphases on the "shaggy heart" sign. *Am J Roentgenol* 84:445–450, 1960.
3. Chang CH, Wittig HJ: Heiner's syndrome. *Radiology* 92:507–508, 1969.
4. Clyde WA Jr, Denny MW: Mycoplasma infections in childhood. *Pediatrics* 40:669–684, 1967.
5. Conte P, Heitzman ER, Markarian B: Viral pneumonia, roentgen pathological correlations. *Radiology* 95:267–272, 1970.
6. Dee P, Winn W, McKee K: *Pneumocystis carinii* infection of the lung: radiologic and pathologic correlation. *Am J Roentgenol* 132:741–746, 1979.
7. Diner WC, Knicker WT, Heiner DC: Roentgenologic manifestations in the lungs in milk allergy. *Radiology* 77:564–572, 1961.
8. Eggleston PA, Ward BH, Pierson WE, Bierman CW: Radiographic abnormalities in acute asthma in children. *Pediatrics* 54:442–449, 1974.
9. Felman AH: Neurogenic pulmonary edema: observations in 6 patients. *Am J Roentgenol* 112:393–396, 1971.
10. Glauser FL, Smith WR: Pulmonary interstitial fibrosis following near-drowning and exposure to short-term high oxygen concentrations. *Chest* 68:373–375, 1975.
11. Gwinn JL, Lee FA: Radiological case of the month (Dermatomyosis of Lung). *Am J Dis Child* 129:703–704, 1974.
12. Heiner DC, Sears JW, Knicker WT: Multiple precipitins to cow's milk in chronic respiratory disease. A syndrome involving poor growth, gastrointestinal symptoms, evidence of allergy, iron deficiency anemia, and pulmonary hemosiderosis. *Am J Dis Child* 103:634–654, 1962.
13. Heitzman ER, Ziter FM, Markarian B, McClennan BL, Sherry HS: Kerley's interlobar septal lines: roentgen pathologic correlation. *Am J Roentgenol* 100:578–582, 1967.
14. Herbert DH: The roentgen features of Eaton agent pneumonia. *Am J Roentgenol* 98:300–304, 1966.
15. Hoenig PJ, Pasquariello PS Jr, Stool SE: *H. influenzae* pneumonia in infants and children. *J Pediatr* 83:215–219, 1973.
16. Kaplan SL, Gnepp DR, Katzenstein A, Feigin RD: Miliary pulmonary nodules due to aspirated vegetable particles. *J Pediatr* 92:448–450, 1978.
17. Kirkpatrick JA, Fleisher DS: Roentgen appearance of chest in acute glomerulonephritis in children. *J Pediatr* 64:492–498, 1964.
18. Levin DC: The P.I.E. syndrome—pulmonary infiltrates with eosinophilia: a report of 3 cases with lung biopsy. *Radiology* 89:461–465, 1967.
19. Macpherson RI, Banerjee AJ: Acute glomerulonephritis: a chest film diagnosis? *J Can Assoc Radiol* 25:58–64, 1974.
20. Matsaniotis N, Karpouzas J, Apostolopoulou E, Messaritakis J: Idiopathic pulmonary hemosiderosis in children. *Arch Dis Child* 43:307–309, 1968.
21. Merten DF, Kirks DR, Grossman H: Pulmonary sarcoidosis in childhood. *Am J Roentgenol* 135:673–679, 1980.
22. Moss G: The role of the central nervous system in shock: the centroneurogenic etiology of the respiratory distress syndrome. *Crit Care Med* 4:181–185, 1974.
23. Neuhauser EBD, Griscom NT: Aspiration pneumonitis in children. *Prog Pediatr Radiol* 1:265–293, 1967.
24. Osborne D: Radiologic appearance of viral disease of the lower respiratory tract in infants and children. *Am J Roentgenol* 13:29–33, 1978.
25. Park S, Nyhan WL: Fatal pulmonary involvement in dermatomyositis. *Am J Dis Child* 129:723–726, 1975.
26. Patel AR, Shah PC, Rhee HL, Sassoon H, Rao K: Cyclophosphamide therapy and interstitial pulmonary fibrosis. *Cancer* 38:1542–1549, 1976.
27. Putman CE, Curtis A McB, Simeone JF, Jensen P: Mycoplasma pneumonia: clinical and roentgenographic patterns. *Am J Roentgenol* 124:417–422, 1975.
28. Reed MH, Pagtahan RD, Zylak C, Berg T: Radiologic

features of miliary tuberculosis in children and adults. *J Can Assoc Radiol* 28:175–181, 1977.

29. Repetto G, Lisboa CM, Emparanza E, Ferretti R, Neira N, Etchart M, Maneghello J: Idiopathic pulmonary hemosiderosis. *Pediatrics* 40:24–32, 1967.
30. Rosenow EC, O'Connell EJ, Harrison EG, Jr.: Desquamative interstitial pneumonia in children. *Am J Dis Child* 120:344–348, 1970.
31. Rowen M, Thompson JR, Williamson RA, Wood BJ: Diffuse pulmonary hemangiomatosis. *Radiology* 127:445–451, 1978.
32. Scanlon GA, Unger JD: The radiology of bacterial and viral pneumonias. *Radiol Clin North Am* 11:317–338, 1973.
33. Serlin SP, Rimsza ME, Gay JH: Rheumatic pneumonia: the need for a new approach. *Pediatrics* 56:1075–1077, 1975.
34. Swischuk LE, L'Heureux P: Unilateral pulmonary vein atresia or stenosis (diagnostic roentgenographic and clinical features). *Am J Roentgenol Radium Ther Nucl Med* 136:667–672, 1980.
35. Unger GF, Scanlon GT, Fink JN, Unger JD: A radiologic approach to hypersensitivity pneumonias. *Radiol Clin North Am* 11:339–356, 1973.
36. Zinkham WH: Visceral larva migrans. *Am J Dis Child* 132:627–633, 1978.

PULMONARY VASCULARITY

In the normal individual, the pulmonary artery and its branches diminish in caliber as they travel from their origin in the hilar regions to the outer periphery of the lungs. Indeed, in the outer third of the lung fields, they become so small that, generally, they are invisible (Fig. 1.72A). Proximal to this zone, the vessels have reasonably distinct walls, and are relatively straight. In addition, it might be added that the vessels one sees are the pulmonary arteries and not the pulmonary veins. Obviously, the veins are present, but usually they are not visualized as discrete structures. Most likely, this is because the pulmonary arteries

have thicker walls. Any deviation from the foregoing pattern of pulmonary vascularity should suggest abnormality, and the abnormal patterns which can be encountered are: (*a*) increased vascularity or vascular congestion, (*b*) decreased vascularity or lung oligemia, (*c*) prominent central arteries with diminutive peripheral branches or pulmonary hypertension, and (*d*) unequal blood flow to the two lungs (Table 1.17). The latter pattern has been discussed earlier in the section dealing with unequal lung size (see p 7), and is not discussed here.

Table 1.17 Pulmonary Vascular Patterns

Increased vascularity	
Active	
Left-to-right shunt	Commonest
Cardiac admixture lesion	
Systemic AV fistula	Rare
Passive	
Left heart failure (myocardial disease)	Commonest
Acute glomerulonephritis (fluid overload)	
Left heart failure (valvular or valvular disease)	Moderately common
Fluid overload (iatrogenic, chronic renal failure)	
Neurogenic pulmonary edema	
Decreased vascularity	
Right outflow tract obstruction (congenital)	Commonest
Acidosis-hypoxia	Common
Hypovolemia (dehydration)	
Obstructive emphysema	
Right outflow tract obstruction (acquired)	Rare
Hypovolemia (blood loss)	

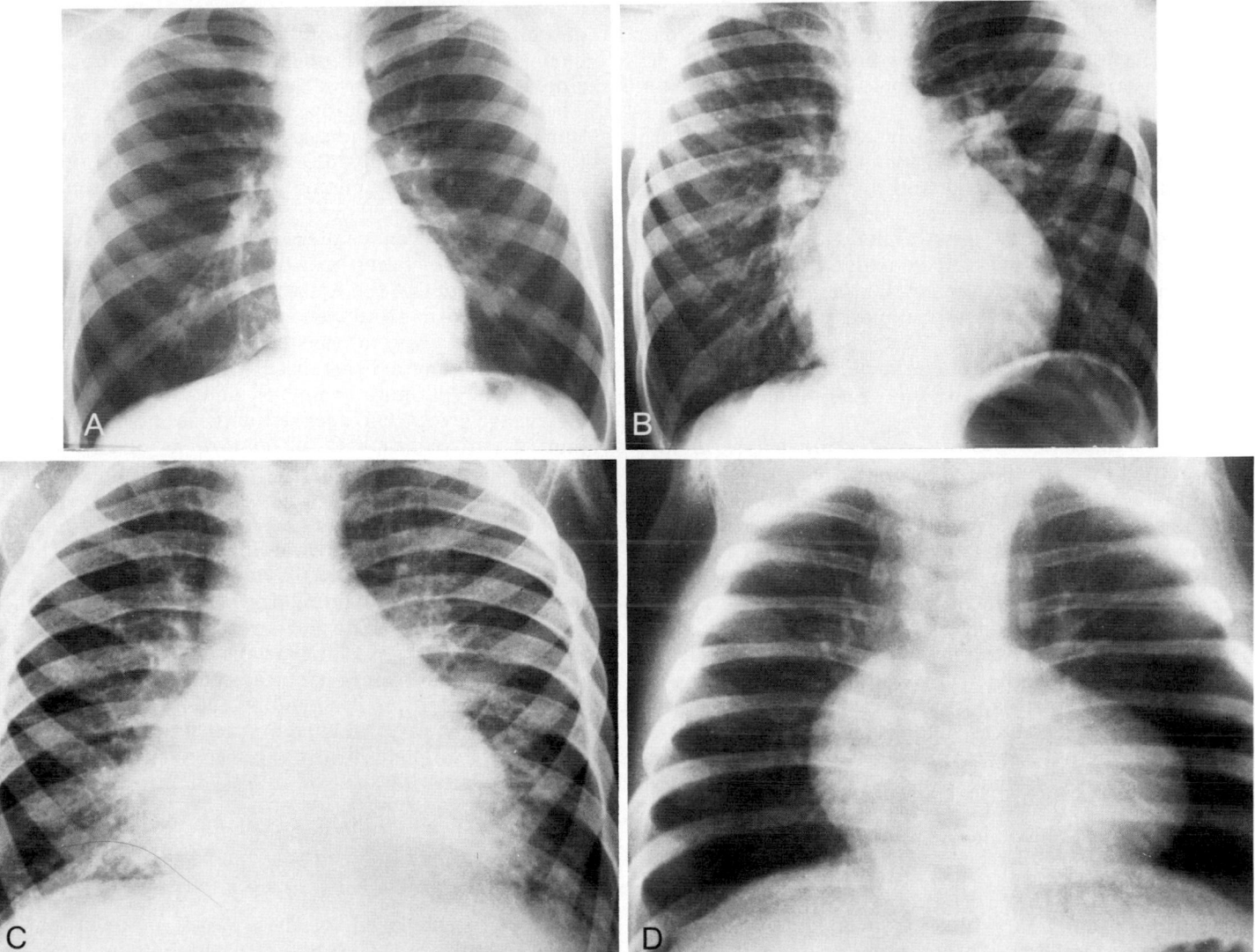

Fig. 1.72. Pulmonary vascularity. A. Normal pulmonary vascularity. Note that the vessels taper uniformly and become invisible in the outer third of the lung fields. **B. Increased vascularity; active congestion.** Note how much larger the individual vessels (pulmonary artery branches) appear. They also are more nodular, and are visible into the outer third of the lung fields. This patient had an ASD. **C. Increased vascularity; passive congestion.** Note the hazy or fuzzy appearance of the pulmonary vascularity. Individual vessels are not visualized and streaks of interstitial fluid are seen. This patient had myocarditis. **D. Decreased pulmonary vascularity.** Note marked radiolucency of the lungs. Also note that individual pulmonary artery branches are hard to find; they are thin and stringy. This patient had tetralogy of Fallot.

Increased Vascularity or Vascular Congestion

The term "vascular congestion," as applied roentgenographically, probably conjures different images for different individuals. The reason for this is that it is used to describe both active and passive congestion, and this is unfortunate for the two appear quite different and have a different etiologic basis. **Active vascular congestion** results from more blood than usual passing through the pulmonary circulation. For this to occur, there must be a communication between the systemic and pulmonary circulations. Because systemic pressures are higher than pulmonary pressures, some of the blood from the systemic circulation is diverted to the pulmonary circulation. Most classically, this occurs with congenital heart lesions in which a left-to-right shunt (i.e., VSD, ASD, PDA, AP-window), or cardiac admixture lesion (i.e., transposition, truncus arteriosus, single ventricle, total anomalous pulmonary venous return, etc.) is present.

Roentgenographically, with active congestion, the pulmonary artery branches become visualized well out into the outer third of the lung fields (Fig. 1.72B), and at the same time, they lose some of their straightness and become more tortuous and meandering. Their walls, however, remain relatively distinct. It is interesting, however, that even though the pulmonary veins clearly also must enlarge and dilate, seldom are they seen as distinct structures. Most likely this occurs because their walls are thinner than those of the arteries. Finally, it might be added that it requires a 2.5 to 1 shunt or greater for the roentgenogram to be able to detect increased pulmonary blood flow. In other words, there must be two-and-one-half times more blood flowing through the pulmonary circulation before one can appreciate increased pulmonary blood flow (1, 2, 4).

With **passive vascular congestion**, excessive flow of blood through the lungs does not occur, but rather, there is obstruction to the passage of blood through the lungs. This can result from obstructing lesions of the pulmonary veins, left side of the heart, or proximal aorta, (i.e., the various types of aortic stenosis, mitral stenosis, aortic or mitral valve insufficiency, coarctation of the aorta), and myocardial disease (i.e., myocarditis, and the cardiomyopathies). In the neonatal period, severe passive congestion can occur with pulmonary vein atresia, total anomalous pulmonary venous return below the diaphragm (type III), and the hypoplastic left heart syndrome (including premature closure of the foramen ovale).

In any given case, the roentgenographic findings are similar, for as blood backs up in the pulmonary veins, it causes intraluminal pressures to rise, and transudation of fluid into the interstitium. This results in haziness of the medial lung fields and a general fuzziness or indistinctness of the pulmonary artery walls. Thereafter, as more fluid accumulates in the interstitium, fuzziness and indistinctness become more profound, and eventually, fluid seeps into the alveolar spaces and classic pulmonary edema is seen (Fig. 1.72C).

If pulmonary venous pressures rise slowly (i.e., over a long period of time), redistribution of blood flow to the upper lobes of the lungs occurs. Most classically, this occurs with mitral stenosis, and commonly is seen in adults. However, mitral stenosis is not the common lesion of rheumatic heart disease in childhood (mitral insufficiency is more common), and thus, in the pediatric age group, one does not witness the phenomenon of redistribution of blood flow as often as in adulthood. This is not to say that it does not occur, but only to indicate that it is seen far less frequently in children than in adults.

Other causes of passive vascular congestion of the lungs, on a noncardiac basis, include iatrogenic fluid overload, neurogenic pulmonary edema, chronic or acute renal failure, acute glomerulonephritis (fluid and electrolyte retention), inappropriate ADH (antidiuretic hormone) secretion, and systemic arteriovenous fistulae. In addition, it should be noted that any left-to-right shunt or cardiac admixture lesion can cause the heart to fail, and in so doing, lead to superimposed passive congestion on an initial picture of active congestion.

Decreased Pulmonary Vascularity

When pulmonary blood flow to the lungs is decreased, the lungs become more radiolucent (or blacker) than normal. The reason, of course, is that the "solid tissue to air" ratio of the lungs is altered in favor of air. Most commonly, of course, this occurs because of an obstructing lesion on the right side of the heart. Such a lesion can be located anywhere from the tricuspid valve to the pulmonary artery, and usually takes the form of a congenital problem such as infundibular pulmonary stenosis, pulmonary atresia, tricuspid atresia, etc. Acquired obstruction also can occur, and most often is seen with reactive pulmonary arteriolar spasm secondary to hypoxia and acidosis. Pulmonary embolus is uncommon in the pediatric age group, and so is obstruction of the pulmonary artery by an adjacent tumor, mass, or mediastinal inflammatory process. In all of these cases, however, the lungs are quite hyperlucent, and the pulmonary arteries difficult to visualize. This is especially true of the lung periphery where the vessels are very thin and stringy (Fig. 1.72D).

Decreased pulmonary blood flow also is seen with obstructive emphysema of the lungs (i.e., asthma, cystic fibrosis, and centrally obstructing endotracheal or paratracheal lesions). In these patients, hypoxia and acidosis often also coexist, and these factors, as they induce vascular spasm, further decreased pulmonary blood flow. Hypovolemia is another cause of decreased pulmonary blood flow in the pediatric age group, and is especially common in infants. Most often, it is secondary to severe vomiting or diarrhea (3), but massive blood loss also is a cause.

Pulmonary Hypertension

Pulmonary hypertension, when demonstrable roentgenographically, presents with markedly enlarged central pulmonary arteries and relatively diminutive pulmonary artery branches. The breakoff point is between the inner and outer two-thirds of the lung fields (see Fig. 1.52B). Pulmonary hypertension usually develops in patients with long-standing left-to-right shunts or cardiac admixture lesions, and does so because of the continuous flow of excessive volumes of blood through the pulmonary circulation. It is, in fact, a protective device wherein the peripheral pulmonary arterial musculature becomes hypertrophied, and clamps down on the flow of blood through the lungs. Pulmonary hypertension also can be seen with chronic overdistention of the lungs, such as occurs in asthma, cystic fibrosis, and alpha-1 antitrypsin deficiency. It also can be seen with multiple pulmonary emboli, but the commonest cause, by far, is an underlying congenital heart lesion with a left-to-right shunt or cardiac admixture problem.

References

1. Chen JTT, Capp MR, Johnsonrude IS, Goodrich JK, Lester RG: Roentgen appearance of pulmonary vascularity in the diagnosis of heart disease. *Am J Roentgenol Radium Ther Nucl Med* 112:559–570, 1971.
2. Simon M: The pulmonary vasculature in congenital heart disease. *Radiol Clin North Am* 6:303–318, 1968.
3. Swischuk LE: Microcardia: uncommon diagnostic problem. *Am J Roentgenol* 103:115–118, 1968.
4. Swischuk LE: *Plain Film Interpretation in Congenital Heart Disease,* ed 2. Baltimore, Williams & Wilkins, 1979, pp 16–28.

GREAT VESSEL CONFIGURATIONS

Although the aorta and pulmonary artery usually are clearly visible in the child, in the infant they often are obscured by the overlying thymus gland. Nonetheless, much as in the adult, either great vessel can be too large or too small (2, 10), and the aorta can be on the left or on the right (Tables 1.18 and 1.19). When it is on the right, it can provide a significant clue to the presence of certain congenital heart problems.

Table 1.18 Aortic Configurations

Large aorta	
Aortic stenosis (valvular) Patent ductus arteriosus	Commonest

Coarctation of aorta
   Systemic hypertension
   Tetralogy of Fallot
   Persistent truncus
	Moderately common

Pseudocoarctation
   Aortitis (see text)
   Aortic aneurysm
   Aorticopulmonary window
	Rare

Small aorta
   Ventricular septal defect
   Atrial septal defect
   AV communis (endocardial cushion)
	Commonest

Supravalvular aortic stenosis
   Interrupted aortic arch (infant)
   Hypoplastic left heart (neonate)
   TAPVR and other intracardiac L→R shunts
	Relatively rare

Right aortic arch Isolated anomaly (no ring, no heart disease)	Commonest

With vascular ring
   With tetralogy of Fallot
   With truncus arteriosus
	Moderately common

With other congenital heart disease	Relatively rare

Table 1.19 Pulmonary Artery Configurations

Large (convex) pulmonary artery	

Pulmonary valve stenosis
   Left-to-right shunts
   Cardiac admixture lesions
	Commonest

Pulmonary hypertension	Moderately common

Pulmonary insufficiency
   Hypoplastic left heart (neonate)
   Interrupted aortic arch (infant)
   Infantile coarctation aorta (infant)
   Idiopathic dilation (adolescent)
   Post-TOF repair
	Relatively rare

Aneurysm Absent pulmonary valve	Very rare
Small (concave or flat) pulmonary artery Infundibular pulmonary stenosis (TOF)	Commonest

Hypoplastic right heart syndrome (neonate)
   Ebstein's anomaly
   Transposition of great vessels
   Truncus arteriosus
	Moderately common

Tricuspid insufficiency Uhl's disease	Rare

Unequal pulmonary artery branches
   Tetralogy of Fallot
   Truncus arteriosus
   Hypoplastic pulmonary artery & lung
	Commonest

Acquired hypoplastic lung (Swyer-James)	Moderately common
Pulmonary valve stenosis (in childhood)	Relatively rare
Unilateral pulmonary vein atresia Hemitruncus arteriosus	Rare

Large Aorta

Before proceeding with a discussion of a large aorta in children, it should be noted that the normal aorta in a child is relatively smaller than its counterpart in an adult. As a consequence, one's index of suspicion for increased size of the aorta must be higher in the child. For the most part, this pertains to the aortic knob, for this is the portion of the aorta most readily visualized on a chest roentgenogram. However, the aorta also can enlarge in its ascending and descending portions, and as far as the latter is concerned, causes include systemic hypertension, some form of aortitis, aneurysm, and coarctation of the aorta.

The commonest cause of enlargement of the ascending and transverse (aortic knob) portions of the aorta is congenital valvular aortic stenosis. Subvalvular aortic stenosis generally is not associated with an enlarged aorta, but occasionally, the aorta may dilate with membranous subvalvular aortic stenosis. In such cases, the position of the hole in the subvalvular membrane is such that it acts as if it were a stenosed aortic valve. In either case, the resultant jet of blood, under pressure, causes the aorta to dilate. With supravalvular aortic stenosis, the aorta is underdeveloped and small.

Less commonly, the aorta enlarges because of aortic insufficiency or systemic hypertension, and in the latter instance, the aorta dilates because of increase peripheral vascular resistance. With aortic insufficiency, enlargement is due to the propulsion of increased volumes of blood into the aorta from the left ventricle. The volume of blood ejected from the left ventricle is increased because, during diastole, blood which would ordinarily pass out, into the systemic circulation, is dumped back into the left ventricle. This, of course, causes the left ventricle to dilate, but at the same time, as the extra blood is ejected into the aorta, it causes the aorta to dilate.

Still another cause of aortic enlargement is increased blood flow associated with a left-to-right shunt at the great vessel level. Most often, the problem is patent ductus arteriosus, but it also can be seen with the much rarer aortico-pulmonary window. In both of these lesions, the excessive volumes of blood flowing through the lungs (because of the left-to-right shunt) are delivered back to the left side of the heart, and since in most cases, there are no associated intracardiac communications, this same increased volume is ejected out the aorta, and causes it to enlarge.

The aorta also enlarges in persistent truncus arteriosus. In this condition, since the pulmonary artery originates from the aorta, it does not drain the right ventricle. The right ventricle empties through an associated VSD, into the left ventricle, and then all of the heart's blood goes out the persistent truncus (aorta) and causes it to enlarge (Fig. 1.73A).

The aorta also can enlarge when the pulmonary artery is obstructed to a profound degree. Classically, this occurs in severe tetralogy of Fallot (see Fig. 1.77), where, in essence, the aorta must handle the output from both ventricles. Enlargement of the aorta due to aortic wall disease is relatively rare in children, but when seen, usually is due to Marfan's syndrome, homocystinuria, Takayshu's aortitis, traumatic or mycotic aortic aneurysm (Fig. 1.73B), or the mucocutaneus lymph node syndrome. The aorta also can dilate, both in its prestenotic and poststenotic portions in

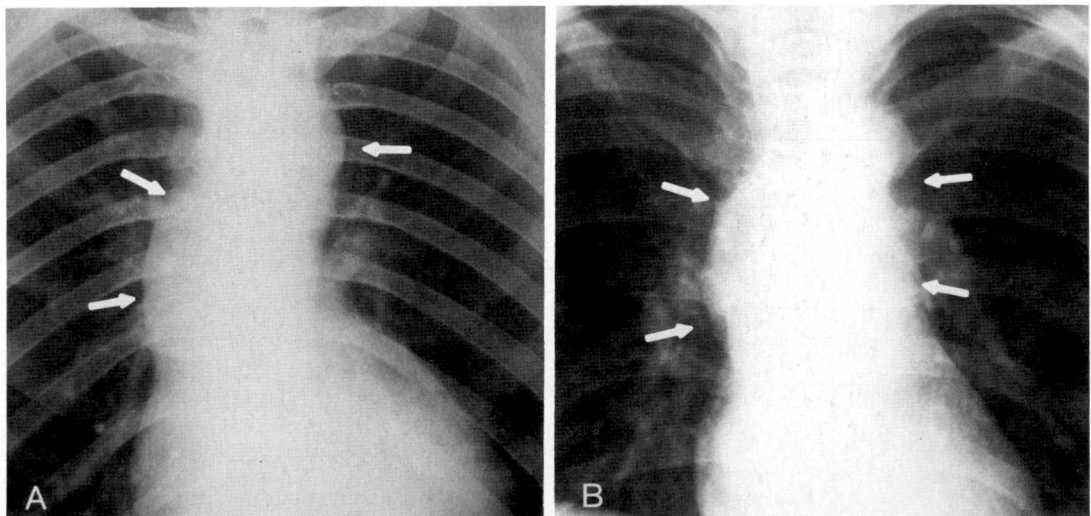

Fig. 1.73. Large aorta. A. Patient with persistent truncus arteriosis. Arrows denote the very large aorta (actually the persistent truncus). Also note the concave pulmonary artery, and in this case, decreased pulmonary vascularity. More commonly, such aortic enlargement is seen with aortic stenosis, aortic insufficiency, and systemic hypertension. B. Dilated aorta due to mycotic aneurysm (arrows).

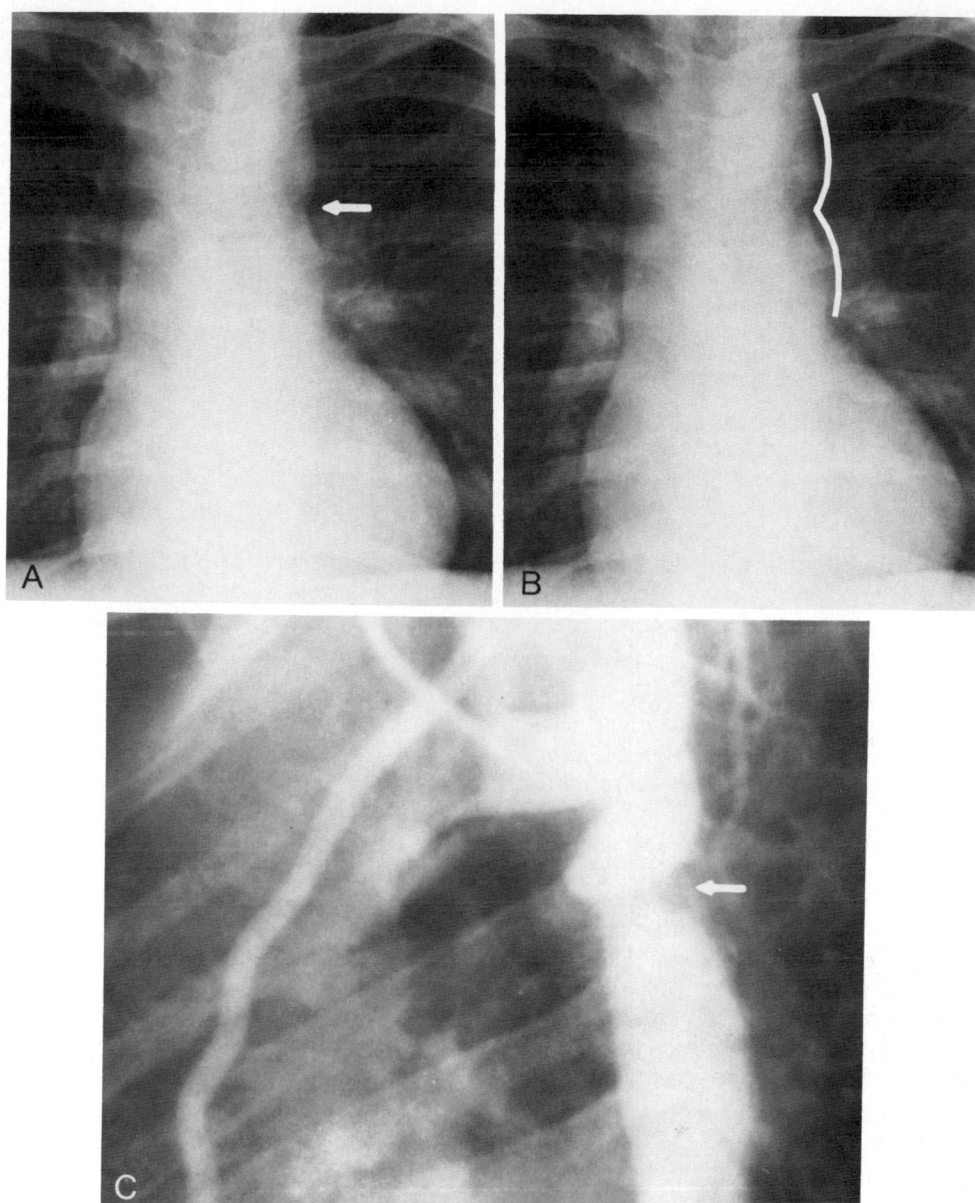

Fig. 1.74. Coarctation of the aorta. A. Note the notch and figure "3" sign (arrows) caused by the prominent pre- and poststenotic portions of the descending aorta. B. Diagrammatic representation of the figure "3" sign. C. Aortogram demonstrating the coarctation (arrow) which produces the figure "3" sign. Also note the collateral circulation.

coarctation of the aorta (Fig. 1.74, A and B), and in the condition known as "pseudo-coarctation" or "congenital kinking" of the aorta (5). In these latter cases, the aorta is dilated, somewhat higher in position than normal, and severely kinked. During cardiac catheterization, no pressure gradient across the apparent narrowing is demonstrable, and the kinking becomes clearly visible with aortography. With true coarctation, of course, actual stenosis and a pressure gradient are present.

Small Aorta

A small aorta can be seen with hypoplasia or underdevelopment of the aorta, or with lesions where less than normal volumes of blood flow through the aorta. The latter cause is much more common, and for the most part, results from the presence of intracardiac left-to-right shunts (i.e., atrial septal defect and ventricular septal defect). In both conditions, since systemic pressures are higher than pulmonary pressures, a left-to-right shunt results, and because it is intracardiac, blood is shunted to the right side of the heart

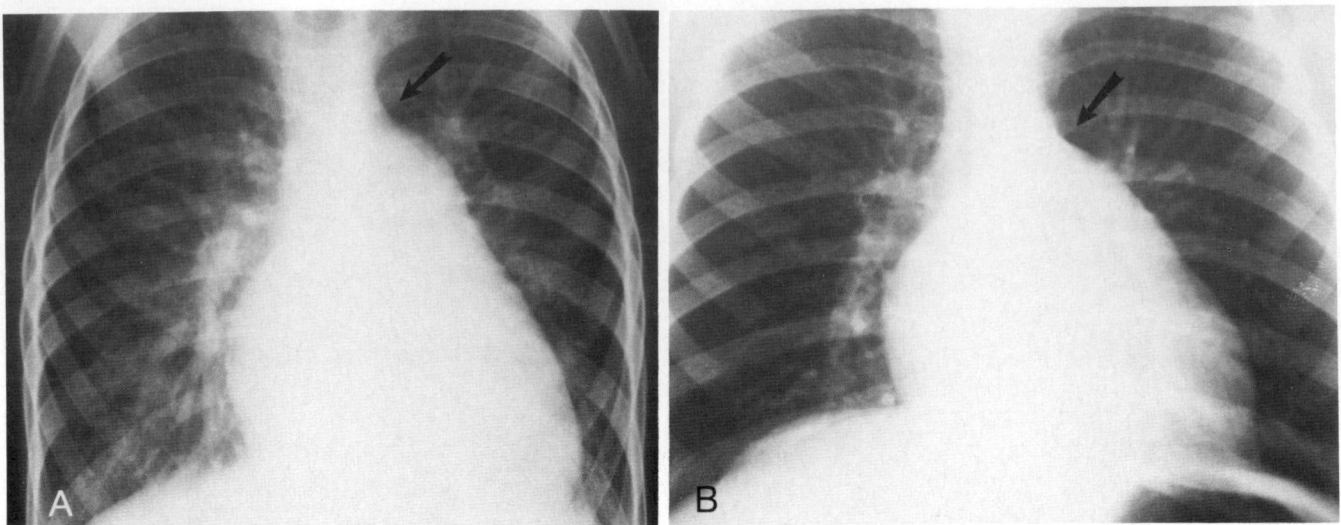

Fig. 1.75. Small aorta. A. Note the small aorta (arrow) in this patient with an ASD. The pulmonary artery, just below it, is enlarged (usual for this condition). B. Note the almost invisible aorta (arrow), secondary to hypoplasia as a part of supravalvular aortic stenosis. This patient had the infantile hypercalcemia syndrome.

before it reaches the aorta. For this reason, even though the shunt causes extra volumes of blood to be returned to the left side of the heart, the aorta is never required to handle this blood, and thus, remains diminutive (Fig. 1.75A). Contrarily, if the left-to-right shunt occurs at the great vessel level (i.e., patent ductus arteriosus, aorticopulmonary window), the aorta is of normal size or enlarged. In these cases, no intracardiac shunt is present, and thus all of the extra blood leaving the left side of the heart must pass through the aorta.

Smallness of the aorta due to actual hypoplasia is relatively uncommon, and when seen, usually occurs in the infant with lesions such as the hypoplastic left heart syndrome (i.e., mitral atresia, aortic atresia), interrupted aortic arch (4, 7), and supravalvular aortic stenosis. This latter condition usually is associated with the infantile hypercalcemia syndrome (William's syndrome) (6), and is about the only one of these lesions which can be seen beyond infancy (Fig. 1.75B). Smallness of the aorta also occurs in long-standing mitral stenosis, but since it takes many years for this to develop, and since mitral stenosis is not the primary childhood lesion in rheumatic heart disease (mitral insufficiency is), it is not commonly seen in children. Smallness of the aorta, in these cases, probably is related to inhibition of blood flow through the left side of the heart.

Right Aortic Arch

A right aortic arch can exist under three conditions: as an isolated anomaly, with a true vascular ring, or with an underlying congenital heart lesion. The commonest situation is for it to exist as an isolated anomaly, and next most common is for it to exist with a congenital heart lesion. In the latter case, the most commonly associated conditions are tetralogy of Fallot (in about 25% of cases) and persistent truncus arteriosus (in about 33% of cases). The presence of a right side aortic arch in these conditions is a valuable clue to their diagnosis, for the incidence of right aortic arch in any other congenital heart lesion is less than 5%. Least common is right aortic arch as part of a vascular ring, and in these cases, the two most common rings (indeed, almost the only) are double aortic arch and

right side aorta with aberrant left subclavian artery and an encircling ductus arteriosus or ligamentum arteriosum (10).

Roentgenographically, a right side aortic arch should be suspected when there is absence of the normal left aortic knob, and right paratracheal fullness, or a definite bulge (bump), on the right (see Fig. 1.82B). In most cases, the bump (aortic knob) is located just a little above where it would be if it were normal and on the left. On barium swallow, there is concomitant right side indentation on the esophagus, and both the trachea and esophagus can also be compressed from behind. In most cases, barium swallow reveals a reverse "S" or opposing double indentations of the esophagus (see Fig. 1.2C).

Large Pulmonary Artery

A large pulmonary artery can be seen with valvular pulmonary stenosis, pulmonary insufficiency, left-to-right shunts, cardiac admixture lesions, severe obstructions of the aorta or left side of the heart, pul-

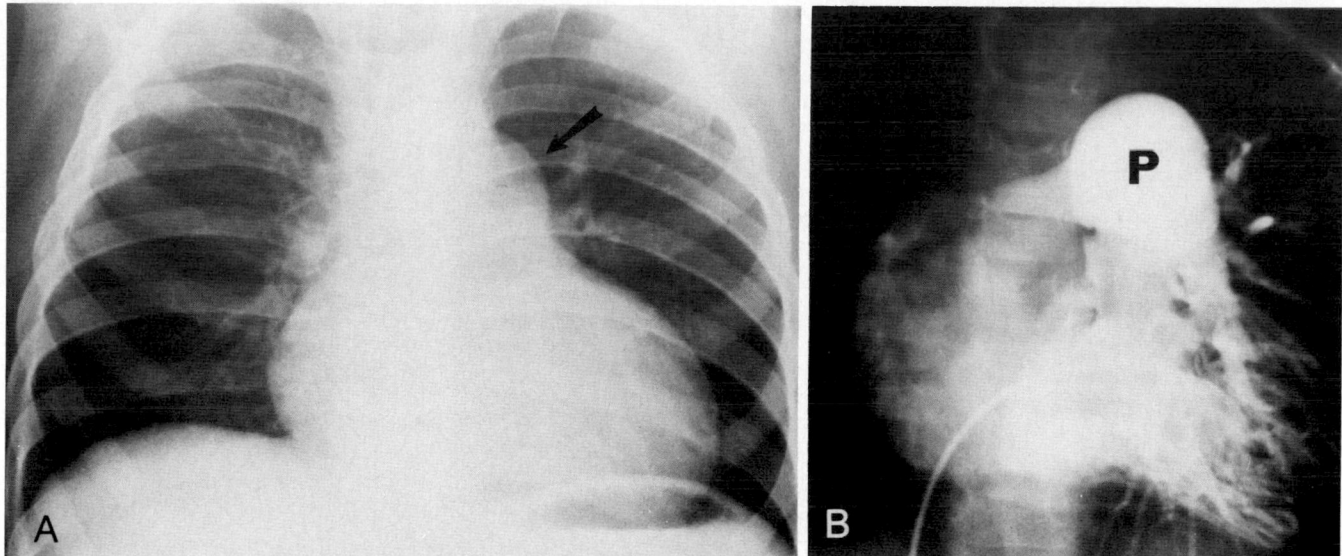

Fig. 1.76. Large pulmonary artery. A. Note the large pulmonary artery (arrow) in this patient with pulmonary valve stenosis and an atrial septal defect (i.e., trilogy of Fallot). B. Pulmonary angiogram showing the large size of the poststenotically dilated pulmonary artery (P). Also see Figure 1.75A for a large pulmonary artery secondary to a left-to-right shunt (i.e., increased flow).

monary hypertension, idiopathic pulmonary artery dilatation, pulmonary valve insufficiency, and primary diseases of the pulmonary artery wall (Table 1.19). The commonest, however, are pulmonary valve stenosis and increased blood flow.

Increased pulmonary blood flow usually occurs with left-to-right shunts or cardiac admixture lesions where intracardiac communications allow abnormal shunting of blood from the left to the right side of the heart (see Fig. 1.75A). However, it also occurs (although far less often) with pulmonary valve insufficiency because blood regurgitated into the right ventricle during diastole results in greater than normal volumes of blood being ejected into the pulmonary artery during systole. As a consequence, the pulmonary artery enlarges, and can become especially large when insufficiency is due to absence of the pulmonary valve. Tetralogy of Fallot commonly is associated with this latter lesion, and in most cases, the proximal right and left pulmonary artery branches also enlarge (1, 8, 9). Indeed, they may erroneously suggest the presence of hilar masses (see Fig. 1.52C).

A final cause of increased flow of blood through the pulmonary artery is severe left side obstruction. However, the lesions producing this problem are not overly common, and tend to present in the neonate or young infant. They include the hypoplastic left heart syn-

drome (mitral atresia, aortic atresia), interrupted aortic arch, and infantile coarctation of the aorta.

After dilation due to excessive blood flow as seen with left-to-right shunting or cardiac admixture, the next most common cause of pulmonary artery dilation is pulmonary valve stenosis. In these cases, in addition to the main pulmonary artery, its left branch also can enlarge, for the jet of blood directed through the stenotic valve, is aimed both at the main pulmonary artery and the left branch (10). This point not withstanding, however, in most cases, the jet hits the main pulmonary artery primarily, and thus it alone is seen to enlarge (Fig. 1.76).

The pulmonary artery also commonly dilates with pulmonary hypertension (see Fig. 1.52B), and rarely with mycotic aneurysms of the pulmonary artery. The pulmonary artery also can dilate after repair of tetralogy of Fallot; in some cases due to iatrogenically induced pulmonary insufficiency, and in others due to dilation of the patch used for correction of infundibular stenosis (see Fig. 1.83C). Idiopathic pulmonary artery dilation is uncommon in the pediatric age group, except in adolescent females. Consequently, if one sees a dilated pulmonary artery in an infant or young child, it is quite unlikely that it is due to idiopathic pulmonary artery dilation, and one should look for some other cause.

Small Pulmonary Artery

A small pulmonary artery occurs because of primary underdevelopment, decreased blood flow through it, or apparent smallness because of its being located in an abnormal position. For the most part, this latter

problem occurs with complete transposition of the great vessels and persistent truncus arteriosus. In the latter lesion, especially, the pulmonary artery may appear quite small (see Fig. 1.73A). Primary under-

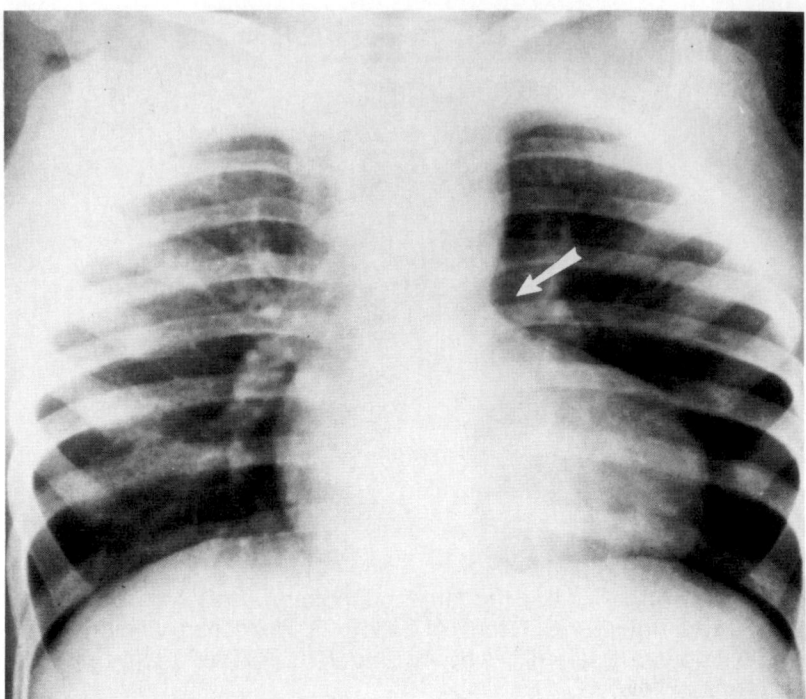

Fig. 1.77. Small pulmonary artery. Note the small pulmonary artery (arrow) producing the so-called concave pulmonary artery segment. This patient had tetralogy of Fallot with infundibular pulmonary stenosis. The aorta is left sided and a little enlarged.

development occurs with infundibular pulmonary stenosis (i.e., tetralogy of Fallot) (Fig. 1.77), the hypoplastic right heart syndrome (i.e., pulmonary valve atresia, tricuspid atresia, tricuspid stenosis), or Ebstein's anomaly. It also can occur with tricuspid insufficiency and Uhl's disease.

Unilateral Pulmonary Artery Size Discrepancy

This problem, for the most part, has been dealt with in the section on unequal aeration of lungs (see p 7). Basically, however, one pulmonary enlarges when the other is absent or hypoplastic, and the phenomenon can occur on a congenital basis or with acquired pulmonary disease such as the Swyer-James lung. In addition, as has been noted earlier, a large left pulmonary artery can be seen in some cases of pulmonary valve stenosis, and a small left pulmonary artery often is seen with tetralogy of Fallot. Smallness of either pulmonary artery is quite common in persistent truncus arteriosus, and finally, the pulmonary artery may be small, along with its lung, on an isolated congenital basis. In this condition, both the pulmonary artery and ipsilateral lung are hypoplastic. Such hypoplasia also occurs in the rare condition known as unilateral pulmonary vein atresia.

References

1. Bove EL, Shaher RM, Alley R, McKneally M: Tetralogy of Fallot with absent pulmonary valve and aneurysm of the pulmonary artery: report of two cases presenting as obstructive lung disease. *J Pediatr* 81:339–343, 1972.
2. Castellanos A, Hernandez FA: Size of ascending aorta in congenital cardiac lesions and other heart diseases. *Acta Radiol* 6:49–64, 1967.
3. Garcia RE, Friedman WF, Kaback MM, Rowe RD: Idiopathic hypercalcemia and supravalvular aortic stenosis. Documentation of a new syndrome. *N Engl J Med* 271:117–120, 1964.
4. Gokcebay TM, Batillas J, Pinck RL: Complete interruption of the aorta at the arch. *Am J Roentgenol Radium Ther Nucl Med* 114:362–370, 1972.
5. Hoeffel JC, Henry M, Mentre B, Louis JP, Pernot C: Pseudocoarctation or congenital kinking of the aorta: radiologic consideration. *Am Heart J* 89:428–436, 1975.
6. Jones KL, Smith DW: The Williams elfin facies syndrome. *J Pediatr* 86:718–723, 1975.
7. Moller JH, Edwards JE: Interruption of aortic arch: anatomic patterns and associated cardiac malformations. *Am J Roentgenol Radium Ther Nucl Med* 95:557–572, 1965.
8. Pernot C, Hoeffel JC, Henry M, Worms AM, Stehlin H, Louis JP: Radiological patterns of congenital absence of the pulmonary valve in infants. *Radiology* 102:619–622, 1972.
9. Osman MZ, Meng CCL, Girdany BR: Congenital absence of the pulmonary valve: report of eight cases with review of the literature. *Am J Roentgenol Radium Ther Nucl Med* 106:58–69, 1969.
10. Swischuk LE: *Plain Film Interpretation in Congenital Heart Disease*, ed 2. Baltimore, Williams & Wilkins, 1979, pp 23–28, 205–221.

CARDIAC SIZE ABNORMALITIES

Obviously, the heart either can be too large or too small (Table 1.20), and when it is too large, a cardiac abnormality is most likely. When it is too small, however, disease other than cardiac is more likely. In addition, it should be noted that a normal size heart does not exclude the presence of heart disease.

Table 1.20 Cardiac Size Abnormalities

Large cardiac silhouette	
Congenital heart disease }	Commonest
Acquired heart disease	
Pericardial fluid }	Moderately common
Extracardiac causes }	Relatively uncommon
Cardiac or pericardial tumors }	Rare
Small cardiac silhouette (microcardia)	
Dehydration }	Commonest
Stretched mediastinum (emphysema) }	Moderately common
Severe blood loss }	Relatively rare
Cardiac atrophy }	Rare

Large Cardiac Silhouette

Usually, if one can exclude a large thymus gland and/or a poor inspiratory effort causing apparent cardiomegaly, a large heart infers the presence of cardiac disease. It can be pericardial, myocardial, or valvular, and in the pediatric age group, most often, is congenital. Next would come a variety of acquired myocardial or valvular abnormalities, and leading the list are rheumatic heart disease and viral myocarditis. Tumors are a rare cause of cardiomegaly, and often are associated with eccentric enlargement or bumps projecting off the cardiac silhouette. Cardiac enlargement, on a noncardiac basis, can result from fluid and electrolyte retention (chronic renal disease, acute glomerulonephritis, inappropriate ADH secretion), peripheral arteriovenous fistulae, severe anemia, and metabolic diseases such as hypothyroidism, hypocalcemia, etc.

As far as pericardial effusions are concerned, the commonest are those seen with rheumatic fever and viral infection. However, pericardial fluid also can be seen with bacterial or fungal infections, generalized body fluid retention (anasarca), chronic or acute renal diseases with fluid retention, the collagen vascular diseases, and metastatic disease to the pericardium. This latter situation, of course, is quite rare, and so are effusions secondary to tuberculosis and fungal infections. Other bacterial infections are more common. Hemopericardium also is relatively rare in children, except when associated with chest trauma. It can, however, occur with bleeding disorders and metastases to the pericardial sac, but these situations are uncommon. Similarly, chyle in the pericardium is very rare.

Distinguishing cardiac enlargement due to pericardial fluid collections from enlargement due to actual cardiomegaly, can be accomplished on plain chest films, but usually is best detected with ultrasonography. On chest films, with pericardial effusions, the heart is rather globular, the vascularity not congested, and the superior mediastinum wider than normal. This is due to the accumulation of fluid in the pericardial sac, as it envelops the roots of the great vessels (Fig. 1.78A). With true cardiac enlargement, the superior mediastinum often is not as wide, and the vessels congested, either on a passive or active basis.

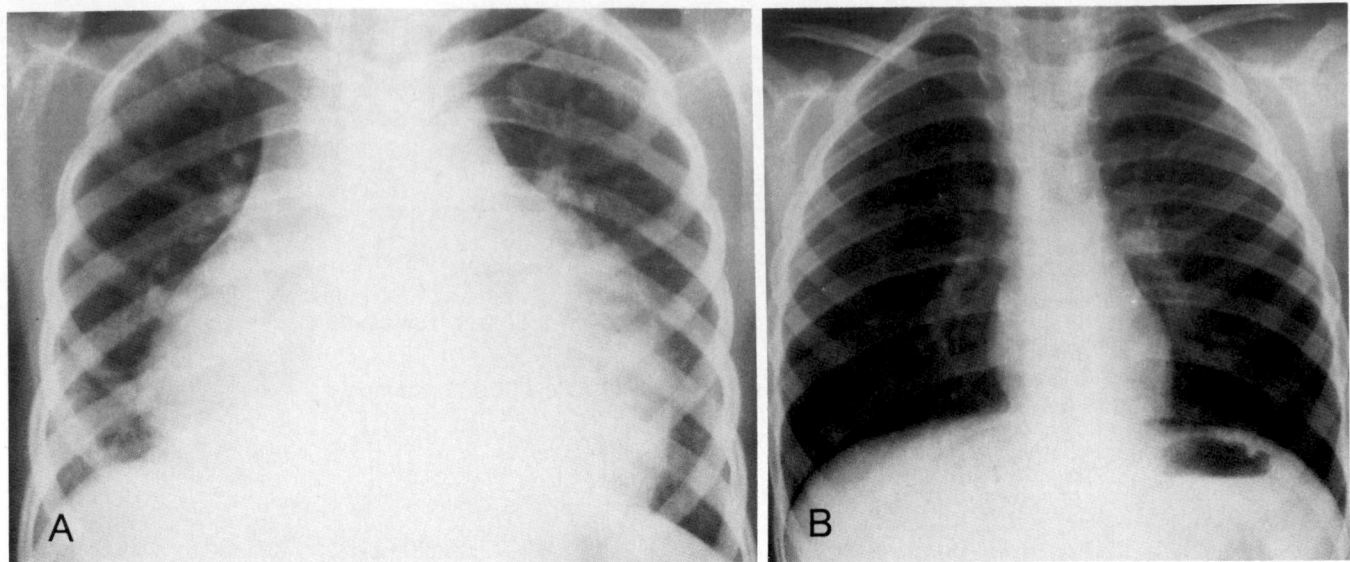

Fig. 1.78. Cardiac silhouette size abnormalities. A. Enlargement. In this patient, enlargement is nonspecific and the heart is globular in shape. However, note that the superior mediastinum is widened due to pericardial fluid accumulating in that portion of the pericardial sac which extends to the bases of the great vessels. Small bilateral pleural effusions also are present in this patient with lupus erythematosus. **B. Microcardia.** Note the very small heart in this child who had severe burns. Microcardia resulted from hypovolemia. For microcardia secondary to overdistention of the lungs, see Figure 1.1.

Small Cardiac Silhouette

A small cardiac silhouette, or so-called microcardia, is surprisingly common in the pediatric age group. For the most part, three causes of microcardia exist: (*a*) markedly decreased intravascular fluid volume, (*b*) stretching and compression of the mediastinum, and (*c*) cardiac atrophy (1). Fluid loss is by far the commonest cause and most frequently is seen with vomiting, diarrhea, and dehydration (Fig. 1.78B). A much less common cause is severe blood loss. After hypovolemia due to profound fluid or blood loss, the next most common cause of a small cardiac silhouette is stretching and compression of the mediastinum by diffuse obstructive emphysema. Most commonly, this is encountered in asthma and cystic fibrosis, but it can be seen with other causes of overaeration (see p 1). Actual cardiac atrophy is relatively rare and seen with the cachexia associated with malignant tumors or chronic infections (1). In addition, some degree of cardiac atrophy occurs with adrenal insufficiency (Addison's disease), but this is quite uncommon in the pediatric age group. The cause probably is disuse atrophy of the cardiac muscle because of the prolonged hypotension present in these patients.

References

1. Swischuk LE: Microcardia: an uncommon diagnostic problem. *Am J Roentgenol* 103:115–118, 1968.

SUPERIOR MEDIASTINAL WIDENING

Superior mediastinal widening can be bilateral or unilateral (Table 1.21), and often the same conditions cause either configuration. In all cases, however, superior mediastinal widening is due to increased soft tissue bulk, and can result from dilated vascular structures, inflammatory diseases of the mediastinum, or primary or secondary tumors.

Table 1.21 Superior Mediastinal Widening

Bilateral and relatively symmetric	
Normal thymus gland	Commonest
Adenopathy (inflammatory, tumoral)	
Mediastinal tumor	Moderately common
Dilated aorta	
Persistent LSVC	
Vein of Galen aneurysm	
TAPVR—type I (snowman or figure 8)	
Mediastinitis	
Thyroiditis	Relatively rare
Mediastinal hematoma	
Goiter	
Mediastinal fat	
Dilated esophagus	
Bilateral upper lobe agenesis	
Aneurysm of great veins	Very rare
Unilateral	
Thymus, normal (R or L)	Commonest
Superior vena cava (R)	
Dilated ascending aorta (R)	
Upper lobe atelectasis (R)	
Adenopathy (R or L)	Moderately common
Mediastinal tumor, cyst (R or L)	
Right side aorta	
Dilated esophagus (R or L)	
Persistent LSVC*	
Mediastinal hematoma (R or L)	
Goiter (R or L)	Rare
Mediastinal fat (R or L)	

a Usually causes bilateral widening because of normal IVC on right.

Bilateral Superior Mediastinal Widening

In infancy, and up to the age of 2 or 3 years, the commonest cause of bilateral superior mediastinal widening, by far, is the normal thymus gland. The configurations of the normal thymus gland are endless, and it would be impossible to illustrate all of them. Furthermore, the subject is covered in a number of other places (2, 10). After the normal thymus gland, some type of tumor or mediastinal lymph node enlargement should be considered (Fig. 1.79, A and B), and in regards to the latter, the causes can be either inflammatory or tumoral (i.e., lymphoma, leukemia, or metastatic disease). Primary tumors in the mediastinum include thyroid neoplasms, teratoma, thymoma, cystic hygroma, neurofibroma, neuroblastoma (ganglioneuroma), and hemangioma, and all occur far less frequently than do the other causes of superior mediastinal widening.

Vascular abnormalities producing mediastinal widening are rather common, but most often, the widening they produce is unilateral. Nonetheless, when the aorta dilates in both its ascending and descending portions, superior mediastinal widening can result, and this occurs most commonly with aortic stenosis or aortic insufficiency. However, it also occurs with persistent truncus arteriosus (see Fig. 1.73A), and aortic wall disease as seen in Marfan's syndrome, homocystinuria, and Takayashu's disease. Occasionally, similar widening can be seen with systemic hypertension, but more often it is the aortic knob and descending aorta which dilate in this condition.

Another uncommon, but characteristic, cause of superior mediastinal widening resulting from dilation of blood vessels is the "snowman" or "figure 8" heart of total anomalous pulmonary venous return (4, 6, 9). In this form of the condition, the so-called vertical vein on the left, the innominate vein on top, and the superior vena cava on the right produce an abnormal U-shaped vessel which causes the widening (Fig. 1.79, C and D). Other venous conditions producing superior mediastinal widening include persistence of the left superior vena cava (3), vein of Galen or other intracranial arteriovenous aneurysms in neonates and in-

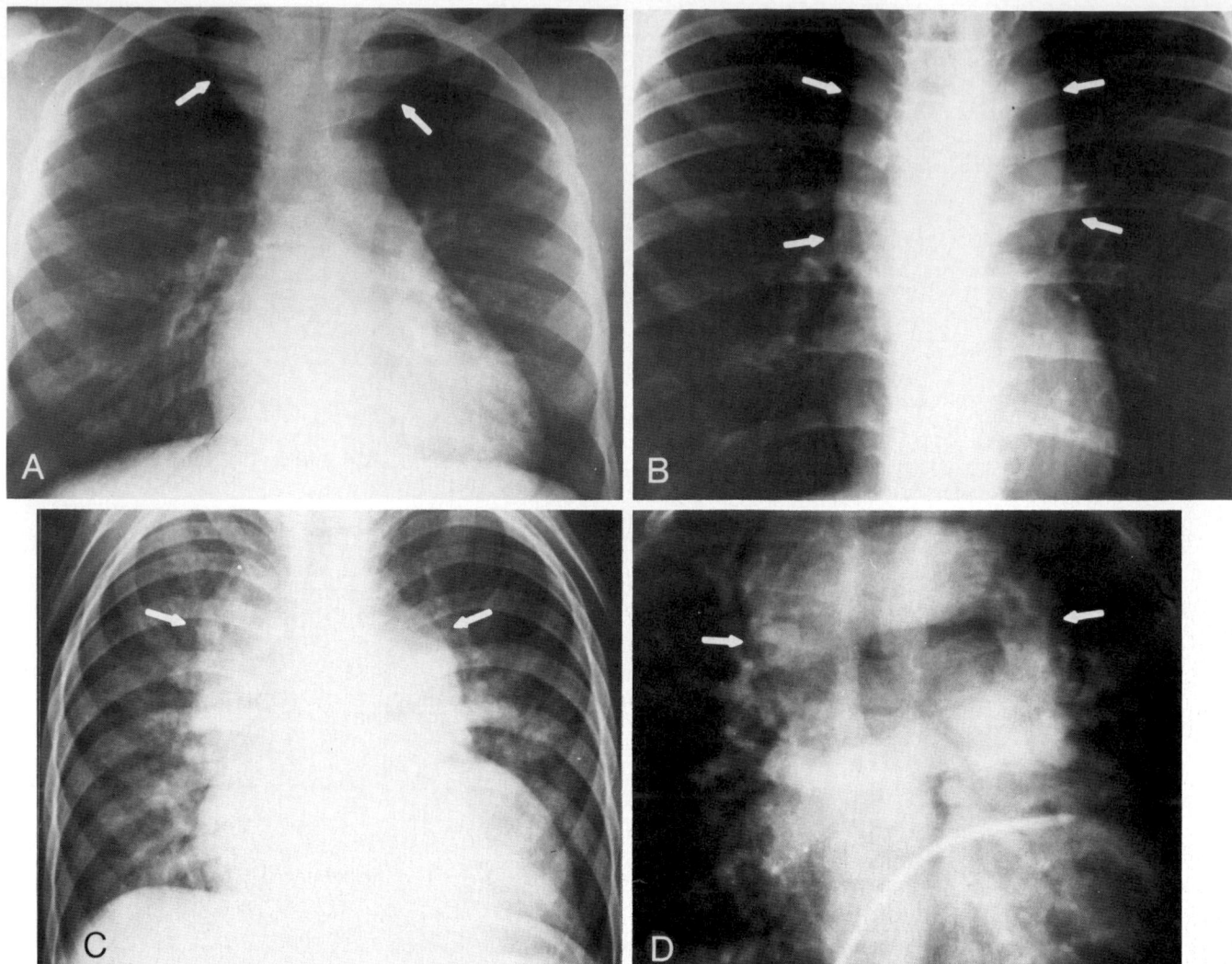

Fig. 1.79. Superior mediastinal widening. A. Note marked superior mediastinal widening due to an **enlarged thyroid gland** (arrows). There is associated tracheal compression. B. Mediastinal widening due to **lymphoma** (arrows). C. Mediastinal widening due to **anomalous pulmonary venous return** (arrows). Also note that the heart is enlarged and the vascularity engorged. D. Cardioangiogram demonstrating the abnormal **inverted U-shaped vessel** which causes the superior mediastinal widening (arrows). All of the blood from both lungs is collected by this vessel and then emptied into the superior vena cava. The vessel lies anterior to the trachea.

fants (i.e., both the carotid arteries and draining jugular veins dilate because of increased blood flow) (11), and aneurysms of the great veins. This latter problem, however, is quite rare.

Inflammatory mediastinitis, thyroiditis, benign goiter, mediastinal hematoma (i.e., trauma, bleeding dis-order, iatrogenic), mediastinal fat accumulation with steroid therapy, a dilated, obstructed esophagus, and the very rare bilateral upper lobe pulmonary agenesis (9), complete the causes of superior mediastinal widening of childhood.

Unilateral Superior Mediastinal Widening

Overall, unilateral superior mediastinal widening is more common on the right. The reason for this is that the superior vena cava is on the right, and can dilate idiopathically (1, 5, 7) (Fig. 1.80, A and B), with heart failure (i.e., increased central venous pressure), with increased blood flow as occurs with total anomalous pulmonary venous return to the superior vena cava, and with obstruction secondary to thrombosis, mediastinal tumors, or intracardiac tumors. Obviously, primary intracardiac tumors are rare, and indeed, more commonly the problem is metastasis from a Wilm's tumor of the kidney. In addition to the fore-

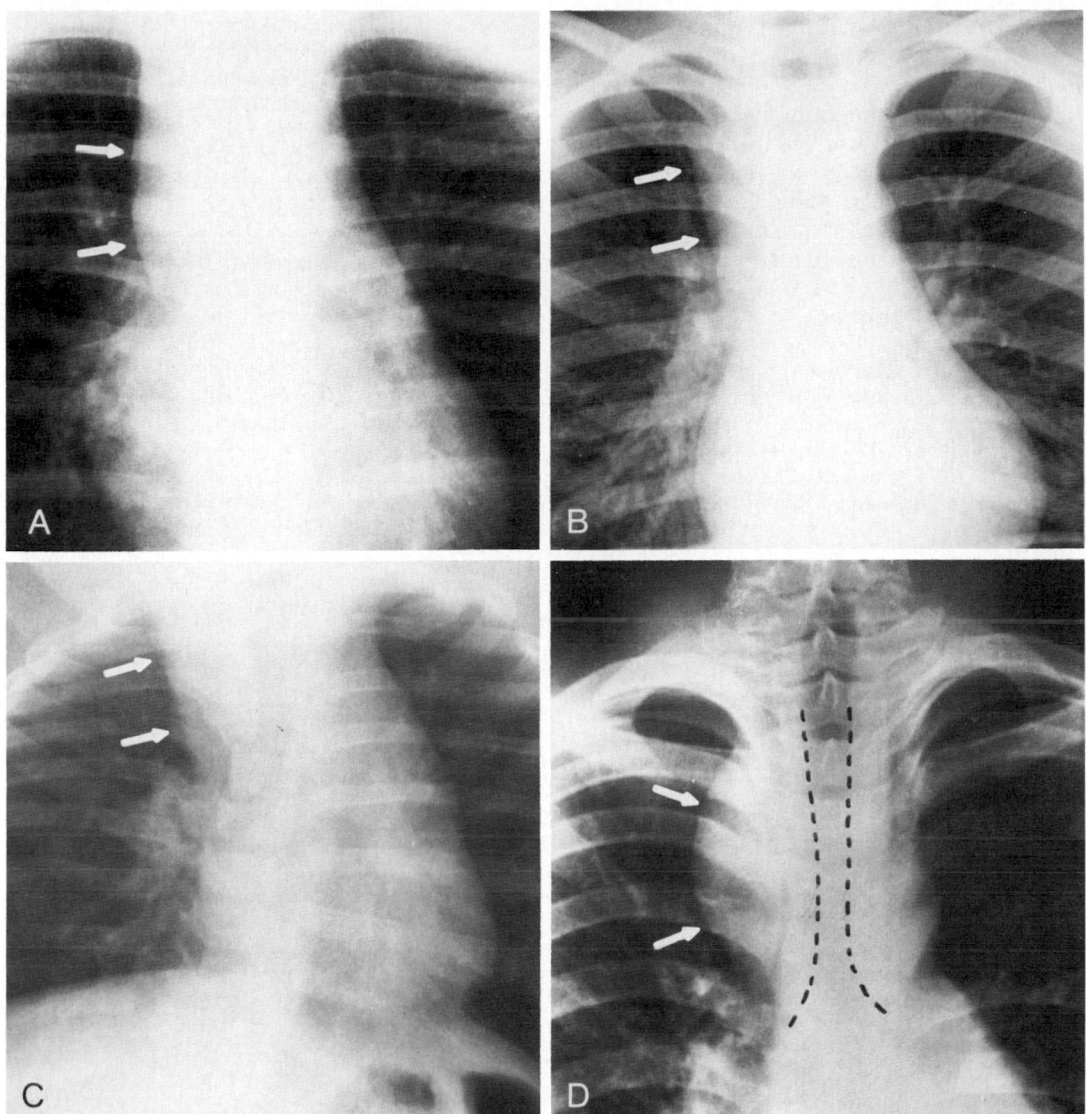

Fig. 1.80. Unilateral superior mediastinal widening. A. Unilateral right side widening due to **idiopathic dilation of the superior vena cava** (arrows). B. Another patient with the same problem showing a somewhat different configuration of right superior mediastinal widening. C. Right side widening due to **right upper lobe collapse** (arrows) associated with surgically proven tracheal bronchus. D. Right side widening due to an **asymptomatic duplication cyst** (arrows).

going causes of superior vena caval prominence, the superior vena cava can be displaced to the right by an enlarged ascending aorta, a right side aortic arch, or a tumor or cyst located between the vena cava and the trachea.

Other common causes of unilateral right side superior mediastinal widening include a unilaterally prominent thymus gland, adenopathy, and right upper lobe atelectasis. Such atelectasis can occur secondary to aspiration, or in association with the rather uncommon tracheal or anomalous apical bronchus (8, 12) (Fig. 1.80C). Rounding out the causes of right side superior mediastinal widening are dilation of the as-

cending aorta as seen in aortic stenosis, aortic insufficiency, and the primary aortic wall diseases, and unilateral mediastinal tumors and cysts (Fig. 1.80D).

On the left, since there is no superior vena cava (except for the rather uncommon anomalous persistence of the left superior vena cava), and because the left upper lobe does not collapse in a fashion similar to that of the right upper lobe, the most common causes of left side mediastinal widening are a unilaterally prominent thymus gland and unilateral adenopathy. Even here, however, a prominent left side thymic lobe is slightly less common than a right side lobe. Left side prominence also can be seen with dilation of the aorta above a coarctation, or occasionally with a mycotic aneurysm.

Finally, it is possible that any of the tumors, cysts, or tumor-like conditions producing bilateral superior mediastinal widening could produce unilateral widening on either side. In differentiating such lesions from the thymus gland, it should be noted that the thymus gland usually does not deviate the trachea, while tumors and tumor-like conditions usually do.

References

1. Bell MJ, Guiterrez JR, DuBoise JJ: Aneurysm of the superior vena cava. *Radiology* 95:317, 1970.
2. Caffey J: *Pediatric X-Ray Diagnosis,* ed 6. Chicago, Year Book Medical Publishers, 1972, pp 443–457.
3. Cha EM, Khoury GH: Persistent left superior vena cava. Radiologic clinical significance. *Radiology* 103:375–381, 1972.
4. Darling RC, Rothney WB, Craig JM: Total pulmonary venous drainage into the right side of the heart: report of 17 autopsied cases not associated with other major cardiovascular anomalies. *Invest* 6:44–65, 1957.
5. Heil BJ, Felman AH, Talbert JL, Hawkins IF, Garmica A: Idiopathic dilatation of the superior vena cava. *J Pediatr Surg* 13:193, 1978.
6. Lester RG, Mauck HP, Grubb WL: Anomalous pulmonary venous return to the right side of the heart. *Sem Roentgenol* 1:102–119, 1966.
7. Polansky S, Gooding CA, Potter B: Idiopathic dilatation of the superior vena cava. *Pediatr Radiol* 2:167, 1974.
8. Siegel MJ, Shackelford GD, Francis RS, McAlister WH: Tracheal bronchus. *Radiology* 130:353–355, 1979.
9. Swischuk LE: *Plain Film Interpretation in Congenital Heart Disease,* ed 2. Baltimore, Williams & Wilkins, 1979, pp 91–97, 235.
10. Swischuk, LE: *Radiology of the Newborn and Young Infant,* ed 2. Baltimore, Williams & Wilkins, 1980, pp 27–36.
11. Swischuk LE: Large vein of Galen aneurysms in the neonate (a constellation of diagnostic chest and neck radiologic findings). *Pediatr Radiol* 6:4–9, 1977.
12. Young LW, Fujioka M: Radiological case of the month, anomalous apical bronchus of the right upper lobe. *Am J Dis Child* 134:615–616, 1980.

MEDIASTINAL BUMPS

Mediastinal bumps usually first are recognized on frontal views of the chest, and in assessing these bumps, it is helpful to consider them by location (Fig. 1.81). Basically, these locations include: (1) right paratracheal, (2) left paratracheal, (3) upper left cardiac border, (4) lower left cardiac border, (5) entire right cardiac border, and (6) paraspinal gutters (Table 1.22). Lumps caused by hilar masses are discussed elsewhere (see p 51).

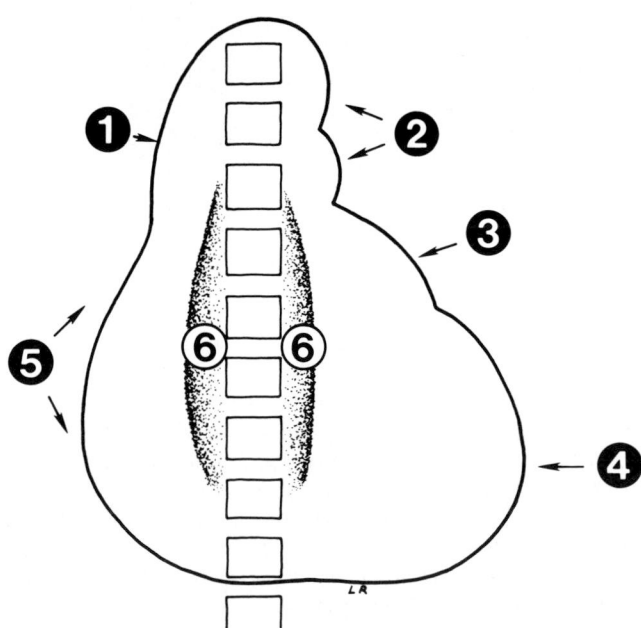

Fig. 1.81. Mediastinal bumps and bulges: diagrammatic representation. Lumps, bumps, and bulges along the mediastinum can be considered according to location: location 1—right paratracheal; location 2—left paratracheal; location 3—high left upper cardiac border; location 4—lower left cardiac border; location 5—entire right cardiac border; and location 6—paraspinal areas.

Table 1.22 Discrete Mediastinal Bumps[a]

Location 1			Tumor (cardiac, pericardial)	}	Rare
Normal azygos vein Lymph node	}	Commonest	Congenital aneurysm of heart		

Right side aorta
  Tumor, cyst
	}	Moderately common	**Location 5**
			  Enlarged right atrium
				}	Commonest

Dilated azygos vein Compressed thymus with anterior pneumothorax	}	Relatively rare	Displacement of RA by large heart	}	Moderately common

Location 2
  Large aorta
  Ductus bump in neonate
	}	Commonest	Mesoversion
			Large thymus
				}	Relatively rare

Tumor, cyst	}	Moderately common	Tumor (cardiac or pericardial) Congenital aneurysm of the heart Coronary artery aneurysm (upper border) Pericardial defect (upper border)	}	Rare
Compressed thymus with anterior pneumothorax	}	Relatively rare			

Post Coarct patch
  Hemiazygos vein enlarged
  Aorta, P.A., ductus aneurysm
	}	Rare	**Location 6**
			 A. Long stripes
			    Normal aorta
				}	Commonest

Location 3
  Thymus
  Left atrial appendage
	}	Commonest	Fluid, tumor, pus
			    Dilated aorta
				}	Moderately common

Cong. corrected trans
  Ebstein's anomaly
	}	Relatively rare	B. Localized bulge
			    Paraspinal abscess
			    Compression fx with hematoma
				}	Commonest

Partial absence pericardium
  Single ventricle with trans.
  Coronary artery aneurysm
  Juxtaposition of R atrial append
  Post Op conduits
  Dilated patch of repaired TOF
	}	Rare	Spinal or paraspinal tumor
			    Adenopathy; inflame, tumor
				}	Relatively rare

Location 4
  Left ventricular hypertrophy
  Right ventricular hypertrophy
	}	Commonest	Extramedullary hematopoiesis
			    Neuroenteric cyst
				}	Rare

[a] Discrete bumps only; for mediastinal widening, see Table 1.21.

Location 1: Right Paratracheal

A lump in this location most commonly is caused by an enlarged lymph node or a vascular structure (Fig. 1.82). Adenopathy usually is inflammatory in nature and most often caused by tuberculous or fungal infection. Next most common is adenopathy secondary to metastatic disease, and least common is isolated adenopathy due to lymphoma or leukemia. When these latter diseases involve the mediastinal lymph nodes, involvement usually is massive and presentation is that of a frank superior mediastinal mass. As far as vascular structures are concerned, the two which regularly produce lumps in this area are a right side aortic arch and the azygos vein (Fig. 1.82B). The right aortic arch bump is located higher than the one caused by the azygos vein, and the azygos vein bump, when normal, is rarely over 1 cm in diameter. When it becomes enlarged, however, it can be very prominent, and most often this occurs with total anomalous pulmonary venous return to the azygos vein (17), or absence of the inferior vena cava with azygos continuation (1, 3, 4, 6, 19). In these latter cases, since systemic blood cannot get back to the heart via the inferior vena cava, it does so through the azygos vein, by way of the paravertebral plexus. On lateral view of the chest, absence of the normal inferior vena cava, just at the bottom of the cardiac silhouette, can provide a valuable clue to diagnosis. Acquired obstruction of the inferior vena cava can produce similar enlargement of the azygos vein, and occasionally the vein can enlarge with heart failure. Remaining causes of a bump in this region include a variety of mediastinal tumors or cysts.

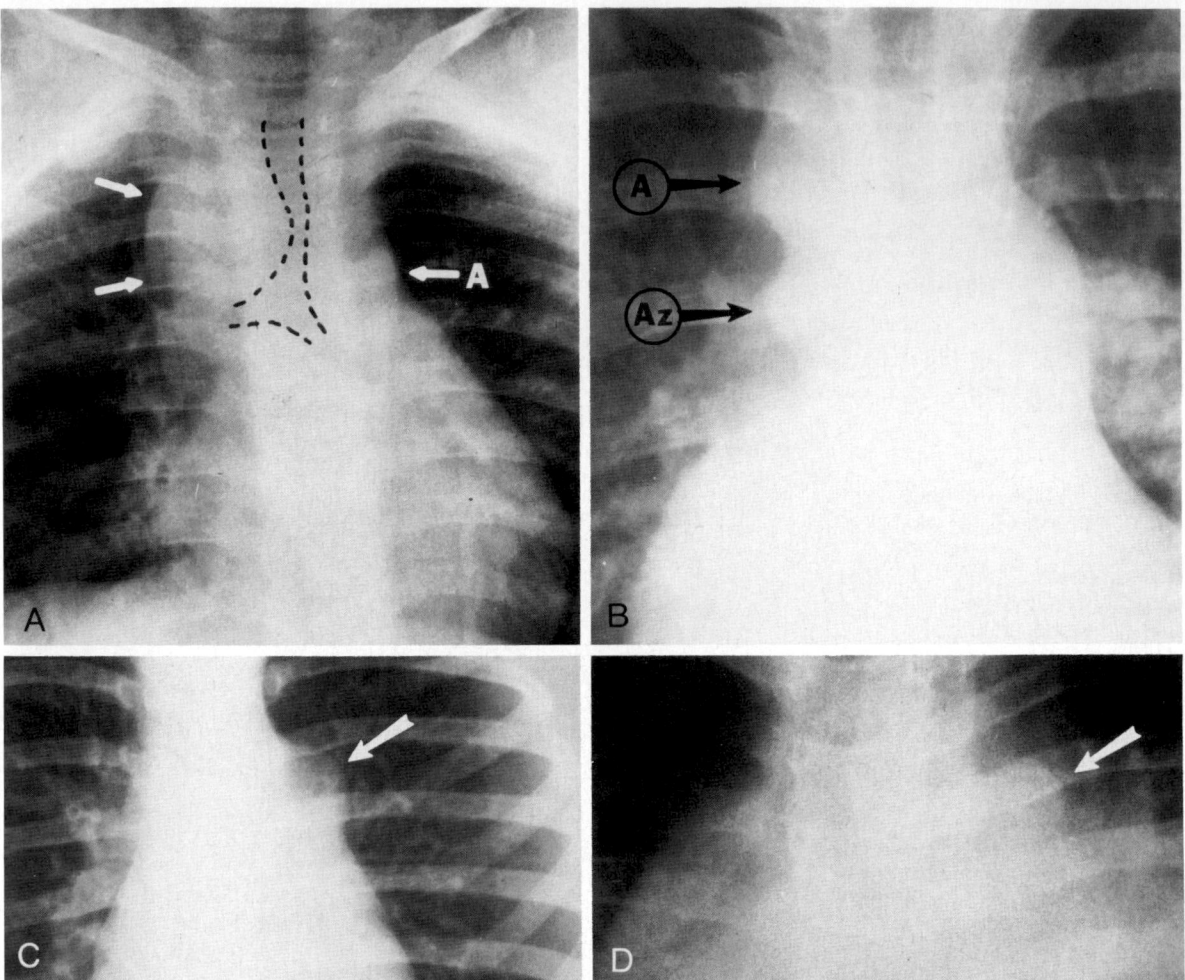

Fig. 1.82.   Mediastinal bumps: locations 1 and 2—right and left paratracheal. A. Note the large right paratracheal lump produced by enlarged lymph nodes (arrows). On the left, note the normal aortic knob (A). B. Right aortic arch and azygos vein. Note typical appearance of a right aortic arch (A) and just below it, the normal azygos vein (Az). C. Large lymph node on the left (arrow). Histoplasmosis skin test positive. A large pulmonary artery would look the same. D. Dilated hemiazygos vein (arrow) in patient with congenital absence of the inferior vena cava and hemiazygos continuation.

Location 2: Left Paratracheal

Vascular structures account for most of the bumps seen in this area for both the aortic knob and main pulmonary artery are located here. Enlargement of both of these structures has been covered previously (see Figs. 1.73 and 1.76), and the only other vascular structure which can enlarge here with any frequency is the patent ductus arteriosus. However, beyond the neonatal period, seldom is it seen as an isolated structure, and indeed, usually it blends with the concomitantly enlarged aorta and pulmonary artery to form the so-called aortico-ductal infundibular complex (16). In the neonate, the dilated infundibular ductal remnant (after spontaneous closure), commonly is seen as the normal ductus bump (5). However, it disappears after the first month or so of life, and thereafter, if

ductal dilation is suspected, one should consider the rather rare ductal aneurysm (12, 15).

Other causes of a lump in this region include lymph node enlargement (Fig. 1.82C), mediastinal tumors (less common), and the very rare, dilated hemiazygos vein (Fig. 1.82D). This latter structure can enlarge if the inferior vena cava is absent or obstructed (6), and the problem is the same as that which occurs when blood is diverted into the azygos vein on the right. However, overall, the hemiazygos problem is quite uncommon. Mediastinal tumors, lymph nodes, aortic or pulmonary artery aneurysms, and dilated post coarctation patch repairs round out other lumps in this area.

Location 3: Upper Left Cardiac Border

In this area, one can encounter discrete bumps or just a generalized fullness, and the commonest cause of the latter is normal thymus, and then an enlarged left atrial appendage. Most commonly, this occurs with rheumatic mitral valve disease (Fig. 1.83A), for although left atrial enlargement also occurs with ventricular septal defect and patent ductus arteriosus, associated enlargement of the left atrial appendage is not as common. However, fullness in this area, not due to enlargement of the left appendage, does occur with certain other congenital heart lesions. For example, in congenitally corrected transposition of the great vessels, the bulge is due to the abnormal left side position of the inverted aorta and right ventricle (Fig. 1.83B). A similar configuration can be seen with single ventricle, where congenitally corrected transposition of the great vessels is a common associated lesion.

Fullness along the left upper cardiac border also can

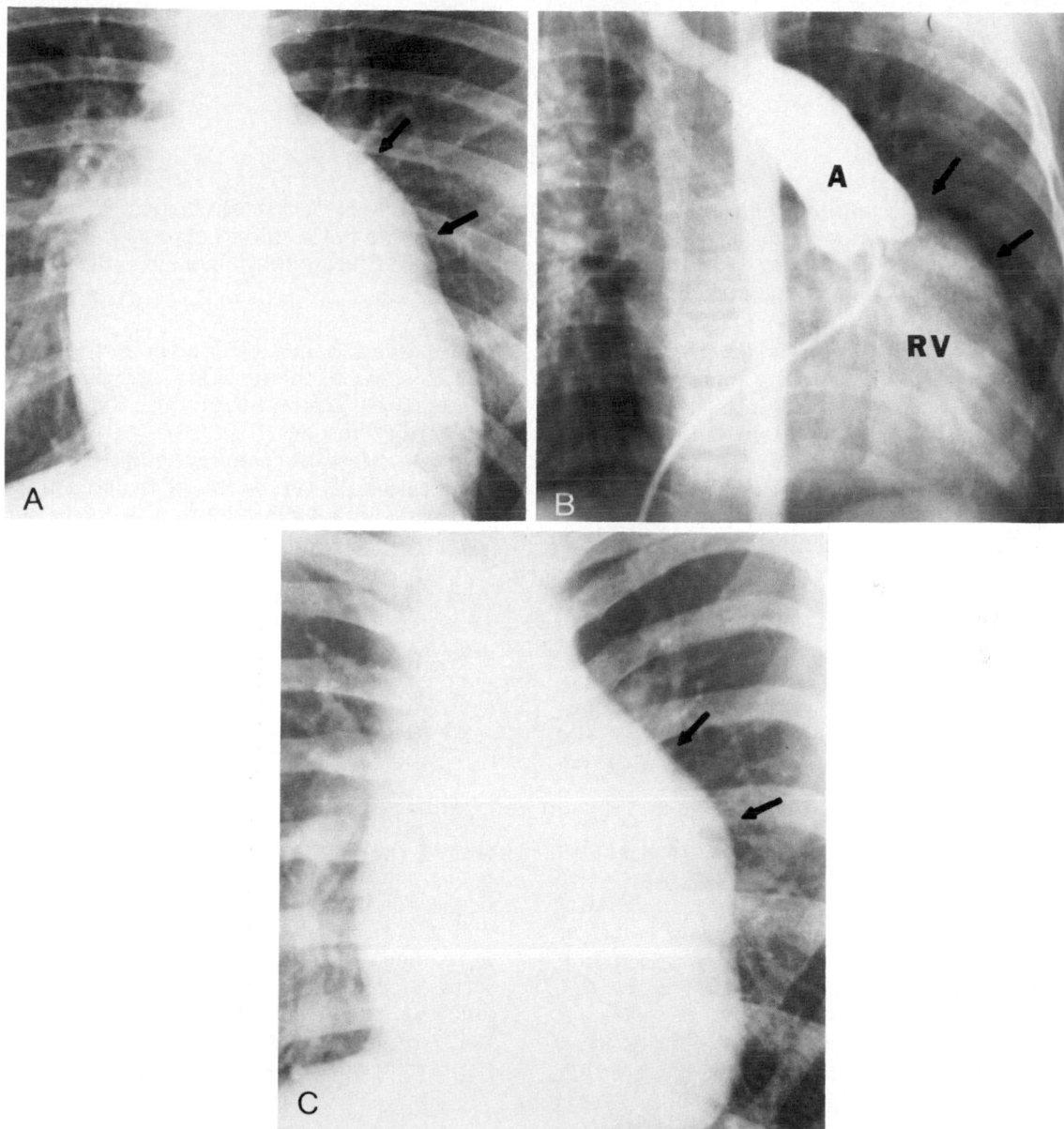

Fig. 1.83. Location 3: upper left cardiac border: generalized fullness. A. Note fullness of the upper left cardiac border due to left atrial appendage enlargement (arrows) in rheumatic heart disease. B. Congenitally corrected transposition of the great vessels. Note position of the right ventricle (RV), and the aorta (A). The aorta is inverted, and together the aorta and right ventricle produce fullness of the upper left cardiac border (arrows). A similar bump can be seen in Ebstein's anomaly (see Fig. 1.86A). C. Note bulging of the upper left cardiac border due to the dilated patch used for correction of infundibular stenosis in tetralogy of Fallot.

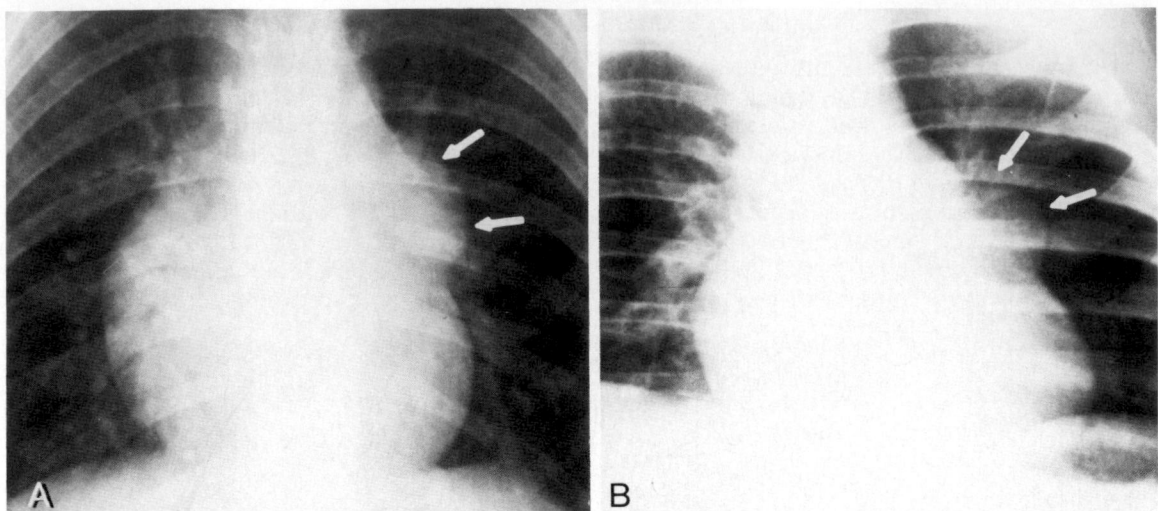

Fig. 1.84. Location 3: upper left cardiac border: discrete bulges. A. Note discrete bulge produced by left atrial appendage herniated through partial left pericardial defect. B. Localized bulge due to coronary artery aneurysm in mucocutaneous lymph node syndrome. B from Cook A, L'Heureux P: Radiographic findings in the mucocutaneous lymph node syndrome. Am J Roentgenol 132:107–109, 1979.

be produced by the rudimentary right ventricle seen in Ebstein's anomaly. In Ebstein's anomaly, the tricuspid valve is displaced forward, into the right ventricle, and most of the right ventricle is incorporated into the right atrium. That which remains, usually is located high, along the upper left cardiac border, and in many cases, produces a discrete bump or step-like fullness of the upper left cardiac border (see Fig. 1.86A).

Other relatively rare causes of generalized fullness along the upper left cardiac border include dilation of the patch utilized for correction of infundibular stenosis is tetralogy of Fallot (Fig. 1.83C) and juxtapositioning of the right and left atrial appendages. Normally, the right atrial appendage lies on the right, but in certain complicated congenital heart lesions, it be-

comes inverted, and lies on the left, just above, or in juxtaposition to the normal left atrial appendage. Together, these structures produce bulging of the upper left cardiac border.

A **discrete bump** along the upper left cardiac border occasionally can be caused by left atrial appendage enlargement, but more often it is due to herniation to the left atrial appendage through a partial pericardial defect (7, 13, 18, 22) or an aneurysm of the coronary artery (Fig. 1.84). Obviously, both conditions are rather rare, and in children, aneurysms of the coronary artery most often occur with the mucocutaneous lymph node syndrome (8, 21) or periarteritis nodosa (11). More recently, post operative pulmonary artery conduits also have been seen to produce bulges here.

Location 4: Lower Left Cardiac Border

Fullness or bulging in this location is due, almost always, to a cardiac abnormality, and usually is caused by left or right ventricular hypertrophy. The latter tends to produce a more discrete or nose-like bulging (i.e., coeur en sabot), and the former, a more generalized bulging or frank fullness (Fig. 1.85, A and B). The coeur en sabot figuration, of course, is classic for tetralogy of Fallot (but not seen in all cases), while left ventricular hypertrophy is seen with lesions producing obstruction to the flow of blood from the left

side of the heart. Rarely, bumps or fullness in this region can be caused by cardiac tumors or aneurysms (Fig. 1.85C).

It also should be noted that generalized bulging or prominence of the left cardiac border occurs with any form of cardiomegaly, and is not limited to right or left ventricular hypertrophy. However, in these cases, the heart is enlarged generally, and prominence of the left cardiac border is less specific.

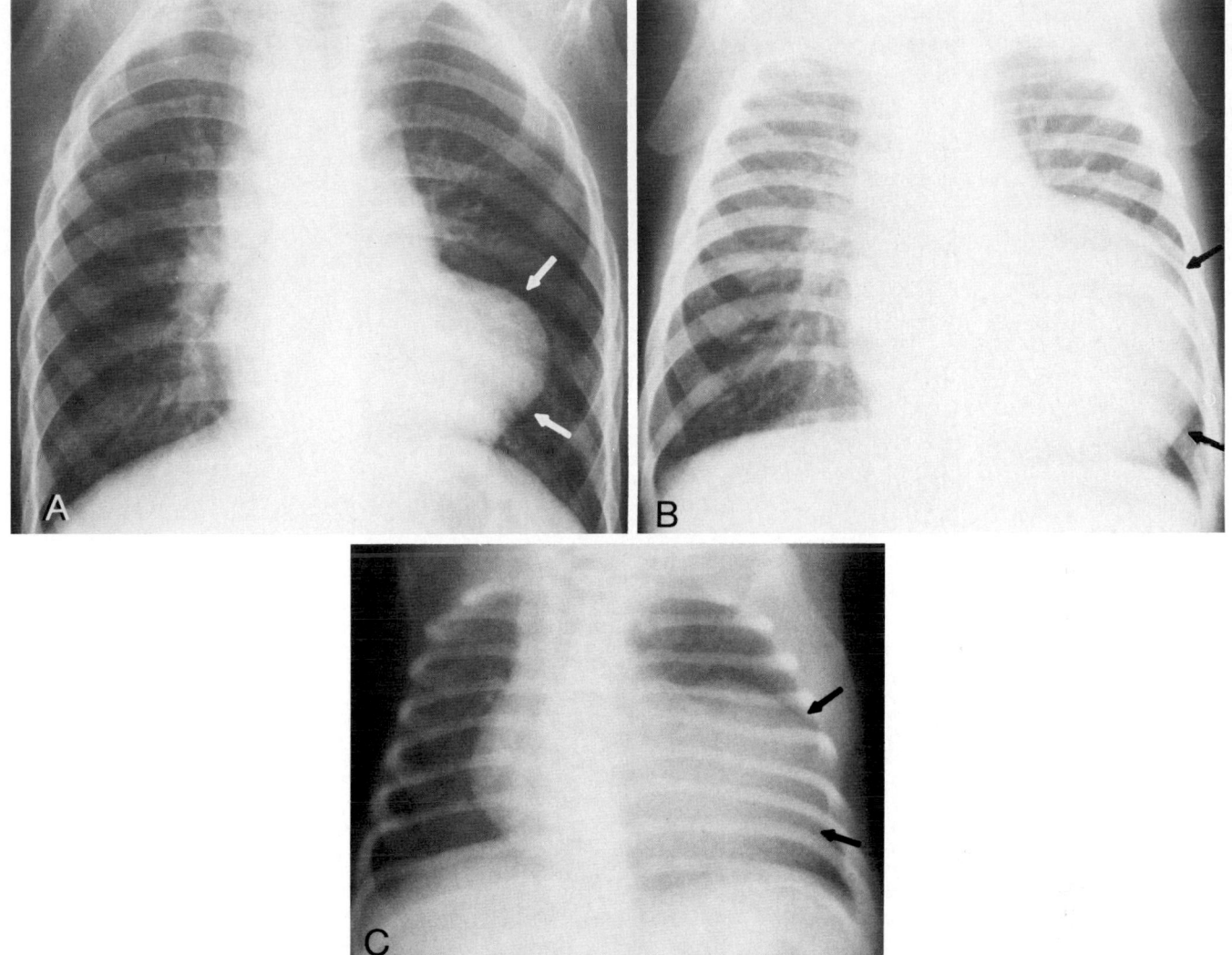

Fig. 1.85. Mediastinal bumps: location 4—lower left cardiac border. A. Note typical cour en sabot configuration of right ventricular hypertrophy (arrows) in tetralogy of Fallot. B. Profound roundness and generalized bulging of the left cardiac border (arrows) due to marked left ventricular hypertrophy. Patient had coarctation of the aorta. C. Very marked bulging of the left lower cardiac border (arrows) due to a cardiac tumor. C courtesy of M. Wagner, M.D., and E. B. Singleton, M.D., Houston, Texas.

Location 5: Right Cardiac Border

Localized bulging of the upper portion of the right cardiac border is uncommon, for isolated right atrial appendage enlargement, herniation of the right atrial appendage through a focal defect of the pericardium, and coronary artery aneurysms all are rare. Overall, then, it is bulging of the lower right cardiac border which is of most concern, and in this regard, the commonest cause of such bulging is enlargement of the right atrium (Fig. 1.86A). This can result from tricuspid insufficiency, tricuspid stenosis, tricuspid atresia, or from the delivery of extra volumes of blood to the right atrium. The latter problem occurs with atrial septal defect and anomalous pulmonary venous

return to the right atrium (either total or partial). Tricuspid valve stenosis or atresia usually are a part of the hypoplastic right heart syndrome, while tricuspid valve insufficiency, although occasionally occurring on an isolated basis, usually is seen with pulmonary valve atresia (type II, with relatively large right ventricle remaining), Ebstein's anomaly, Uhl's disease of the myocardium, and trilogy of Fallot. When massive, the right atrial curve extends high into the mediastinum (Fig. 1.86A).

The right atrium also is displaced to the right, even though it is not itself enlarged, when the remainder of the heart enlarges. This can occur even if it is the left

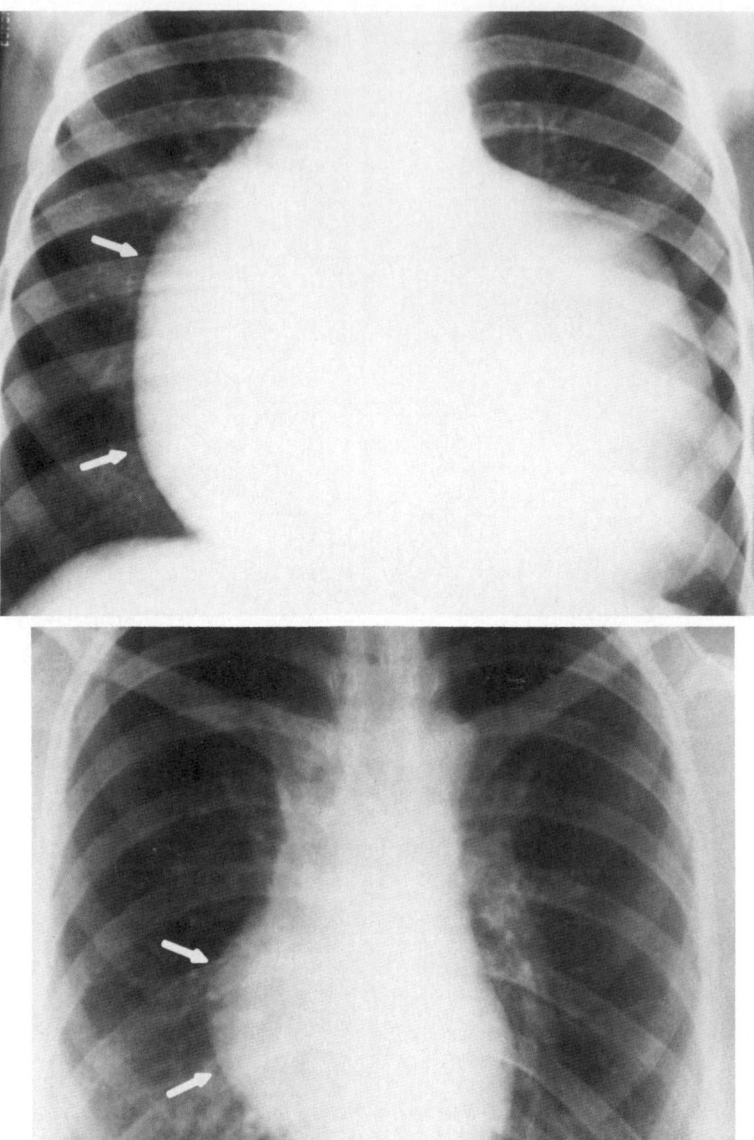

Fig. 1.86. Mediastinal bumps: location 5—right cardiac border. A. Marked right atrial enlargement (arrows) in patient with tricuspid insufficiency secondary to Ebstein's anomaly of the tricuspid valve. Note how high the right atrial curve extends into the superior mediastinum. Also note the typical shoulder or bump along the upper left cardiac border (a location 3 bulge). The pulmonary vascularity is decreased and the pulmonary artery is small and concave. B. Apparent bulging of the right cardiac border (arrows) suggesting right atrial enlargement, but due, in fact, to partial cardiac rotation to the right (i.e., mesocardia).

side of the heart which enlarges, and an excellent example of this is prominence of the right cardiac border caused by hypertrophy of the left ventricle in conditions such as aortic stenosis. Similar pseudoenlargement of the right atrium occurs with the cardiac malposition known as mesocardia. Mesocardia represents a lesser degree of dextroversion of the heart (i.e.,

lesser degree of rotation of the heart to the right), and the result is that the heart seems to sit exactly midline. This causes the right atrial region to appear more prominent than usual (Fig. 1.86B). Rarely, the right cardiac border can be made prominent by a pericardial or cardiac tumor, and even more rarely, by a cardiac aneurysm.

Location 6: Paraspinal Lumps and Thickenings

The only normal stripe, on upright view, regularly visualized in the pediatric age group is the one caused by the descending aorta on the left (Fig. 1.87A). Usually it is normal, but can become more prominent with systemic hypertension or poststenotic dilation in coarctation of the aorta (Fig. 1.87B). When the aorta is right-sided and descends on the right, a similar stripe, but perhaps a little more slanted, occurs on the right. The presence of this stripe provides a significant clue to the presence of the right side aortic arch (see Fig. 1.36A). The next most common paraspinal stripe also usually occurs on the left and is caused by the accumulation of pleural fluid against the spine (Fig.

1.87C). It must be differentiated from a normal, left, paraspinal stripe which can be seen in the recumbent (supine) position. Other causes of diffuse paraspinal widening of the soft tissues is that which occurs with underlying pathologic processes of the spine such as osteomyelitis (pus), fractures, spinal and spinal cord tumors, paraspinal lymphoma or leukemia (Fig. 1.87D), and paraspinal pleural fibrosis (Fig. 1.87E). In many of these cases, however, thickening is more localized than diffuse, and indeed, such localized bumps or areas of thickening along the spine usually are accounted for by the presence of paraspinal accumulations of pus, fluid, blood (Fig. 1.87F), or tumor.

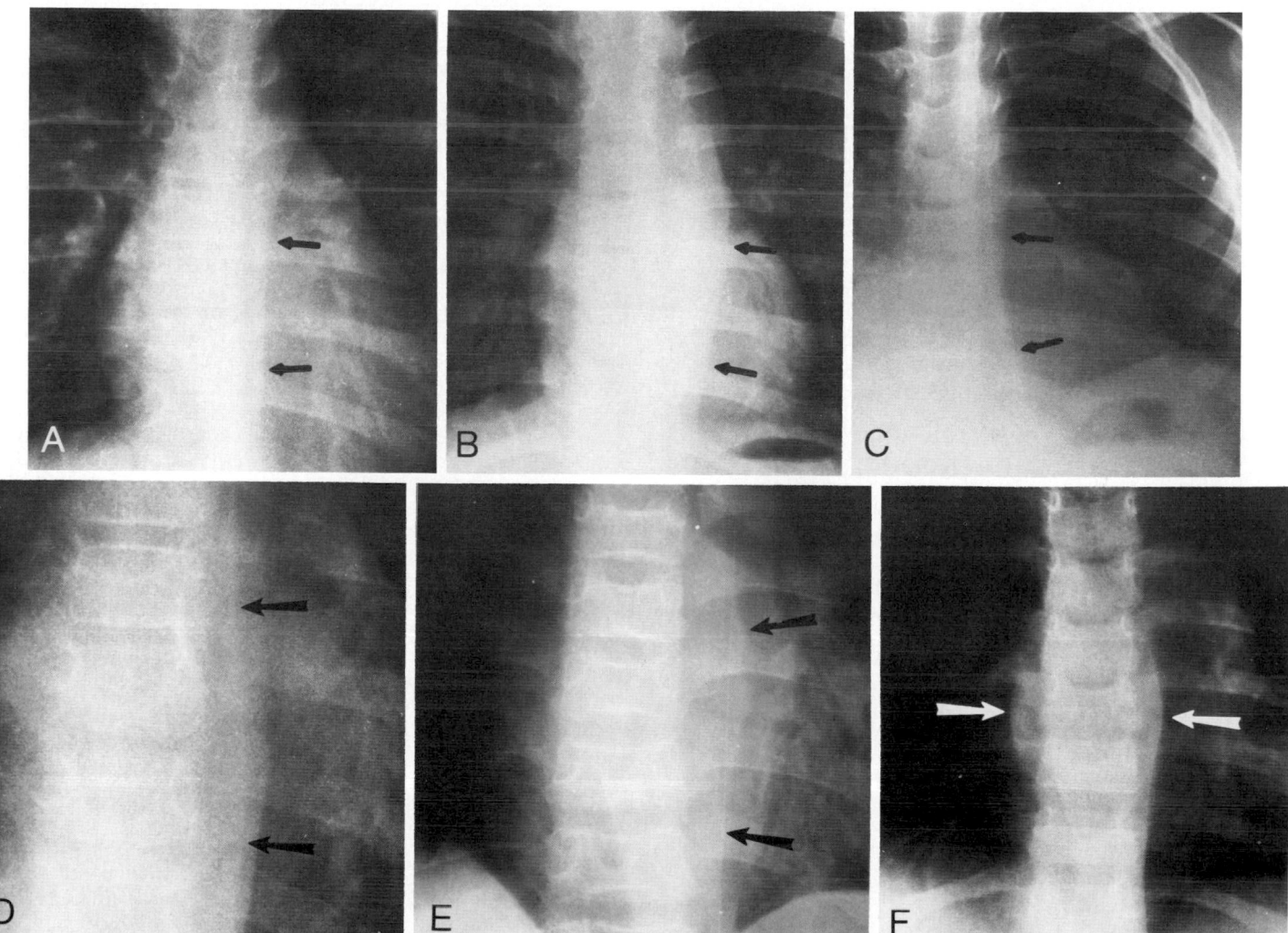

Fig. 1.87. Paraspinal stripes and bumps: location 6. A. Note the normal left paraspinal stripe (arrows) produced by the normal descending aorta. B. Markedly dilated descending aorta (arrows) in patient with coarctation. C. Left paraspinal stripe (arrows) secondary to fluid accumulation in a patient with nephrotic syndrome. A subpulmonic effusion also was present on the left, and an extensive effusion was present on the right. D. Paraspinal stripe due to lymphoma (arrows). This disappeared after treatment. E. Paraspinal stripe (arrows) due to pleural thickening in patient with sickle cell disease and repeated pneumonias with empyema. F. Bilateral localized paraspinal bulging (arrows) secondary to bleeding from a pathologic fracture of a verbetra involved with eosinophilic granuloma.

In such cases, it is essential that one inspect the adjacent vertebral bodies and intervening disc spaces for clues to the proper diagnosis. This is facilitated best on lateral view, and when both vertebrae and disc are destroyed, osteomyelitis is the best bet. With most other problems, the disc spaces remain intact, but with infection, other than that due to some fungal agents, the disc space is narrowed.

Paraspinal blood accumulations most commonly are seen with some form of thoracic spine injury, but it should be recalled that accidental trauma to the thoracic spine is not particularly common in childhood. Indeed, more often than not, trauma takes the form of a pathologic compression fracture of the vertebral body(ies) and this occurs with conditions such as metastatic disease, histiocytosis-X (Fig. 1.87F), leukemia, and lymphoma. It also occurs with the demineralized spine of rickets, steroid therapy, Cushing's syndrome, osteogenesis imperfecta, and hyperparathyroidism.

Other causes of paraspinal bulging include primary bony tumors of the spine (somewhat rare in childhood) and neurogenic tumors such as neuroblastoma, ganglioneuroma, and neurofibroma. The latter is the least common of the three. Other less common causes of widening of the paraspinal stripe include extramedullary hematopoiesis, neurenteric cysts (usually associated with anterior vertebral body defects), aneurysms of the aorta, and dilated azygos or hemiazygos veins with obstruction of the superior vena cava after repair of transposition of the great vessels (20).

References

1. Abrams HL: Vertebral and azygos venous systems, and some variations in systemic venous return. *Radiology* 69:508–526, 1975.
2. Amplatz K, Lester RG, Schiebler GL, Adams P Jr, Anderson RC: The roentgenologic features of Ebstein's anomaly of the tricuspid valve. *Am J Roentgenol Radium Ther Nucl Med* 81:788–794, 1959.
3. Anderson RC, Adams P Jr, Burke B: Anomalous inferior vena cava with azygos continuation (infrahepatic interruption of inferior vena cava): report of 15 cases. *J Pediatr* 59:370–383, 1961.
4. Berdon WE, Baker DH: Plain film findings in azygos continuation of the inferior vena cava. *Am J Roentgenol Radium Ther Nucl Med* 104:452–457, 1968.
5. Berdon WE, Baker DH, James LS: The ductus bump (a transient physiologic mass in chest roentgenograms of newborn infants). *Am J Roentgenol* 95:91–98, 1965.
6. Brodelius A, Johansson BW, Sievers J: Anomalous inferior vena cava with azygos and hemiazygos continuation. *Acta Paediatr Scand* 51:331–336, 1962.
7. Chang CV, Leigh TF: Congenital partial left pericardial defect associated with herniation of the left atrial appendage. *Am J Roentgenol Radium Ther Nucl Med* 86:517–520, 1961.
8. Cook A, L'Heureux P: Radiographic findings in the mucocutaneous lymph node syndrome. *Am J Roentgenol* 132:107–109, 1979.
9. Deutsch V, Wexler L, Blieden LC, Yahini, JH, Neufeld HN: Ebstein's anomaly of tricuspid valve: critical review of rotengenological features and additional angiography signs. *Am J Roentgenol* 125:395–411, 1975.
10. Elliott LP, Hartmann AF Jr: The right ventricular infundibulum in Ebstein's anomaly of the tricuspid valve. *Radiology* 89:694–700, 1967.
11. Glanz S, Bittner SJ, Berman MA, Dolan TF Jr, Talner NS: Regression of coronary-artery aneurysms in infantile polyarteritis nodosa. *N Engl J Med* 249:939–941, 1976.
12. Heikkinen ES, Similä S: Aneurysm of ductus arteriosus in infancy: report of two surgically treated cases. *J Pediatr Surg* 7:392–397, 1972.
13. Hoeffel JC, Henry M, Pernot C, Vaillant G: A new case of congenital partial pericardial defect with preoperative diagnosis. *J Canad Assoc Radiol* 24:261–264, 1973.
14. Kato H, Koike S, Yamamoto M, Ito Y, Yano E: Coronary aneurysms in infants and young children with acute febrile mucocutaneous lymph node syndrome. *J Pediatr* 86:892–898, 1975.
15. Kirks DR, McCook TA, Serwer GA, Oldham, NH Jr: Aneurysm of the ductus arteriosus in the neonate. *Am J Roentgenol* 134:573–576, 1980.
16. Klatte EC, Burko H: The roentgen diagnosis of patent ductus arteriosus. *Sem Roentgenol* 1:87–101, 1966.
17. Möes CAF, Fowler RS, Trusler CA: Total anomalous pulmonary venous drainage into the azygos vein. *Am J Roentgenol* 98:378–387, 1966.
18. Nogrady MB, Nemec J: Partial congenital percardial defect in childhood: report of four cases. *J Canad Assoc Radiol* 21:116–119, 1970.
19. Petersen RW: Infrahepatic interruption of inferior vena cava with azygos continuation (persistent right cardinal vein). *Radiology* 84:304–307, 1965.
20. Polansky SM, Culham JAG: Paraspinal densities developing after repair of transposition of the great arteries. *Am J Roentgenol* 134:394–396, 1980.
21. Swischuk LE: *Plain Film Interpretation in Congenital Heart Disease*, ed 2. Baltimore, Williams and Wilkins, 1979, pp 76–77, 197, 133–134, 202.
22. Tabakin BS, Hanson JS, Tampas JP, Caldwell EJ: Congenital absence of left pericardium. *Am J Roentgenol Radium Ther Nucl Med* 94:122–128, 1965.
23. Weerasena M, Jayasinghe M de S: Anomalous inferior vena cava with dilated azygos vein. *Aust Radiol* 17:32–35, 1973.

MISCELLANEOUS MEDIASTINAL ABNORMALITIES

Mediastinal Shift

The commonest cause of mediastinal shift is volume loss or gain on one or the other of the lungs. This whole problem has been discussed earlier (see p 7), but basically, with volume loss, the mediastinum shifts towards the involved lung, while with volume gain, it shifts away from the involved lung. The commonest cause of volume loss is atelectasis, and the commonest cause of volume gain is obstructive emphysema. However, volume gain also can be seen with large pleural fluid collections and large unilateral chest masses and volume loss with unilateral pulmonary hypoplasia or agenesis (Table 1.23).

Table 1.23   Mediastinal Shift

Unilateral atelectasis	
Unilateral obstructive emphysema	Commonest
Unilateral pleural fluid	
Unilateral mediastinal mass	
Unilateral pulmonary hypoplasia	Relatively rare
Pectus excavatum	
Absence of pericardium (unilateral)	
Agenesis of one lung	Rare

Other causes of mediastinal shift include pectus excavatum and absence of the left pericardium (1, 3). The latter condition, of course, is rather rare, but when seen, often is associated with increased prominence of the aorta and pulmonary artery. There is, however, no evidence of primary lung volume discrepancy, and the same situation exists with a pectus excavatum deformity of the chest. This latter condition is much more common than is absence of the left pericardium, and roentgenographically, the findings are rather characteristic. In addition to shift of the mediastinal structures, there is increased prominence of the right side vascular markings, especially those just against the spine, a more horizontal posture of the posterior ribs, and deeply slanted anterior ribs (Fig. 1.88).

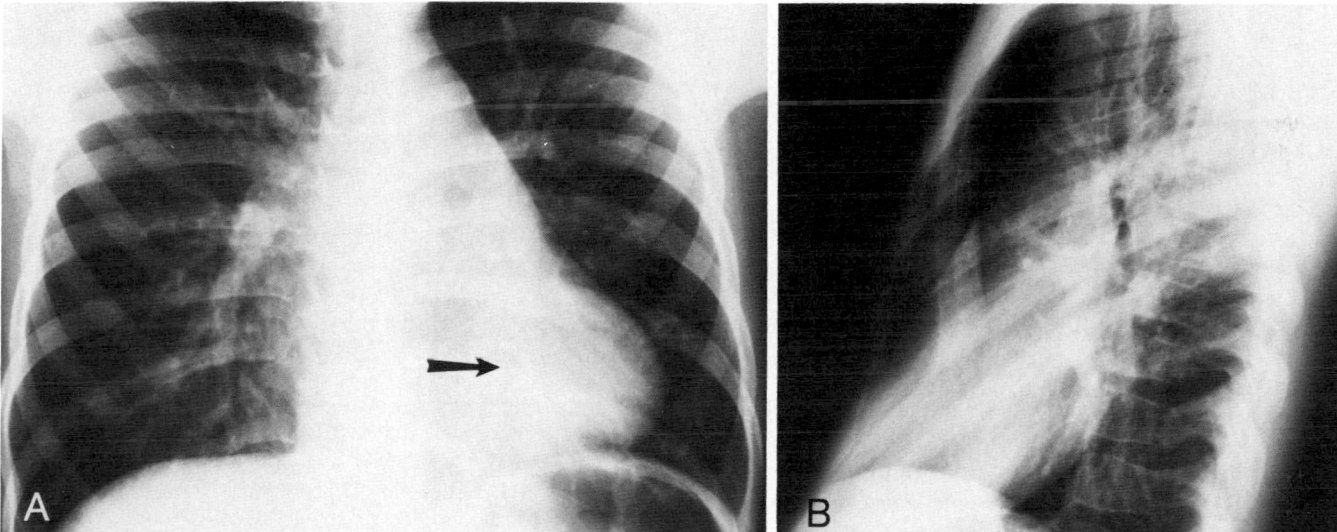

Fig. 1.88.   Mediastinal shift. A. Pectus excavatum. Note typical shift of the mediastinal structures to the left (arrow), accentuation of the right lung vascularity, nonvisible cardiac silhouette to the right of the spine, horizontally oriented posterior ribs, and deeply slanting anterior ribs. **B.** Lateral view showing degree of pectus excavatum deformity. Similar shift can be seen with absence of the pericardium, but on lateral view, the "depressed sternum" deformity, of course, is not present. In addition, the aorta and pulmonary artery usually appear more discrete and prominent on frontal view.

Indistinctness or Obliteration of the Mediastinal Silhouette Edge

Indistinctness or obliteration of the mediastinal silhouette edge is termed the silhouette sign (2), and most commonly results from the presence of adjacent pneumonia or atelectasis. The reason for it occurring is that the involved portion of the lung then becomes the same density (water) as the normal heart, and together, these densities cause obliteration of the normal heart-lung interface (Fig. 1.89). The same phenomenon can occur along the diaphragmatic leaflets. Other causes of indistinct mediastinal edges include pulmonary contusion, a wide variety of infiltrates, and some neoplasms.

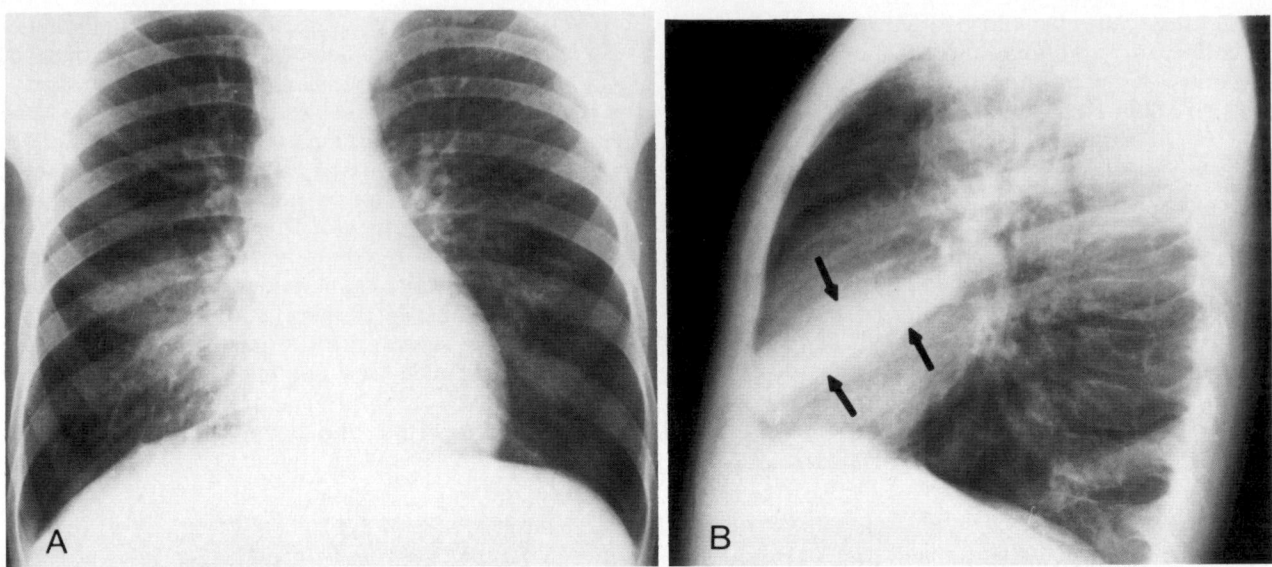

Fig. 1.89. Silhouette sign. Note obliteration of the right cardiac border (i.e., positive silhouette sign). Normally, it should appear as sharp as that on the left. Atelectasis of the right middle lobe (arrows in B) is the cause. This patient had asthma and a mucous plug. Similar cardiac border obliteration occurs with pneumonias and contusions.

Increased Density Behind the Heart

As far as this finding is concerned, most commonly it is seen on the left. The main reason is that there is more heart on the left, and the commonest causes of the finding are pneumonia or atelectasis. Depending on the extent of the problem, the density can be focal, or diffuse and even involve the entire cardiac silhouette (Fig. 1.90, A and B). When left lower lobe collapse is the problem, the edge of the collapsed lung frequently can be seen through the cardiac silhouette (Fig. 1.90C).

Other causes of increased density behind the heart include hiatus hernia (usually on the left), pulmonary sequestration (on either side, but usually on the left), pleural fluid behind the heart (usually on the left), and other posterior mediastinal masses (either side). With sequestration, one may see vessels supplying

and/or draining the lesion (Fig. 1.93, D and E). Very rarely, pleural fluid accumulations or masses anterior to the heart can produce increased density of the cardiac silhouette.

References

1. Dimich I, Grossman H, Bowman FD Jr, Griffith SP: Congenital absence of the left pericardium. *Am J Dis Child* 110:309–314, 1965.
2. Felson B, Felson H: Localization of intrathoracic lesions by means of the posteroanterior roentgenogram. The silhouette sign. *Radiology* 55:363–374, 1950.
3. Tabakin BS, Hanson JS, Tampas JP, Caldwell EJ: Congenital absence of the left pericardium. *Am J Roentgenol Radium Ther Nucl Med* 94:122–128, 1965.

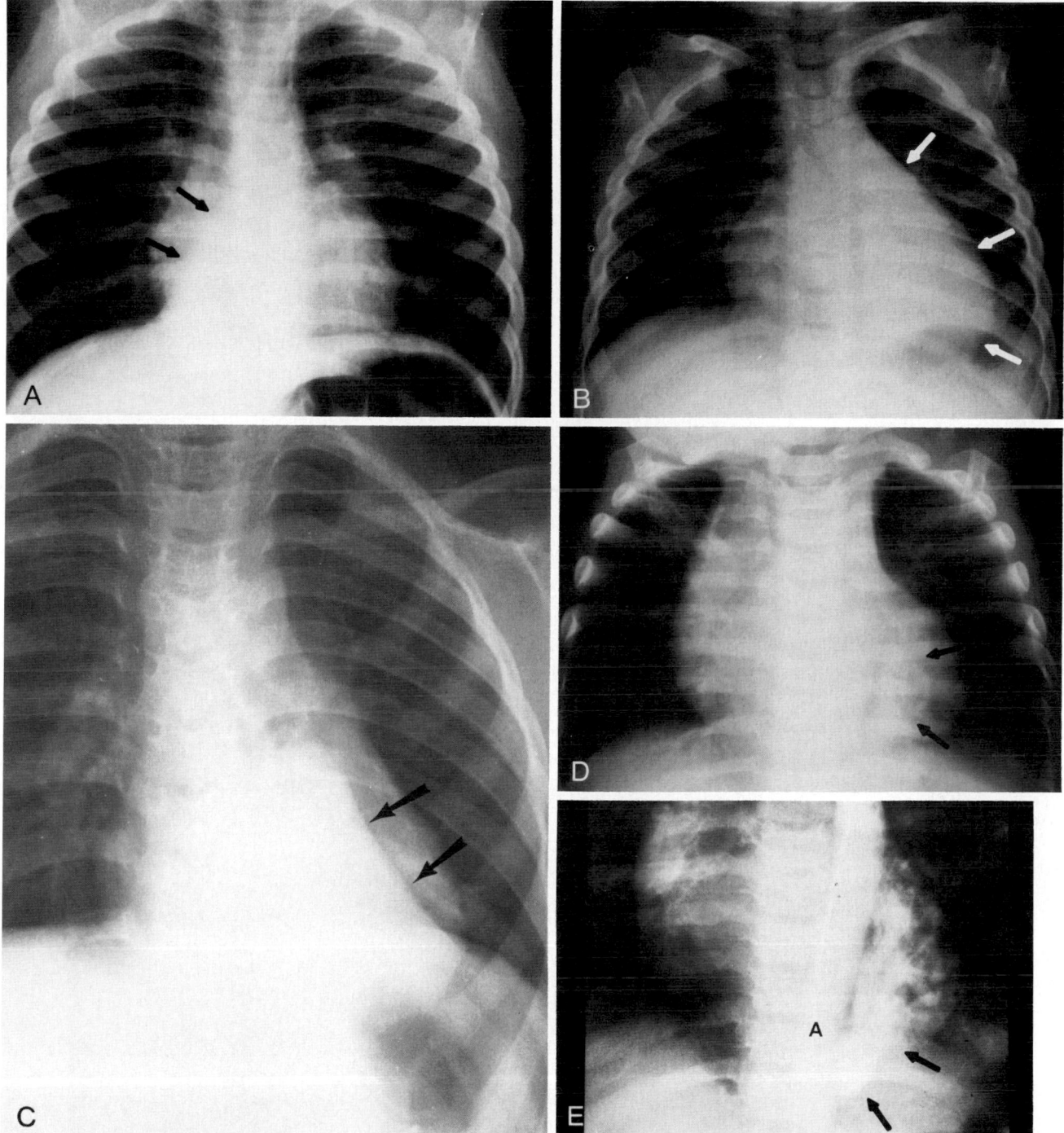

Fig. 1.90. Retrocardiac densities. A. Note the irregular density behind the right side of the heart (arrows), due to an early consolidating pneumonia. B. Generalized increase in density of the entire left side of the heart (compare to normal radiolucency of right side) due to an extensive consolidating pneumonia, completely hidden by the heart. C. Typical configuration of left lower lobe atelectasis, producing a triangle of increased density behind the left side of the heart (arrows). D. Note irregular density behind the left side of the heart (arrows). Draining or supplying vessels also appear to be present, and this suggests a sequestration. E. Aortogram in same patient demonstrating aorta (A) and the systemic vessels (arrows) to the sequestration. Also see Figure 1.93D for a retrocardiac density due to a hiatus hernia.

LUNG MASSES

For the most part, this section deals with masses occurring within the lungs, and not in the mediastinum or along the chest wall. In other words, they are true intrapulmonary masses, and in childhood, they are not particularly common (Table 1.24). Actually, the commonest mass is a pseudomass, and is due to consolidating pneumonia (3). In these cases, the consolidation is caught just at the stage where it mimicks a mass (Fig. 1.91A). Next most common, as a cause of a pulmonary mass, is a solid pulmonary abscess, and then less commonly, one can encounter a number of acquired or congenital pulmonary cysts. Cysts tend to have a sharp edge to their outer circumference, while abscesses are more apt to have a fuzzy one. Of course, when a lung cyst becomes infected, it may look just as an abscess.

Rounding out the causes of intrapulmonary mass are loculated pleural effusions and postinflammatory pseudotumors. Postinflammatory pseudotumors result from previously consolidating infections (4), but generally are uncommon in the pediatric age group. However, they can occur with atypical measles pneumonia (1, 2, 5, 6), and occasionally with other pneumonias. Loculated pleural effusions can be quite large, but in most cases, they are of somewhat oblong or oval configuration. In addition, their usually tapering, spindle-shaped ends attest to their interlobar fissure location (Fig. 1.91B). Because they tend to disappear on their own, they often are referred to as vanishing tumors.

References

1. Margolin FR, Gandy TK: Pneumonia of atypical measles. *Radiology* 131:653–655, 1979.
2. Mitnick J, Becker MH, Rothberg M, Genieser NB: Nodular residua of atypical measles pneumonia. *Am J Roentgenol* 134:257–260, 1980.
3. Rose RW, Ward BH: Spherical pneumonias in children simulating pulmonary and mediastinal masses. *Radiology* 106:179–182, 1973.
4. Schwartz EE, Katz SM, Mandell GA: Post-inflammatory pseudotumors of the lung: fibrous histiocytoma and related lesions. *Radiology* 136:609–613, 1980.
5. Wood BP, Bernstein RM: Pulmonary nodular "pneumonia" during the acute atypical measles illness. *Ann Radiol* 21:193–198, 1978.
6. Young LW, Smith DI, Glasgow LA: Pneumonia of atypical measles, residual nodular lesions. *Am J Roentgenol Radium Ther Nucl Med* 110:439–448, 1970.

Table 1.24 Lung Masses

Pneumonia pseudomass	}	Commonest
Pulmonary abscess Cysts (acq. or cong.)	}	Moderately common
Loculated pleural fluid Pulmonary tumor Postinflammatory pseudotumor	}	Relatively rare

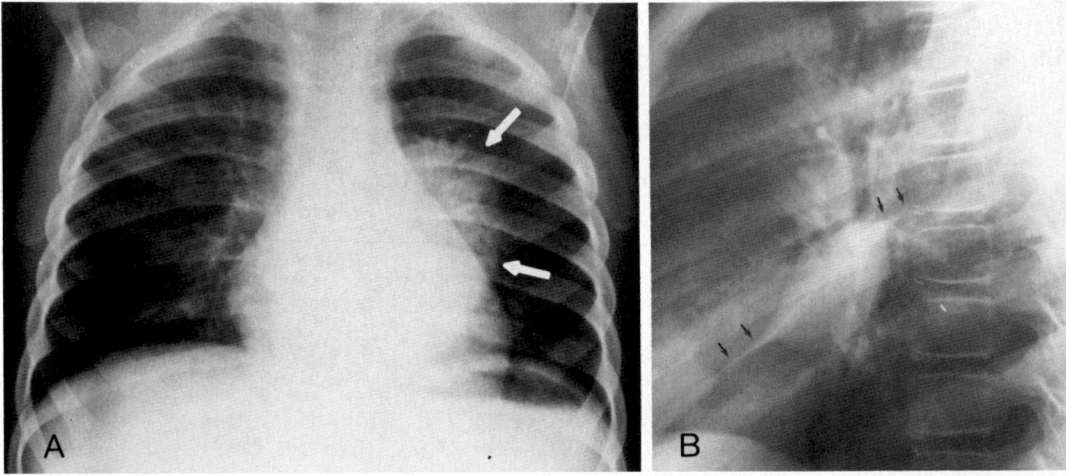

Fig. 1.91. Pulmonary masses. A. Apparent mass (arrows) due to consolidating pneumonia. B. Interlobar effusion producing pulmonary mass. Note the characteristic tapering edges (arrows).

DIAPHRAGMATIC LEAFLET POSITION AND CONTOUR ABNORMALITIES

Normally, the right diaphragmatic leaflet is a little higher than the left. Occasionally, the left can be elevated because of an underlying distended stomach or splenic flexure, but generally, the right remains higher than the left. In addition, it should be noted that normally the diaphragmatic leaflets have a sharp outline, and if the outline becomes fuzzy at all, an adjacent infiltrate or areas of atelectasis should be suspected. The insertion of the normal major fissures can cause similar obliteration, but usually the cause is pneumonia or atelectasis. Position and contour ab-

normalities of the diaphragmatic leaflets are best considered on a unilateral and bilateral basis (Table 1.25).

Table 1.25 Diaphragmatic Leaflet Position Abnormalities

Unilateral elevated Atelectasis Splinting Distended stomach or splenic flexure (L) Subpulmonary effusion	}	Commonest	Ascites Peritonitis Hemoperitoneum Abdominal mass Neuromuscular disease	}	Moderately common
Paralysis Eventration Abdominal mass Abdominal abscess	}	Moderately common	Bilateal eventration Laryngotracheal foreign body	}	Rare
			Agenesis (newborn)	}	Very rare
Diaphragmatic hernia (except neo- nate where common) Diaphragmatic tumor Agenesis or hypoplasia of lung	}	Rare	Bilateral depressed Asthma Viral infection (broncholitis)	}	Commonest
			Cystic fibrosis Overaeration with acidosis	}	Moderately common
Unilateral flattened Empyema or other fluid Obstructive emphysema	}	Commonest	Air hunger (see text) Bilateral tension pneumothorax Bilateral pleural fluid Other obstruct emphysema (see text)	}	Rare
Tension pneumothorax	}	Moderately common			
Bilateral elevated Poor inspiration	}	Commonest	Localized bulging Diaphragmatic hernia Eventration	}	Commonest

Unilaterally Elevated Diaphragmatic Leaflet

The commonest causes of a unilaterally elevated diaphragmatic leaflet are atelectasis of the ipsilateral lung or splinting of the diaphragmatic leaflet secondary to pneumonia, rib injury, or subdiaphragmatic injuries and inflammations. On the left, a distended stomach or splenic flexure also are common causes of an elevated diaphragmatic leaflet, but on the right, since the liver lies directly beneath the diaphragm, such causes are uncommon.

Other moderately common causes of unilateral elevation of a diaphragmatic leaflet are phrenic nerve palsy, eventration, an underlying abdominal mass or abscess, and a subpulmonic effusion. With subpulmonic effusions, the diaphragmatic leaflet often, but not always, appears somewhat flat medially and

squared off laterally (Fig. 1.92, A and B). On lateral view, in these cases, one usually can see a fluid meniscus in the posterior costophrenic angle, and decubitus views clearly demonstrate the presence of such fluid. These subpulmonic effusions occur most commonly with the nephrotic syndrome, acute glomerulonephritis, and intrathoracic or intraabdominal lymphoma. Relatively rare causes of a unilaterally elevated diaphragmatic leaflet include congenital or acquired (posttraumatic) diaphragmatic hernia (except in the neonate where the congenital form is common), diaphragmatic tumor, hypoplasia or aplasia of the diaphragm, and hypoplastic lung. In this latter condition, the diaphragmatic leaflet is elevated because of loss of volume in the hypoplastic lung.

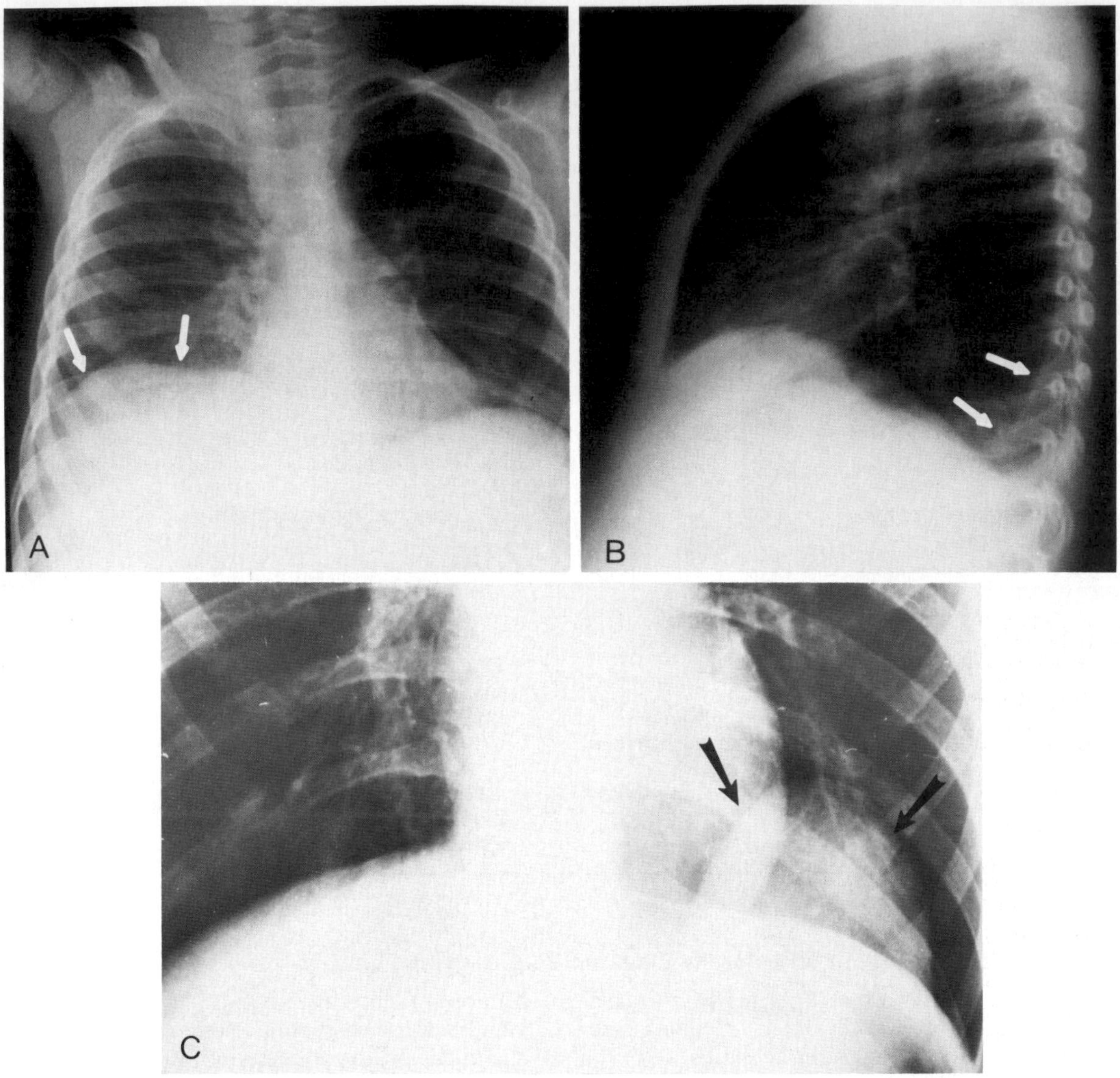

Fig. 1.92. Elevated diaphragmatic leaflets. A. **Subpulmonic effusion.** Note characteristic squared-off and somewhat flat appearance of the apparently elevated right diaphragmatic leaflet. This is characteristic of a subpulmonic effusion. A subpulmonic effusion also is present on the left, but the apparently elevated diaphragmatic leaflet appears near normal in configuration. Note, however, that there is a paraspinal collection of fluid (i.e., left paraspinal stripe). B. Lateral view in same patient demonstrating typical posterior menisci of pleural fluid (arrows). This patient had nephrotic syndrome. C. **Diaphragmatic leaflet bump.** This bump (arrows) was due to a kidney projecting through a congenital posterior diaphragmatic opening.

Unilaterally Depressed Diaphragmatic Leaflet

A diaphragmatic leaflet becomes depressed because of some space occupying problem in the ipsilateral hemithorax. For this reason, it almost always is a secondary finding, and can be seen with conditions such as unilateral obstructive emphysema, tension pneumothorax, and massive pleural fluid accumulations. With fluid or air (pneumothorax) accumulations, if the volume is massive, the diaphragmatic leaflet not only is depressed, but also is inverted.

Bilaterally Elevated Diaphragmatic Leaflets

Undoubtedly the commonest cause of bilaterally elevated diaphragmatic leaflets is simple underaeration of the chest secondary to a poor inspiratory effort. Thereafter, intraabdominal space occupying problems such as ascites, peritonitis, large abdominal masses, etc., lead to elevation of the diaphragmatic leaflets, and then, one should consider diaphragmatic weakness with neuromuscular disease, bilateral eventration, or the very rare, diaphragmatic agenesis (a neonatal problem). Another uncommon cause of bilaterally elevated leaflets is a central, tracheal, or laryngeal obstructing foreign body. These foreign bodies usually are located at or below the level of the larynx, but above the carina. Because they produce inspiratory obstruction, the lungs never are fully inflated, and the diaphragmatic leaflets constantly are higher in position than normal. However, it requires an astute observer, and one who has knowledge of the problem to appreciate the finding.

Bilaterally Depressed Diaphragmatic Leaflets

As with the unilaterally depressed diaphragmatic leaflet, some intrathoracic space occupying problem must exist to produce this phenomenon. Most commonly, this occurs with obstructive emphysema as seen with asthma and viral lower respiratory tract infections (especially bronchiolitis in the infant). However, it is also seen with other causes of obstructive emphysema, and these include cystic fibrosis, alpha-1 antitrypsin deficiency, congenital cutis laxa, central or bilateral foreign bodies, vascular rings and anomalies, intratracheal lesions, and paratracheal masses and cysts.

Overaeration of the lungs with bilateral leaflet depression also is commonly seen with acidosis and dehydration. In these cases, in an attempt to blow off CO_2, the lungs become hyperinflated and the leaflet becomes depressed. The findings can mimic obstructive emphysema for at the same time, dehydration leads to loss of fluid, hypovolemia, and diminished pulmonary vascularity. Air hunger, as seen with severe cyanotic congenital heart disease, and even noncyanotic heart disease, can lead to similar overaeration of the lungs. Bilateral pleural fluid or air (pneumothorax) collections of a degree large enough to produce bilateral diaphragmatic leaflet depression, are not particularly common, but can occur. The cause for diaphragmatic depression, in these cases, is obvious.

Localized Bulges on Diaphragmatic Leaflets

The commonest discrete bulge of a diaphragmatic leaflet is a focal diaphragmatic hernia with some organ protruding through the defect (Fig. 1.92C). Posteriorly, this occurs with the kidney, while anteriorly it can occur with the spleen, liver, or omentum. In any of these cases, the bulge is located towards midline. Smaller eventrations also can produce somewhat localized bulging of the diaphragmatic leaflets, but other than these two conditions, localized bulging of the diaphragmatic leaflets is uncommon in children. Certainly, diaphragmatic tumors are rare, and so are pleural tumors which would originate in this area and cause a lump.

MEDIASTINAL MASSES: DIAGNOSTIC APPROACHES

In considering mediastinal masses, it is customary to consider them as occurring in the anterior, middle, and posterior mediastinal compartments. In the **anterior compartment**, the most common mass is the normal thymus gland, and one of its distinguishing features is that it does not displace the trachea. Only when the gland is unusually high in position or especially if it is associated with a thymic cyst does displacement occur. Thymic tumors are quite rare, but other masses occurring in the anterior mediastinum include thyroid tumors, goiter, inflamed thyroid glands, teratoma (often with calcification and usually in infants), cystic hygroma (usually extending from neck), and lymphoma. Actually, lymphomatous involvement of the anterior mediastinum is quite common in children (see Fig. 1.79B), and represents an extension of the same process originating in the middle mediastinum. Such mass formation can take the form of lymph node enlargement or infiltration of the thymus gland by the lymphoma or leukemia. Mediastinal cysts are rare in the anterior mediastinum, and another relatively uncommon anterior superior mediastinal mass is the one resulting from the snowman or "figure 8" heart of type I total anomalous pulmonary venous return (see Fig. 1.79, C and D). Finally, it might be noted that destructive or tumoral lesions of the sternum can result in retrosternal masses projecting into the superior mediastinum.

Inferiorly, in the anterior mediastinum, one can encounter diaphragmatic hernias, and occasionally these can extend into the pericardial sac. Those located just to one or other side of midline are termed Morgagni hernias.

In the **middle mediastinum,** the commonest mass is that associated with lymphoma or leukemia and as noted in the preceding paragraph, these masses frequently extend into the anterior mediastinum. Enteric (duplication) cysts of the esophagus also occur in this compartment (Fig. 1.93, A and B), and can be seen anywhere along the course of the esophagus. Bronchogenic cysts, on the other hand, tend to occur in the upper middle compartment, and very often, just around the carina. Enlarged vessels such as the SVC, aorta, or pulmonary artery also can produce middle mediastinal masses, and in addition, enlarged lymph nodes, either inflammatory or tumoral in nature, should be considered. In this latter regard, the problem, as noted earlier, most often is lymphoma or leukemia.

In the **posterior mediastinal compartment,** one

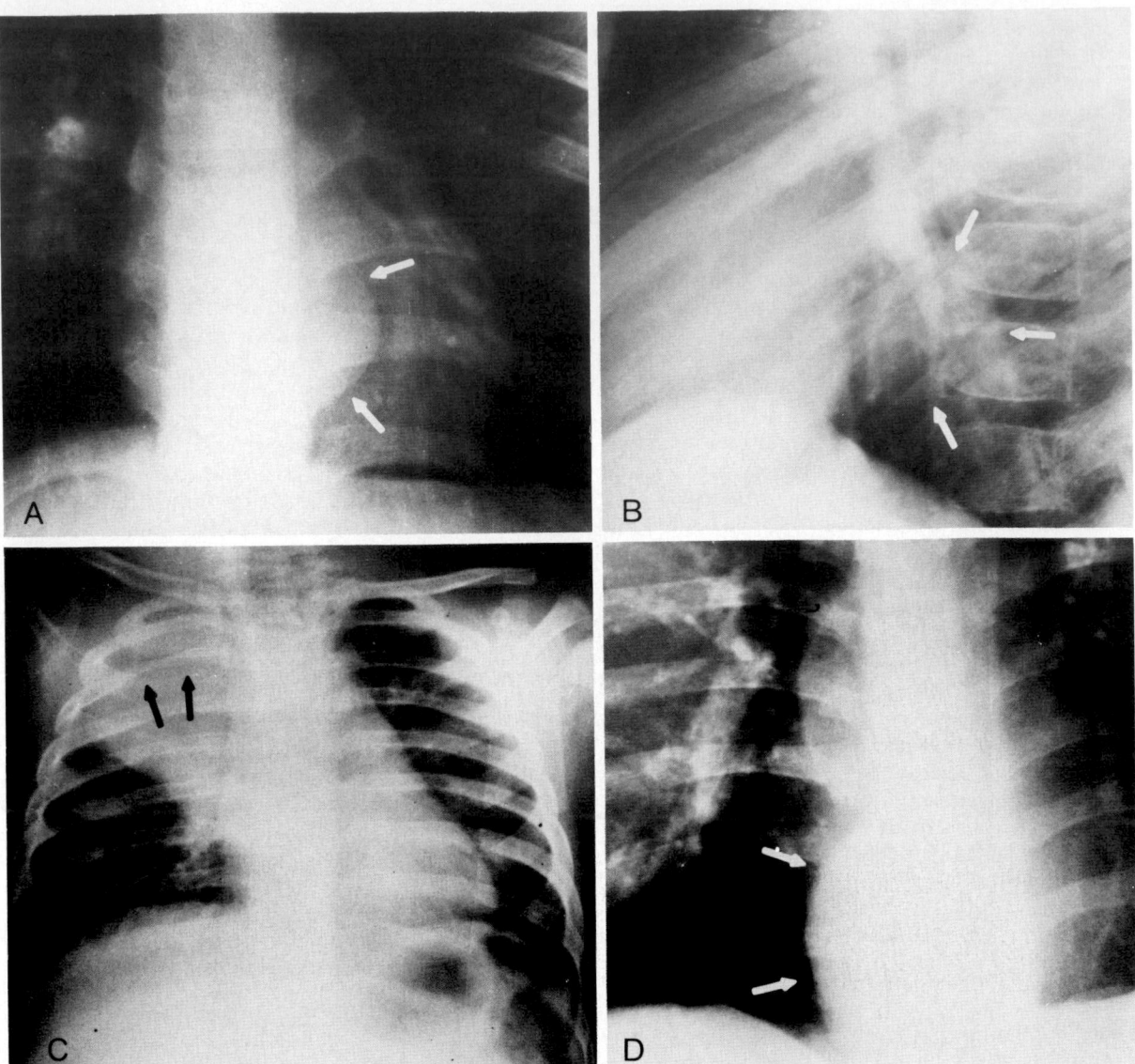

Fig. 1.93. Mediastinal masses. A. Spherical retrocardiac mass (arrows) due to a **duplication cyst.** B. Lateral view shows the retrocardiac (middle mediastinum) position of the mass (arrows). C. Posterior mediastinal mass due to **neuroblastoma.** Without the presence of rib erosion (arrows), it would be more difficult to diagnose this mass as being posterior mediastinal. D. Nonspecific retrocardiac mass (arrows) which on barium swallow turned out to be a **hiatus hernia.** More often, masses due to hiatus hernias are more central or left-sided.

is dealing primarily with neurogenic tumors and cysts, and very often associated erosive changes in the vertebrae and ribs provide clues to the proper diagnosis (Fig. 1.93C). In this regard, most often one is dealing with a neuroblastoma or ganglioneuroma, for these tumors can produce adjacent rib erosion, and even involve the spine in a dumb-bell fashion. In such cases, pedicular widening and posterior vertebral bodies scalloping along with calcification of the tumor can be seen. Neurofibromas, occurring alone or as part of generalized neurofibromatosis, are rather uncommon

in children, but once again, produce changes similar to those outlined for neuroblastoma and ganglioneuroma. Neuroenteric cysts and lateral or anterior meningoceles also are rare, but when seen, are associated with anterior vertebral body defects and abnormal spinal curvatures. Other primary tumors such as teratoma, sarcoma, etc., are quite uncommon in the posterior mediastinum.

In the **lower portion of the posterior mediastinum,** one can encounter foramen of Bochdalek hernias, enteric cysts, hiatus hernias (Fig. 1.93D), pancreatic pseudocyst extensions into the chest, and pulmonary sequestrations. In the neonate, Bochdalek hernias are most common, but in the older child, pulmonary sequestration and hiatus hernia are the most common. In addition to these problems, one may see a posterior mediastinal mass arising as part of, or secondary to, infection, trauma, or tumoral growth of the spine or spinal cord.

Chapter 2

FACE, SINUSES, MASTOIDS, AND NECK

NECK—UPPER AIRWAY

Tongue Size Abnormalities

Determination of the size of the tongue, roentgenographically, is not always practical, but still, one should appreciate those conditions where tongue size changes are an important point in diagnosis (Table 2.1). In this regard, a small tongue is rare and usually is part of underdevelopment of the mandible. Enlargement of the tongue is more common and most often occurs with hypothyroidism. Thereafter, one should consider trisomy-21 (mongolism), and then rare conditions such as the Beckwith-Wiedemann syndrome (1, 2, 5), a variety of developmental cysts of the tongue (4), and tumors such as hemangiomas, lymphangiomas, rhabdomyomas, and rhabdomyosarcomas (3, 6).

References

1. Cohen MM Jr, Gorlin RJ, Feingold M, ten Bensel RW: The Beckwith-Wiedemann syndrome. Seven new cases. *Am J Dis Child* 122:515–519, 1971.
2. Filippi G, McKusick VA: Beckwith-Wiedemann syndrome; exomphalos-macroglossia—report of two cases and review of literature. *Medicine* 49:279–298, 1970.
3. Liebert PS, Stool SE: Rhabdomyosarcoma of the tongue in an infant. Results of combined radiation and chemotherapy. *Ann Surg* 178:621, 1973.
4. Lister J, Zachary RB: Cystic duplications in the tongue. *J Pediatr Surg* 3:491–493, 1968.
5. McNamara TO, Gooding CE, Kaplan SL, Clark RE: Exomphalos-macroglossia-gigantism (visceromegaly) syndrome; (the Beckwith-Wiedemann syndrome). *Am J Roentgenol* 114:264–267, 1972.
6. Solomon MP, Tolete-Velcek F: Lingual rhabdomyoma (adult variant) in a child. *J Pediatr Surg* 14:91–94, 1979.

Table 2.1 Tongue Size Abnormalities

A. Large tongue		
Hypothyroidism	}	Commonest
Trisomy-21		
Beckwith-Wiedemann syndrome	}	Relatively rare
Tumor	}	Rare
Cyst		
B. Small tongue		
Aglossia	}	Relatively rare
Hypoglossia		

Nasopharyngeal Soft Tissues

Specifically, these tissues are located next to the roof of the mouth, and the commonest cause of thickening of these tissues is normal adenoidal lymphoid hypertrophy (Fig. 2.1). It might be noted, however, that before the age of 3 months, adenoidal tissue is sparse, and indeed, invisible roentgenographically (1). After 3 months, however, it becomes progressively thicker, and it is not unusual to see ½-to-1-inch thicknesses of tissue in this region in older, normal adolescents. In infants and young children, this degree of normal thickening can produce airway obstruction. In older children, airway obstruction often is less pronounced, but can be a cause of mouth breathing etc. In any of these cases of more than normal adenoidal hypertrophy, the underlying problem usually is repeated respiratory tract infection in a patient prone to produce an overabundance of lymphoid tissue.

A less common cause of increased thickness of the nasopharyngeal soft tissues, but certainly one not rare, is the so-called juvenile angiofibroma (2–4, 8). This tumor, a lesion of adolescent males, usually presents with epistaxis and/or sinusitis, and the soft tissue mass virtually fills the nasopharynx (Fig. 2.2A). In other words, the air gap which exists between the anterior surface of the normal adenoids and the pterygomaxillary plate is obliterated. The main reason for this is that the tumor starts in this area, and thus, obliterates the space early. With adenoidal hypertrophy, only occasionally is the space obliterated, for it requires very massive enlargement of the adenoids to

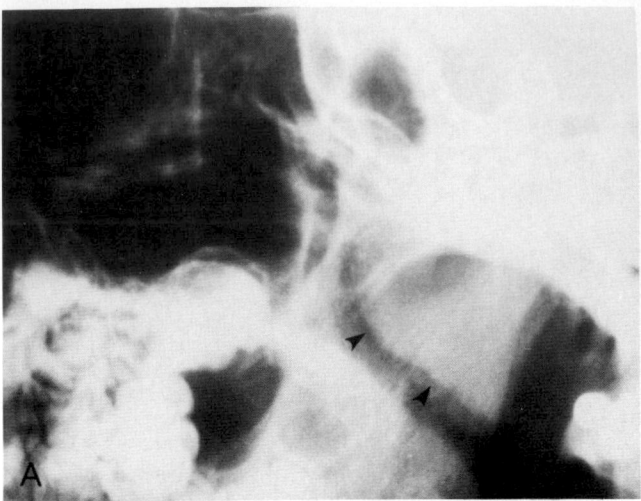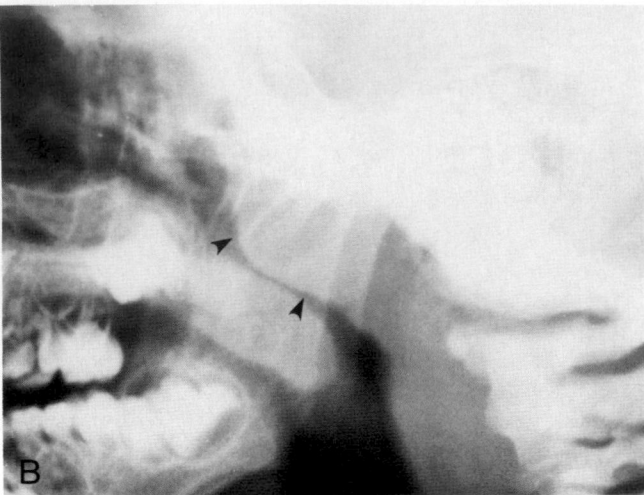

Fig. 2.1. Normal adenoids and retropharyngeal lymphoid tissue. A. Note abundant adenoidal tissue in the nasopharynx (arrows). Also note the normal air gap between the anterior surface of the adenoidal mass and the posterior wall of the maxillary sinuses. B. Another patient demonstrating adenoidal and retropharyngeal lymphoid tissue enlargement (arrows) erroneously suggesting a pathologic retropharyngeal mass. The uvula is a little enlarged in this patient because of associated pharyngitis.

Table 2.2   Nasopharyngeal Soft Tissues

A. Increased thickness		
Normal adenoids	}	Commonest
Infection		
Nasopharyngeal tumors	}	Moderately, common
Basal encephalocele	}	Relatively rare
Base of skull tumors		
B. Decreased thickness		
Small, normal (under 3 months)	}	Commonest
Surgical removal	}	Moderately common
Hypo or agammaglobulinemia	}	Relatively rare
Ataxia telangiectasia syndrome		

produce this finding. Angiography and contrast-enhanced computerized tomography vividly demonstrate the hypervascularity and angiomatous nature of a juvenile angiofibroma (Fig. 2.2B). Rounding out the list of causes of increased thickness of the nasopharyngeal soft tissues are lymphoma (Fig. 2.2C), the rather rare lymphoepithelioma, and a smattering of tumors such as neurofibroma, neuroblastoma, teratoma, cystic hygroma, chordomas of the clivus (5), and basal encephaloceles (Table 2.2).

Decreased thickness of the nasopharyngeal soft tissues, as has been noted earlier, is normal under the age of 3 months, but when lymphoid tissue is absent in older children one should consider surgical removal of the adenoids (moderately common), or underdevelopment with immunologic deficiency states such as agammaglobulinemia (hypogammaglobulinemia) and the ataxia telangiectasia syndrome (6). These latter conditions, of course, are relatively rare.

References

1. Capitanio MA, Kirkpatrick JA: Nasopharyngeal lymphoid tissue. Roentgen observations in 257 children two years of age or less. *Radiology* 96:389–391, 1970.
2. Fitzpatrick PJ: The nasopharyngeal angiofibroma. *Clin Radiol* 18:62–68, 1967.
3. Gonsalves CG, Briant TDR: Radiologic findings in nasopharyngeal angiofibromas. *J Can Assoc Radiol* 29:209–215, 1978.
4. Holman CB, Miller WE: Juvenile nasopharyngeal fibroma: roentgenologic characteristics. *Am J Roentgenol* 94:292–298, 1965.
5. Nolte K: Malignant intracranial chordoma and sarcoma of the clivus in infancy. *Pediatr Radiol* 8:1–6, 1979.
6. Ozonoff MB: Ataxia-telangiectasia: chronic pneumonia sinusitis, and adenoidal hypoplasia. *Am J Roentgenol* 120:297–299, 1974.
7. Pick T, Maurer HM, McWilliams NB: Lymphoepithelioma in childhood. *J Pediatr* 84:96–100, 1974.
8. Sessions RB, Wills PI, Alford BR, Harrell JE, Evans RA: Juvenile nasopharyngeal angiofibroma: radiographic aspects. *Laryngoscope* 86:2–17, 1976.
9. Swischuk LE: *Radiology of the Newborn and Young Infant,* ed 2. Baltimore, Williams & Wilkins, 1980, pp 201–202.

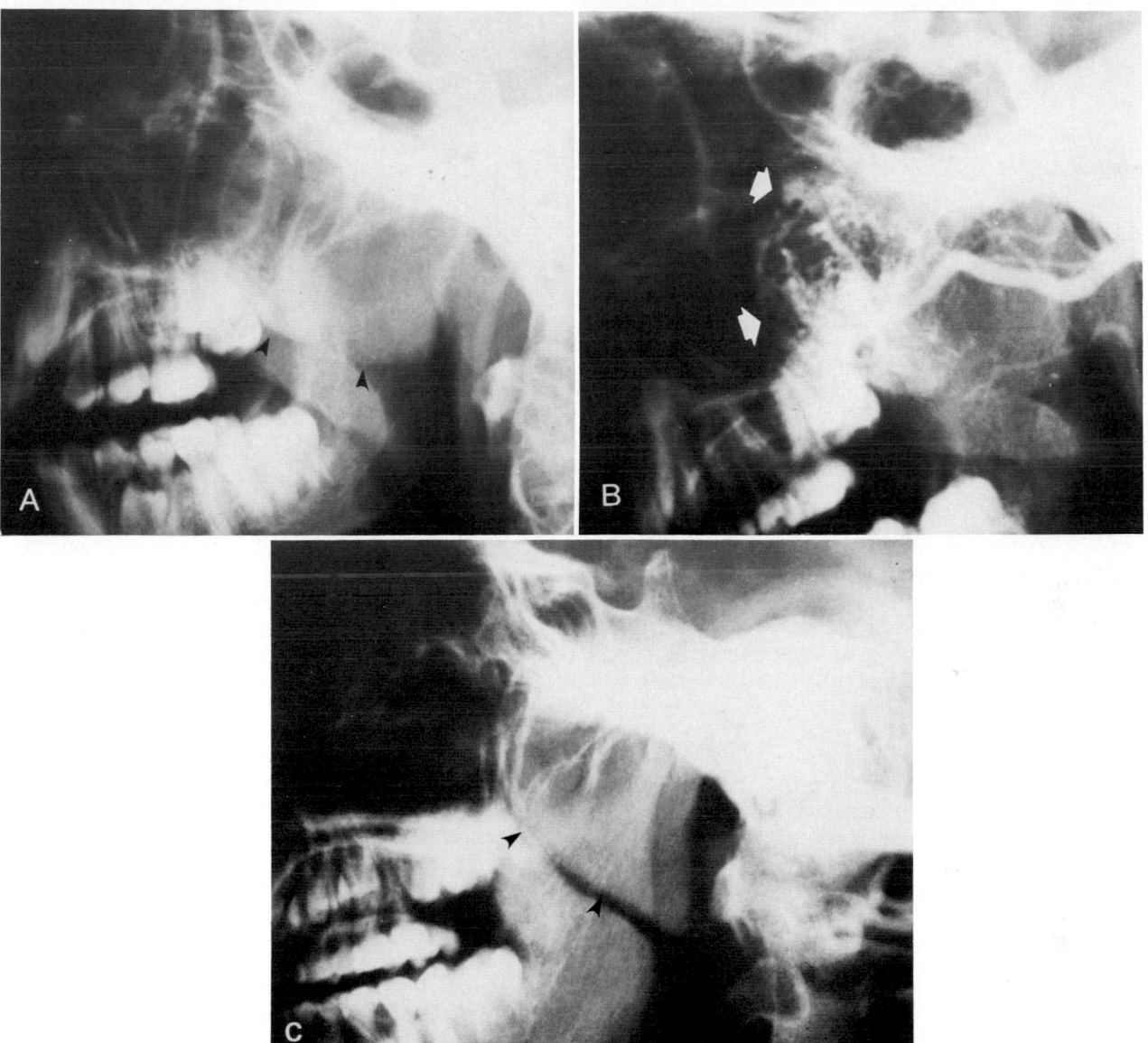

Fig. 2.2. Nasopharyngeal masses. A. Juvenile angiofibroma. Note the mass (arrows) filling the nasopharynx. Also note that there is no air gap in front of the mass (compare with normal adenoidal enlargement in Fig. 2.1A). B. Angiogram demonstrating vascularity typical of a juvenile angiofibroma (arrows). C. Enlargement of the adenoidal tissue mass secondary to lymphoma (arrows). Again note that the anterior air gap has been obliterated. Such obliteration occurs with simple adenoidal hyperplasia in a few very severe cases only.

Uvula and Hard Palate Abnormalities

Underdevelopment of the uvula, and occasionally, the hard palate, are seen with congenital cleft palate. The small uvula is readily demonstrable roentgenographically, and during phonation, will not assume its normal right angle posture of apposition against the posterior pharyngeal wall (2) (see Fig. 2.3A). Enlargement of the uvula most commonly is due to pharyngitis (see Fig. 2.1B), but occasionally can be seen with angioneurotic edema, and very rarely, with a tumor or cyst of the palate. The hard palate can be deformed or deviated secondary to a tumor arising above it, but this is an uncommon situation (1).

References

1. Frech RS, McAlister WH: Teratoma of the nasopharynx producing depression of the posterior hard palate. *J Can Assoc Radiol* 20:204–205, 1969.
2. Swischuk LE, Smith PC, Fagan CJ: Abnormalities of the pharynx and larynx in childhood. *Semin Roentgenol* 9:283–300, 1974.

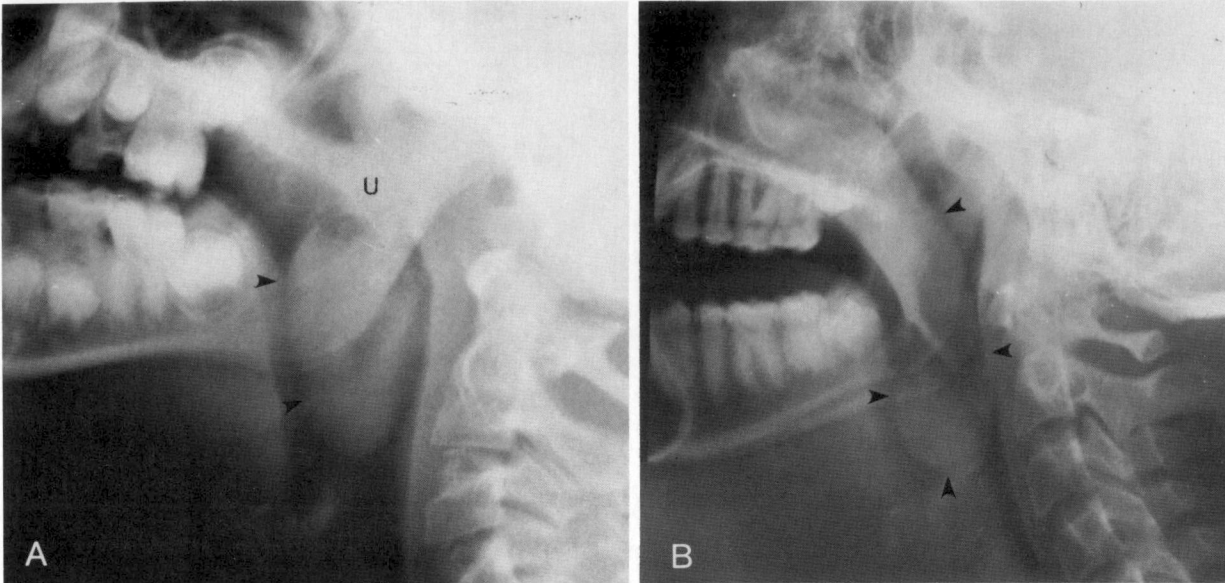

Fig. 2.3. Nasopharyngeal masses. A. Note the **enlarged palatine tonsils** (arrows). Such tonsilar enlargement is common in children, with or without tonsilar infection, and thus, cannot be used as a barometer of tonsilitis. Also note the position and size of the normal uvula (U). It is in a phonating position (i.e., crying) and characteristically assumes a right angle bend to the adenoidal pad along the posterior pharyngeal wall. B. Nasopharyngeal mass due to an **antrochoanal polyp** (arrows). These polyps originate in the maxillary sinus and dangle into the nasopharynx.

Hypopharyngeal Masses

Although any mass arising from the glottis, aryepiglottic folds, retropharynx, or nasopharynx, can extend into the hypopharynx, this section deals with those masses which occur in the hypopharynx proper. The most common such mass is the enlarged, inflamed palatine tonsil(s). In most cases, the finding is normal (Fig. 2.3A), but occasionally, the tonsils can be so large that they contribute to airway obstruction. Furthermore, in some chronic cases, calcifications within the tonsils can be seen (1). The next most common cause of a hypopharyngeal mass is that due to projection of the inferior portion of a prominent uvula over the palatine tonsils. This really is a pseudomass, and normal. A rare cause of a mass in the hypopharynx is a tumor or cyst arising in the hypopharynx, and a still rarer cause is an antrochoanal polyp, extending from the maxillary sinus, on a long stalk, into the hypopharynx (Fig. 2.3B). These polyps arise in the maxillary sinuses (2), and as they dangle into the hypopharynx, may cause difficulties with breathing or swallowing.

References

1. Thomas DP: Tonsilloliths—a common cause of pharyngeal calcification. *Aust Radiol* 18:287–291, 1974.
2. Towbin R, Dunbar JS, Bove K: Antrochoanal polyps. *Am J Roentgenol* 132:27–31, 1979.

RETROPHARYNGEAL SOFT TISSUE THICKENING

Thickening of the retropharyngeal space can be due to blood, edema, pus, or tumor (4) (Table 2.3), but the commonest cause is pseudothickening due to buckling of the airway, when the neck is flexed, and the film obtained during expiration. Once this pitfall is appreciated, it becomes obvious that the retropharyngeal soft tissues should be evaluated only with the airway distended in full inspiration, and the neck held in extension (Fig. 2.4). In addition to this misleading configuration of the retropharyngeal soft tissues, one can encounter true, but still innocuous, thickening due to normally overabundant lymphoid tissue. Indeed, the 'thickening' or 'mass' so produced often appears lumpy and worrisome (see Fig. 2.4C), and yet the lumpy configuration favors normal lymphoid tissue. With pathologic thickening, the mass produced usually shows a smooth anterior margin and displaces the airway forward in a continuous arc (Fig. 2.5).

In terms of such pathologic thickening, it can be due to tumor, cyst, inflammation, abscess, edema, or massive lymph node enlargement and, in addition to the arc-like displacement of the airway, there is obliteration of the normal stepoff of the air column at the level of the larynx (Fig. 2.5). Normally, with full inspiration, the soft tissues below the level of the larynx are approximately two times as thick as those

Table 2.3 Retropharyngeal Soft Tissue Thickening

Buckling of airway (pseudothickening) Inflammation (adenopathy) Retropharyngeal abscess	Commonest
Edema with C-spine injury Retropharyngeal tumor	Moderately common
Noninflammatory adenopathy Osteomyelitis of C-spine Tumors of C-spine	Relatively uncommon
Myxedematous thickening Edema with obstructed SVC Vein of Galen aneurysms Enteric cyst Goiter	Rare

above, and the reason for this is that the esophagus is located in this region. Roentgenographically this produces a stepoff of the air column, a finding which is present even in those children with prominent, normal lymphoid tissue (see Fig. 2.4). With a pathologic mass, the stepoff usually is totally obliterated, even in less than florid cases (Fig. 2.5). In these less severe cases, if one is uncertain as to the presence of soft tissue thickening, a barium swallow may be required to demonstrate displacement of the esophagus from the cervical spine.

The commonest cause of pathologic retropharyngeal soft tissue thickening is retropharyngeal inflammatory adenopathy (viral or bacterial) with or without frank abscess formation. If a frank abscess evolves, air can be seen in the thickened soft tissues and, most commonly, such abscesses occur secondary to supurative (pyogenic) adenitis. Occasionally they are seen with perforation of the pharynx by foreign bodies or iatrogenic intubation. The inflammation, in any of these cases, is accompanied by muscle spasm, straightening of the cervical spine and, in some cases, actual hyperflexion of the spine. This leads to a variety of pseudodislocated appearances of C_1 on C_2, and C_2 on C_3. Inflammatory adenopathy in this region also can be seen with tuberculosis (scrofula) and fungal diseases such as histoplasmosis.

Moderately common causes of retropharyngeal soft tissue thickening include prevertebral edema or hematoma secondary to cervical spine injury, and a variety of retropharyngeal tumors. Most common of these is a cystic hygroma (2), but others include neuroblastoma, ganglioneuroma, neurofibroma (5), hemangioma, and even an occasional teratoma. Other causes of noninflammatory adenopathy include: histiocytosis X (Fig. 2.5B), leukemia, lymphoma, and sinus histiocytosis (1).

Thickening of the retropharyngeal space also is seen, but less often, with underlying cervical spine osteomyelitis, primary cervical spine tumors, retropharyngeal goiter, myxedematous thickening in hypothyroid infants (3), duplication cysts, edema secondary to obstruction of the superior vena cava (6), and enlargement of the jugular veins and carotid arteries in vein of Galen or other large intracranial arteriovenous malformations (7). In these latter cases, the sheer size of the blood vessels causes forward displacement of the airway.

References

1. Bankaci M, Morris RF, Stool SE, Paradise JL: Sinus histiocytosis with massive lymphadenopathy: report of its occurrence in two siblings with retropharyngeal involvement in both. *Ann Otol Rhinol Laryngol* 87:327–331, 1978.
2. Barrand KG, Freeman NV: Massive infiltrating cystic hygroma of the neck in infancy. *Arch Dis Child* 48:523–531, 1973.
3. Grunebaum M, Moskowitz G: The retropharyngeal soft tissues in young infants with hypothyroidism. *Am J Roentgenol* 108:543–545, 1970.
4. McCook TA, Felman AH: Retropharyngeal masses in infants and young children. *Am J Dis Child* 133:41–43, 1979.
5. Steichen FM, Einhorn AF, Fellini A, Feind CR: Congenital retropharyngeal neurofibroma causing laryngeal obstruction in a newborn. *J Pediatr Surg* 6:480–483, 1971.
6. Swischuk LE: *Radiology of the Newborn and Young Infant,* ed 2. Baltimore, Williams & Wilkins, 1980, pp 199–201.
7. Swischuk LE, Crowe JE, Mewborne EB Jr: Large vein of Galen aneurysms in the neonate. A constellation of diagnostic chest and neck radiologic findings. *Pediatr Radiol* 6:4–9, 1977.

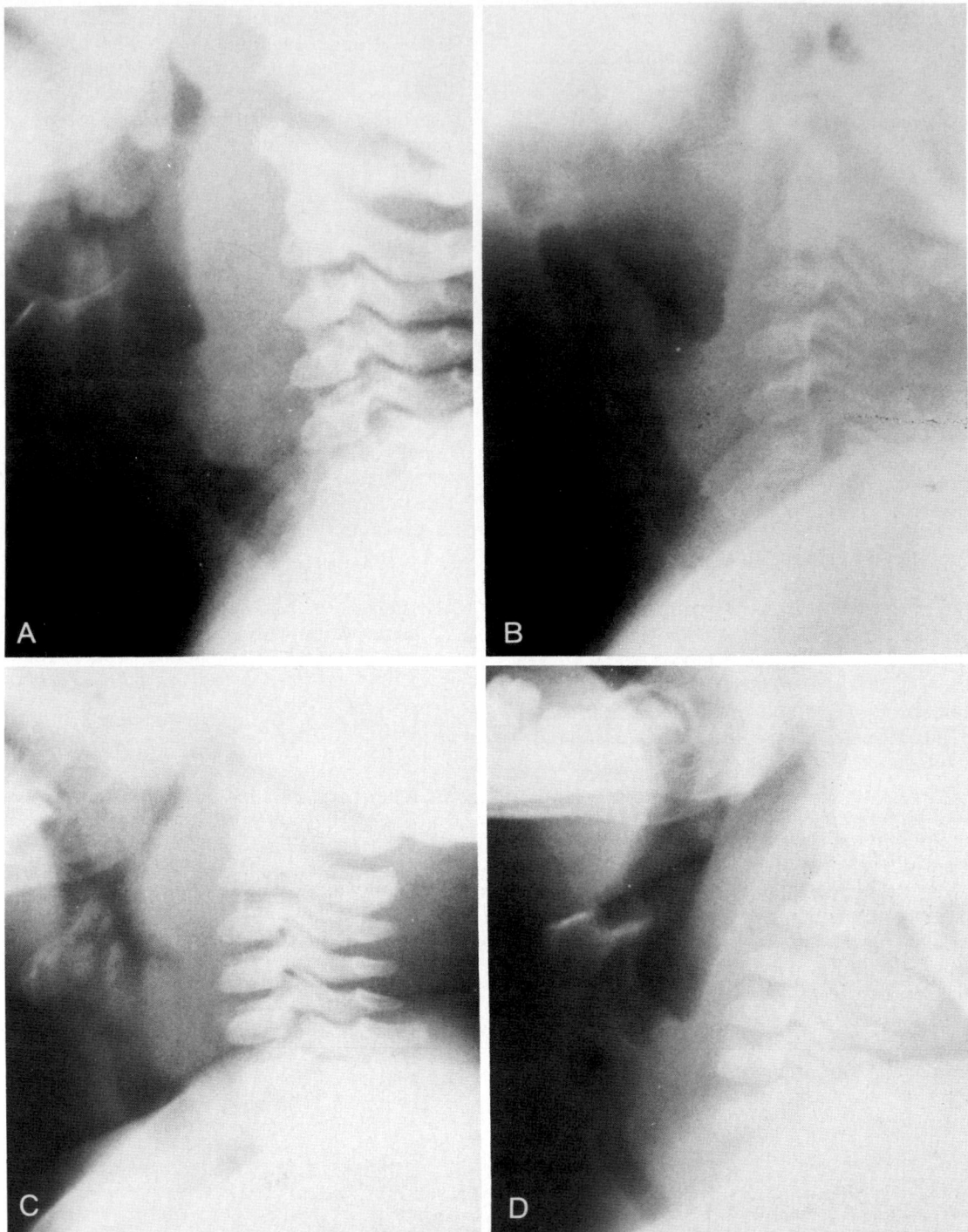

Fig. 2.4. Normal retropharyngeal pseudomasses and thickenings. A. Note **lymphoid tissue** producing mass-like findings in the retropharyngeal space. These were remarkably persistent until a deep inspiratory effort was obtained. **B.** With deep inspiration the airway is fully distended and the previously noted findings have disappeared. **C.** Another infant with retropharyngeal thickening suggesting a lumpy retropharyngeal mass. The lumpiness rules in favor of lymphoid tissue, but is not absolutely diagnostic. **D.** With proper technique, note that the mass has all but disappeared; only the central pad of lymphoid tissue still projects into the posterior aspect of the distended hypopharynx. Note, however, that the lateral recesses of the hypopharynx are normally distended, and that because of this, the normal stepoff between the posterior hypopharyngeal wall and the upper trachea is retained. When a true retropharyngeal mass is present, the lateral recesses usually are not distended and the stepoff obliterated.

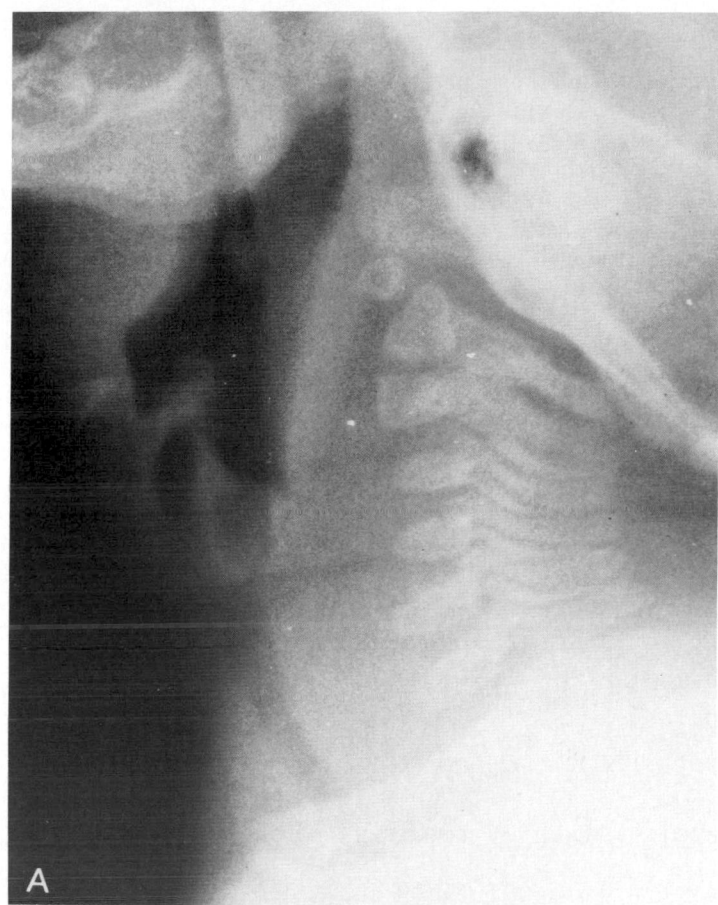

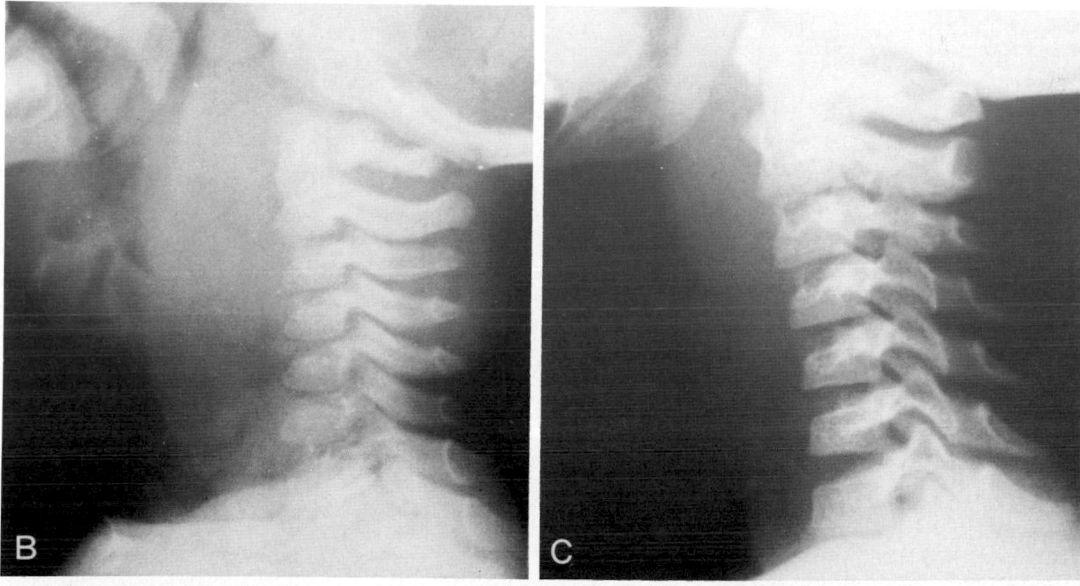

Fig. 2.5. Abnormal retropharyngeal masses and thickenings. A. Young child with **retropharyngeal cellulitis** (i.e., preabscess) producing marked anterior displacement of the airway (arrows). Compare the findings with those seen in the infant shown in Figure 2.4D. In contrast to that infant, the infant at hand demonstrates the upper trachea to be displaced further from the spine and the stepoff between the posterior pharyngeal air column and upper tracheal air column to be obliterated. The end result is that the entire airway is pushed forward in a continuous arc, a configuration not usually seen with normal lymphoid tissue. B. Similar findings, but more marked, in a patient with **massive adenopathy in Letterer-Siewe's disease.** C. **Retropharyngeal cellulitis and adenitis** produce straightening of the spine, anterior displacement of the upper trachea, thickening of the retropharyngeal soft tissues, and obliteration of the stepoff between the hypopharyngeal and tracheal air columns.

ABNORMALITIES OF THE EPIGLOTTIS AND ARYEPIGLOTTIC FOLDS

For the most part, abnormalities of the epiglottis consist of enlargement, for only occasionally will one see it to be smaller than normal (hypoplastic) or deformed. The usual cause of deformity is scarring after corrosive agent (usually lye) burn and, as far as enlargement is concerned, the commonest cause, by far, is epiglottitis (Table 2.4) (1–4). With this infection, usually caused by the bacterium *H. influenzae*, the epiglottis can become very thick and swollen (Fig. 2.6, A and B). In most cases, in addition to the epiglottis becoming thickened, there is thickening of the aryepiglottic folds. Milder cases must be differentiated from the so-called omega epiglottis, a normal variation wherein the lateral flaps of the epiglottis bend down so far that, on lateral view of the neck, they make the epiglottis appear thickened (Fig. 2.6C). Symptoms associated with epiglottitis center around dysphagia and some respiratory distress. Occasionally, the epiglottis can become swollen with angioneurotic edema (5), and during the acute phase of corrosive agent ingestion (i.e., chemical burns). Tumors and cysts of the epiglottis are virtually unheard of.

As far as the aryepiglottic folds are concerned, with the hypopharynx well distended, normal ones appear very thin and have a stout, triangular base (see Fig. 2.7A). Under certain circumstances, however, the thin portions of the folds can become thickened, and the commonest cause of such thickening is epiglottitis (1–4). This finding, together with a thickened epiglottis, virtually is pathopneumonic of the condition, and only rarely is mimicked by angioneurotic edema (5). A very rare cause of thickening of the aryepiglottic folds is an aryepiglottic fold cyst (1).

The aryepiglottic folds can appear somewhat thickened (pseudothickening) if the hypopharynx is incompletely distended with air, and with buckling of the folds in the condition known as laryngomalcia (1, 4). However, in neither of these cases are the folds truly thickened, for they only appear thickened because of their distorted configuration.

Table 2.4 Epiglottic and Aryepiglottic Fold Abnormalities

A. Enlarged epiglottis		
Epiglottitis	}	Commonest
Angioneurotic edema	}	
Lye burns		Relatively rare
Tumor, cyst	}	Very rare
B. Thickened aryepiglottic folds		
Buckling with poor insp.	}	
Epiglottitis		Commonest
Buckling with laryngomalacia	}	Moderately common
Aryepiglottic cyst	}	Relatively rare

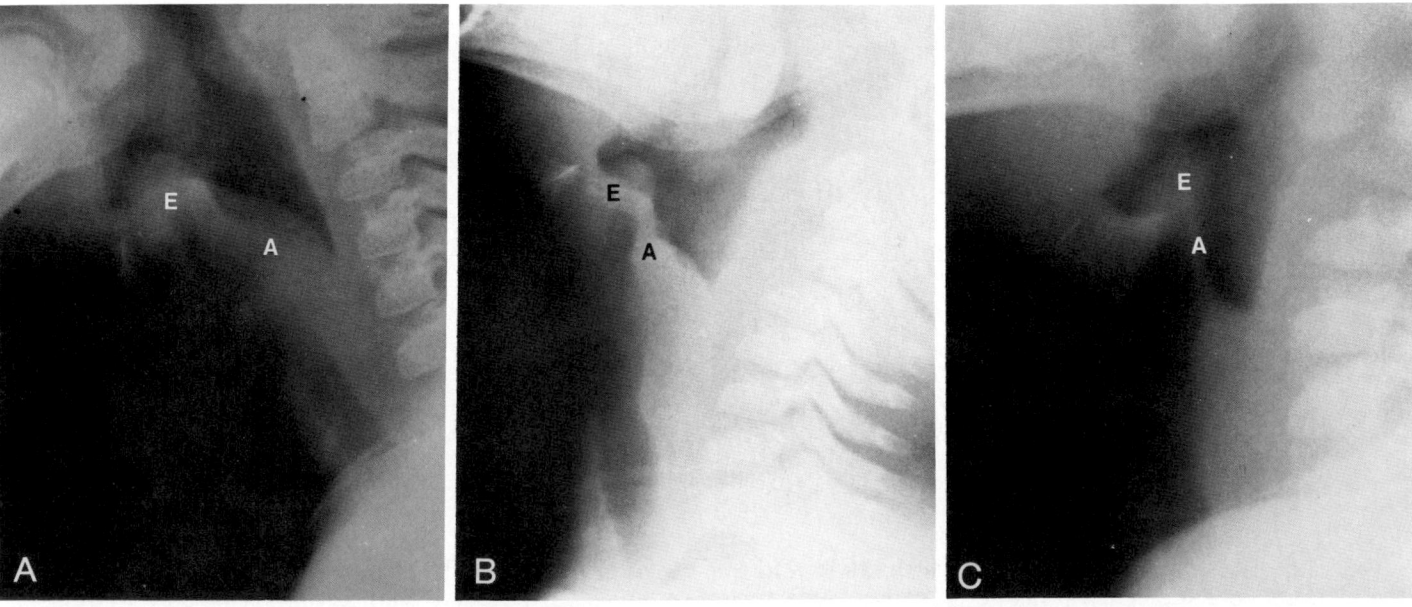

Fig. 2.6. Epiglottic thickening. A. Typical thickening of the epiglottis (E) and aryepiglottic folds (A) in epiglottitis. Compare with the normal epiglottis and aryepiglottic folds in Figure 2.7A. B. Moderate epiglottic (E) and aryepiglottic fold (A) swelling in another patient with less severe epiglottitis. C. **Normal omega epiglottis.** Note the falsely thickened epiglottis (E). Even if one were to interpret this finding as being representative of true epiglottic thickening, the fact that the aryepiglottic folds (A) are thin, should dissuade one from the diagnosis. The findings in this patient are normal, for with epiglottitis the folds usually are thickened.

References

1. Dunbar JS: Upper respiratory tract obstruction in infants and children. *Am J Roentgenol* 109:225–247, 1970.
2. Poole CA, Altman DH: Acute epiglottitis in children. *Radiology* 80:798–805, 1963.
3. Rapkin RH: Diagnosis of epiglottitis: Simplicity and reliability of radiographs of neck in differential diagnosis of croup syndrome. *J Pediatr* 80:96–98, 1972.
4. Swischuk LE, Smith PC, Fagan CJ: Abnormalities of the pharynx and larynx in childhood. *Semin Roentgenol* 9:283–300, 1974.
5. Watts FB Jr, Slovis TL: The enlarged epiglottis. *Pediatr Radiol* 5:133–136, 1977.

VOCAL CORD ABNORMALITIES

The vocal cords are readily visible on both lateral and frontal views of the neck, and indeed, frequently are visible at the top of regular chest films. Abnormalities of the vocal cords include indistinctness of their margins, thickening or increase in their bulk, fixation in the midline, and nodular growths. Any of these can be bilateral or unilateral (Table 2.5).

Table 2.5 Vocal Cord Abnormalities

A. Indistinct, fuzzy on lateral view	
Croup	Commonest
Paralysis	Moderately common
Trauma Storage diseases Lipoid proteinosis	Relatively rare
B. Bilateral cord thickening and/or fixation	
Croup	Commonest
Trauma (iatrogenic) Paralysis Epiglottitis	Moderately common
Trauma (noniatrogenic)	Relatively uncommon
Storage diseases Lipoid proteinosis Laryngeal web	Relatively rare
C. Unilateral thickening and/or fixation	
Paralysis	Commonest
Iatrogenic trauma Subglottic hemangioma	Moderately common
Laryngeal web (unilateral)	Rare
D. Nodules	
Papillomatosis	Commonest
Posttracheostomy granuloma	Relatively uncommon

Indistinct-Thickened Cords on Lateral View

The vocal cords can appear indistinct and thickened because of edema or spasm and in some cases, both problems are present together. This certainly is true in croup, the commonest cause of indistinct vocal cords visible on lateral view (Fig. 2.7A). A similar appearance can be seen with vocal cord paralysis, vocal cord infiltration (see next section), and laryngeal trauma. In regards to trauma, it more often is iatrogenic (secondary to intubation) than noniatrogenic. Rarely the cords can have a similar appearance with laryngeal webs. Such webs, however, must involve the cords proper to cause any degree of fixation. Most laryngeal webs do not involve the cords directly.

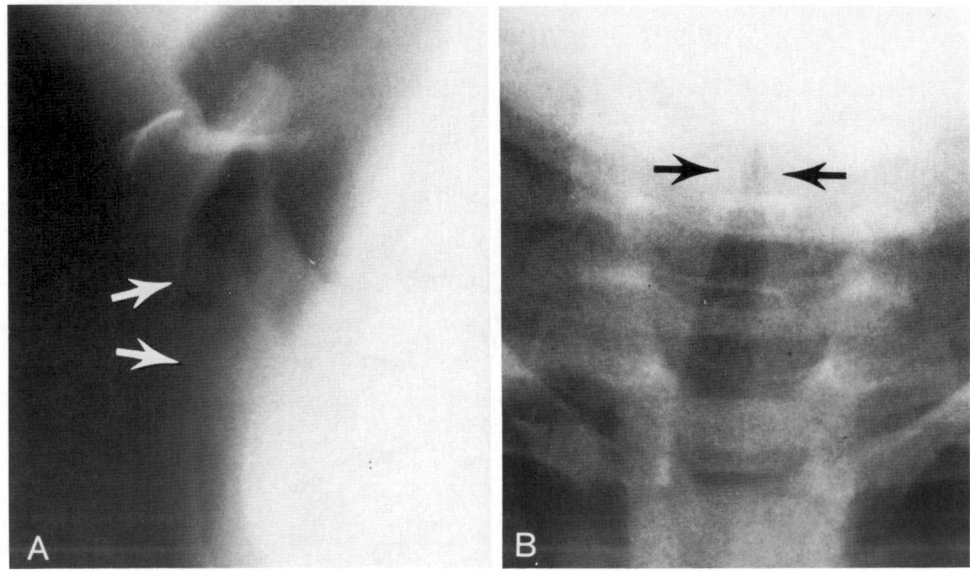

Fig. 2.7. Indistinct vocal cords on lateral view. A. Note the indistinct vocal cords (arrows) in this patient with croup. The prominent, airfilled ventricle is common in croup. Similar cord indistinctness can be seen with edema secondary to trauma and fixation of the cords with vocal cord paralysis. Note the normal, thin aryepiglottic folds and their stout triangular base. B. Frontal view, in same patient, demonstrating typical funnel-shaped configuration of the inferior aspect of the vocal cords and subglottic portion of the trachea (arrows). This finding is rather characteristic of croup, but can be seen in some cases of epiglottitis.

Thickened or Fixed Cords on Frontal View

Once again, croup is the commonest cause of this finding, and the spastic, edematous cords form a funnel or slit-like glottic opening (Fig. 2.7B). Similar fixation of the cords occurs with some cases of epiglottitis (3) and with vocal cord paralysis (Fig. 2.8, A, B). The latter problem usually occurs with neurologic conditions such as the Arnold-Chiari malformation, cerebral agenesis, and posterior fossa meningoceles (1, 4, 8). In the neonatal period, however, the most common cause is anoxic damage to the brain stem.

Trauma to the larynx also can cause the vocal cords to appear thickened and fixed on frontal view, and often the cords are lumpy and asymmetric. Other causes of thickening of the vocal cords include the various storage diseases and lipoid proteinosis (7). Tumors of the cords are quite rare, except for juvenile laryngeal papillomatosis and infantile subglottic hemangioma, but in these conditions, thickening, most often, is unilateral. Laryngeal webs, when they involve the vocal cords directly, also can produce fixation of the cords mimicking the findings of vocal cord paralysis.

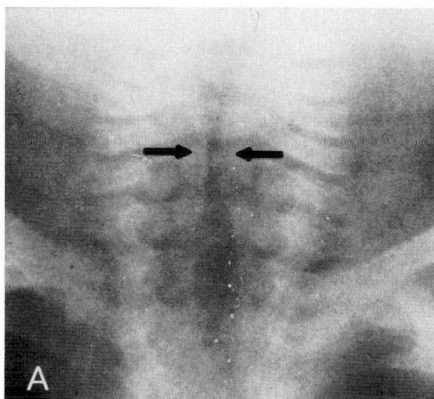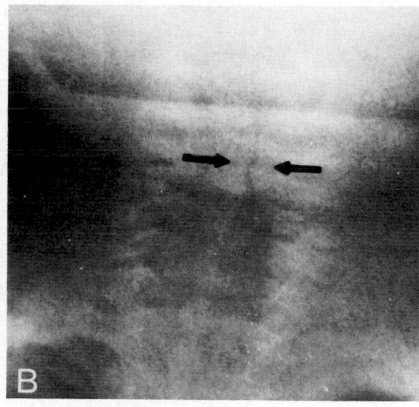

Fig. 2.8. Vocal cord fixation. A. Inspiratory view demonstrating bilateral vocal cord fixation (arrows). Normally, the vocal cords should fall away from midline and result in the glottic opening being of nearly the same width as the trachea. B. Expiration (phonation) view demonstrating slightly wavy (corrugated), but still fixed vocal cords (arrows), and over distention of the obstructed trachea. The degree of cord excursion between resting and phonation is far below normal and signifies cord fixation. On lateral view, the findings in this patient were very similar to those of the infant with croup in Figure 2.7A.

Unilateral Thickening or Fixation of the Vocal Cords

The commonest cause of unilateral fixation, or apparent thickening, of the vocal cords is vocal cord paralysis, and the commonest cause of such paralysis is stretching of the recurrent laryngeal nerve by an aneurysm, or anomaly of position, of the aorta or pulmonary artery. Similar stretching, however, can be caused by critically located cysts or masses in the mediastinum, and in the neonatal period, injury to this nerve can occur with stretching of the neck during difficult deliveries. The findings are rather characteristic, as on frontal view, the involved cord pouts towards midline both with quiet breathing and phonation. The other cord moves freely, and in time, may hypertrophy in a compensatory fashion. Unilateral thickening of the vocal cords also can occur when a subglottic hemangioma extends into the cords (see Fig. 2.11C), and in some cases of juvenile papillomatosis of the cords (2, 3, 6). In addition, rarely, when a laryngeal web involves one cord only, unilateral fixation can occur.

Nodules of Vocal Cords

By far, the commonest, and almost exclusive, cause of nodular bumps on the vocal cords is the condition known as juvenile papillomatosis (2). The etiology of this condition is unknown, but presumed to be viral (i.e., viral warts). It presents with insidious onset of hoarseness and cough in young children (usually males). Demonstration of nodules on or around the vocal cords is characteristic and usually best visualized on lateral view (Fig. 2.9). A much less common cause of vocal cord nodules is a postinflammatory granuloma secondary to chronic tracheostomy tube placement.

References

1. Holinger PC, Holinger LD, Reichert TJ, Holinger PH: Respiratory obstruction and apnea in infants with bilateral abductor vocal cord paralysis, meningomyelocele, hydrocephalus, and Arnold-Chiari malformation. *J Pediatr* 92:368–373, 1978.
2. Oleske JM, Kushnick T: Juvenile papilloma of the larynx. *Am J Dis Child* 121:417–419, 1971.
3. Slovis TL, Arcinue E: Subglottic edema in acute epiglottitis in children. *Am J Roentgenol* 132:500–504, 1979.
4. Snow JB Jr, Rogers KA: Bilateral adductive paralysis of vocal cords secondary to Arnold-Chiari malformation and its management. *Laryngoscope* 25:316, 1965.
5. Sutton TJ, Nogrady MB: Radiologic diagnosis of subglottic hemangioma in infants. *Pediatr Radiol* 1:211–215, 1973.
6. Swischuk LE: *Emergency Radiology of the Acutely Ill or Injured Child.* Baltimore, Williams & Wilkins, 1979, pp 122–124.
7. Weidner WA, Wenzi JE, Swischuk LE: Roentgenographic findings in lipoid proteinosis: a case report. *Am J Roentgenol Radium Ther Nucl Med* 110:457–461, 1970.
8. Williams JL, Capitanio MA, Turtz MG: Vocal cord paralysis; radiologic observations in 21 infants and young children. *Am J Roentgenol* 128:649–651, 1977.

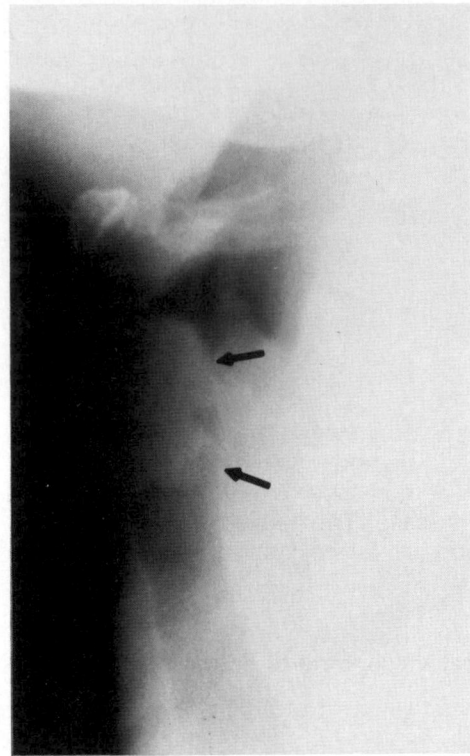

Fig. 2.9. Vocal cord nodules: juvenile papillamotosis. Note the lumpy, nodular appearing vocal cords (arrows). The findings are rather characteristic of juvenile papillomatosis.

SUBGLOTTIC TRACHEAL NARROWING

This section deals with narrowing of the trachea just below the level of the glottis. The length of such narrowing seldom is over 1.5 cm, and the narrowing can be circumferential or eccentric (Table 2.6).

Table 2.6   Subglottic Tracheal Narrowing

A. Circumferential	
Croup	} Commonest
Subglottic stenosis Paradoxic collapse with other obstruction	} Moderately common
B. Eccentric	
Anterior trachea (normal)	} Commonest
Subglottic hemangioma Posttracheostomy tube inflame-fibrosis	} Moderately common

Intratracheal thyroid
    Subglottic mucocele
    Histiocytoma
	} Rare

Circumferential Subglottic Tracheal Narrowing

The commonest cause of such narrowing is that which occurs with croup (Fig. 2.10, A and B). It might be noted, however, that if the hypopharynx is not well distended, such narrowing may not develop, and then, all one may see is thickening of the vocal cords (see Fig. 2.7). The reason for this is that most of the narrowing is due to paradoxical collapse of the subglottic portion of the trachea during inspiration. It has been shown that with any glottic or paraglottic obstruction, during inspiration, intratracheal pressures fall into the negative range, and because of this, the tracheal wall collapses (4). As a result, with expiration, the area of apparent narrowing frequently opens up, even to the point of being totally normal. If, however, considerable edema is associated, some narrowing will persist and the finding is most common

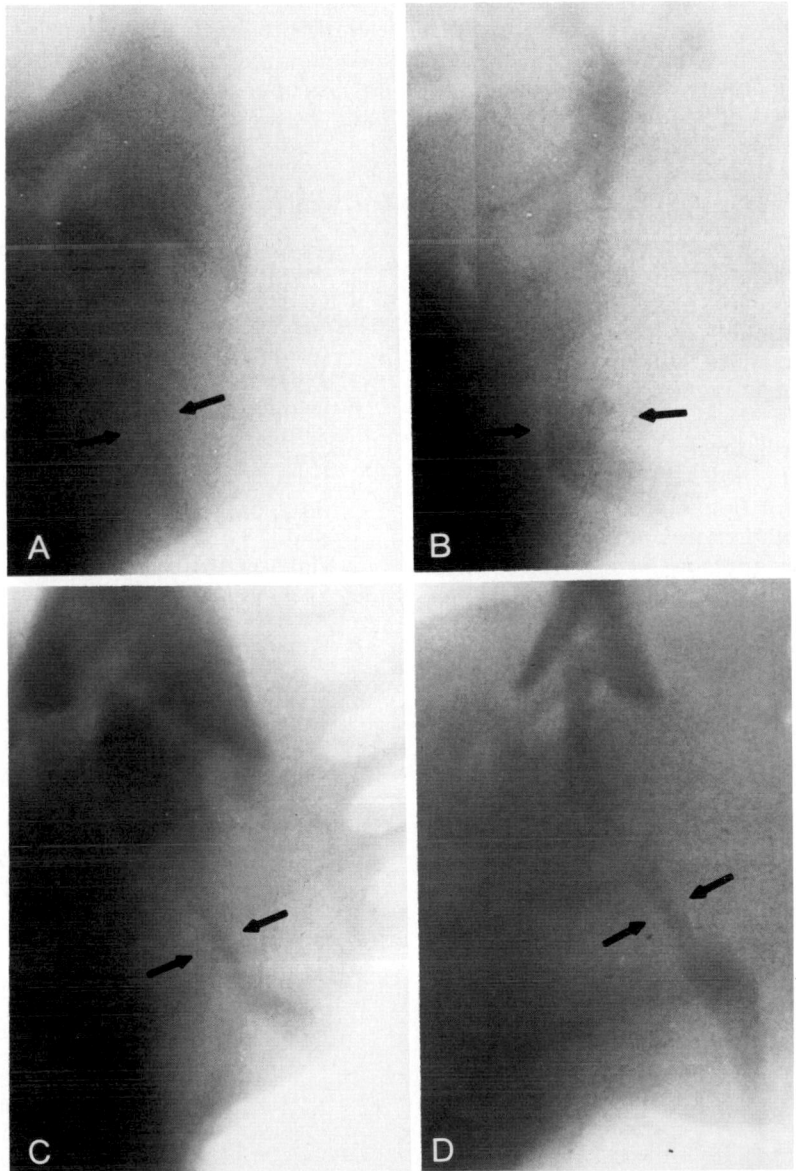

Fig. 2.10. Subglottic tracheal narrowing. A. **Croup.** Inspiratory view demonstrating typical subglottic narrowing (arrows), overdistention of the hypopharynx, fuzziness of the vocal cords, and a prominent ventricle. B. Expiratory view demonstrates overdistention of the trachea and opening of the previously narrowed subglottic portion of the trachea to almost a normal diameter (arrows). This is common in croup. C. **Subglottic stenosis.** Inspiratory view. Note typical subglottic narrowing (arrows) indistinguishable from that seen in croup. D. Expiratory view, however, demonstrates the subglottic narrowing to persist (arrows). This is characteristic of subglottic stenosis.

with bacterial croup. Most often, of course, croup is viral in origin, but occasionally it can be the result of bacteria infection, and in such cases, also may be associated with inflammatory membranes visible just below the cords (5).

Mimicking the findings of croup, but not being nearly as common, is congenital subglottic stenosis (1, 3, 7). On the inspiratory view, the findings are indistinguishable from those of croup, but differentiation can be accomplished on the expiratory view. As opposed to croup, with subglottic stenosis, subglottic narrowing remains fixed on expiration (Fig. 2.10, C and D). Acquired subglottic stenosis can produce a similar configuration, and is becoming more common as tracheostomy and neonatal intratracheal tube placements become more common. It might be noted, however, that not all cases of acquired subglottic stenosis (7–9) are smooth and circumferentially stenotic.

Indeed, membranes, granulomas, and a variety of eccentric narrowings also occur.

A relatively rare cause of circumferential narrowing is paradoxical, inspiratory subglottic collapse due to an obstructing laryngeal web, and once again differentiating the findings from croup is difficult. Indeed, as far as the subglottic narrowing is concerned, it appears virtually the same both on inspiration and expiration. However, on frontal view, as opposed to croup, the vocal cords move normally with most laryngeal webs. The reason for this is that most webs are located away from the cords; the majority lie above, a few below, and only a very few lie at the level of the cords proper. In these latter cases, vocal cord motion is impaired and it is then that the findings can mimic those of croup or vocal cord paralysis, on frontal view too.

Eccentric Subglottic Tracheal Narrowing

The commonest cause of eccentric subglottic tracheal narrowing usually is overlooked, but consists of a small anterior indentation of the trachea seen mostly in infants (Fig. 2.11A). Usually it occurs during inspiration and is of unknown cause. Only once have I seen it mimicked by a subglottic hemangioma, a very rare situation. The reason for this is that most hemangiomas are posterior or lateral (11) and indeed, in infancy, a posterior or lateral subglottic indentation almost always is due to a hemangioma (Fig. 2.11, B and C). Other less common causes of eccentric subglottic tracheal narrowing include iatrogenic stenosis after intubation, extension of juvenile papillomas below the cords, ectopic intratracheal thyroid tissue (6), subglottic mucoceles (2), and postinflammatory histiocytomas (10).

References

1. Cundy RL, Bergstrom LB: Congenital subglottic stenosis. *J Pediatr* 82:282–284, 1973.
2. Dagan R, Leiberman A, Strauss R, Bar-Ziv J, Hirsch M: Subglottic mucocele in an infant. *Pediatr Radiol* 8:119–121, 1979.
3. Grunebaum M: The roentgenologic investigation of congenital subglottic stenosis. *Am J Roentgenol* 125:877–880, 1975.
4. Gyepes MT, Desilets DT: The submentovertical projection: a new approach to the study of laryngeal and pharyngeal function in infants. *Radiology* 92:758–762, 1969.
5. Han BK, Dunbar JS, Striker TW: Membranous laryngotracheobronchitis (membranous croup). *Am J Roentgenol* 133:53–58, 1979.
6. Hardwick DF, Cormode EJ, Riddell DG: Respiratory distress and neck mass in a neonate intratracheal thyroid. *J Pediatr* 89:591–605, 1976.
7. Holinger PH, Brown WT: Congenital webs, cysts, laryngoceles, and other anomalies of the larynx. *Ann Otol Rhinol Laryngol* 76:744–752, 1967.
8. Paparo GP, Smychych PS: Postintubation subglottic stenosis and cor pulmonale. *J Pediatr* 90:97–98, 1977.
9. Scott JR, Kramer SS: Pediatric tracheostomy: I. Radiographic features of normal healing. *Am J Roentgenol* 130:887–891, 1978.
10. Siegel MJ, McAlister WH: Tracheal histiocytoma; an inflammatory pseudotumor. *Can Assoc Radiol* 29:273–274, 1978.
11. Sutton TJ, Nogrady MB: Radiologic diagnosis of subglottic hemangioma in infants. *Pediatr Radiol* 1:211–215, 1973.

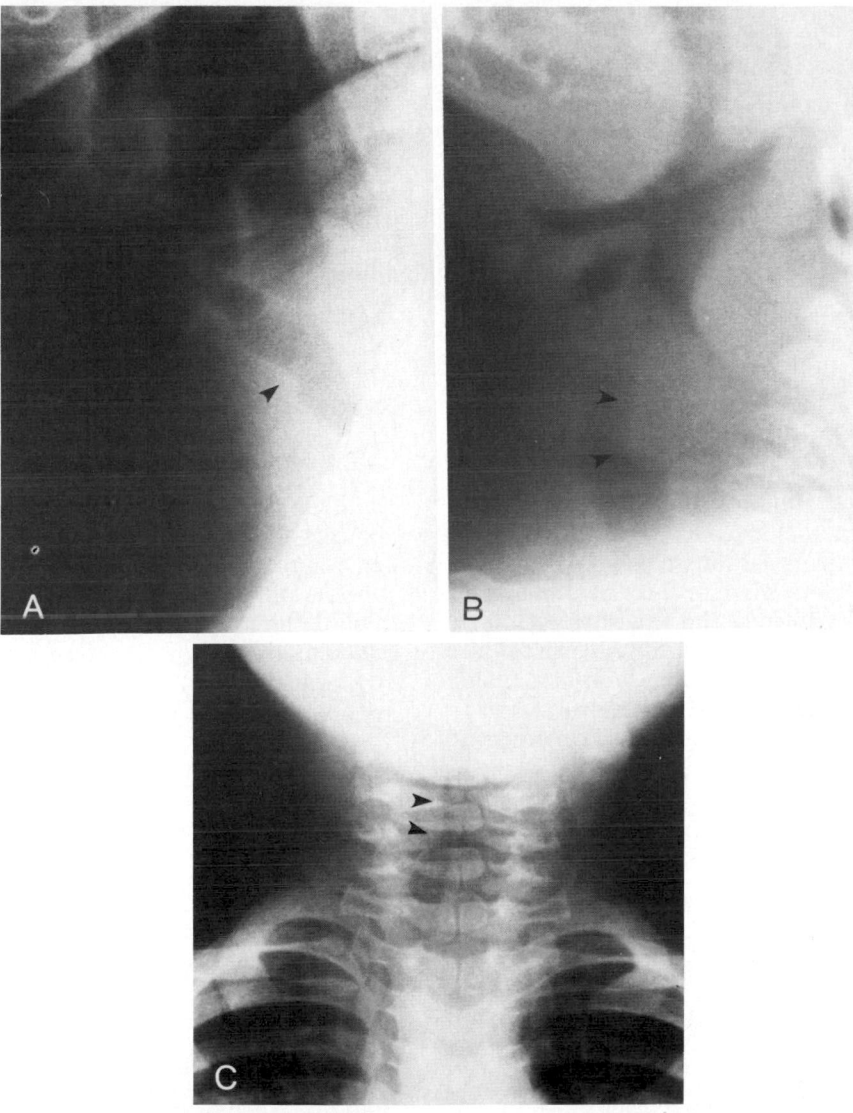

Fig. 2.11. Eccentric subglottic masses and narrowings. A. Normal anterior tracheal pseudomass (arrows). The exact etiology of this finding is unknown, but it is common. B. Posterior subglottic mass secondary to subglottic hemangioma (arrows). C. Another patient with a subglottic hemangioma producing eccentric lateral wall narrowing of the subglottic portion of the trachea (arrows).

CALCIFICATION OF UPPER AIRWAY CARTILAGE

Perhaps the commonest cause of calcification of the upper airway cartilages is that which is idiopathic (1). However, calcification also can be seen with chondrodysplasia punctata (stippled epiphyses) and idiopathic hypercalcemia (2, 3).

References

1. Russo PE, Coin CG: Calcification of the hyoid, thyroid, and tracheal cartilages in infancy. *Am J Roentgenol* 80:440–442, 1958.
2. Shiers JA, Neuhauser EBD, Bowman JR: Idiopathic hypercalcemia. *Am J Roentgenol* 78:19–29, 1957.
3. Swischuk LE: *Radiology of the Newborn and Young Infant*, ed 2. Baltimore, Williams & Wilkins, 1980, p 213.

MANDIBULAR ABNORMALITIES
Small Mandible (Micrognathia)

A small mandible usually is seen as part of the following syndromes: Pierre Robin syndrome, Goldenhar syndrome, Weyers mandibulofacial dysostosis, Treacher Collins mandibulofacial dysostosis, trisomy 17–18 and 13–15, and the cri-du-chat syndrome. In these conditions, mandibular hypoplasia involves both sides, but when it involves one side, the term hemifacial microsomia often is applied. A small mandible also can be seen with aglossia, cleidocranial dysostosis, pyknodysostosis, and some chondrodystrophies.

Large Mandible

The commonest cause of isolated enlargement of the mandible is fibrous dysplasia, or so-called cherubism (see Fig. 2.13B). The mandible also can enlarge with gigantism, but of course, such enlargement is not isolated to the mandible. Enlargement of the mandible also can occur with primary bony tumors, lymphoma (Burkett's), metastatic disease, histiocytosis-X, and cysts in the mandible.

Destructive Lesions of the Mandible

Destruction of the mandible can be seen with infection (Fig. 2.12A), histiocytosis-X, and tumor. Bone destruction in histiocytosis-X may be so widespread and "clean" that the teeth seem to float in an invisible matrix. This has been termed the floating teeth sign (Fig. 2.12B) and is seen, but less commonly, with other destructive lesions such as leukemia, lymphoma, and metastatic disease. A rarer cause of floating teeth is mandibular destruction secondary to hemangioma or lymphangioma of the mandible. Primary bone malignancies such as fibrosarcoma, osteosarcoma, and Ewing's sarcoma of the mandible are rare. Reparative granulomas (3) also can produce nonspecific destruction of the mandible, but more often, produce a multiloculated cystic lesion (see Fig. 2.13C). In addition to these findings, the teeth often also are destroyed with any of these lesions.

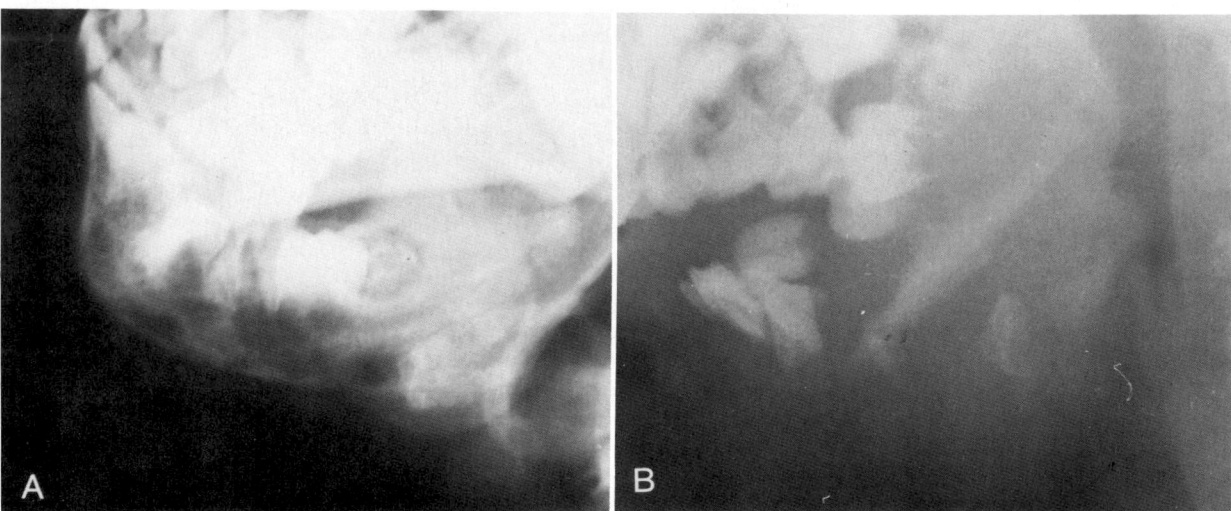

Fig. 2.12. Destructive lesions of the mandible. A. Widespread destruction due to osteomyelitis. B. Typical floating teeth due to widespread destruction in histiocytosis-X. From Swischuk LE: *Radiology of the Newborn and Young Infant*, ed 2. Baltimore, Williams and Wilkins, 1980.

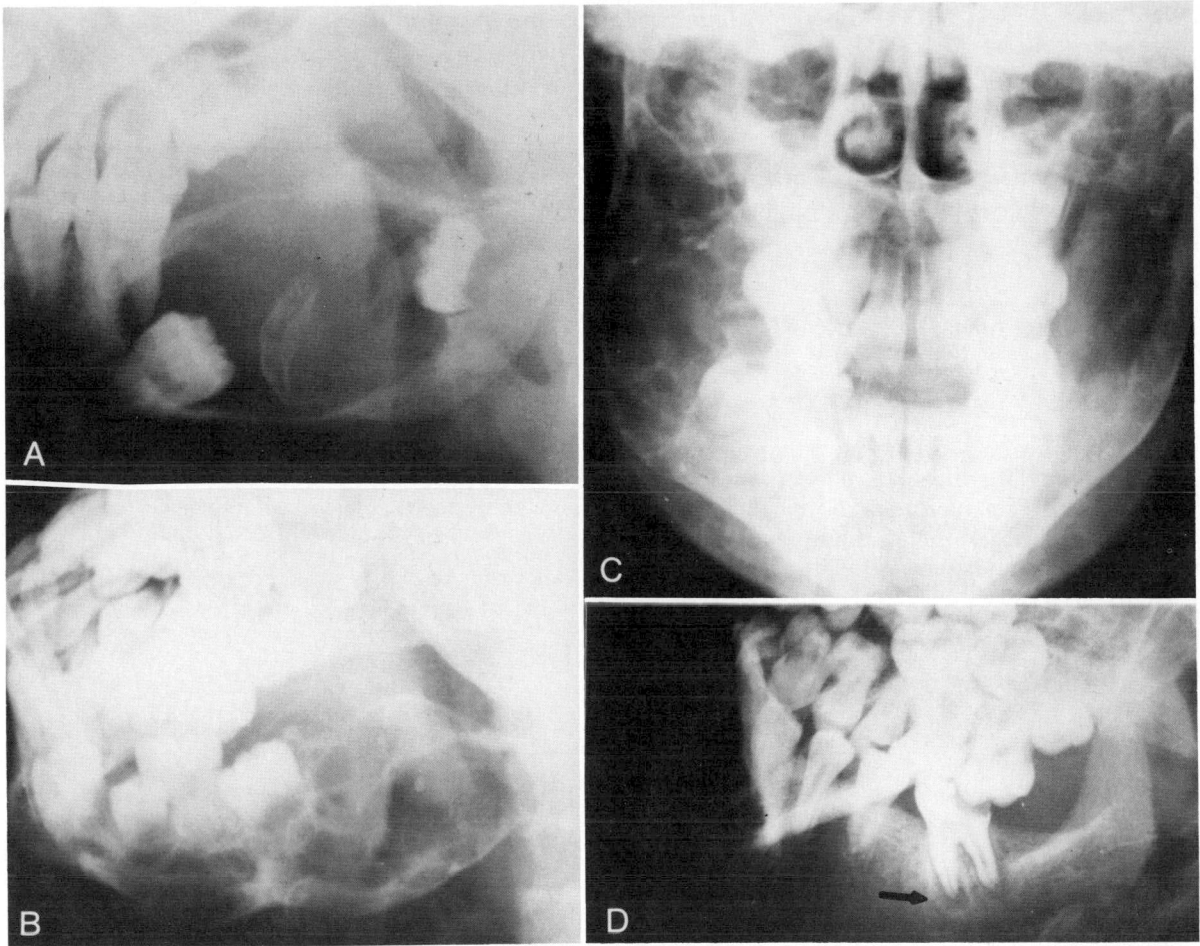

Fig. 2.13. Cystic lesions of the mandible. A. Typical, well demarcated, large dentigerous cyst in an 11-year-old child. Note the characteristic, ectopic tooth anteriorly. The posterior tooth is a normal, unerupted molar. B. Multiloculated lesion due to reparative granuloma of jaw in an 8-year-old. This lesion often also is called a giant cell tumor. Similar multiloculation can be seen with ameloblastomas. C. Fibrous dysplasia producing a multiloculated lesion on the right, and a more diffusely lytic lesion on the left. Note that the mandible is enlarged (cherubism). D. Periapical abscess or so-called radicular cyst (arrow) of a molar with a large carie.

Cysts of the Mandible

The most common cyst of the mandible is the dentigerous cyst. It is solitary, of variable size, demarcated by a sharp sclerotic margin, and associated with an ectopic tooth (Fig. 2.13A). It also has a clear-cut association with the basal cell naevus syndrome (2, 4). Other cysts are rather uncommon (5), except, perhaps, the so-called radicular cyst. This is not a true cyst, but rather an abscess cavity around a tooth root. Usually it is small and has indistinct margins (Fig.

2.13D). Occasionally, an ameloblastoma, or reparative granuloma (1, 3), can produce a near solitary cystic lesion, but most often both of these lesions produce multilocular cysts (Fig. 2.13B). The commonest cause of a multilocular cyst, however, is fibrous dysplasia (Fig. 2.13C). Giant cell tumors also produce multiloculated cystic lesions, but currently, most of these are believed to be reparative granulomas (3).

Increased Sclerosis of the Mandible

The commonest cause of **diffuse increased sclerosis** of the mandible is Caffey's disease, or infantile cortical hyperostosis (periosteal new bone deposition). However, sclerosis also can be seen with osteoblastic bone dysplasias such as osteopetrosis, pycnodysostosis, infantile hypercalcemia, and fibrous dysplasia.

Fibrous dysplasia also can produce **focal sclerosis** and other causes of focal sclerosis include histiocytosis-X (healing phase), chronic osteomyelitis, reactive periostitis with adjacent soft tissue infection (i.e., adenitis), and sclerosing tumors such as hemangiomas and odontomas.

Abnormalities of the Maxilla

For the most part, causes of cysts, tumors, destruction, increased sclerosis, etc., of the maxilla are the same as for the mandible. By the same token, a small or large maxilla occurs for the same reasons as does a small or large mandible, and consequently, almost anything that can be said for the mandible can be said for the maxilla.

References

1. Bhaskar SN: Oral tumors of infancy and childhood: a survey of 293 cases. *J Pediatr* 63:195–210, 1963.

2. Gorlin RJ, Goltz RN: Multiple nevoid basal-cell epithelioma, jaw cysts and bifid ribs: syndrome. *New Engl J Med* 262:908, 1960.
3. Jaffe HL: Giant cell reparative granuloma, traumatic bone cyst, and fibrous (fibro-osseous) dysplasia of the jaw bones. *Oral Surg* 6:159–175, 1953.
4. Rater CJ, Selke AC, Van Epps EF: Basal cell nevus syndrome. *Am J Roentgenol* 103:589–594, 1968.
5. Shafer WG: Cysts, neoplasms, and allied conditions of odontogenic origin. *Seminars Roentgenol* 6:403–413, 1971.

Hypoplasia of the Teeth

Hypoplasia or absence of the teeth can occur with the aglossia-adactylia syndrome, cliedocranial dysostosis, pyknodysostosis, ectodermal dysplasia (anhidrotic type) (1, 2), the otopalatodigital syndrome, hypoparathyroidism, and osteogenesis imperfecta (odontogenesis imperfecta) (3).

References

1. Capitanio MA, Chen JTT, Arey JB, Kirkpatrick JA:

Congenital anhidrotic ectodermal dysplasia. *Am J Roentgenol* 103:168–172, 1968.
2. Gwinn JL, Lee FA: Radiological case of the month (congenital anhidrotic ectodermal dysplasia). *Am J Dis Child* 128:215–216, 1974.
3. Taybi H: *Radiology of Syndromes.* Chicago, Year Book Medical Publishers, 1975.

Lamina Dura Abnormalities

The normal lamina dura is seen as a thin white line surrounding the tooth root or bud. In some children it is exceptionally dense, but yet normal (Fig. 2.14A.). It also may become more dense in hypoparathyroidism.

When it is indistinct, the most likely problems are hyperparathyroidism or severe rickets (Fig. 2.14B), but it also becomes somewhat indistinct with any cause of severe demineralization.

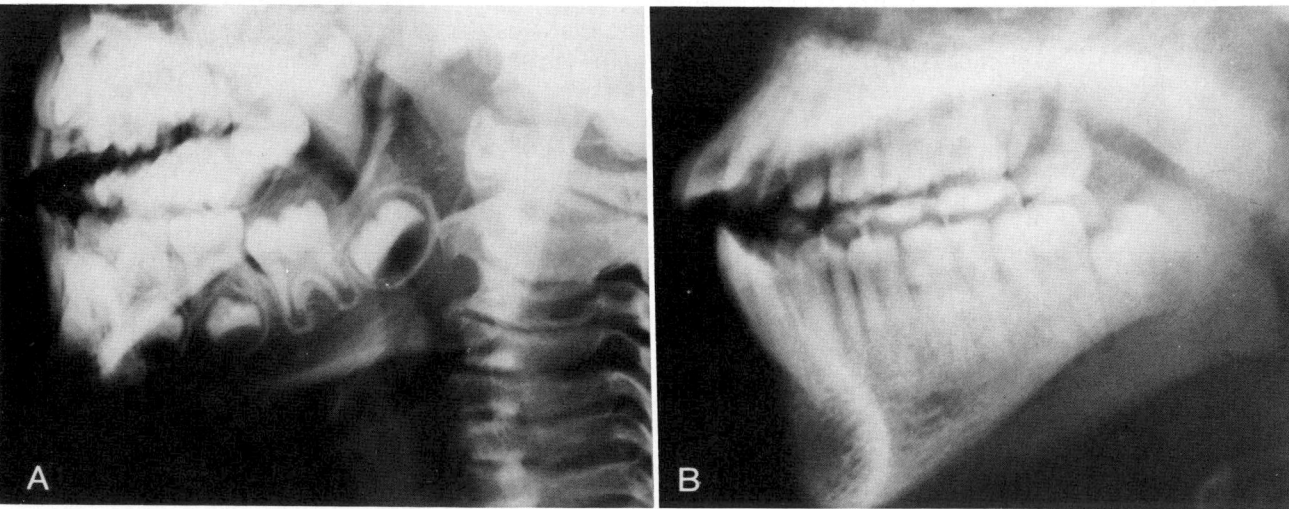

Fig. 2.14. Lamina dura abnormalities. A. Extremely dense lamina dura, occasionally seen in a normal child. B. Virtually invisible lamina dura in a patient with severe rickets.

PARANASAL SINUSES

The paranasal sinuses develop at different times, but ethmoid and maxillary sinus development occurs first. In this regard, these sinuses are present at birth, but of course, difficult to visualize and assess. Closely behind ethmoid and maxillary sinus development is sphenoid sinus development, and then, at about the age of 7 to 10 years, come the frontal sinuses. All of these facts are important in the assessment of sinus disease in children, but it is especially important to appreciate that maxillary and ethmoid sinus development occurs early, and that because of this, sinusitis under the age of 6 months is not uncommon at all.

Opacification of the Sinuses

Normally, the paranasal sinuses are aerated and radiolucent, and when they become opacified, they are diseased (1, 5). Opacification can be due to mucosal thickening, fluid accumulation (i.e., pus, blood), or tumor growth. It is highly unlikely that mucosal edema, from crying, can fill the sinus cavities so as to mimic abnormal opacification. Overall, the commonest causes of sinus cavity opacification are mucosal thickening and fluid accumulation (Fig. 2.15, A and B). The commonest fluid is the inflammatory exudate associated with acute sinusitis, while mucosal thickening most commonly occurs with allergy, infection,

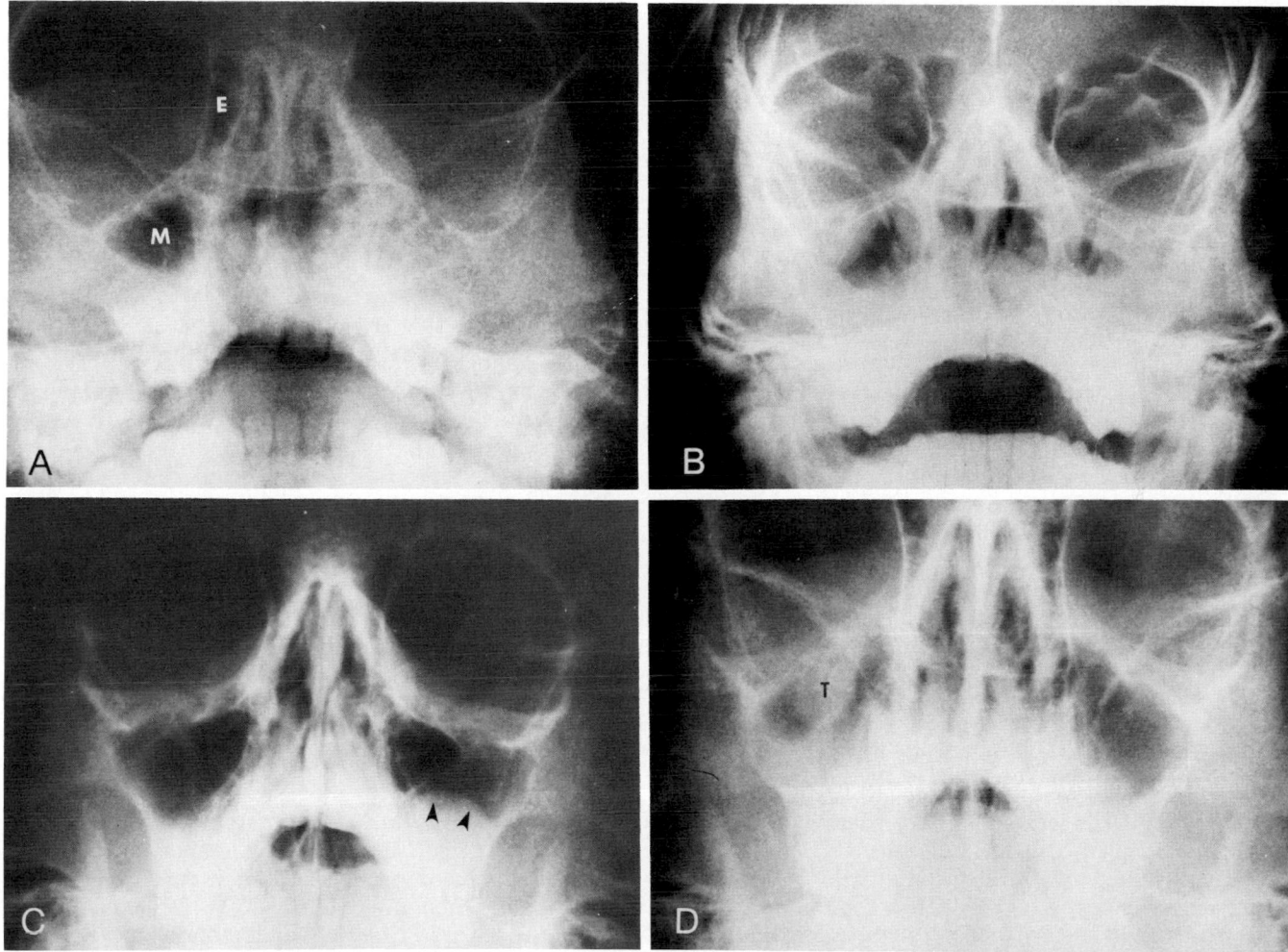

Fig. 2.15. Paranasal sinus obliteration and intrasinuosidal masses. A. The maxillary (M) and ethmoid (E) sinuses on the right are normal. On the left they are totally obliterated by inflammatory change. If they were obliterated on both sides there would be a tendency to say that they did not exist because "the patient is too young to have sinuses." Under such circumstances the roentgenographic diagnosis of sinusitis never would be made. B. Note mucosal thickening of the right maxillary sinus and an air fluid level on the left. C. Note retention cyst (arrows) rising from the floor of the left maxillary sinus. D. Partially obliterated right maxillary sinus and teardrop (T) configuration of blowout fracture.

or cystic fibrosis. Very often, with allergy, mucosal thickening is circumferential (i.e., small area of aeration in the center remains), while with acute sinusitis, on upright view, airfluid levels may be seen. Opacification of the sinuses also can occur with polyps, either on a sporadic allergic basis, or in association with cystic fibrosis (2). Rarely one can encounter the so-called antrochoanal polyp (6), a polyp which arises in the maxillary sinus, causes it to be opacified, and then extends, indeed dangles, as a mass, into the nasopharynx (see Fig. 2.3B).

Opacification by blood usually occurs with trauma to the face and nose, but occasionally can be seen with a bleeding disorder, or even a severe infection. Opacification of the sinuses by tumors arising within them is quite rare in children, and actually, it is more common for the tumor to arise from the bones around the sinus cavity. This is especially true of the maxillary and sphenoid cavities, and such tumors often turn out to be extensions of some soft tissue sarcoma, or a tumor of the lymphoma-leukemia group. Metastatic disease also might be considered, and rarely, the tumors may be odontogenic in origin.

Angiofibromas of the nasopharynx also can involve the sinuses, and depending on the size of the lesion, the maxillary, ethmoid, and sphenoid sinuses may be involved. These tumors may present with sinusitis and epistaxis, and the roentgenographic findings (especially the angiographic ones) are rather characteristic (see Fig. 2.2, A, B). After angiofibroma, the next most common tumor arising in the nasopharynx is the lymphoepithelioma, but sinus involvement with this tumor is less common. Opacification of the sinuses also can occur with mucoceles (4), and with the rare, Wegener's granulomatosis (3).

Sinus Wall Destruction

Destruction of the paranasal sinus walls occurs primarily with infection and tumor, and of course, most often the sinus cavity itself is opacified. Tumor destruction probably is more common, for infection of the order which would lead to osteomyelitis and bone destruction is not that common these days. Tumors which destroy the paranasal sinus walls usually turn out to be some sort of sarcoma, lymphoma, leukemia, or metastatic disease. Rarely, hemangiomas, lymphangiomas, or odontogenic tumors can produce destruction. Destruction also can occur with mucoceles (4), but these generally are uncommon in children, and sinus destruction also occurs with Wegener's granulomatosis (3), and histiocytosis-X.

Masses in the Paranasal Sinuses

The commonest mass seen in a paranasal sinus is a postinflammatory retention cyst and, most commonly, this cyst occurs in the maxillary sinuses, often along the floor (Fig. 2.15C). These cysts usually are smooth-edged, round, or half-moon shaped, and not associated with bony destruction. They result from the postinflammatory blockage or mucous glands. Less commonly, one can encounter mucoceles of the paranasal sinuses, either inflammatory or posttraumatic in origin. These lesions result from the blockage of the main draining ducts of the sinuses and, actually, more often than producing intrasinusoidal masses, they produce sinusoidal opacification and expansion. In this regard, ethmoid and sphenoid sinus involvement is most common in children (4). Masses due to tumors and polyps of the sinus cavities are less common than those due to retention cysts.

Finally, a very specific mass occurring in the maxillary sinus is that associated with a blowout fracture of the orbit. In these cases, blunt trauma to the orbit forces intraorbital contents through the thin floor of the orbit (i.e., roof or maxillary sinus), and the soft tissues so displaced, project as a mass (i.e., tear drop) from the roof of the maxillary sinus (Fig. 2.15D). Laminography often is most helpful in demonstrating these and other mass lesions of the sinus cavities.

Asymmetry of Sinus Cavities

Asymmetry can involve size, density, or configuration. Normally, the frontal sinuses are very asymmetric both in terms of size and radiolucency. The sphenoid sinus cavities also tend to be a little asymmetric as far as size is concerned, but the ethmoid and maxillary sinus cavities (especially the maxillary) usually are symmetric in all respects. With the frontal sinuses, unequal, but normal, unilateral thickening of the bone overlying the sinus cavities can lead to apparent asymmetry of aeration, but with the other sinus cavities, if asymmetry of density exists, underlying disease should be suspected (i.e., infection with exudate or mucosal edema, trauma with blood, tumors, polyps, etc).

A pitfall to avoid in the assessment of sinus size asymmetry, especially with the maxillary sinus cavities, is not to interpret a sinus cavity as being congenitally small, when actually it just appears that way because it is incompletely aerated or encroached upon by mucosal thickening (Fig. 2.15B). Indeed, since in most of these cases, associated demineralization of the sinus wall (common with infection and inflammation) renders it indistinct, it is difficult not to think that the sinus cavity simply is not there. For these reasons, then, it is easy to make the erroneous interpretation that the small central triangle of remaining radiolucency is the true sinus cavity.

Enlargement of a sinus on one or another side can be seen with intrasinusoidal expanding lesions such as mucoceles (4), large polyps, and occasionally, intrasinusoidal tumors. Distortion of sinus shape can be seen with trauma, neurofibromatosis, or less commonly, with deforming tumors of the face.

References

1. Kogutt MS, Swischuk LE: Diagnosis of sinusitis in infants and children. *Pediatrics* 52:121–124, 1973.
2. Ledesma-Medina J, Osman MZ, Girdany BR: Abnormal paranasal sinuses in patients with cystic fibrosis of the pancreas. Radiological findings. *Pediatr Radiol* 9:61–64, 1980.
3. Orlowski JP, Clough JD, Dyment PG: Wegener's granulomatosis in the pediatric age group. *Pediatrics* 61:83–90, 1978.
4. Siegel MJ, Shackelford GD, McAlister WH: Paranasal sinus mucoceles in children. *Radiology* 133:623–626, 1979.
5. Swischuk LE: *Emergency Radiology of the Acutely Ill or Injured Child.* Baltimore, Williams & Wilkins, 1979, pp 131–134.
6. Towbin R, Dunbar JS, Bove K: Antrochoanal polyps. *Am J Roentgenol* 132:27–31, 1979.

SOFT TISSUES OF THE NECK

The soft tissues of the anterior and lateral parts of the neck seldom are examined roentgenographically, but **generalized increased soft tissue bulk, or an actual mass,** are not uncommon and can be seen with cervical adenopathy and a variety of soft tissue tumors. Clear-cut masses anterior, or lateral, to the trachea can be seen with lesions such as thyroid cysts, sublingual thyroid (Fig. 2.16), and branchial cleft cysts.

Some of these cysts can be injected via communicating sinus tracts opening into the skin, but probably are best demonstrated with ultrasound or CT scans. **Calcifications of the soft tissues of the neck** most often occur in inflamed lymph nodes, but occasionally can be seen with chronic infections of the salivary glands. Very rarely, they may be seen in an underlying cervical teratoma.

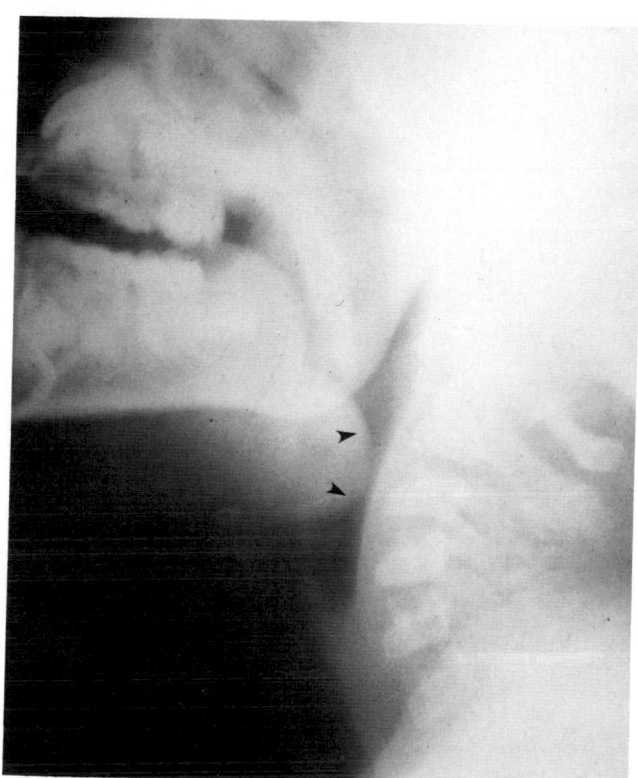

Fig. 2.16. Neck masses. Note the large sublingual thyroid (arrows) projecting into the hypopharynx (courtesy M. H. Schreiber, M.D., Galveston, Texas).

Chapter 3

ABDOMEN

ABDOMINAL MASSES

Childhood abdominal masses are common, and currently, a number of investigative modalities are available for their detection. A complete dicussion of each of these is beyond the scope of this book, but in Figure 3.1, a summary of mass location, its most likely organ of origin, and the most productive investigative studies for its investigation is presented. This, or a similar, orientation is helpful as it facilitates a more rapid and efficient investigation. In the past, the intravenous pylogram was the mainstay of one's radiologic workup, but now, ultrasonography usually is the first screening procedure. It has the advantage of not having to use ionizing radiation and also that it is totally noninvasive. Its main drawbacks are that it is operator dependent (especially realtime scanning) and that abdominal gas can interfere with the obtaining of satis-factory images. However, these problems usually are circumvented, and overall, ultrasonography has had a major impact on investigation of abdominal masses in children. Indeed, much more so than computerized tomography (CT scanning). In the future, however, NMR probably will play a greater role than CT does today. A summary of ultrasound and CT findings is presented in Table 3.1A.

Information immediately available with ultrasonography includes (a) location of the mass and (b) whether it is solid or cystic. In many cases, for purely diagnostic purposes, the investigation could stop at this point, but for one reason or another, valid or not, another study almost always is obtained. Just which study this is depends on the location of the mass. For example, if the mass is in the right upper quadrant, isotope

ABDOMINAL MASSES

ZONES

⑥ ANYWHERE

ZONE	MOST LIKELY CAUSE OR ORGAN OF ORIGIN		MOST PRODUCTIVE STUDIES (after plain films)	
1	Liver	(++++)	Ultrasound – CAT[a]	(++++)
	Gallbladder	(++++)	Isotopes	(++++)
	Bile Duct	(++++)	Angiography	(+++)
	Duodenum	(++)	GI Series	(++)
	Adrenal	(+)	IVP	(+)
2	Spleen	(++++)	Ultrasound	(++++)
	Stomach	(++++)	GI Series – CAT[a]	(+++)
	Adrenal	(+)	Angiography	(+++)
			Isotopes	(++)
			IVP	(+)
3	Adrenal	(++++)	Ultrasound–CAT[a]	(++++)
	Pancreas	(++++)	IVP	(++++)
	Liver	(++++)	GI Series	(++)
	Stomach	(++++)	Angiography	(++)
	Kidney	(++)	Isotopes	(+)
4	Kidney	(++++)	IVP	(++++)
	Adrenal	(++)	Ultrasound –CAT[a]	(++++)
	Retroperit Tumor	(++++)	Angiography	(++++)
5	Bladder	(++++)	Cystogram	(++++)
	Uterus·Vagina	(++++)	IVP	(++++)
	Ovaries	(++++)	Ultrasound–CAT[a]	(++++)
	Presacral Masses	(++++)	Barium Enema	(++)
			Angiography	(+++)
			Myelography	(++++)
6	Mesenteric Cysts	(++++)	Ultrasound–CAT[a]	(++++)
	Omental Cysts	(++++)	GI Series	(++)
	Duplication Cysts	(++++)	Barium Enema	(++)
			Angiography	(++)

[a]NMR should be useful where CT is useful.

Fig. 3.1. Abdominal masses: roentgenographic approach. The abdomen has been divided into zones and, then, for each zone the most likely glands of origin and most productive investigative procedures are outlined.

Table 3.1A   Abdominal Masses

Tissue or Organ	Ultrasound			Computed Tomography			
	Sonolucent, anechoic	Echoic	Mixed complex	Muscle density (gray)	Bone density calcium (white)	Air, fat, fluid density (Dk gray-black)	Enhancement with contrast
Free fluid^e	+	0	0	0	0	+	0
Blood CNS (fresh)	+	0	0	0	+ (most)	0	0
Blood CNS (old)	0	+	+	+	0	0 (most)	0
Blood in vessels and organs	+	0	0	+	0	0	+
Abscess, empyema (fresh)	+	0	0	±	0	0 (most)	+ (rim)
Abscess, empyema (old)	0	+	+	±	0	+	+ (rim)
Muscle	+	0	0	+	0	0	+
Fat	0	+	+	0	0	+	0
Calcium (fine parenchymal)	0	+^a	0	0	+	0	0
Calcium (calculi)	0	+^a	0	0	+	0	0
Bone	0	+^a	0	0	+	0	0
Fibrosis, cirrhosis	0	+	0	+	0	0	±
Hemachromatosis	0	+	0	0	+	0	±
Air and gas	0	+	0	0	0	+	0
Hematoma—new	+	0	0	+	+	+	0
Hematoma—old	0	+	+	+	0	+	0
Thrombus	0	+^b	+^b	+	0	+	0
Neoplasm (solid)	0^c	+	+	+	0	+ (most)	+ (most)
Neoplasm (cystic)	+	0	±	+	0	0	0
Adenopathy	+^c	0	+	+	0	0	0
Lymphangioma	0	+	+^d	+	0	+	0
Hemangioma	0	+	+^d	+	0	+	+
Cyst (simple)	+	0	0	0	0	+	0
Multiple cysts (large)	0	0	+^d	+	0	+	0
Multiple cysts (small-micro)	0	+	+	+	0	0	0
Pseudocysts	+	0	+ (old)	0	0	+	+ (rim)

^a Causes shadowing.
^b Organized.
^c If gain too high, especially lymphoma.
^d With septations or loculations.
^e Blood, serous, chyle, urine, bile.

studies are most productive (i.e., the most likely organs of origin are the liver or biliary tract) but if the mass is suspected to be of renal origin, an IVP and, often, a voiding cystogram are obtained. The voiding cystogram is obtained when reflux or lower urinary tract obstruction are suspected as causes of hydronephrosis. The IVP can be augmented by total body opacification, a phenomenon occurring within the first 1 or 2 min after infection. During this time, as the organs blush, one can determine how well they or a mass are being perfused. In other words, one obtains some idea of whether the mass is vascular or avascular and, in effect, total body opacification is just a poor man's arteriogram. However, with the advent of ultrasonography, CT scanning, and nuclear magnetic resonance, it is being relied on less and less for this purpose. In addition to augmentation of the IVP by total body opacification, an inferior vena cavagram can be obtained, but once again, many times the inferior vena cava can be visualized with one or more of the new modalities. Information which can be obtained regarding the inferior vena cava includes displacement, compression, and intraluminal obstruction (i.e., thrombus, Wilm's tumor extension from the kidney, etc.).

If a mass in retroperitoneal, but nonrenal, the IVP is of lesser value and, currently, contrast-enhanced computerized tomography, NMR, and ultrasound are more the choices for retroperitoneal masses. In many of these cases, CT and NMR might be preferred over ultrasonography, for they offer more precise delineation of tumor extent (i.e., in neuroblastoma, retroperitoneal lymphoma, and other retroperitoneal sarcomas).

If a mass is believed to be in the gastrointestinal tract, a barium enema or upper GI series can be obtained, but if the lesion is believed to be in the mesentery, CT scanning and NMR are more productive. Pelvic masses can be investigated with CT scanning and NMR if ultrasonographic studies are inconclusive. Cystograms and intravenous pylograms usually provide indirect information only.

Angiography usually is relegated to those masses where delineation of the vascular supply of the mass is critical to its diagnosis and/or treatment. In this regard, it has its greatest role in the investigation of

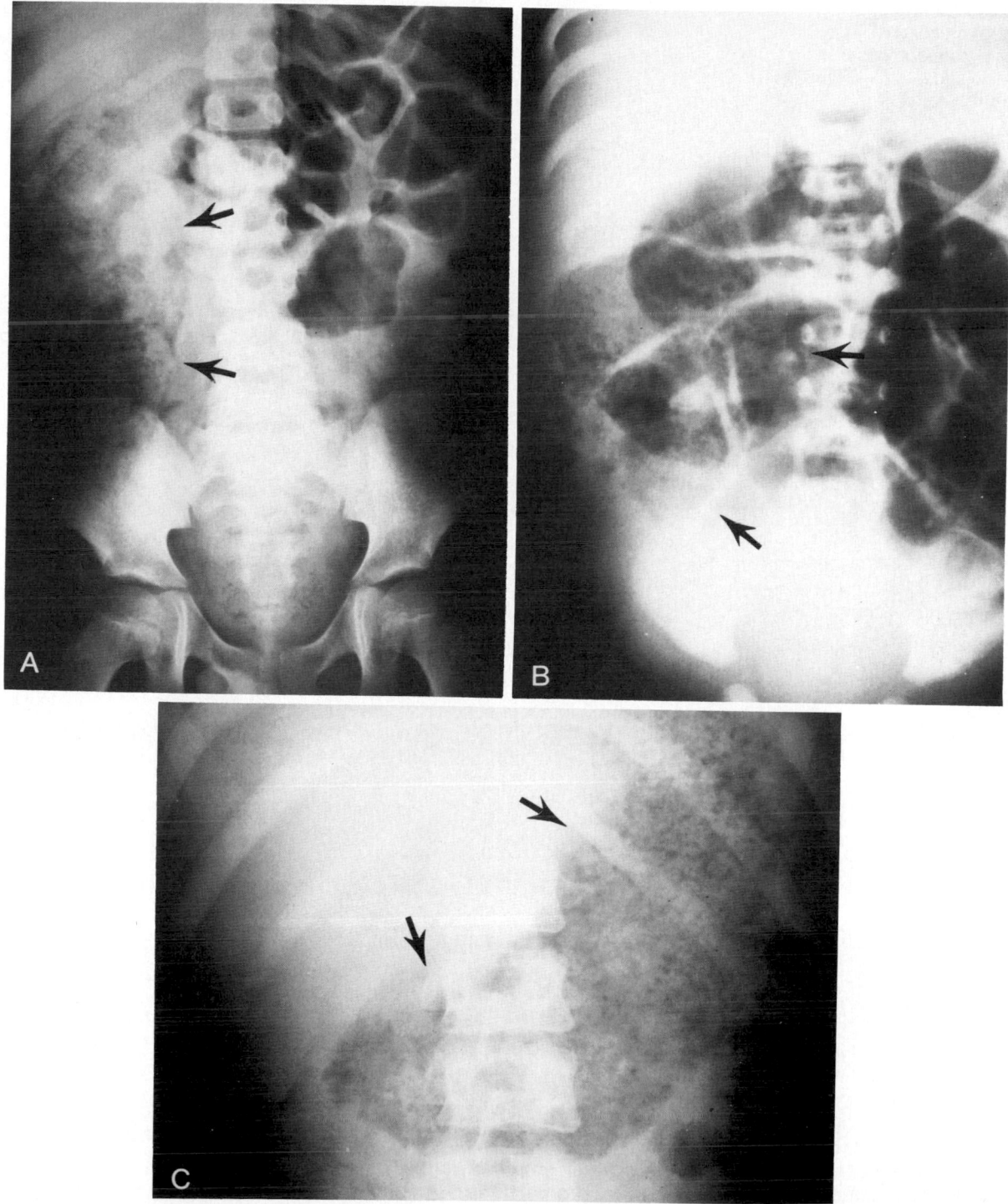

Fig. 3.2. Granular masses. A. Feces in colon (arrows). B. Abdominal abscess (arrows) secondary to idiopathic (ischemic) small bowel perforation in infant. C. Granular appearing food in stomach (arrows). Bezoars have a similar appearance.

Table 3.1B Abdominal Masses

Granular abdominal masses		
Food in stomach	}	Commonest
Feces in colon		
Intra-abdominal abscess	}	Moderately common
Bezoar	}	Relatively rare
Localized pneumatosis		
Large diverticulum		
Abdominal pseudomasses		
Urinary bladder	}	Commonest
Fluid-filled stomach		
Umbilical hernia	}	Moderately common
Meningomyelocele		
Fluid-filled intestine		
Large skin lesion	}	Relatively rare

liver masses, especially tumors. It is utilized less often with other tumors in the abdomen, especially now that ultrasonography, CT scanning, and nuclear magnetic resonance are available.

On **plain films**, the **roentgenographic identification of an abdominal mass** depends on noting (*a*) actual enlargement of the involved organ, (*b*) secondary displacement of gas-filled portions of the gastrointestinal tract, (*c*) displacement or obliteration of other organs or structures by the mass, and (*d*) occasionally, bone erosion or destruction (i.e., rib, vertebral body, pelvis). In addition, some masses may show calcification, some may show increased density, and others appear granular (Fig. 3.2). Calcifications and density abnormalities are dealt with in later sections, and as far as granularity of a mass is concerned, it usually indicates that air is mixed with some solid material (Table 3.1B). Basically, the solid material can be food,

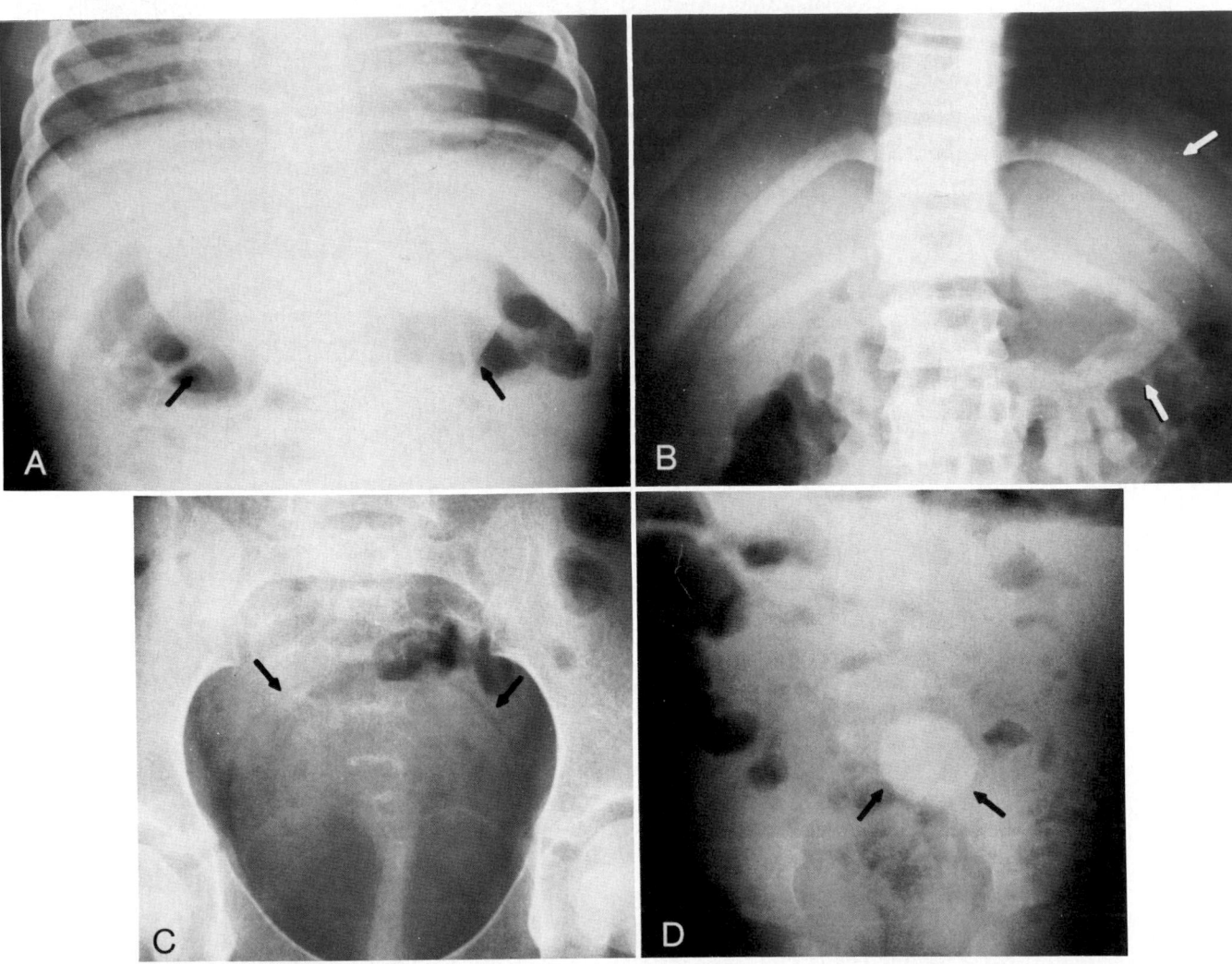

Fig. 3.3. Abdominal pseudotumors. A. Fluid-filled stomach (arrows), in upright position, producing a pseudomass. B. pseudomass produced by food in fundus of stomach (arrows) C. Pseudomass produced by distended normal urinary bladder (arrows). D. Pseudomass produced by umbilical hernia (arrows). A similar pseudomass can be seen with meningoceles.

feces, or purulent exudate (pus), but most commonly, it is a pseudomass due to food in the stomach or fecal material in the colon (Fig. 3.2). In either of these cases, it may be impossible, on roentgenographic grounds alone, to differentiate the findings from those of an intra-abdominal abscess, the next most common cause of a granular appearing adominal mass (Fig. 3.2B). Less commonly, a granular mass can be the result of a bezoar (3, 4), a lesion usually occurring in the stomach, but occasionally, both in the stomach and small intestine. At either site, obstruction can result and, in addition, bleeding from associated ulceration can occur. A relatively rare cause of a granular appearing abdominal mass is an area of localized pneumatosis cystoides intestinalis (i.e., intramural gas). Such localized pneumatosis cystoides intestinalis is most commonly seen in the neonatal period with necrotizing enterocolitis. A final, and rare, cause of a

large granular mass is a large, impacted, diverticulum. Most often this occurs in infancy with a Meckel's diverticulum.

In addition to considering true masses in the abdomen, one also must be aware of certain common pseudomasses (Table 3.1B). The commonest of these are the fluid-filled urinary bladder and fluid-filled stomach (Fig. 3.3). However, another common pseudomass usually seen in infancy is an umbilical hernia (Fig. 3.3D); and when the hernia contains air-filled intestine, the mass appears bubbly. A similar central pseudomass can be seen in infants with a meningocele or meningomycele, and in neonates with an umbilical stump. Other less common causes of pseudomasses include fluid-filled loops of intestine, colostomy or ileostomy openings, and over-lying skin lesions such as hemangiomas and neurofibromas.

ABDOMINAL CALCIFICATIONS AND OTHER OPACITIES

Abdominal calcifications are not rare in children, and basically can be (a) irregular, amorphous, or flocculent; (b) curvilinear; (c) punctate; (d) stone or stone-like; and (e) formed (i.e., bones, teeth, etc.) (Table 3.2).

Table 3.2 Intra-Abdominal Calcifications and Opacities

Irregular—Flocculent		
Tumors (especially neuroblastoma) (1)	Commonest	
Idiopathic adrenal (2)		
Foreign material (pica) (1)	Moderately common	
Venous thrombi (2)		
Liver, postabscess, postthrombus (2)		
Papillary necrosis kidney (2)	Relatively rare	
Lymph nodes (2)		
Infarct spleen, liver, kidney, intestine, etc.		
Bladder (schistosomiasis, cytoxan)		
Oxalosis (kidney)		
Hamartoma (2)		
Prostate		
Necrotic bowel—old (2)	Rare	
Infarcted ovary (2)		
Infarcted abdominal testes (2)		
Pancreatitis (1)		
Curvilinear		
Cystic tumors		
Posthemorrhagic outline of adrenal gland	Moderately common	

Residual meconium peritonitis from neonate		
Hydronephrosis	Relatively rare	
Cystic kidney or other cyst		
Renal cortical necrosis		
Stones or stone-like densities		
Fecalith in appendix	Commonest	
Urinary tract stones		
Gall stones	Moderately common	
Ingested pebbles		
Granulomas in spleen, liver		
Phleboliths		
Medullary sponge kidney	Rare	
Ingested mercury, chromium salts		
Formed calcification		
Teratoma-dermoid	Commonest	
Staghorn calculi	Rare	
Fetus in fetu	Very rare	
Miscellaneous—diffuse of organ		
Milk of calcium gallbladder or hydronephrotic kidney		
Diffuse kidney, oxalosis, RTA, chronic glomerulo	Rare	
Wolman's disease of adrenal gland		
Hemochromatosis liver		

(1), generalized or focal; (2), focal.

Irregular Amorphous or Flocculent Calcifications

For the most part, this type of calcifications is seen with tumor necrosis, infection, inflammation, venous thrombosis, hemorrhage, or infarction. Necrosis within a tumor, however, probably is most common, and most often is seen with a neuroblastoma (Fig. 3.4A). These calcifications can be finely granular or more irregular and flocculent, and actually, sooner or later can be seen with almost any intra-abdominal tumor (i.e., hepatoblastoma, hepatic hemangioma, teratoma, dermoid (Fig. 3.4B), Wilm's tumor, other adrenal tumors, etc.). None, however, demonstrate irregular calcifications as often as does neuroblastoma or its more mature relative, the ganglioneuroma.

Postinflammatory irregular calcifications can occur in lymph nodes (Fig 3.4D) and in the liver (13) and spleen. Less commonly, they occur in the kidney, and rarely in the prostate gland (19). In the liver, postinflammatory or catheterization-induced calcifications can remain after the neonatal period (1, 3, 33). Posthemorrhagic calcifications can occur in any organ, but most commonly are seen in the adrenal gland. Such hemorrhage occurs at birth, and since the residual calcification often is discovered as an incidental finding, it has been termed idiopathic adrenal gland calcification (20). In truth, however, it is posthemorrhagic in nature and, in some cases, the calcification can be peripherally curvilinear and in the triangular shape of the adrenal gland. These features, (especially on the right) together with the characteristic location, make these calcifications rather pathognomonic (Fig. 3.4C). Other irregular calcifications can be seen in conditions such as renal papillary necrosis (sepsis,

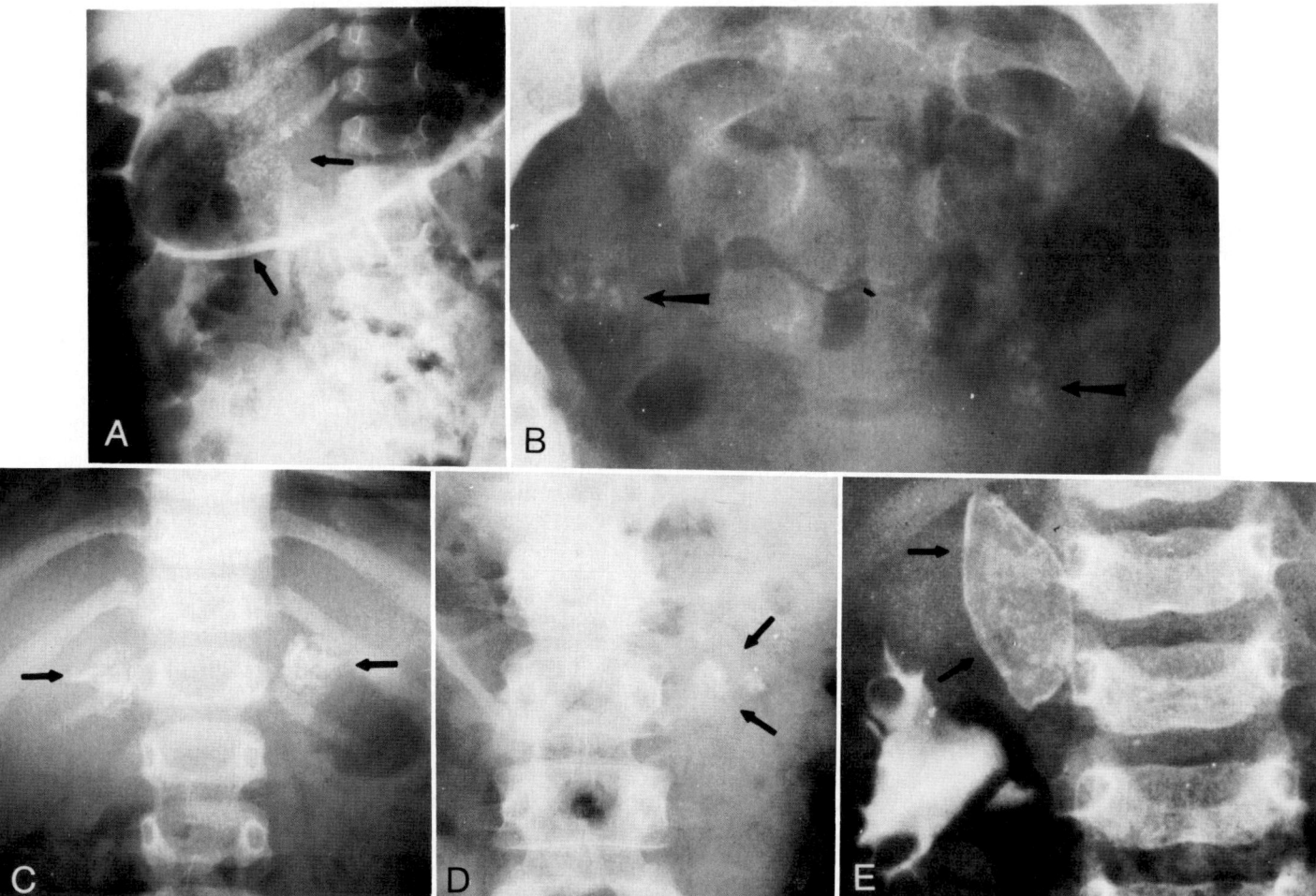

Fig. 3.4. Irregular abdominal calcifications. A. Irregular amorphous calcifications within a ganglioneuroblastoma (arrows). B. Irregular calcifications in bilateral ovarian dermoids (arrows). C. Typical idiopathic (posthemorrhagic) adrenal calcifications (arrows). Note the almost triangular shape of the right gland. D. Irregular calcifications in old inflammed abdominal lymph nodes (arrow). E. Typical bullet-shaped calcification of venous thrombus in the inferior vena cava (arrows). From: Kassner EG, Baumstark A, Kinkhabwala MN, Ablow RC, Haller JO: Pediatr Radiol 4:167–171, 1976.

dehydration, collagen vascular disease, sickle cell disease, diabetes), renal tubular acidosis (distal tubular type), and oxalosis (Fig. 3.5, A and B) (8, 22, 27, 37, 40, 42). In addition, intrarenal calcifications can occur with any number of hypercalcemia states including hyperparathyroidism, hypervitaminosis D, severe osteoporosis, steroid therapy, the milk-alkali syndrome, ileal dysfunction (22), and sarcoidosis (4, 10).

Rarely, focally regular calcifications can be seen with hamartomas of the liver or spleen, or as residual calcifications from perinatal intestinal ischemia, perforation, or meconium peritonitis. Migrating calcifications can occur with idiopathically amputated ovaries in girls (7, 26), and infarcted intra-abdominal testes in young male infants also can produce focal irregular calcifications. Similar calcifications also can occur after infarction in organs such as the liver,

spleen, kidney, intestine, etc. Irregular calcifications, of a more diffuse nature, occur with chronic pancreatitis (18). However, the situation is quite rare in children but can occur alone or in association with cystic fibrosis (81). The pancreatic distribution of the calcifications is a clue to their diagnosis (Fig. 3.5C). Calcifications secondary to thrombi of the portal vein, inferior vena cava, or renal vein are a little more common (13, 14, 21, 32, 34, 35, 39, 43) and often are bullet-shaped. Indeed, their appearance is quite diagnostic (Fig. 3.4D). Calcifications of the urinary bladder secondary to inflammations or infections such as schistosomiasis, and cytoxan cystitis also can be encountered, but all are rare.

Although not true intra-abdominal calcifications, certain other intra-adominal opacities can mimic calcifications. For the most part, these are opacities in

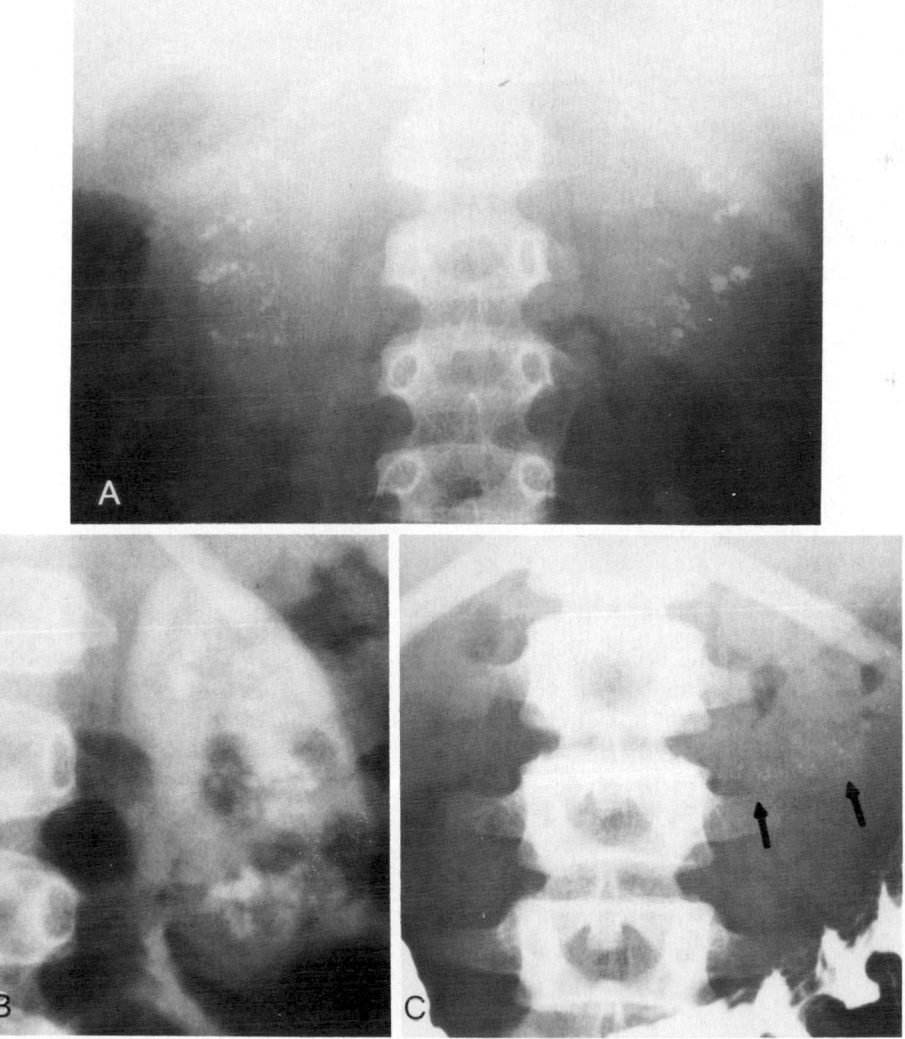

Fig. 3.5.   Irregular abdominal calcifications. A. Typical irregular calcifications in both kidneys due to renal tubular acidosis. B. Similar irregular calcifications in patient with oxalosis. Also, note diffuse, homogeneous parenchymal calcification of both kidneys. This was a scout film. C. Small scattered calcifications in the pancreas (arrows) in this 12-year-old girl with chronic pancreatitis.

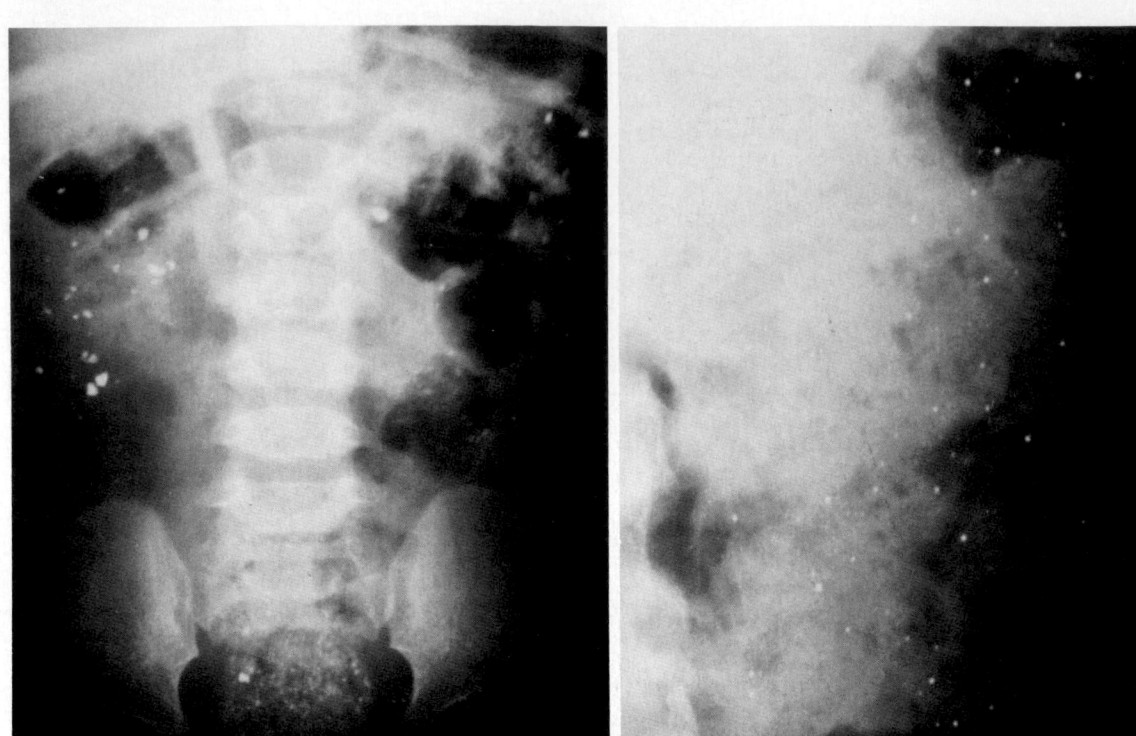

Fig. 3.6. Scattered abdominal opacities. A. Diffuse opacities (dirt) scattered throughout the colon in this "dirt eater." Similar densities can be seen with lead ingestion and bismuth containing medications. B. Small globules in the G.I. tract secondary to mercury ingestion.

the intestinal tract, and one of the most common causes is dirt eating or pica (2, 9) (Fig. 3.6A). Similar densities can be seen with lead ingestion (i.e., paint chips), bismuth-containing medications, mercury, and chromium compounds. The latter two tend to form small globules within the gastrointestinal tract (Fig. 3.6B). Of all of these, dirt eating is most common, but ingestion of bismuth-containing medications is not rare because they commonly are used to treat gastroenteritis. Neither one, however, leads to serious problems; but, with chromium compounds, dire sequellae, including death, are common.

Curvilinear Calcifications

These calcifications, apart from those seen with meconium periotonitis in the neonatal period, are quite rare. They can, however, be seen in the periphery of contracting adrenal gland hemorrhages, and on rare occasions, in hydronephrotic or multicystic kidneys (24) (Fig. 3.7A). They also can be seen with renal cortical necrosis (25, 44) (Fig. 3.7C) and cystic, abdominal tumors. Although the tumor can be of any type, there is a certain propensity for it to be a neonatal adrenal cortical carcinoma (37) (Fig. 3.7B). With renal cortical necrosis, if calcification is incomplete, it may appear irregular. By the same token, when it is very complete and surrounds the kidney, diffuse calcification of the renal parenchyma can be mimicked (Fig. 3.7C).

Very rarely, curvilinear calcifications can be seen in the wall of a urinary bladder with schistosomiasis or hemorrhagic cystitis after cytoxan therapy. Clearly, these latter two situations are rather rare, and by the same token, so are curvilinear calcifications within the blood vessels of the abdomen.

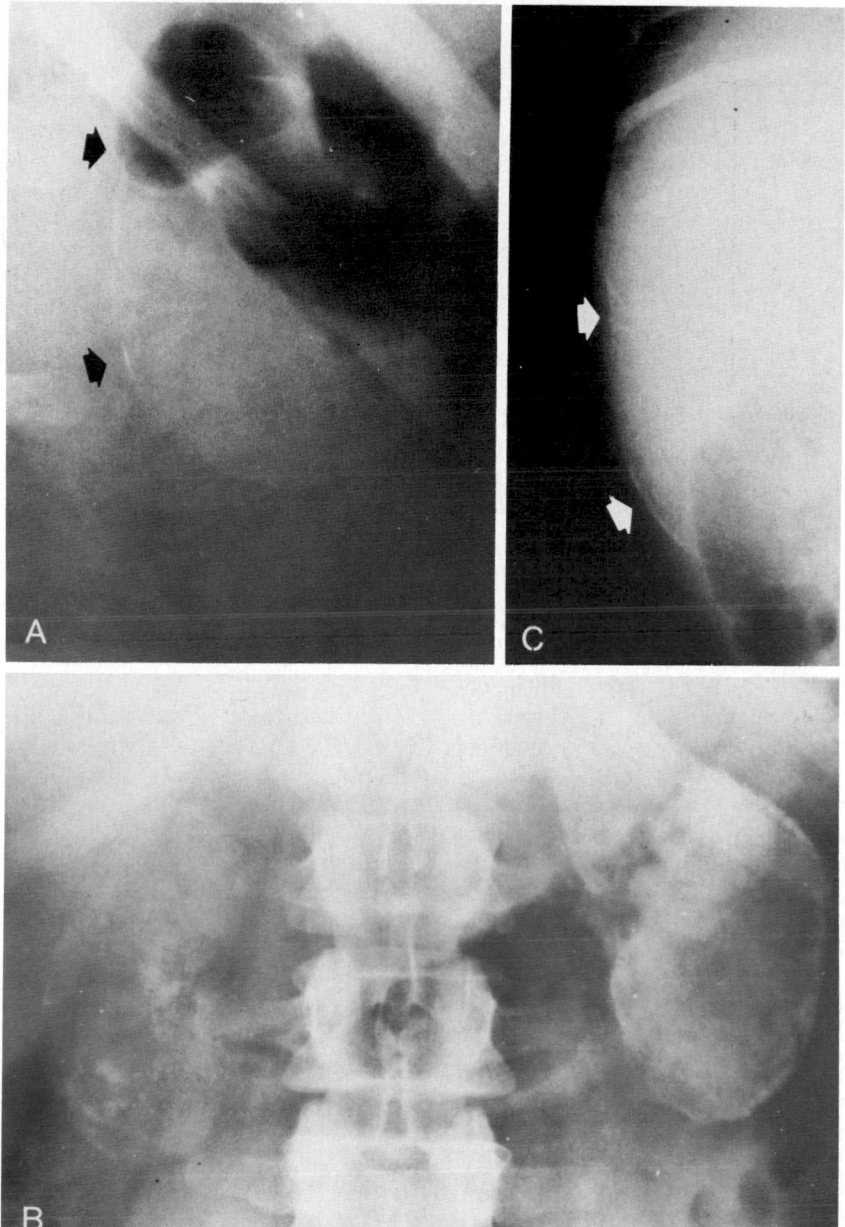

Fig. 3.7. Curvilinear calcifications. A. Curvilinear calcification in cystic kidney (arrows); 13-year-old child. B. Cuvilinear rim-like calcification in the periphery of an adrenal cortical carcinoma in a neonate (arrows). C. Curvilinear calcifications outlining the kidney in renal cortical necrosis. On the right the calcification is less complete and appears somewhat fragmented and irregular. On the left it is more complete and, because it surrounds the entire kidney, appears somewhat homogeneous. Fig. B Courtesy Dr. Charles Hendrick, Amarillo, Texas.

Stones, Stone-Like, and Punctate Calcifications

Calcified stones occur in the urinary tract, biliary tract, appendix (12, 41), and Meckel's diverticula (17). Those in the appendix (fecaliths) are most common (Fig. 3.8A), and those in Meckel's diverticula are least common. After appendiceal fecaliths, urinary tract stones come next (Fig. 3.8B), and of these, renal and ureteral stones are more common than bladder stones (27, 40). Actually, bladder stones tend to occur, almost

exclusively, in chronically immobilized children (10), and as a rule are quite large (Fig. 3.8C). Those in the upper tract, on the other hand, usually are small and, for this reason, just as difficult to detect as in the adult.

In children, most renal stones have been said to be associated with urinary tract infection, obstruction, or hypercalcemic, metabolic states such as idiopathic

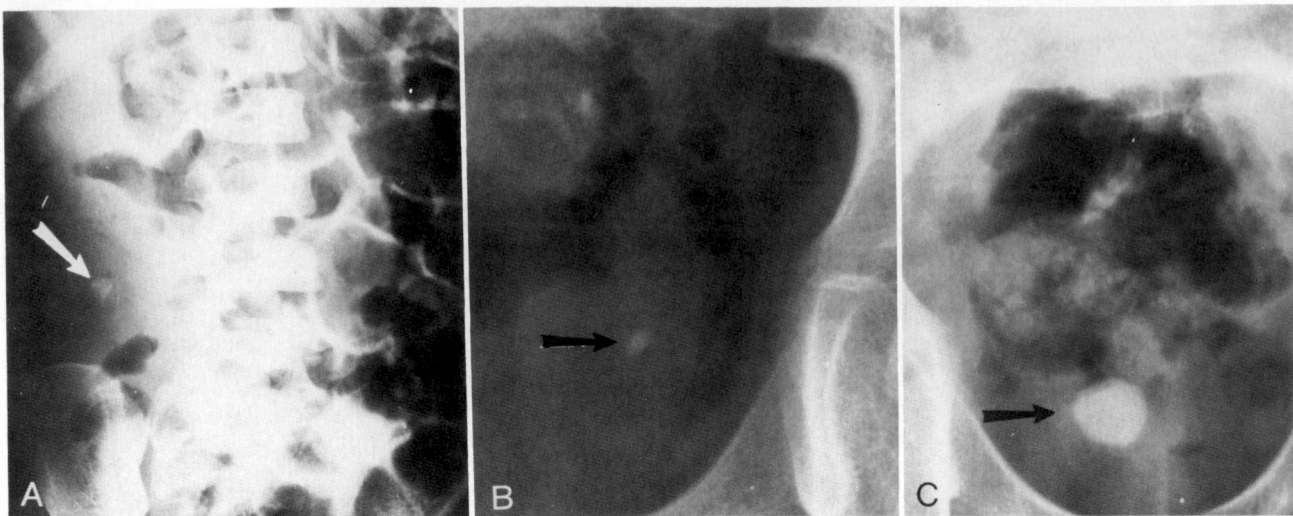

Fig. 3.8. **Stone and stone-like calcifications.** A. Fecalith (arrow) in patient with perforated appendicitis. Note the surrounding soft tissue abscess and associated small bowel obstruction. B. ureteral stone (arrow) in a young male with renal colic. C. Large bladder stone (arrow) in a chronically immobilized (neurogenic disease) child.

hypercalcemia, hyperparathyroidism, hypervitaminosis D, severe osteoporosis, the milk-alkali syndrome, oxalosis (8, 42), and cystinosis. However, it is becoming increasingly apparent that idiopathic stone formation in childhood is more common than generally appreciated and indeed it should no longer surprise one to see children with the problem. Intratubular calcifications associated with renal tubular ectasia are almost unheard of in children.

Stones in the biliary tract most often are seen in patients with hemolytic anemias, but if one is in an area where sickle cell disease is not common, idiopathic gallstone formation becomes more prevalent. Rarely, they are seen with chronic ileal disease (22). The characteristic location (anterior part of right upper quadrant), multiplicity, and often faceted nature of the stones is the key to their diagnosis (Fig. 3.9A). They also are readily demonstrable with ultrasonog-

raphy. Calcified pelvic phleoliths, so common in the adult female, rarely are seen in childhood (28), and actually, when a phleobolith is visualized, it most likely is in a hemangiomatous tumor or AV malformation (Fig. 3.9C). The round, somewhat bullseye appearance of these stones is a strong clue to their origin.

Finally, it should be noted that ingested pebbles can mimic stones (Fig. 3.9B), and so can ingested iron and calcium tablets (36). Iron tablets, when ingested in overdose, are especially important to detect for they can be associated with a severe gastritis and hemorrhage. Solitary, punctate calcified granulomas of the liver or spleen, usually due to healed tuberculosis or histoplasmosis, can be mistaken for some other interabdominal opacity, but when they are numerous, no such problem exists (Fig. 3.9D).

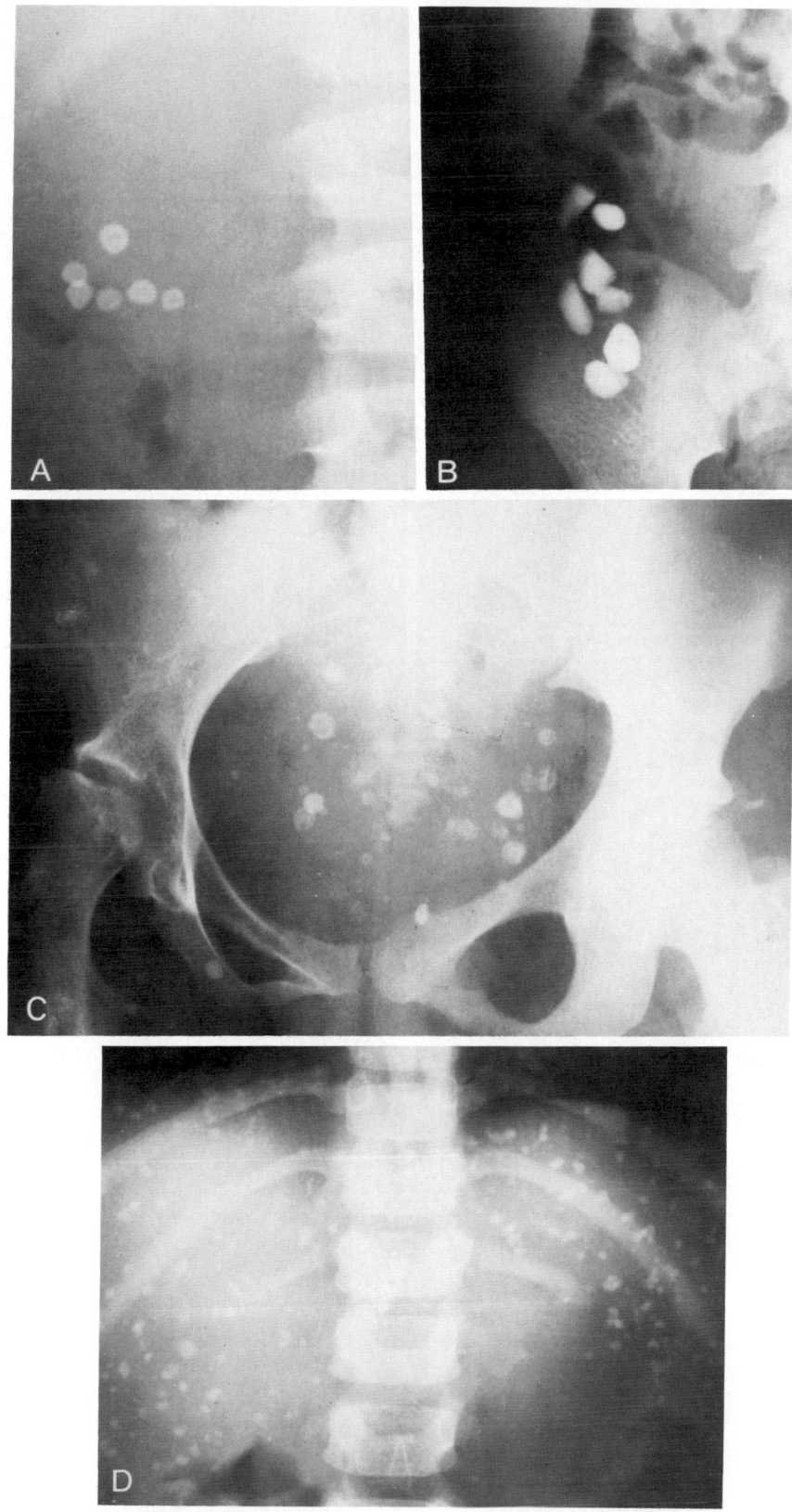

Figure 3.9. Stone, stone-like, and punctate calcifications. A. Typical gallstones in a patient with sickle cell disease. B. Pebbles in the cecum mimicking pathologic calcifications. This patient was a dirt eater. C. Multiple phleboliths in an extensive hemangiomatous lesion (Hasselbalch-Merritt syndrome). Some of these calcifications have a typical "bullseye" appearance. Also note associated bony deformity of the pelvis. This is characteristic of hemangiomatous-lymphangiomatous tumors. D. Typical punctate calcifications in both the liver and spleen in patient with healed histoplasmosis.

Formed Calcifications

These calcifications are not particularly common in childhood, but do occur in dermoids or teratomas (30). Most are located in the pelvis of females, and arise from the ovaries (Fig. 3.10, A and B), but they also can be presacral or higher in the retroperitoneum (Fig. 3.10C). Many times they also contain teeth or fat, and then the diagnosis can be established with complete confidence. The teeth are easily visualized on plain films, but the fat is better visualized with CT scanning. Similar calcifications, but usually more differentiated into actual, and recognizable, bony structures (i.e., femur, humerus, spine, etc.) occur in the rare abdominal tumor known as fetus in fetu. These tumors, previously considered related to teratomas now are believed to be aborted monozygotic twins. Staghorn calculi, mimicking formed calcifications, are rare in children (5), and almost always occur in chronically immobilized patients or those with other severe hypercalcemic states.

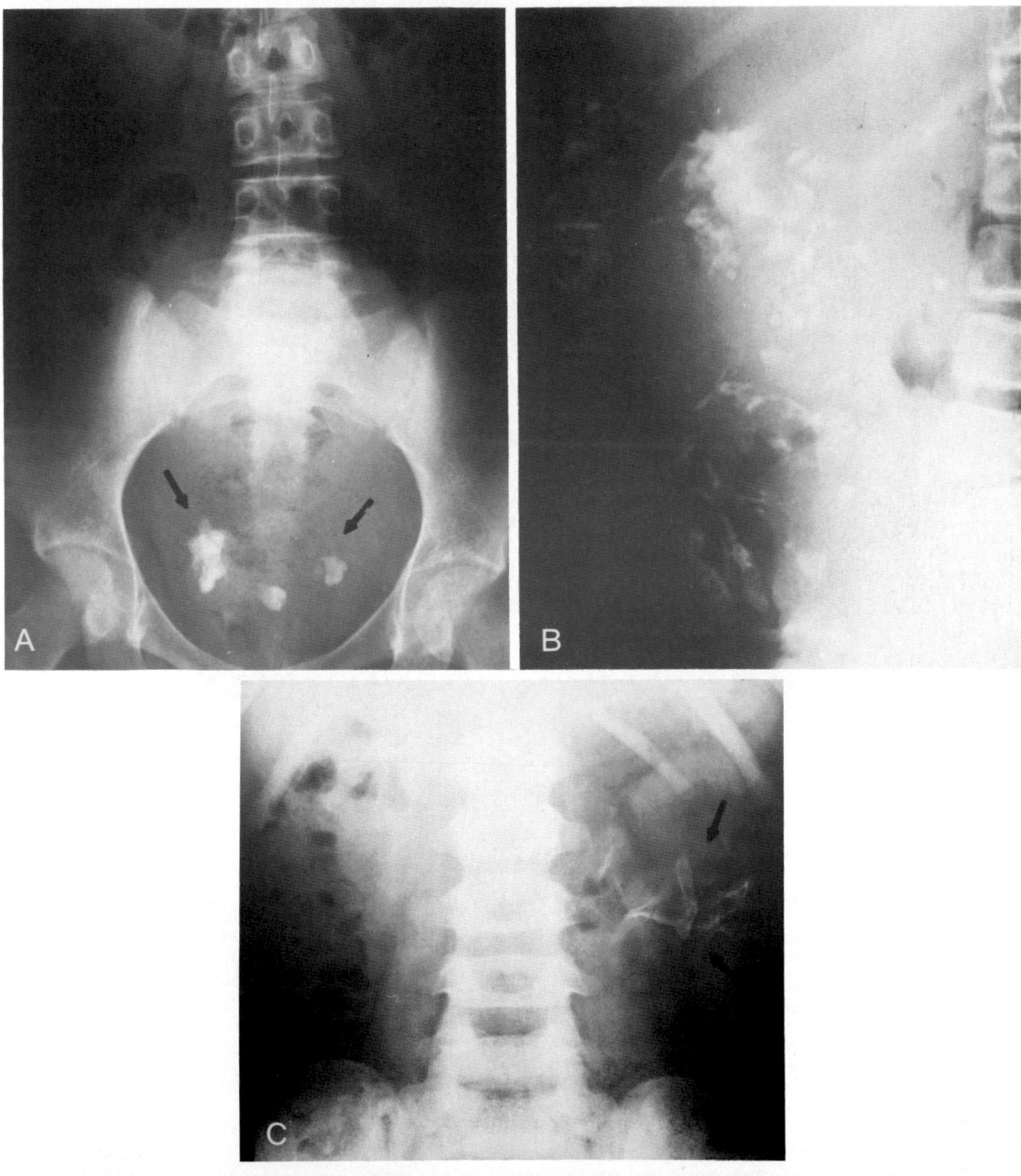

Figure 3.10. Formed calcifications. A. Note quite well-formed teeth in a teratoma of the ovary (arrows). Also note the soft tissue mass of the tumor rising out of the pelvis. B. Lateral view in another patient with a very large teratoma containing both formed bone and teeth. C. Formed calcification (bone) in a retroperitoneal teratoma (arrows).

Miscellaneous Calcifications

Occasionally, rather than calcifications being irregular, curvilinear, stone-like, or formed, they are very fine, diffuse, and virtually homogeneous. Rarely, this occurs with milk of calcium in an obstructed, diseased gallbladder (6), and even more rarely, with milk of calcium in a hydronephrotic kidney. Fine, diffuse, and homogeneous parenchymal calcifications of the kidney can be seen with oxalosis (see Fig. 3.5). A final, peculiar calcification, often very dense, is that which occurs in the enlarged adrenal glands of the storage disease known as Wolman's disease (16, 29, 31).

References

1. Ablow RC, Effman EL: Hepatic calcifications associated with umbilical vein catheterization in the newborn infant. *Am J Roentgenol* 114:380–385, 1972.
2. Alexander WJ, Kadish JA, Dunbar JS: Ingested foreign bodies in children. In Kaufmann HJ (ed): *Progress in Pediatric Radiology*. Chicago, Year Book Medical Publishers, 1969, pp 256–285.
3. Ansari BM, Davies DB, Jones MR: Report of calcification in the liver of a male infant with known congenital cytomegalic inclusion disease. *J Pediatr* 90:661–662, 1977.
4. Barratt TM, Simmonds HA, Cameron JS, Potter CF, Rose GA, Arkell DG, Williams DI: Complete deficiency of adenine phosphoribosyltransferase: a third case presenting as renal stones in a young child. *Arch Dis Child* 54:25–31, 1979.
5. Bartone, FF, Johnston JH: Staghorn calculi in children. *J Urol* 118:76–79, 1977.
6. Beauregard WG, Ferguson WT: Milk of calcium cholecystitis. *J Pediatr* 96:876–877, 1980.
7. Bedros AA, Fritzsche PJ, Heldinger HE, Young LW: Radiological case of the month—mobile calcified spontaneously amputated ovary. *Am J Dis Child* 135:467–468, 1981.
8. Carsen GM, Radkowski MA: Calcium oxalosis. A case report. *Radiology* 113:165–166, 1974.
9. Clayton RS, Goodman PH: Roentgenographic diagnosis of geophagia (dirt eating). *Am J Roentgenol* 73:203, 1955.
10. Conley SB, Shackelford GD, Robson AM: Severe immobilization hypercalcemia renal insufficiency and calcification. *Pediatrics* 63:142–145, 1979.
11. Daeschner CW, Singleton EB, Curtis JC: Urinary tract calculi and nephrocalcinosis in infants and children. *J Pediatr* 57:721–732, 1960.
12. Faegenburg D: Fecaliths of the appendix: incidence and significance. *Am J Roentgenol* 89:752–759, 1963.
13. Franken EA Jr, Smith WL, Siddique A: Noninvasive evaluation of liver disease in pediatrics. *Radiol Clin North Am* 18:239–252, 1980.
14. Gammill SL, Nice CM: Calcification in the inferior vena cava. *Radiology* 92:1288–1290, 1969.
15. Gwin JL, Lee FA: Radiological case of the month—thrombus calcification in the inferior vena cava. *Am J Dis Child* 124:385–386, 1972.
16. Harrison RB, Francke P Jr: Radiographic exhibit: radiographic findings in Wolman's disease. *Radiology* 124:188, 1977.
17. Hirschy JC, Thorpe JJ, Cortese AF: Meckel's stones: a case report. *Radiology* 119:19–20, 1976.
18. Iannaccone G, Antonelli M: Calcification of the pancreas in cystic fibrosis. *Pediatr Radiol* 9:85–89, 1980.
19. Izzidien AY: Prostatic calcification in a 4 year old boy. *Arch Dis Child* 55:963–968, 1980.
20. Jarvis JL, Seaman WB: Idiopathic adrenal calcification in infants and children. *Am J Roentgenol* 82:510–520, 1959.
21. Kassner EG, Baumstark A, Kinkhabwala MN, Ablow RC, Haller JO: Calcified thrombus in the inferior vena cava in infants and children. *Pediatr Radiol* 4:167–171, 1976.
22. Kirks DR: Lithiasis due to interruption of the enterohepatic circulation of bile salts. *Am J Roentgenol* 133:382–288, 1979.
23. Knox AJS, Webb AJ: The clinical features and treatment of fetus in fetu; two case reports and a review of the literature. *J Pediatr Surg* 10:483–489, 1975.
24. Kutcher R, Schneider M, Gordon DH: Calcification in polycystic disease. *Radiology* 122:77–80, 1977.
25. Leonidas JC, Berdon WE, Griebetz D: Bilateral renal cortical necrosis in the newborn infant; roentgenographic diagnosis. *J Pediatr* 79:623–627, 1971.
26. Lester PD, McAllister WH: A mobile calcified spontaneously amputated ovary. *J Can Assoc Radiol* 21:143–145, 1970.
27. Malek RS, Kelalis TP: Nephrocalcinosis in infancy and childhood. *J Urol* 114:441–448, 1975.
28. Marquis JR: The incidence of pelvic phleboliths in pediatric patients. *Pediatr Radiol* 5:211–212, 1977.
29. Marshall WC, Ockenden BG, Fosbrooke AS, Cummings JN: Wolman's disease; rare lipodosis with adrenal calcification. *Arch Dis Child* 44:331–341, 1969.
30. Partlow WF, Taybi H: Teratomas in infants and children. *Am J Roentgenol* 112:155–166, 1971.
31. Queloz JM, Capitanio MA, Kirkpatrick JA: Wolman's disease. Roentgen observations in 3 siglings. *Radiology* 104:357–359, 1972.
32. Schullinger JN, Santulli TV, Berdon WE, Wigger HJ, MacMillan RW, Demartini PD, Baker DH: Calcific thrombi of the inferior vena cava in infants and children. *J Pediatr Surg* 13:429–434, 1978.
33. Shackelford GD, Kirks DR:Neonatal hepatic calcification secondary to transplacental infection. *Radiology* 122:753–757, 1977.
34. Silverman NR, Borns PF, Goldstein AH, Greening RR, Hope JW: Thrombus calcification in the inferior vena cava; a specific roentgenologic entity. *Am J Roentgenol* 106:97–102, 1969.
35. Singleton EB, Rosenberg HS: Intralumenal calcification of the inferior vena cava. *Am J Roentgenol* 86:556–560, 1961.
36. Staple TW, McAlister WH: Roentgenographic visualization of iron preparation in the gastrointestinal tract. *Radiology* 83:1051, 1964.
37. Swischuk LE: *Radiology of the Newborn and Young Infant,* ed 2. Baltimore, Williams & Wilkins, 1980, p 610.
38. Tada S, Yasukochi H, Ohtaki C, Fukuta A, Takanashi R: Fetus in fetu. *Br J Radiol* 47:146–148, 1974.
39. Tseng CH, Chang GKJ, Lora F: Congenital calcified thrombosis of inferior vena cava, bilateral renal veins, and left spermatic vein. *Pediatr Radiol* 6:176–177, 1977.
40. Wenzl JE, Burke EC, Stickler GB, Utz DC: Nephrolithiasis and nephrocalcinosis in children. *Pediatrics* 41:57–61,1968.

41. Williams HH: Coproliths in children: recognition and significance. *Pediatrics* 34:372–377, 1964.
42. Young LW: Radiological case of the month-nephroxlaosis. *Am J Dis Child* 132:517–518, 1978.
43. Young LW: Radiological case of the month, calcification IVC and renal veins. *Am J Dis Child* 132:921–922, 1978.
44. Young LW: Radiological case of the month, bilateral renal cortical necrosis and calcification in a surviving child. *Am J Dis Child* 133:203–204, 1979.

ABNORMAL ORGAN AND TISSUE DENSITIES

Normally, each organ or tissue in the abdomen has a specific density, i.e., air-containing structures are relatively black, fatty structures gray or radiolucent, and muscles and solid organs relatively white (i.e., water density). If any of these organs or tissues appear whiter or denser than normal, it is because they are enlarged (i.e., more tissue mass) or infiltrated with calcium or iron salts. The former, of course, is most common.

Diffuse excess calcium deposition usually affects the kidneys and can occur with any number of hypercalcemic states (i.e., hyperparathyroidism, severe osteoperosis, steroid therapy-induced osteoperosis, excess calcium intake, milk alkali syndrome, idiopathic hypercalcemia, hypervitaminosis D, hyperparathyroidism-like states in hormonally active bone tumors, oxaluria, renal tubular acidosis). Generalized increased density of the liver usually occurs because of increased iron deposition, and most often this takes the form of secondary hemochromatosis after repeated transfusions (1, 7). Often this increase in density is best demonstrated with CT scanning. Similar excessive iron deposition has been described in abdominal lymph nodes after multiple transfusions in thalassemia (10), but idiopathic or primary hemochromatosis in children is very rare.

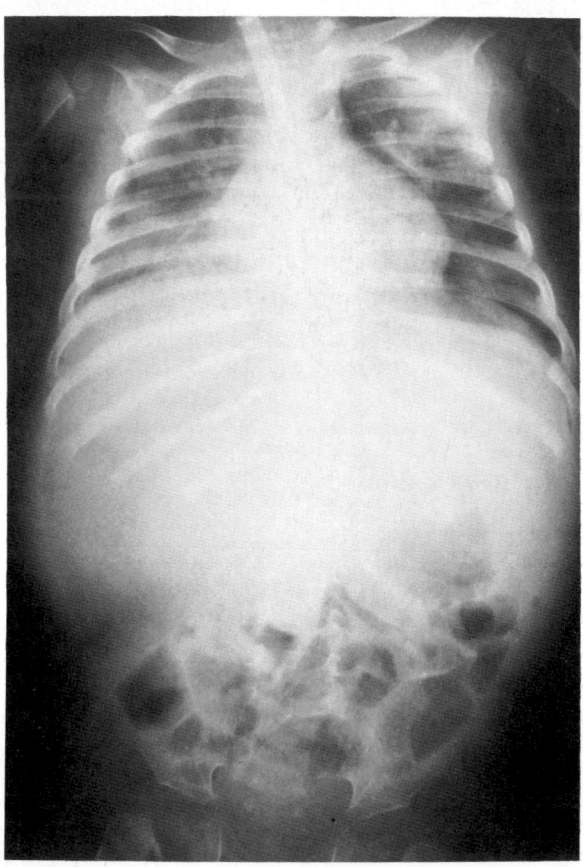

Figure 3.11.   Fatty liver. Typical radiolucent appearance of a fatty liver. The liver also is enlarged and is displacing the intestines downward. Note that the spleen is whiter than the liver (they should have the same density) and that the abdominal wall, on the right, also is whiter than the liver. Ordinarily, it also should be of the same density as the liver. In addition, in normal individuals, the liver is separated from the abdominal wall by the radiolucent properitoneal fat line. In fatty liver the line disappears and blends with the radiolucent liver.

Decreased density, or abnormal radiolucency of an organ, is rather uncommon, except in the liver where, with marked fatty replacement, the liver can appear quite radiolucent (4, 6, 8, 9, 12). Most commonly, such fatty degeneration occurs with severe protein malnutrition in cystic fibrosis or kwashiorkor. However, it also can be seen with toxic insult to the liver, Reye's syndrome, and diabetes mellitus (6). The finding of fatty liver, in such cases, often is readily demonstrable with plain films (Fig. 3.11), but usually is more vivid on CT scans.

A generalized increase in abdominal fat leads to radiolucency of the entire abdomen, and can be seen with lipomas of the abdomen (3, 11), or excessive accumulation of fat in the omentum, mesentary (5), or retroperitoneal space. The latter situation most commonly occurs with exogenous obesity, but steroid therapy utilized for conditions such as the nephrotic syndrome (2), regional enteritis, etc., is probably just as common. More rarely, increased fatty tissue can be seen with the Prader-Willi syndrome, Cushing's syndrome, and the Laurence-Moon Biedl syndrome. Increased radiolucency in the abdomen, because of excessive fat content, also is said to occur with chylous ascites and with chylous cysts, but the finding is difficult to appreciate on plain films.

Finally, it should be noted that fat frequently is present in dermoids or teratomas in the abdomen, and this finding, together with the frequently present formed bone or teeth assures the diagnosis. Fat in these lesions, once again, is more readily demonstrable with CT scanning, and although some of these lesions can occur in the retroperitoneal space, most occur in the pelvis, in ovaries. In infancy, a fair number also occur in the presacral area.

References

1. Franken EA Jr, Smith WL, Siddiqui A: Noninvasive evaluation of liver disease in pediatrics. *Radiol Clin North Am* 18:239–252, 1980.
2. Gilsanz V, Brill PW, Wolf BS: Increased retroperitoneal fat: a sign of corticosteroid therapy. *Radiology* 123:147–148, 1977.
3. Giubilei D, Cicia S, Nardia P, Patane E, Villani RM: Radiographic exhibit: lipoma of the omentum in a child. *Radiology* 137:357–358, 1980.
4. Griscom NT, Capitanio MA, Wagoner ML, Culham G, Morris L: The visibly fatty liver. *Radiology* 117:385–389, 1975.
5. Hernandez R, Poznaski AK, Holt JF, Weintraub W: Abnormal fat collections in the omentum and mesocolon of children. *Radiology* 122:193–196, 1977.
6. Melhem RE: The radiolucent liver. *Pediatr Radiol* 4:153–156, 1976.
7. Smith WL, Quattromani F: Radiodense liver in transfusion hemochromatosis. *Am J Roentgenol* 128:316–317, 1977.
8. Swischuk LE: A new and unusual roentgenographic finding of fatty liver in infants. *Am J Roentgenol* 122:159–164, 1974.
9. Swischuk LE, McConnell RF Jr: The radiographic demonstration of fatty liver in children (a clue to protein malnutrition). *J Pediatr* 88:452–454, 1978.
10. Winchester PH, Cerwin R, Dische R, Canale V: hemosiderin laden lymph nodes: an unusual roentgenographic manifestation of homozygous thalassemia. *Am J Roentgenol* 118:222–226, 1973.
11. Young LW, Severson MV, Burke EC, Hattery RR: radiological case of the month—retroperitoneal lipoma in a child. *Am J Dis Child* 134:83–84, 1980.
12. Yousefzadeh, DK, Lupetin AR, Jackson JH Jr: The radiographic signs of fatty liver. *Radiology* 131:351–355, 1979.

EXTRAINTESTINAL AIR

As in the adult, extraintestinal air can be located in the peritoneal cavity, retroperitoneal space, intestinal wall (i.e., pneumatosis cystoides intestinalis), biliary tract, portal veins, and occasionally, in the kidney. In the latter case, air usually is present in the collecting systems of patients with ureteroileostomies (8). The finding actually is normal for these patients, but in other, very rare cases (usually diabetics), air (gas) in the kidney is the result of severe gas-forming infection. Air in the biliary tract is very uncommon in the pediatric age group, and usually the result of reflux into the biliary tract secondary to duodenal obstruction. Portal vein gas most commonly is seen in the neonate, either iatrogenically introduced by umbilical vein catheterization, or as a complication of necrotizing enterocolitis (1). In older children, it is much less common, but can be seen with any cause of intestinal necrosis (Fig. 3.12A). Air in the liver parenchyma itself usually is the result of a liver abscess.

Intraperitoneal free air is much more common than retroperitoneal free air, and the causes and roentgenographic findings of either are much the same as in the adult. Most commonly, of course, the problem is a perforated viscus, but in the neonate, and occasionally, the older infant, free air can be seen as a complication of positive pressure respirator therapy. It may or may not be associated with visible pneumomediastinum. Intramural air, that is, pneumatosis cystoides intestinalis, is very common in the neonate with necrotizing enterocolitis, but after this age period, it is not common at all. Still, however, it does occur, and can be seen with bowel overdistention, ischemia to the bowel, severe enterocolitis, the collagen vascular diseases, in children on steroid or other immunosuppressive therapy, cystic fibrosis, leukemia, and very rarely, secondary to a pneumomediastinum (2–7, 9–11). Wherever pneumatosis intestinalis is due to simple overdistention of the intestine, air enters the intestinal wall through mucosal tears, but with the other causes of intestinal disease, pneumatosis cystoides intestinalis is a complication of intestinal ischemia and necrosis. The cause in patients with cystic fibrosis

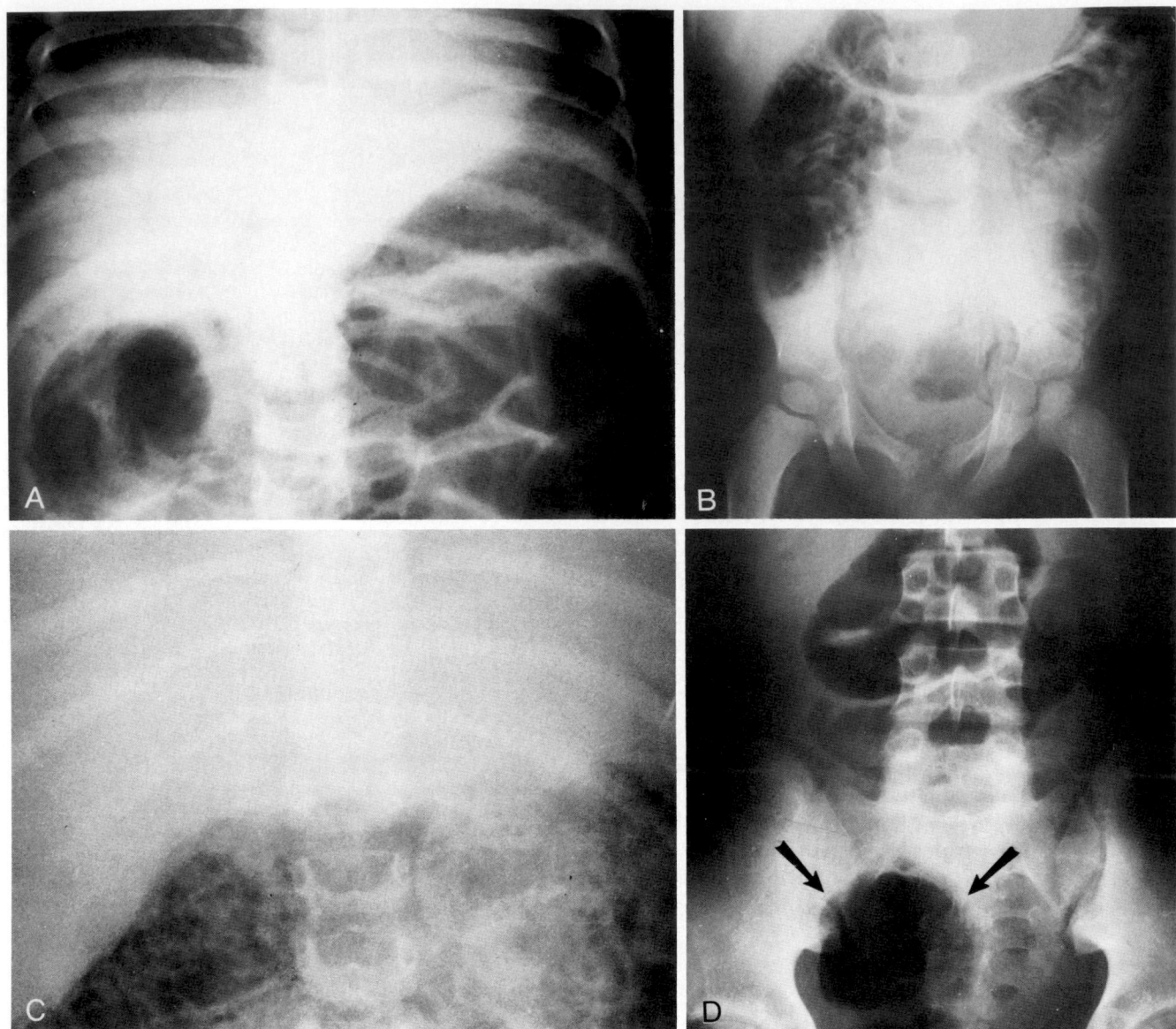

Figure 3.12. Extraintestinal gas. A. Typical appearance of air in the portal veins. This patient, with severe skin burns, had an acute hypotensive episode, bowel ischemia, necrotizing enterocolitis and subsequent portal vein gas. B. **Pneumatosis cystoides intestinalis.** Typical linear and curvilinear collection of gas in the wall of the intestine. C. Bubbly pattern of pneumatosis cystoides intestinalis in patient with acute burn, shock, and hypotension. D. Large collection of gas in a pelvic abscess (arrow), secondary to perforated appendicitis. Also, note small bowel obstruction. On upright view an air-fluid level was present in this abscess cavity.

or immunosuppressive problems is unknown. Roentgenographically, pneumatosis cystoides intestinalis can present as linear, curvilinear, or bubbly collections of gas in the intestinal wall (Fig. 3.12, B and C).

Finally, it should be noted that free extraintestinal air can be seen loculated in abdominal abscesses. In some cases, these abscesses appear surprisingly clean, and the collection of air can be misinterpreted for a cyst or diverticulum (Fig. 3.12D).

References

1. Arnon RG, Fishbein JF: Portal venous gas in pediatric age group: review of the literature and report of 12 new cases. *J Pediatr* 79:255–259,1971.
2. Bornes PF, Johnston TA: Indolent pneumatosis of the bowel wall associated with immune suppressive therapy. *Ann Radiol* 16:163–166, 1973.
3. Djurhuus MJ, Lykkegaard E, Pock-Steen OC: Gastrointestinal radiological findings in cystic fibrosis. *Pediatr*

Radiol 1:113–118, 1973.
4. Fischer TJ, Cipel L, Stiehm ER: Pneumatosis intestinalis associated with fatal childhood dermatomyositis. *Pediatrics* 61:127–129, 1978.
5. Keats TE, Smith TH: Benign pneumatosis intestinalis in childhood leukemia. *Am J Roentgenol* 122:150–152, 1974.
6. Kleinman P, Meyers MA, Abbott G, Kazam E: Necrotizing enterocolitis with pneumatosis intestinalis in systemic lupus erythematosus and polyarteritis. *Radiology* 121:595–598, 1976.
7. Oliveros MA, Herbst JJ, Lester PD, Ziter FA: Pneumatosis intestinalis in childhood dermatomyositis. *Pe-*

diatrics 52:711–712, 1973.
8. Rittenberg GM, Warren D: Air in the pelvicalceal system: a normal finding in patients with ureteroileostomies. *Am J Roentgenol* 128:311–312, 1977.
9. Seaman WB, Fleming RJ, Baker DH: Pneumatosis intestinalis of the small bowel. *Semin Roentgenol* 1:234, 1966.
10. White H, Rowley WF: Cystic fibrosis of the pancreas: clinical and roentgenographic manifestations. *Radiol Clin North Am* 1:539–556, 1963.
11. Wood RE, Herman CJ, Johnson KW, di Sant Agnese PA: Pneumatosis coli in cystic fibrosis. *Am J Dis Child* 129:246–248, 1975.

AIRLESS ABDOMEN

Normal infants and young children usually show considerable gas in the intestinal tract, and thus, when an airless abdomen is encountered, some abnormality should be suspected (Table 3.3). Most often, the problem is severe vomiting, and for the most part, this occurs with acute gastroenteritis or appendicitis. Other causes include neurologic disease with increased intracranial pressure and, so-called, "cyclic" vomiting. In addition, decreased air in the intestinal tract can be seen with decreased or depressed swallowing (i.e., moribund patient, obstructing nasopharyngeal tubes), and high gastro-intestinal obstruction. Only occasionally is a totally airless abdomen an incidental normal finding.

Table 3.3   Abdominal Gas

Airless abdomen	
Vomiting with appendicitis Vomiting with gastroenteritis	Commonest
Vomiting, other causes Decreased swallowing (depressed, moribund)	Moderately common
Normal, incidental High gastrointestinal obstruction	Rare
Distended stomach	
Normal in infants	Commonest
Gastric outlet obstruction	Moderately common
Localized ileus in gastroenteritis Duodenal obstruction Acute gastric dilation	Relatively uncommon

ABNORMAL INTESTINAL GAS PATTERNS

In the normal child one usually can identify gas in the stomch, and scattered in the small bowel and colon. Abnormal gas patterns include (*a*) isolated distension of the stomach, (*b*) distension of stomach and duodenum, (*c*) dilated loops of small bowel, (*d*) dilated colon and small bowel, (*e*) isolated colon dilation, (*f*) dilated transverse colon only, (*g*) one or two isolated loops of bowel (sentinel loops), and (*h*) airless intestine. The latter pattern has been discussed previously with airless abdomen.

Distended Stomach

The commonest cause of a distended stomach (Fig. 3.13), filled with air, is normal air swallowing in infants (Table 3.3). Thereafter, gastric outlet obstruction should be considered, and most often the problem is severe pylorospasm or actual pyloric stenosis. Pylorospasm, without peptic ulcer, is most common in infants and young children, but spasm with ulcer disease is not that uncommon. Pyloric stenosis usually is due to hypertrophy of the circular pyloric muscle, and can occur in both classic and atypical forms (13). Much more rarely it is due to post ulcer stricture; even more rarely it is due to critically located enteric (duplication) cysts, ectopic pancreatic tussue, gastric polps, or gastric tumors. All of these lesions lead to eccentric narrowing of the antropyloric region. With pyloric stenosis, however, narrowing is circumferential. In pyloric stenosis, the area of narrowing can be (*a*) long and associated with the typical muscle mass or olive of pyloric stenosis or (*b*) short and thin. In the latter cases, stenosis may be associated with a small, hypertrophied, nonpalpable muscle mass (i.e., 1–1.5 cm or less in diameter) or just minimal thickening of the pyloric muscle (14). Differentiation from pylorospasm in such cases is difficult but important. Usually it can be accomplished by subjecting the patient to a trial of antispasmodic therapy (14), because if one or the other of these atypical forms of pyloric stenosis is present, antispasmodics do not alleviate the problem. In simple pylorospasm, they do. More recently, ultrasonography has proven valuable in differentiating and defining these various forms of pyloric stenosis because it allows actual visualization of the muscle itself.

Isolated gastric distention also occasionally can oc-

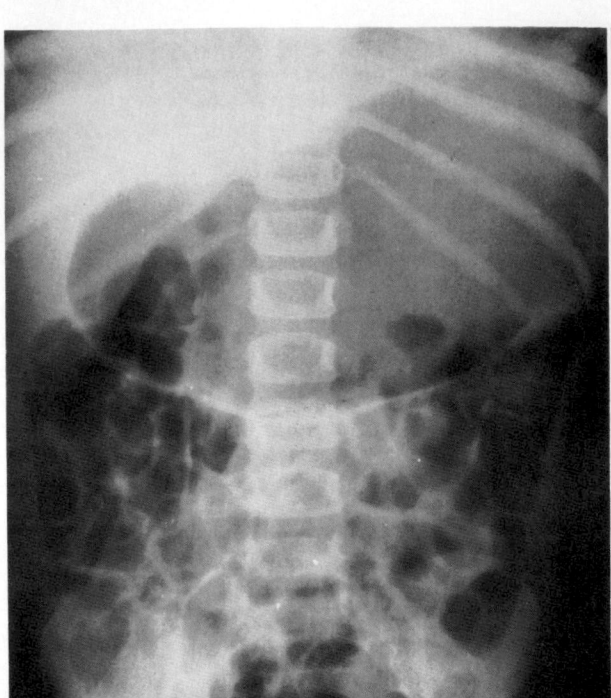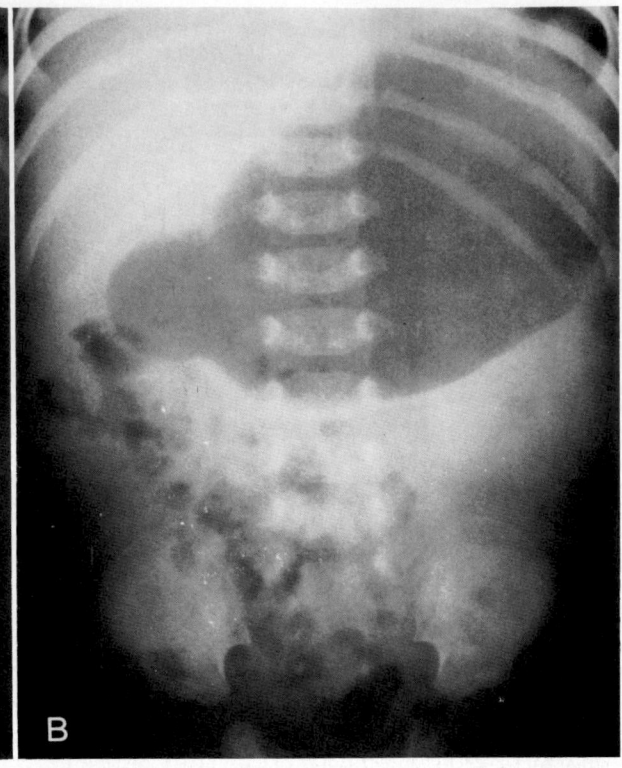

Figure 3.13.   Gastric distension. A. Note what at first appears to be a pathologically overdistended stomach. However, such distention is common in normal infants and is due to air swallowing. This was a normal infant. Also note that the remainder of the gas pattern is normal. B. Another infant with a distended stomach and very little gas in the remainder of the gastrointestinal tract. Such a pattern can be seen with gastric outlet obstruction (i.e., pyloric stenosis) and a few cases of gastroenteritis (i.e., localized paralytic ileus). However, it also can be seen in normal infants and this patient was normal.

cur with gastroenteritis (fortuitous distention of the stomach) and with postoperative paralytic ileus. In the latter instance, distention may be so profound as to cause cardiorespiratory difficulty (probably due to mechanical pressure and vagal overstimulation). Similar acute distention can be seen in severely ill patients (i.e., in sepsis), and occasionally with excessive air swallowing as occurs with severe respiratory distress or large tracheoesophageal fistula. Uncommonly, endotracheal tubes erroneously directed into the esophagus can result in severe gastric distention; indeed, even rupture.

Finally, it might be noted that, in the supine position, duodenal obstruction can present with what appears to be simple gastric overdistention. Because of this, gastric outlet obstruction erroneously is suggested, and the reason for this is that, in the supine position, the descending duodenum is filled with fluid and is invisible. The stomach, of course, being more anterior, is air-filled and visible. Consequently, one erroneously believes that it only, is distended and obstructed. Decubitus or upright views can reveal the true nature of the obstruction in these cases.

Small Bowel Obstruction (Table 3.4)

With small bowel obstruction, just as in the adult, distended intestinal loops tend to assume a more orderly than normal configuration, and on upright views, present as acute, inverted hairpin loops. The number of loops corresponds to the level of obstruction; i.e., if obstruction is located in the third or fourth portion of the duodenum, only the duodenal loop is distended, while if it is located in the jejunum, or ileum, progressively increasing numbers of distended loops are seen. As far as obstructions around the

duodenum are concerned, problems such as duodenal atresia, anular pancreas, duodenal bands (with or without midgut volvulus), and even duodenal diaphragms tend to declare themselves in the neonatal period. However, both duodenal diaphragms and duodenal bands can remain silent until later childhood. Much less commonly, one can have obstruction of the duodenum due to a compressing tumor, cyst, or postoperative adhesion. Compression due to the superior mesenteric artery occurs only in those patients who

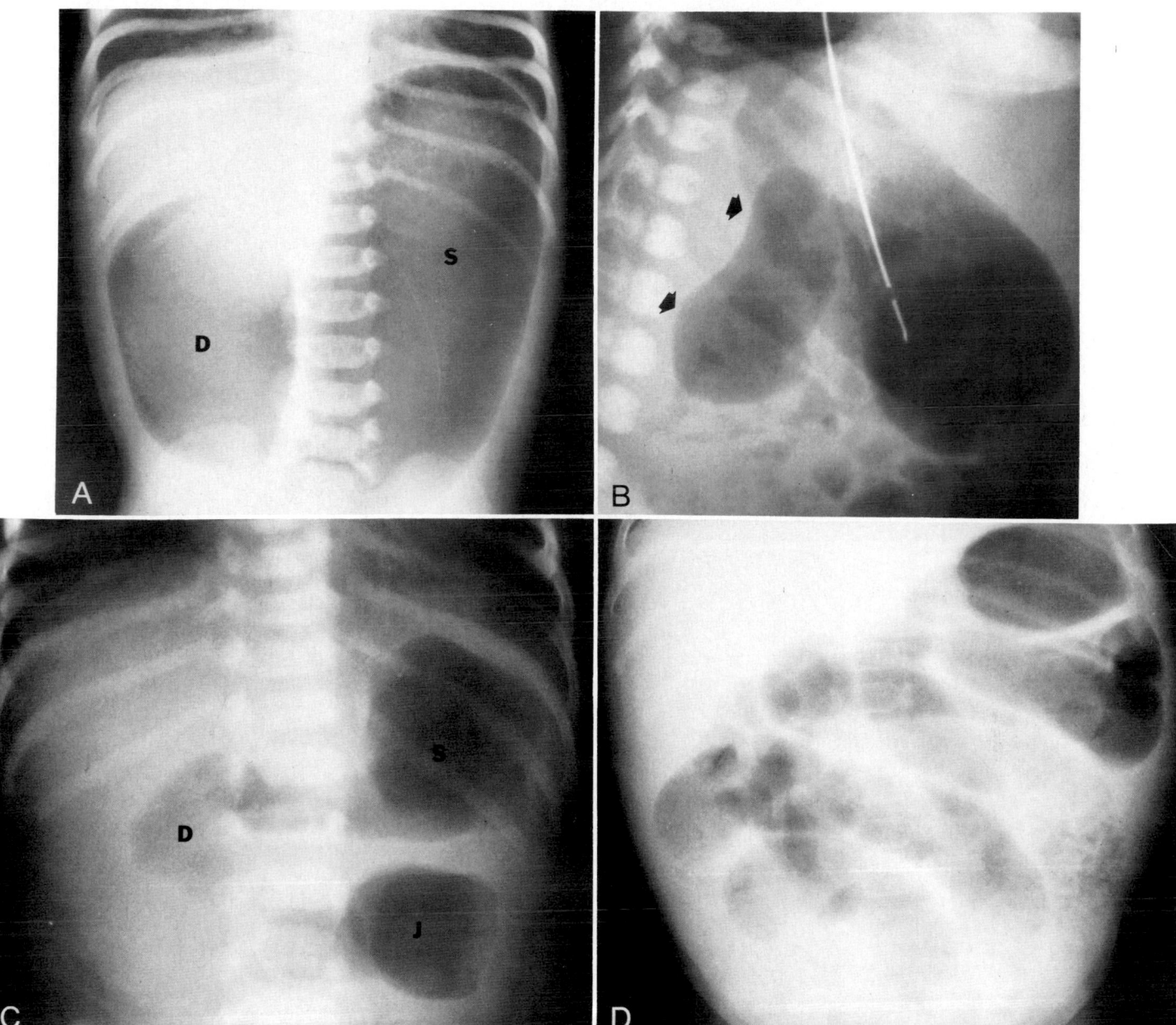

Figure 3.14. Intestinal obstruction; number of loops indicating level of obstruction. A. Typical double bubble of duodenal atresia. High duodenal obstruction, stomach (S), duodenum (D). B. Distended stomach and duodenal loop (arrows) indicating obstruction at the third and fourth portions of the duodenum. Usually this is due to a duodenal band, with or without associated midgut volvulus. C. Triple bubble representing the distended stomach (S), duodenum (D), and early jejunum (J). This is seen with high jejunal obstruction. D. Low small bowel obstruction presenting with numerous distended loops of intestine. This patient had an incarcerated inguinal hernia.

Figure 3.14 (Cont'd). E. Low, small intestinal obstruction. Note organized loops of small bowel, in a somewhat stepladder configuration typical of small bowel obstruction. Obstruction was secondary to perforated appendicitis, a common cause of small bowel obstruction in childhood. F. Upright view in some patient demonstrating numerous inverted U-shaped loops with short air-fluid levels. G. Infant with intussusception showing early small bowel obstruction (numerous distended loops of intestine), and typical paucity of gas on the right side (i.e., empty right lower quadrant or flank sign).

are quite thin and who remain in the supine position for prolonged periods of time. These include chronically ill children, neurologically impaired children, and those in total body casts (i.e., body cast syndrome).

With duodenal atresia and anular pancreas, the duodenal bulb is markedly dilated, and leads to the classic double bubble sign (Fig. 3.14A). Contrast studies usually are not required in these patients, but with similar level obstructions due to duodenal stenosis or diaphragms, since air will be seen distal to the distended bulb, contrast studies usually are required. They, of course, demonstrate the level of obstruction, and in addition, the large duodenal bulb, or so-called megabulbia.

When the entire duodenal loop is distended, and obstruction seems to be present at the junction of the third and fourth portions of the duodenum (Fig. 3.14B), one should consider a duodenal band. Less often the problem is a duodenal diaphragm, a compressing adjacent tumor or cyst, a postoperative adhesion, or compression by the superior mesenteric artery. In most cases, however, the problem is a duodenal band, a problem associated with poor fixation of the small bowel (i.e., malrotation). Midgut volvulus may or may not be present in these patients, but always is a threat. If the problem is compression by the superior mesenteric artery, the clinical setting noted in the previous paragraph should provide one with the major clue to proper diagnosis. If one notes three bubbles, one can assume that obstruction is present in the upper jejunum (Fig. 3.14C), and thereafter one simply derives a general idea as to the level of obstruction by noting the number of distended loops present (Fig. 3.14D).

The commonest cause of low small bowel obstruction in children is perforated appendicitis (4, 7–9, 11). In these cases, postperforation inflammation causes a partial mechanical obstruction (Fig. 3.14, E and F). Closely following perforated appendicitis is intussusception, and actually, under 3 to 4 years of age is more common. The degree of obstruction in intussusception depends on the length of time the intussusception has been present, and to some extent, how far it has progressed into the colon. In up to half the cases, the head of the intussusception can be seen on plain films. More often, however, absence of gas and loss of visualization of the liver edge, on the right side of the abdomen can provide further helpful clues (Fig. 3.14G). In infancy, intussusception usually is considered idiopathic, but may be related to nonspecific inflammatory mucosal thickening or lymph node enlargement. In older children, however, a leading lesion such as a polyp, tumor, or diverticulum usually is present.

Other less common causes of small bowel obstruction in children include regional enteritis, psuedo-obstruction (paralytic ileus) with gastroenteritis, obstruction secondary to postoperative adhesions, late presenting peritoneal bands, compressing cysts, small bowel tumors, delayed meconium ileus in cystic fibrosis (1), and late presenting, midgut volvulus. Lesions such as jejunal or ileal atreasia, of course, present in the neonatal period, and so do most congenital stenoses.

Colon Obstruction

The commonest cause of colon obstruction in childhood is functional megacolon, and the second Hirschsprung's disease (Table 3.4). Functional megacolon often is secondary to the muscle spasm seen with anal fissures, but also can be psychogenic. Other causes of large bowel obstruction are rather rare, but include compression of the colon by adjacent cysts, colonic tumors, aberrant peritoneal or fibrous bands, volvulus, postinflammatory stricture, a small bony pelvis, Chaga's disease, and functional obstruction such as might occur with fecal impaction or hypothyroidism.

Table 3.4 Abdominal Gas

Paralytic ileus			Peritoneal bands		
Gastroenteritis	Commonest		Compressing cysts		Rare
			Midgut volvulus		
Peritonitis			Small bowel tumors		
Sepsis	Moderately common		Large bowel obstruction (beyond neonatal period)		
Moribund patient			Functional megacolon	Commonest	
Vascular insult					
Drug depression	Rare		Hirschsprung's disease	Moderately common	
Hypokalemia					
Small bowel obstruction (beyond neonatal period)			Volvulus		
Perforated appendicitis	Commonest		Compressing cysts		Rare
Intussusception			Colon tumor		
			Small pelvis		
Postoperative adhesions					
Regional enteritis	Moderately common				
Pseudo-obstruction in gastroenteritis					

Paralytic Ileus (Table 3.4)

Paralytic ileus presents with numerous distended loops of both large and small bowel, and the picture is not nearly as orderly as that which is seen with mechanical ileus or obstruction. As a result, on upright view numerous "sluggish" loops of intestine with long, air-fluid levels, are seen. This is quite different from the acute hairpin, rather organized pattern seen with mechanical obstruction (Fig. 3.15). In the pediatric age group, the commonest cause of paralytic ileus is gastroenteritis, and thereafter, one should consider problems such as hypokalemia, hypocalcemia, peritonitis, meningitis, sepsis, prolonged bedriddeness, drugs such as valium or glucagon, and cutis laxa (3). Vascular insult to the intestines, producing paralytic ileus is rather uncommon in children.

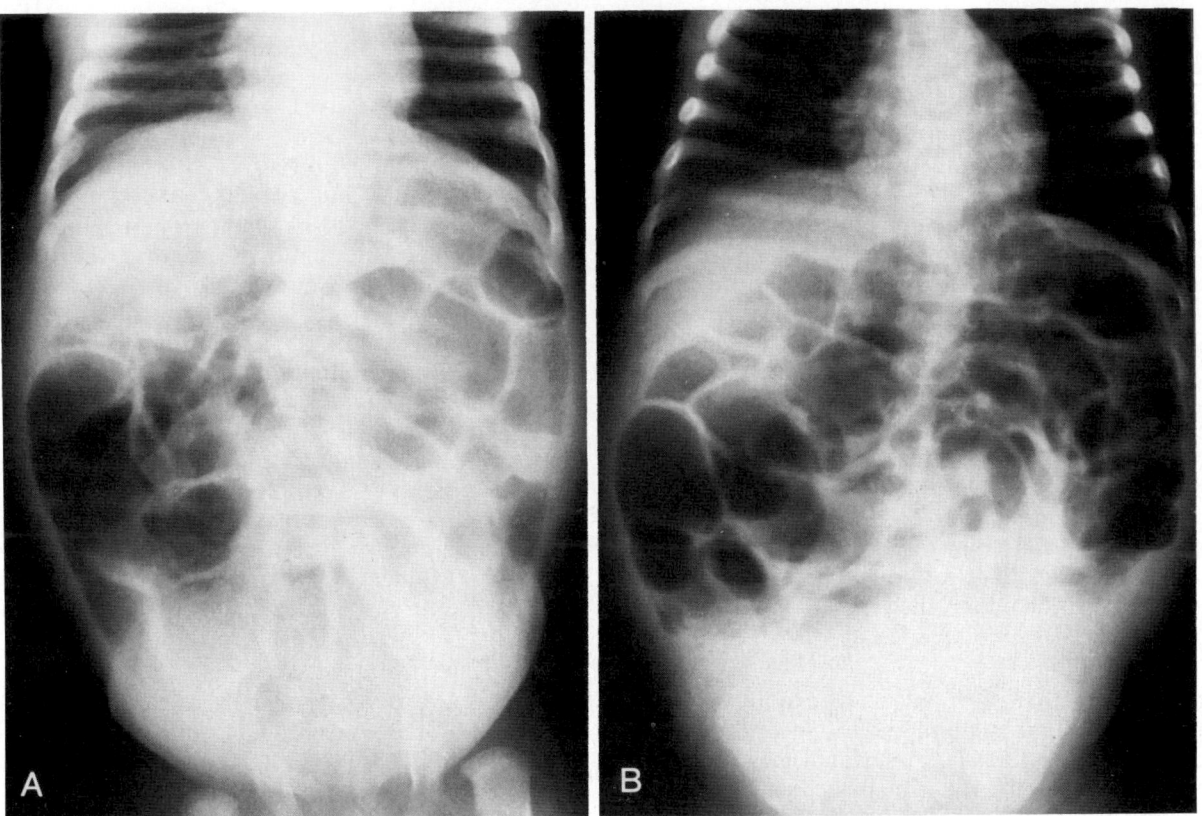

Figure 3.15. Gastroenteritis. A. Note numerous loops of distended intestine. Both large and small bowel are involved and both are proportionately distended. This is characteristic of paralytic ileus. With obstruction, the obstructed loops are dilated out of proportion to the remainder of the gastrointestinal tract. B. Upright view showing numerous air-fluid levels but less orderliness than that seen with small bowel obstruction depicted in Figure 3.14.

Dilated Transverse Colon (Table 3.5)

The transverse colon, being uppermost in the abdomen, often normally is filled with air when the patient is examined in the supine position (Fig. 3.16A). However, it also can be distended, on a reflex basis, with adjacent pancreatic inflammation or injury (2, 10, 16, 17). In these cases, the colon overlying the diseased pancreas is paralyzed and focally dilated, and the term "colon cut-off" often is applied to the configuration. A somewhat similar finding, and actually, one seen more often, occurs with perforated appendicitis (Fig. 3.16B). However, as opposed to the cut-off of the colon being on the splenic flexure side in pancreatitis (11, 12), in appendicitis, the cut-off is on the hepatic flexure side. In these cases, the finding is believed to result from a combination of nonspecific, paralytic ileus of the transverse colon and lack of air in the cecum and asecnding colon due to spasm. Dilation of the transverse colon due to ischemic disease or toxic megacolon in Hirschsprung's disease, regional enteritis, or amebic colitis is relatively rare. However, it does occur, and often is associated with mural edema manifesting in thumbprinting.

Table 3.5   Abdominal Gas

Dilated transverse colon (colon cut-off)		
Normal	}	Commonest
Perforated appendicitis	}	Moderately common
Pancreatitis	}	Relatively uncommon
Ischemia, infarct	}	Rare
Toxic megacolon		
Sentinal loops		
Appendicitis	}	Commonest
Closed loop obstruction	}	Moderately common
Paralytic ileus with other infections		
Isolated loop in gastroenteritis	}	Relatively rare
Normal, fortuitous		
Intestinal trauma	}	Rare
Infarction		
Volvulus		

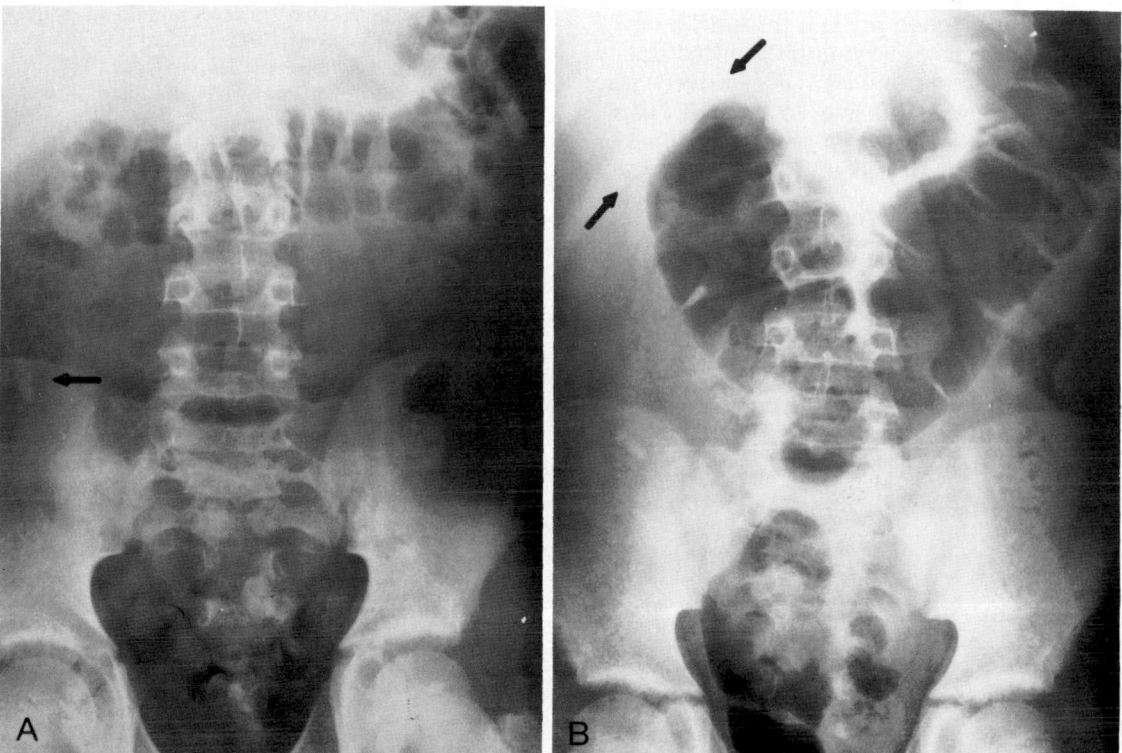

Figure 3.16.   Dilated transverse colon. A. The transverse colon is normal in this patient. The patient had an acute abdomen and a fecalith on the right (arrows). Ordinarily surgery would ensue, but symptoms resolved quickly and no surgery was performed in this patient. B. Two years later the patient presented with more severel abdominal symptoms, a markedly dilated transverse colon and now a right side colon cutoff sign (arrow). Note, specifically, that there is no air or fecal material in the cecum and ascending colon. This is quite different from the situation depicted in A and should signify perforation. This patient did, indeed, have perforation at this time. Note that scoliosis, slight indistinctness of the ipsilateral psoas shadow, and early small bowel obstruction also are present. Also note that the fecalith is still present.

Sentinel Loops (Table 3.5)

Sentinel loops are focally distended loops of intestine which are distended because they (a) overlie inflamed or injured abdominal contents, (b) are involved in a closed loop obstruction, (c) are the first loops to be seen early in the course of regular intestinal obstruction, or. (d) have suffered an ischemic insult. Sentinel loops overlying inflamed or injured abdominal viscera are most common and, of these, those occurring in the right flank or right lower quadrant, secondary to appendicitis, are commonest. They represent the dilated terminal ileum and cecum (Fig. 3.17) (4, 15). Sentinel loops seen elsewhere can result from infections such as cholecystitis, pancreatitis, pyelonephritis, cystitis, etc., (15). Fortuitous, false sentinel loops can be seen in some normal individuals, and also with gastroenteritis. They tend to disappear from one view to another, while truly pathologic sentinel loops remain more fixed. Focally distended loops secondary to local intestinal ischemia are rather uncommon in the pediatric age group, except as seen in necrotizing enterocolitis of infancy.

Distention of the sigmoid colon mimicking sigmoid volvulus is quite common in normal children (Fig. 3.18, A and B). Indeed, such normal distention of the sigmoid colon is much more common than that due to sigmoid volvulus. Sigmoid volvulus is relatively rare in children, and cecal volvulus is even rarer (5). However, as in the adult, when seen it usually presents as a large distended cecum in the mid-abdomen or left upper quadrant.

References

1. Edge WEB, Nuss D, Loening WEK: Late onset intestinal obstruction in cystic fibrosis—meconium ileus equivalent. *S Afr Med J* 52:271–274, 1977.
2. Grollman AI, Goodman S, Fine A: Localized paralytic ileus: an early roentgen sign in acute pancreatitis. *Surg Gynecol Obstet* 91:65–70, 1950.
3. Harris RD: Small bowel dilatation in Ehler's-Danlos syndrome—an unreported gastrointestinal manifestation. *Br J Radiol* 47:623–627, 1974.
4. Isdale JM: The radiological signs of acute appendicitis in infancy and childhood. *S Afr Med J* 53:363–364, 1978.
5. Kirks DR, Swischuk LE, Merten DF, Filston HC: Cecal volvulus in children. *Am J Roentgenol* 136:419–422, 1981.
6. May LM, O'Neill FE, Allen SW: Cecal ileus: an undescribed and helpful sign in acute appendicitis. *Texas J Med* 54:92, 1958.
7. Mayson PB Jr, Rosenthal SJ: Roentgen findings in delayed diagnosis of appendicitis. *Am J Roentgenol* 103:347–350, 1968.
8. Melamed M, Melamed JL, and Rabushka SE: Appendicitis: "functional" bowel obstruction associated with perforation of the appendix. *Am J Roentgenol* 99:112–117, 1967.
9. Riggs W, Parvey LS: Perforated appendix presenting with disproportionate jejunal distention. *Pediatr Radiol* 5:47–49, 1976.
10. Schwartz S, Nadelhaft J: Simulation of colonic obstruction at the splenic flexure by pancreatitis: roentgen features. *Am J Roentgenol* 78:607–616, 1957.
11. Swischuk, LE: *Emergency Radiology of the Acutely Ill or Injured Child.* Williams & Wilkins, Baltimore, 1979, pp 136–144.
12. Swischuk LE, Hayden CK Jr: Appendicitis with perforation: the dilated transverse colon sign. *Am J Roentgenol* 135:687–690, 1980.
13. Swischuk LE, Hayder CK Jr, Tyson KR: Atypical muscle hypertrophy in pyloric stenosis. *Am J Roentgenol* 134:481–484, 1980.
14. Swischuk LE, Hayder CK Jr, Tyson KR: Short segment pyloric narrowing; pylorospasm or pyloric stenosis? *Pediatr Radiol* 10:201–205, 1981.
15. Young BR: Significance of regional or reflex ileus in roentgen diagnosis of cholecytitis, perforated ulcer, pancreatitis and appendiceal abscess, as determined by survey examination of acute abdomen. *Am J Roentgenol* 78:581–586, 1957.
16. Young LW: Pancreatic and/or duodenal injury from blunt trauma in childhood: radiopaque examinations and radiological review. *Ann Radiol* 18:377–390, 1975.
17. Young LW: Pancreatic and/or duodenal injury from blunt trauma in childhood: radiopaque examinations and radiological review. *Ann Radiol* 18:377–390, 1975.

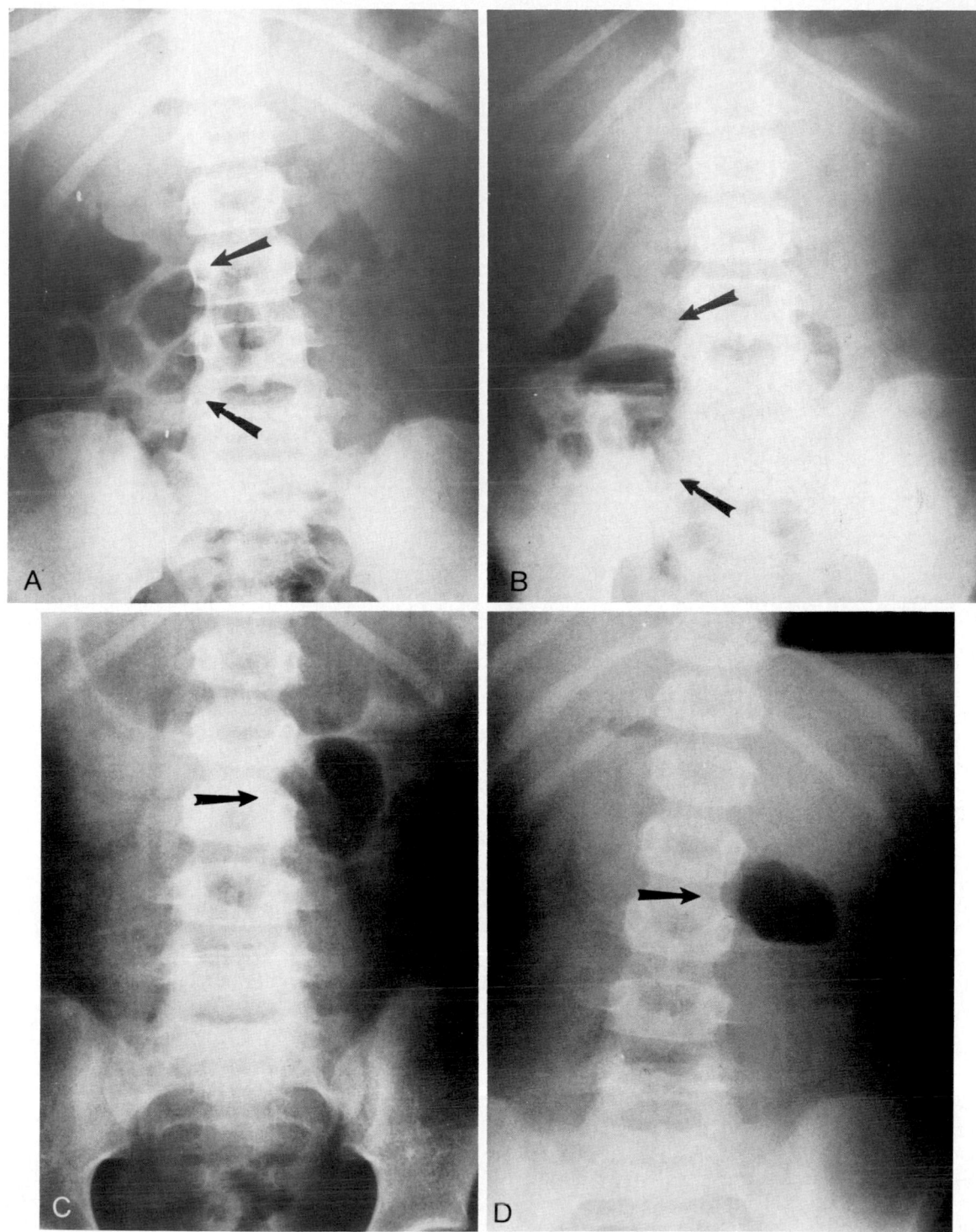

Fig. 3.17. Sentinel loops. A. Typical collection of gas in the cecum and terminal small bowel in a patient with early nonperforated appendicitis (arrows). B. Upright view demonstrates the same findings and also slight indistinctness of the ipsilateral psoas shadow. C. Localized loops of small bowel herald an early small bowel obstruction (arrow). D. Upright view confirms the findings and demonstrates the same loops (arrow). Such fixed loops, no matter how small, should alert one to the presence of an obstruction, either an ordinary obstruction, or a so-called closed loop obstruction.

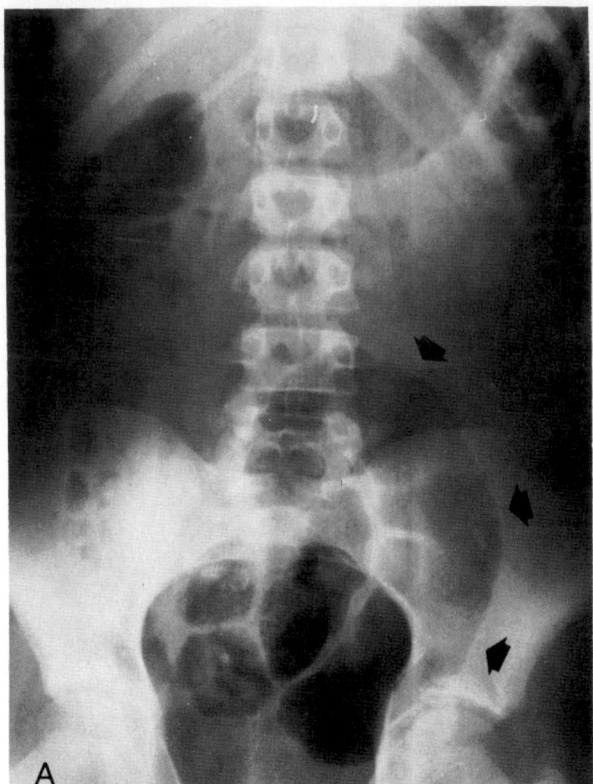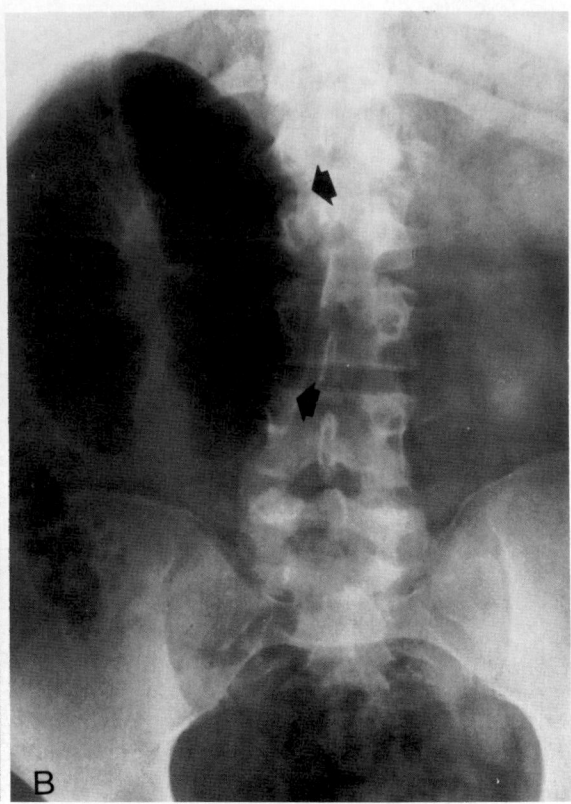

Fig. 3.18. Sigmoid sentinel loop. A. Note what would appear to be a volved sigmoid colon (arrows). Actually this patient did not have volvulus, and such fortuitous distention of the sigmoid colon is common in normal children. B. Another patient with a more ominous appearing, high sigmoid loop (arrows). This patient had abdominal pain and constipation. Symptoms resolved in less than 24 hr. Of course, it would be difficult to say that transient volvulus of the sigmoid colon, of very short duration, was never present, but the clinical findings did not suggest an acute mechanical problem.

THUMB-PRINTING

Thumb-printing can result either from the thickening of the intestinal mucosa and submucosa (i.e., edema or infiltration), or simply from mucosal distortion secondary to intestinal spasm. When it is due to spasm, it is best demonstrated with barium enema, but when due to edema or infiltration, can be appreciated on plain films. Spasm producing thumb-printing can be seen in Hirschsprung's disease and with intestinal inflammatory disease. When the problem is mural edema, ulcerative colitis usually is the cause, but thumb-printing also can be seen with regional enteritis, pseudomembranous colitis, intestinal ischemia, amebic colitis, hemolytic uremic syndrome, eosinophilic (allergic) gastroenteritis (3), Henoch-Schönlein purpura (1), and intramural intestinal bleeding (2). This can occur after trauma or with blood dyscrasias such as hemophilia. In most of these conditions, the finding is better demonstrated with barium studies.

References

1. Byrn JR, Fitzgerald JF, Northway JD, Anand SK, Scott JR: Unusual manifestations of Henoch-Schonlein syndrome. *Am J Dis Child* 130:1335–1337, 1976.
2. Grossman H, Berdon WE, Baker DH: Reversible gastrointestinal sign of hemorrhage and edema in the pediatric age group. *Radiology* 84:33, 1965.
3. Teele RL, Katz AJ, Goldman H, Kettell RM: Radiographic features of eosinophilic gastroenteritis (allergic gastroenteropathy) of childhood. *Am J Roentgenol* 132:575–580, 1979.

OTHER ABDOMINAL FINDINGS

Numerous other abdominal findings are seen on barium and IVP studies and these are summarized in Tables 3.6 to 3.23. They are not discussed in detail because of space limitations, but references are cited where appropriate.

Table 3.6 Esophageal Stenosis

Corrosive esophagitis Peptic esophagitis	Most common
Posttracheoesophageal fistula	Moderately common
Congenital, tracheobronchial remnants Trauma, chronic foreign body Infectious esophagitis Epidermolysis bullosa Barrett's esophagus	Rare

Table 3.7 Indentations of Esophagus

Mediastinal tumors Aberrant right subclavian artery (posterior)	Most common
Vascular ring (bilateral indentation plus posterior) Aberrant left subclavian artery with right aortic arch (posterior) Mediastinal cyst, tumor Lymph nodes Enlarged left atrium (anterior)	Moderately common
Systemic collaterals (congenital or acquired) Pulmonary sling (between trachea and esophagus) Right aortic arch left descending aorta (posterior)	Relatively rare
Left aortic arch, right descending aorta (posterior) Enlarged coronary sinus (anterior) Azygos or hemiazygos dilation	Rare

Table 3.8 Antropyloric Narrowing

Pylorospasm Hypertrophic pyloric stenosis (typical)	Most common
Hypertrophic pyloric stenosis (incomplete hypertrophy) (1)	Moderately common
Pyloric stenosis-atypical short segment (2) Chemical gastritis Tumor Aberrant pancreas Duplication cyst Congenital stenosis-atresia Chronic granulomatosis disease of childhood (neutrophil dysfunction) (3) Regional enteritis	Relatively rare

References

1. Swischuk LE, Hayden CK Jr Tyson KR: Atypical muscle hypertrophy in pyloric stenosis, Am J Roentgenol 134:481–484, 1980.
2. Swischuk LE, Hayden CK Jr, Tyson KR: Short segment pyloric narrowing pylorospasm or pyloric stenosis? Pediatr Radiol 10:201–205, 1981.
3. Griscom DT, Kirkpatrick Jr, Girdany BR, et al: Gastric antral narrowing in chronic granulomatosis of childhood. Pediatrics 54:456–460, 1974.

Table 3.9 Thickened Small Bowel Mucosal Folds

Edema[a]
  Nephrotic syndrome
  Hypoproteinema
  Portal vein obstruction
  Portal hypertension
Gastroenteritis[a]
	Most common

Celiac disease[a] Cystic fibrosis[a] Protein losing enteropathy[a] Regional enteritis (Crohn's disease)[a]	Moderately common
Giardiasis (more common if endemic)[b] Eosinophilic gastroenteritis[a] Intestinal lymphangiectasia[b] Zollinger-Ellison syndrome[a] Constrictive pericarditis[a]	Relatively rare

[a] Thick and straight.
[b] Thick and tortuous.

Reference

1. Swischuk LE: Mucosal patterns in diffuse disease in the small bowel. Med Radiogr Photogr 47:34–40, 1971.

Table 3.10 Thickened Gastric Mucosal Folds

Normal (not as marked as in adults)	Commonest
Gastritis Lymphoma Eosinophilic gastroenteritis Menetrier's disease	Relatively rare

Table 3.11 Colonic Mucosal Ulceration

Ulcerative colitis Crohn's disease (regional enteritis) Necrotizing enterocolitis in infancy	Commonest
Infectious bacterial colitis	Moderately common
Ischemic colitis Postradiation colitis Obstructive (stercoral) colitis Pseudomembranous enterocolitis	Relatively rare

Table 3.12   Megacolon

Functional (psychogenic) megacolon Hirschsprung's disease	Commonest
Anorectal anomalies with stenosis	Moderately common
Congenital stenosis; isolated Hypothyroidism Chagas' disease Chronic immobilization Medication producing hypotonia Neuronal intestinal dysplasia (1) Plexiform neurofibromatosis of colon	Relatively rare

Reference

1. Scharli AF, Meier-Ruge W: Localized and disseminated forms of neuronal intestinal dysplasia mimicking Hirschsprung's disease. J Pediatr Surg 16:164–170, 1981.

Table 3.13   Filling Defects in Intestine

Normal fecal material Lymphoid hyperplasia (1)[a,e]	Commonest
Lymphoid hyperplasia (small bowel)[a,f] Juvenile polyps; inflammatory-sporadic (2)[c,e] Pseudopolyps—ulcerative colitis[b,e] Pseudopolyps—Crohn's disease[b,e] Familial polyposis[a,b,e]	Moderately common

Other polyposis syndromes
    Peutz-Jeghers syndrome (small bowel)
    Canada-Cronkhite syndrome (colon, stomach)
    Gardner's syndrome
Juvenile polyps, inflammatory-familial (2)[c,e]
	Relatively rare

[a] Small cobblestone.
[b] Large cobblestone.
[c] Varying sizes; some with stalks.
[d] Large and small bowel.
[e] Mostly large bowel.
[f] Mostly small bowel.

References

1. Capitanio MA, Kirkpatrick JA: Lymphoid hyperplasia of the colon in children. Radiology 94:323–327, 1970.
2. Schwartz AM, McCauley RGK: Juvenile gastrointestinal polyposis. Radiology 121:441–444, 1976.

Table 3.14   Small Kidneys

Chronic pyelonephritis[a] Chronic glomerulonephritis[a] Congenitally hypoplastic[a]	Commonest
Renal vein thrombosis (chronic with atrophy)[b] Atrophy after obstructive uropathy[a] Renal artery stenosis; occlusion[b]	Moderately common
Postirradiation[b] Papillary necrosis (late)[a] Ask-Upmark kidney[b] Juvenile nephronophthisis (medullary sponge)[a]	Relatively rare

[a] Often or usually bilateral.
[b] Usually unilateral.

Table 3.15   Large Kidneys

Nephrotic syndrome[b] Acute glomerulonephritis[b] Wilm's tumor[a]	Commonest
Compensatory hypertrophy[a] Fused ectopy[a] Infant of diabetic mother[b] Infantile polycystic kidney[b] Adult polycystic kidney[b] Multicystic dysplastic kidney[a] Leukemia-lymphoma[b] Infant of diabetic mother[b]	Moderately common
Intrarenal abscess, hematoma[a] Renal vein thrombosis (acute)[a] Other renal tumors[a] Glycogen storage disease[b] Tuberous sclerosis[b] Beckwith-Wiedemann syndrome[b] Sickle cell disease[b] Nephroblastomatosis[b]	Relatively rare

[a] Usually unilateral.
[b] Usually bilateral.

Table 3.16   Prolonged Nephrogram

Infantile polycystic kidney (streaky) Tamm-Horsfal proteinuria (neonates)	Commonest
Renal vein thrombosis Acute tubular necrosis Acute ureteral obstruction	Moderately common
Papillary necrosis Severe hypotension (tubular necrosis)	Relatively rare

Table 3.17 Megaureter

Distal obstruction Ureterovesical reflux }	Commonest
Diabetes insipidus Prune belly syndrome }	Moderately common
Megaureter, primary Barter's syndrome Chronic water-drinking }	Moderately common

Table 3.18 Pear-Shaped Bladder

Neurogenic }	Commonest
Pelvic Hematoma }	Moderately common
Pelvic lymphoma, leukemia Iliopsoas muscle hypertrophy Inferior vena caval obstruction with collaterals }	Rare
Pelvic lipomatosis }	Very rare

Table 3.19 Large Bladder

Neurogenic Urethral obstruction Psychogenic }	Commonest
Prune belly syndrome Chronic diuretic therapy }	Moderately common
Diabetes insipidus Psychogenic water drinking Megacystis-microcolon syndrome Barter's syndrome }	Relatively rare

Table 3.20 Small Bladder

Spastic neurogenic }	Commonest

Severe cystitis (infection, drug in-
  duced)
Chronic distal obstruction with hy-
  pertrophy
Bladder diversion }
	Moderately common

Congenital small Surrounding tumor }	Rare

Table 3.21 Large Calices—Hydronephrosis

Distal obstruction (calyceal steno- sis, UPJ, lower UT obstruction) }	Commonest
Ureterovesicular reflux }	Moderately common
Papillary necrosis }	Relatively rare
Congenital megacalices }	Rare

Table 3.22 Filling Defects—Urinary Tract

Stones Blood clots Vascular compressions }	Commonest
Ureterocele (ectopic with duplicated kidney) }	Moderately common
Ureterocele—orthopic Polyps Tumors Fungal pyelitis with debris Bacterial pyelitis with debris }	Relatively rare

Table 3.23 Presacral Masses

Sacrococcygeal teratoma Obstructed rectum with fecal mate- rial }	Commonest
Abscess (ruptured appendix, Crohn's disease) }	Moderately common
Hematoma with trauma Rhabdomyosarcoma Neurogenic tumors Chordoma of sacrum Anterior meningocele Duplication cysts }	Rare

Chapter 4

BONES AND SOFT TISSUES

This chapter deals with a great many bony and soft tissue abnormalities, and while some occur alone others occur as part of certain syndromes or dysplasias. To discuss each of these syndromes in detail would defeat the purpose of this book, but yet, they must be mentioned. If more details are desired, however, they can be obtained from a number of currently available textbooks on the subject (1–6).

References

1. Caffey J: *Pediatrric X-Ray Diagnosis,* ed 7. Chicago, Year Book Medical Publishers, 1978.
2. Cremin BJ, Beighton P: *Bone Dysplasias of Infancy.* Berlin, Springer-Verlag, 1978.
3. Smith DW: *Recognizable Patterns of Human Malformation.* Schaffer AJ (consulting ed): *Major Problems in Clinical Pediatrics.* Philadelphia, WB Saunders, 1970, vol 7.
4. Spranger JW, Langer LO, Wiedemann HR: *Bone Dysplasias.* Philadelphia, WB Saunders, 1974.
5. Swischuk LE: *Radiology of the Newborn and Young Infant,* ed 2. Baltimore, Williams & Wilkins, 1980.
6. Taybi H: *Radiology of Syndromes,* ed 2. Chicago, Year Book Medical Publishers, 1982.

GENERALIZED BONE DENSITY CHANGES

For the most part, generalized bone density increase (i.e., whiter bones) infers excess calcium deposition and decreased density, loss, or decreased deposition of calcium. Causes of both are discussed in the following paragraphs and summarized in Tables 4.1 and 4.2.

Table 4.1 Increased Bone Density

Osteopetrosis Chronic renal disease (treated)	Commonest
Idiopathic osteosclerosis of newborn Neonatal intrauterine infections Hypothyroidism Heavy metal intoxication Old periosteal bone deposition	Moderately common
Idiopathic hypercalcemia Mucopolysaccharidosis Mucolipidosis	Relatively rare
Pyknodysostosis Myelofibrosis, leukemia Fluorosis Hypervitaminosis D Van Buchem's disease Kenny-Caffey syndrome[a] Melorheostosis[b] Pachydermoperiostitis[b] Mastocytosis (late stages) Hyperphosphatemia[b] Engelmann's disease[b] Sarcoidosis Robinow-Silverman-Smith syndrome Pyles disease (neonate)[b]	Rare

[a] Medullary canal stanosis—thin bones with thick cortex.
[b] Diaphyseal predominance with or without expanded or wavy cortex (periostium).

INCREASED BONE DENSITY

Excess calcium deposition leading to increased bone density can occur on a metabolic basis, with certain hematologic disorders and, inherently, in some bony dysplasias or syndromes (Table 4.1). In terms of the **dysplasias,** the one best known is osteopetrosis or Albers-Schönberg disease. In this condition, except in very mild cases, the changes of markedly white bones, virtual obliteration of the medullary canal, a bone-within-bone appearance of many of the bones, and transverse fractures of the chalk-like skeleton are easy to detect (Fig. 4.1A). Associated anemia and hepatosplenomegaly are common, and are important in differentiating the condition from other conditions associated with increased bone density. For the most part, these include entities such as pyknodysostosis (19, 25), the idiopathic hypercalcemia (Williams') syndrome, and the Robinow-Silverman-Smith syndrome (16).

In pyknodysostosis, certain clinical (i.e., dwarfism, shortened extremities, frontal bossing) and roentgenographic (terminal phalangeal underdevelopment, pear-shaped frontal calvarial configuration, Wormian bones) features cause confusion with cleidocranial dysostosis. However, in the latter, the clavicles and pubic bones usually are not intact, and no bony sclerosis occurs. Pyknodysostosis also can be confused with osteopetrosis, but with pyknodysostosis, no hematologic disturbances are present, and thus, there is no hepatosplenomegaly. In addition, the "bone-within-bone" appearance and certain metaphyseal growth disturbances, such as splaying and transverse banding, are absent. Williams' syndrome is associated with an abnormal facial appearance (often termed elfin facies) and in many cases, vascular abnormalities, such as supravalvulvar aortic stenosis, peripheral pulmonary artery coarctations, and systemic artery stenoses. The bones, although increased in density, are not deformed or shortened to the point that an obvious dysplasia is suggested. Overall, however, the condition is not that common. Even more rare is the Robinow-Silverman-Smith syndrome, a form of middle segment dwarfism where, in addition to sclerotic bones (16), hypoplastic genitalia and spinal anomalies are seen.

In the neonatal period, all of the three preceding conditions can be confused with a normal, transient form of osteosclerosis (20), and the osteosclerosis of some intrauterine infections. Infants demonstrating the transient form of increased bony density are believed to have, as a normal variation, more compact bone than usual. The finding resolves by 2 or 3 months

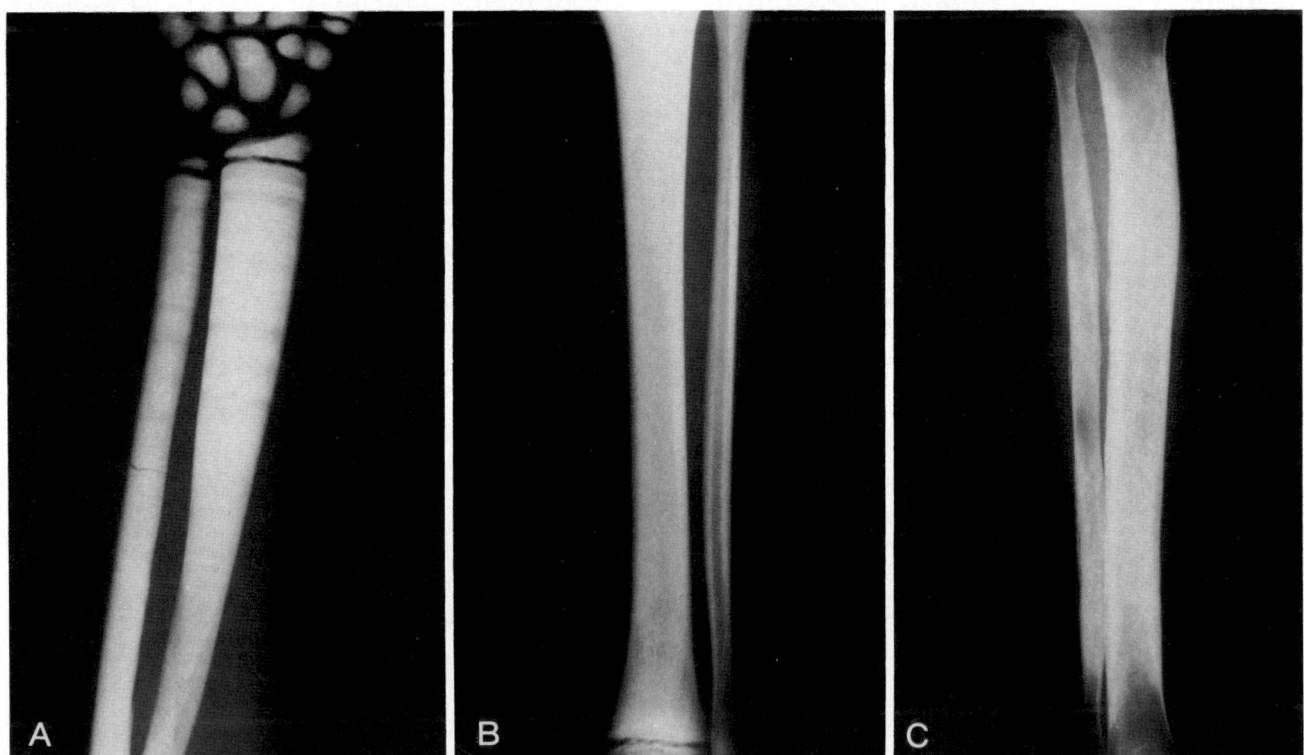

Fig. 4.1. Increased bone density. A. Typical appearance of bony sclerosis in osteopetrosis. Also note some diaphyseal widening and multiple transverse, trophic bands. B. Generalized osteosclerosis in granulocytic leukemia. C. Osteosclerosis due to periosteal new bone deposition in Engelmann-Camurati disease or progressive diaphyseal dysplasia.

of age and usually is considered innocuous. The cause of increased bone density in neonatal infections, primarily rubella (20, 23), is unknown, but there may be impaired turnover of bone in these patients (23).

Increased bone density in **hematologic** disease is uncommon but occasionally can be seen with myelofibrosis, either primary, or secondary to leukemia (21) (Fig. 4.1B). Patchy sclerosis, eventually leading to more uniform sclerosis, as seen after multiple bone infarction in sickle cell disease, is not common in infants and young children. If it is seen, it occurs in older children and young adults. **Metabolic** causes of increased bone density include the previously mentioned idiopathic hypercalcemia or Williams' syndrome, dialyzed patients with chronic renal disease (usually healing phase of renal osteodystrophy), hypervitaminosis D (increased calcium and phosphorus deposition), and hypothyroidism (20). In hypothyroidism, it is not known why the bones appear dense, but it may be because of slow bone growth leading to a lack of normal turnover of calcium in the bones. This, however, is conjecture only, but whatever the cause is, with treatment, density decreases. Other causes of increased bone density include chronic lead intoxication, other heavy metal intoxication, fluorosis, the odd case of sarcoidosis (22), pseudo and pseudopseudohypoparathyroidism, and the Kenny-Caffey syndrome. In the latter condition sclerosis is associated with stenosis of the medullary canals. As a result the bones are quite thin but yet their cortices are thick and dense.

Before leaving the subject of increased bone density, it might be noted that under certain conditions the diaphyses of the bones are dense and yet the metaphyseal regions are of normal density, or indeed demineralized. This occurs with certain bone dysplasias and with profound diaphyseal periosteal new bone deposition from any cause. Bony dysplasias to be considered include progressive diaphyseal dysplasia or Engelmann-Camurati disease (Fig. 4.1C), Pyle's disease in infancy, Van Buchem's generalized osteosclerosis (4, 18), pachydermoperiostosis, and melorheostosis (2). Similar changes also occur with healing Caffey's disease (infantile cortical hyperostosis), healing widespread osteomyelitis, and healing injuries such as those sustained in the battered child syndrome. An unusual cause of increased bone density is work hypertrophy in athletes who overuse an extremity (i.e., forearm in baseball pitching and tennis, etc., and the tibia in ballet). Finally, it should be noted that a relative increase in bone density of the diaphysis occurs when there is rapid demineralization of the metaphyses. This occurs with acute onset osteoporosis and can produce a picture which erroneously suggests that the problem is in the diaphyses, rather than the metaphyses.

DECREASED BONE DENSITY

Decreased bone density results from decreased calcium content of the bones, and the problem occurs both with osteoporosis and osteomalacia (Table 4.2). With osteoporosis, however, there is concomitant decrease in bone matrix (i.e., osteoid), while with osteomalacia, bone matrix is normal. However, the bone matrix in osteomalacia is never adequately mineralized, and in time, actually becomes relatively overabundant. This leads to bone softening, bending, and fracturing. These fractures may be overt, or of the Looser type, that is a green-stick fracture due to chronic bending. With osteoporosis, bone bending is not a particular problem but since the bones are structurally weak they do tend to fracture easily. An exception occurs in familial hyperphosphatemia where the combination of bone overgrowth and overdestruction (severe bone hypermetabolism) precludes the formation of normal bone and, in the more severe cases, causes the osteoporotic bones to become severely ballooned, softened, and bowed.

The decrease in bone matrix in **osteoporosis** can result from a basic lack of its formation or loss after its normal deposition. This latter phenomenon occurs whenever osteoclastic activity surpasses osteoblastic activity and results is bone atrophy. Most often this occurs with immobilization, either acute or chronic, but it also is common with the hyperemia associated with infections, inflammations, trauma, and the occasional AV fistula. Inherently the problem exists in certain bony dysplasias and dystrophies, and also with any cause of bone marrow hypercellularity or impregnation by foreign material (i.e., the storage diseases).

With immobilization of an extremity, or the whole body, normal stresses on bone are removed and osteoblastic activity is depressed. In the face of continued osteoclastic activity, this leads to bone atrophy and osteoporosis; i.e., old bone is not replaced by new bone and slowly bone loss and demineralization occur. Roentgenographically, this is manifest by thinning of the trabeculae and cortices and, with time, disappearance of the smaller trabeculae and increased prominence of the larger ones (Fig. 4.2). Eventually the bone assumes a very glassy appearance with the thin, but white, trabeculae and cortices standing out in prominent relief. Overall the pattern is rather delicate. The same phenomenon occurs with hyperemia and also in the early stages of any bone marrow hypercellularity or foreign material impregnation problem. Hypercellularity usually occurs with the chronic anemias, leukemia, lymphoma, metastatic disease, and mastocytosis, while foreign material impregnation is seen with the various storage diseases. In all of these cases, when the smaller trabeculae disappear altogether, a helter-skelter pattern of large trabeculae remains (Fig. 4.2C).

In osteomalacia, with no matrix or osteoid loss, the trabeculae and cortex do not become thinned, only

Table 4.2   Decreased Bone Density

Osteoporosis
    Disuse (immobilization) ⎫
    Failure to thrive (undernutrition) ⎭ Commonest

    Chronic anemia (14) ⎫
    Osteogenesis imperfecta
    Steroid therapy
    Collagen vascular diseases   Moderately common
    Liver tumors (20)
    Hyperemia with
       Infection, inflammation,
        AV fistula ⎭

    Idiopathic hypocalcemia ⎫
    Cushing's syndrome (10)
    Idiopathic juvenile osteoporosis
       (6, 7)
    Mucopolysaccharidoses   Relatively rare
    Turner's syndrome (3)
    Hyperthyroidism
    Sudeck's atrophy
    Gaucher's disease (12) ⎭

    Scurvy ⎫
    Niemann-Pick disease
    Pseudo or pseudopseudohypo-
       parathyroidism
    Sarcoidosis
    Winchester's syndrome (24)
    Progeria
    Ehler-Danlos syndrome
    Mucolipidoses
    Mastocytosis (9)
    Homocystinuria   Rare
    Phenylketonuria
    Pyle's disease
    Otopalitodigital syndrome
    Other craniometaphyseal dyspla-
       sias
    Lipogranulomatosis (17)
    Hyperphosphatemia
    Diaphyseal dysplasia (Engel-
       mann-Camurati) ⎭

Osteomalacia
    Rickets (all types) ⎫
    Hyperparathyroidism (including   Commonest
       renal osteodystrophy) ⎭

    Hypophosphatasia, pseudohypo- ⎫
       phosphatasia
    Fibrogenesis imperfecta
    Gangliosidosis[a]   Relatively rare
    Jansen's metaphyseal dysosto-
       sis[a]
    Mucolipidosis II (I cell disease)[a] ⎭

[a] In infancy, changes resemble hyperparathyroidism.

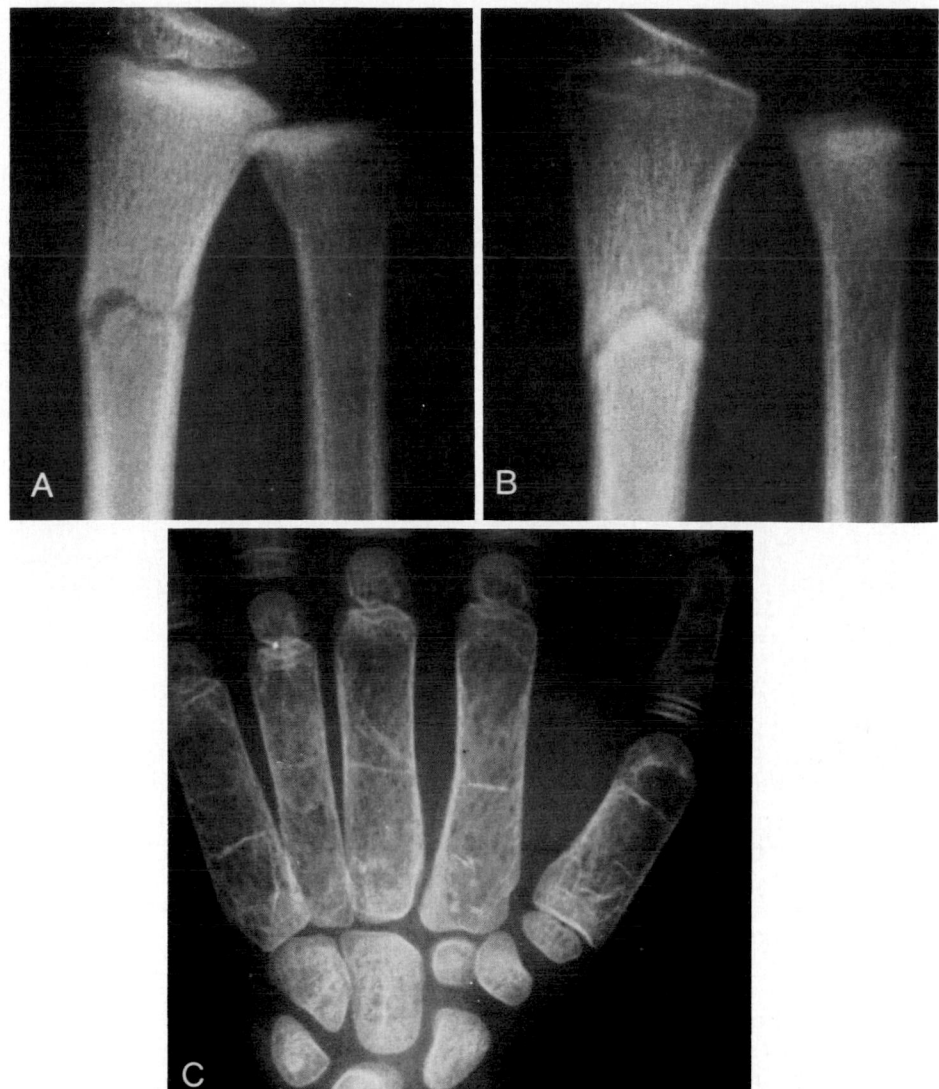

Fig. 4.2. Diminished bone density: osteoporosis. A. Normal, trabecular pattern and bone density in patient with recent fracture. B. Same patient, approximately 2 weeks after the fracture demonstrates loss of smaller trabeculae, and overall demineralization. Note that the cortices remain white and relatively distinct. Also, see Figs. 4.3A and 4.18B. C. Long-standing osteoporosis in patient with Cooley's anemia, demonstrating expanded bones, a helter-skelter pattern of thin remaining trabeculae, and thin, but distinct cortices. The bones have a very glassy appearance.

demineralized. The result is a coarse, indistinct, fuzzy pattern of demineralization, quite different from the delicate, sharp-appearing pattern seen with osteoporosis (Fig. 4.3). Thereafter, as the changes advance, the cortex becomes so poorly defined that it virtually disappears. A more or less complete list of conditions producing osteomalacia is presented in Table 4.2, but the most common are rickets and hyperparathyroidism. Hyperparathyroidism usually is secondary, and seen mostly in, renal osteodystrophy, for primary hyperparathyroidism is rare in childhood. Most of the other conditions listed in Table 4.2 would be expected to produce osteomalacia and are no surprise, but a comment regarding Jansen's metaphyseal dysostosis, gangliosidosis, and mucolipidosis II is in order. These

diseases, unrelated to hyperparathyroidism, for some reason produce changes indistinguishable from it in infancy. Later on, as the patient grows older, the findings become more those of typical osteoporosis. Finally, it should be noted that osteoporosis and osteomalacia can occur together, and then the findings of both are intertwined. Actually, the problem is not so uncommon and the reason for this is that, in many of the conditions producing severe osteomalacia, illness is so severe that the patient becomes bedridden. This leads to disuse (immobilization) osteoporosis. Examples of relatively pure osteoporosis, osteomalacia, and mixed osteomalacia and osteoporosis are presented in Fig. 4.3.

For the most part, the rules just outlined regarding

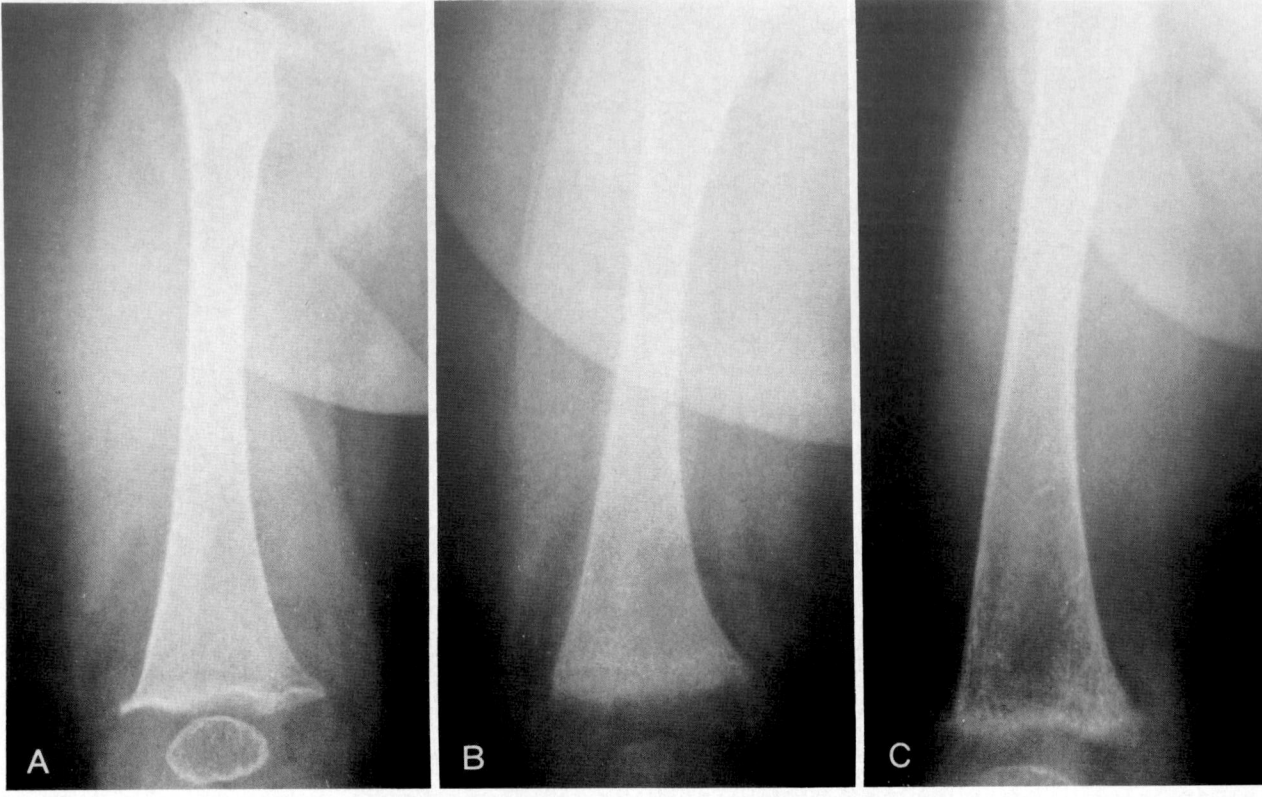

Fig. 4.3. A. **Osteoporosis.** Typical findings of glassy appearing bones, with thin, but distinct cortices. This patient had scurvy. Note the ringed epiphysis. B. **Osteomalacia.** Note indistinctness of the cortex and trabeculae. Also note typical rachitic changes in the metaphysis. Osteomalacia is characteristic of rickets. C. **Mixed osteoporosis and osteomalacia.** Patient with severe mental retardation, immobilization, and nutritional rickets. The findings are a mixture of those seen in the previous two patients.

osteomalacia and osteoporosis can be applied to conditions causing them with fair reliability. However, in hyperphosphatemia a condition characterized by hypermetabolic bone disease, bone formation and subsequent resorption are so rapid that the cortex appears laminated and erroneously suggests osteomalacia. In actual fact, however, the problem is osteoporosis. In these cases, it is the rapidity with which changes in trabecular pattern occur that causes the findings to mimic those of osteomalacia.

References

1. Aschinberg LC, Solomon LM, Zeis PM, Justice P, Rosenthal IM: Vitamin D-resistant rickets associated with epidermal nevus syndrome: demonstration of a phosphaturic substance in the dermal lesions. *J Pediatr* 91:56–60, 1977.
2. Beauvais P, Faure C, Montagne JP, Chigot PL, Maroteaux P: Leri's melorheostosis: three pediatric cases and a review of the literature. *Pediatr Radiol* 6:153–159, 1977.
3. Brown DM, Jowsey J, Bradford DS: Osteoporosis in ovarian dysgenesis. *J Pediatr* 84:816–820, 1974.
4. Cremin BJ: Sclerosteosis in children. *Pediatr Radiol* 8:173–177, 1979.
5. Hollister DW, Rimoin DL, Lachman RS, Cohen AH, Reed WB, Westin GW: The Winchester syndrome: a nonlysosomal connective tissue disease. *J Pediatr* 84:701–709, 1974.
6. Houang MTW, Brenton DP, Renton P, Shaw DG: Idiopathic juvenile osteoporosis. *Skeletal Radiol* 3:17–23, 1978.
7. Jowsey J, Johnson KA: Juvenile osteoporosis: bone findings in seven patients. *J Pediatr* 81:511–517, 1972.
8. Karlin CA, Browner AC: Multiple primary hemangiomas of bone. *Am J Roentgenol* 129:162–164, 1977.
9. Lucaya J, Perez-Candela V, Aso C, Calvo J: Mastocytosis with skeletal and gastrointestinal involvement in infancy; two case reports and a review of the literature. *Radiology* 131:363–366, 1979.
10. McArthur RG, Cloutier MD, Hayles AB, Sprague RG: Cushing's disease in children: findings in 13 cases. *Mayo Clin Proc* 47:318–326, 1972.
11. Mehls O, Willich E, Beduhn D, Schuler HW, Krempien B, Ritz E: Roentgenological findings in the skeleton of dialysed children. *Pediatr Radiol* 1:183–190, 1973.
12. Meyers H, Cremin B, Beighton P, Sacks S: Chronic Gaucher's disease: radiological finding in 17 South African cases. *Br J Radiol* 48:465–469, 1975.
13. Moncrieff MW, Brenton DP, Arthur LJH: Case of tumour rickets. *Arch Dis Child* 53:740–745, 1978.
14. Moseley JE: Skeletal changes in the anemias. *Semin Roentgenol* 9:169–184, July, 1974.

15. Pollack JA, Schuller AL, Crawford JD: Rickets and myopathy cured by removal of non-ossifying fibroma of bone. *Pediatrics* 52:364, 1973.
16. Robinow M, Silverman FN, Smith HD: A newly recognized dwarfing syndrome. *Am J Dis Child* 117:645–649, 1969.
17. Schultz G, Lang EK. Disseminated lipogranulomatosis: early roentgenographic changes. *Radiology* 82:675–678, 1964.
18. Scott WC, Gautby THT: Hyperostosis corticalis generalisata familiaris. *Br J Radiol* 47:500–503, 1974.
19. Srivastava KK, Bhattacharya AK, Galatius-Jensen F, Tamaela LA, Borgstein A, Kozlowski K: Pycnodysostosis (report of four cases). *Australas Radiol* 22:70–78, 1978.
20. Swischuk LE: *Radiology of the Newborn and Young Infant,* ed 2. Baltimore, Williams & Wilkins, 1980, pp 447, 613, 644.
21. Tebbi K, Zarkowsky HS, Siegel BA, McAlister WH: Childhood myelofibrosis and osteosclerosis without myeloid metaplasia. *Radiology* 114:246, 1975 (abstract).
22. Weston M, Duffy P: Osteosclerosis in sarcoidosis. *Australas Radiol* 19:191–193, 1975.
23. Whalen JP, Winchester P, Krook L., O'Donohue N, Dische R, Nunez E: Neonatal transplacental rubella syndrome; its effect on normal maturation of the diaphysis. *Am J Roentgenol* 121:166–172, 1974.
24. Winchester P, Grossman H, Lim WN, Danes BS: A new acid mucopolysaccharidosis with skeletal deformities simulating rheumatoid arthritis. *Am J Roentgenol Radium Ther Nucl Med* 106:128, 1969.
25. Wolpowitz A, Matisonn A: A comparative study of pycnodysostosis, cleidocranial dysostosis, osteopetrosis and acro-osteolysis. *Radiology* 113:758, 1974 (abstract).
26. Wooten WB, de Sants LA, Finkelstein JB: Case report 61, diagnosis; systematic mastocytosis. *Skeletal Radiol* 3:53–55, 1978.

LONG BONE TUBULATION ABNORMALITIES

With tubulation abnormalities of the long bones one can encounter undertubulated (short, squat) or overtubulated (long, thin) bones. Short, squat bones can be classified as follows: (*a*) simple short, squat bones; (*b*) bones which are dumbbell in appearance; (*c*) bones were middle segment (radius-ulna, tibia-fibula), shortening predominates; and (*d*) bones which are so wide that they appear ballooned. With long, thin bones it is not practical to subclassify the configurations because the bones tend to appear much the same from condition to condition.

Undertubulation: Short, Squat Bones (Table 4.3)

Undertubulation can occur on a focal or generalized basis and, whereas focal shortening usually is secondary to injury, infection, or congenital hypoplasia, generalized shortening occurs primarily with bone dysplasias, dwarfing syndromes, and widespread phocomelia such as occurs in thalidamide embryonopathy. In terms of bony dysplasias, the one best known to produce short, squat bones is achondroplastic dwarfism (Fig. 4.4A), a form of dwarfism serving as a prototype for all forms due to impaired enchondral bone formation. In addition to the short long bones, the ribs are short, the iliac wings square and hypoplastic, the acetabular angles flat, the calvarial base underdeveloped and constricted, the vertebra small and cuboid, and the spinal canal itself narrower than normal. At the same time, the foramen magnum is smaller than normal and may lead to obstructive hydrocephalus. Hypochondroplasia probably is related to achondroplasia, but the bone changes are much less pronounced (4, 6, 8).

In the neonatal period, a number of other dwarfs which tend to resemble severely afflicted achondroplasts can be encountered. Most have definite features which distinguish them from true achondroplasia, but to review all of these would be beyond the scope of this book. On the other hand, one might at least be familiar with some of their names; asphyxiating thoracic dystrophy (long bone shortening usually not so severe), achondrogenesis (lower spine is unossified), thanatophoric dwarfism (looks like severe achondroplasia), short rib polydactyly dwarfism (Majewski and Saldino-Noonan types—very short bones), metatrophic dwarfism (have dumbbell-shaped long bones), the Kniest syndrome (resemble metatrophic dwarfs), the severe micromelic form of punctate epiphyseal dysplasia (20), Jansen-type metaphyseal dysostosis (shows changes similar to hyperparathyroidism), and diastrophic dwarfism. In the latter condition, the bones usually are more bowed than in the other syndromes and the spine markedly kyphoscoliotic. In addition, severe clubfoot deformity is present, and actually, is a hallmark of the condition.

Short, but not always squat bones are seen in the condition known as pseudoachondroplasia. Certain features in these children may at first suggest achondroplasia, but the problem is not so much poor enchondral bone formation as epiphyseal maldevelopment. The changes vary in severity and it is the more severe cases which are confused with achondroplasia (Fig. 4.4B). However, if one examines the epiphyses closely, one will note that they are markedly or predominantly involved, whereas in achondroplasia, epiphyseal changes are minimal.

There are two forms of pseudoachondroplasia: multiple epiphyseal and spondyloepiphyseal types. In the latter, severe platyspondyly exists, while in the former it does not. In either case, however, along with marked epiphyseal underdevelopment, there is concomitant metaphyseal growth impairment. As a result, metaphyseal flaring and long bone shortening occur and it

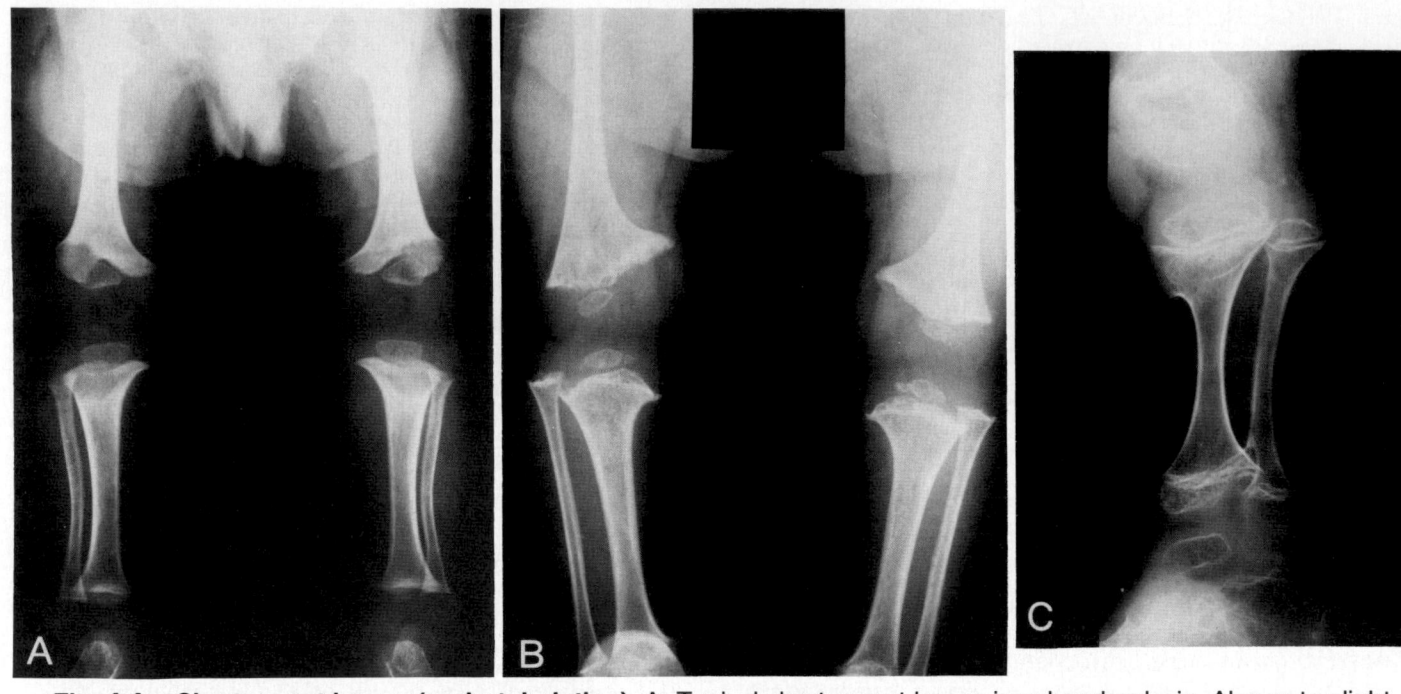

Fig. 4.4. Short, squat bones (undertubulation). A. Typical short, squat bones in achondroplasia. Also note slight degree of bowing and that the fibulae are considerably longer than the tibiae. B. **Pseudochondroplasia.** Note overall similar appearance to achondroplasia, but also note that epiphyseal involvement is marked. In less severe cases, the bones are not as squat, but still quite short. C. **Dumbbell**-shaped bones in metatrophic dwarfism.

is for this reason achondroplasia is misdiagnosed. The term "pseudoachondroplasia" has been applied to these patients, for even though one is reminded of achondroplasia, no other features of the condition exist (i.e., the calvarium is normal, the spinal canal not particularly narrowed, the vertebrae are not cuboid, etc.).

In some conditions where the long bones are short, metaphyseal flaring is so pronounced that a **dumbbell appearance of the bones results**. Only a few conditions produce such a degree of change and, for the most part, include metatrophic dwarfism (Fig. 4.4C), the Kniest syndrome, and the more severe cases of pseudoachondroplasia. Dumbbelling to a lesser degree occurs with many of the dwarfing syndromes noted in the preceding paragraphs, especially the Ellis-Van Creveld syndrome (19) and diastrophic dwarfism. However, the finding usually is not a key to diagnosis. In the first three conditions mentioned, it is.

Conditions where **middle segment** or so-called **mesomelic shortening** predominates are not particularly common but include mesomelic dwarfism (Nievergelt's and Langer types), the nail patella syndrome (hereditary osteoonychodysplasia), dyschondrosteosis or Madelung's deformity (upper extremity predominance), the Ellis-van Creveld syndrome (19), the Robinow-Silverman syndrome (5), and the ulno-fibular dysplasia syndromes of Reinhardt and Pfeiffer. In many of these cases, the bones, in addition to being short, also are curved or bent (Fig. 4.5A) and in dyschondrosteosis or Madelung's deformity, the posteriorly dislocated distal ulna is typical (Fig. 4.5, B and C). In mesomelic dwarfism and the ulnofibular dysplasia syndromes, the involved bones also often are severely hypoplastic.

Before leaving the topic of generalized bone shortening, it might be worth noting that there are a number of conditions where the bones are shortened, but yet not particularly squat. This occurs, for example, in the Turner and Cornelia deLange syndromes, in cleidocranial dysostosis, and in both camptomelic dwarfism and Larsen's syndrome. In these latter cases, in addition to generalized hypoplasia, the ends of the long bones of the upper extremity, especially around the elbow, tend to be hypoplastic. In Larsen's syndrome, multiple joint dislocations coexist and are quite specific for the syndrome.

Bone shortening on an **isolated basis** most often occurs after trauma or infection of a bone. In the battered child syndrome, shortening may be more generalized but still rather asymmetric. Osteogenesis imperfecta, in its congenita form, also can produce asymmetrically short, squat bones. Shortening of the bones in this form of osteogenesis imperfecta occurs

Table 4.3   Undertubulation: Short, Squat Bones

Achondroplasia Storage diseases	} Commonest

Hypothyroidism
Metaphyseal dysostosis
Pseudoachondroplasia[a]
Dyschondrosteosis or Madelung's
   deformity[b]
Turner's syndrome[c]
Cornelia de Lange syndrome[c]
Epiphyseal metaphyseal injury:
   trauma, infection[e]
	} Moderately common

Hypochondroplasia
Neonatal dwarfs[a] (see text)
Rickets (hypophosphatemic; type
   B)
Severe punctate epiphyseal dyspla-
   sia
Hyperphosphatemia
Hypophosphatasia
Metatropic dwarfism[a]
Kniest's syndrome[a]
Campomelic dwarfism
Larsen's syndrome[d]
Phocomelia (thalidamide)[d]
Lipogranulomatosis
Epiphyseal metaphyseal injury: ra-
   diation[e]
Epiphyseal metaphyseal injury: vi-
   tamin A intox.[e]
	} Relatively rare

[a] Bones frequently dumbbell shaped.
[b] Middle segment undertubulation predominates.
[c] Bones short but not necessarily squat.
[d] Bones often hypoplastic at one end or the other.
[e] Problem usually focal or asymmetric.

because of numerous intrauterine factors, hypercallosus, and subsequent remodeling. In the tarda form of the disease, although fractures occur, there is not the same tendency to undertubulation. Indeed, the bones usually are thin and gracile (i.e., overtubulated). A rare cause of focal bone shortening is epiphyseal-metaphyseal injury after vitamin A intoxication (15).

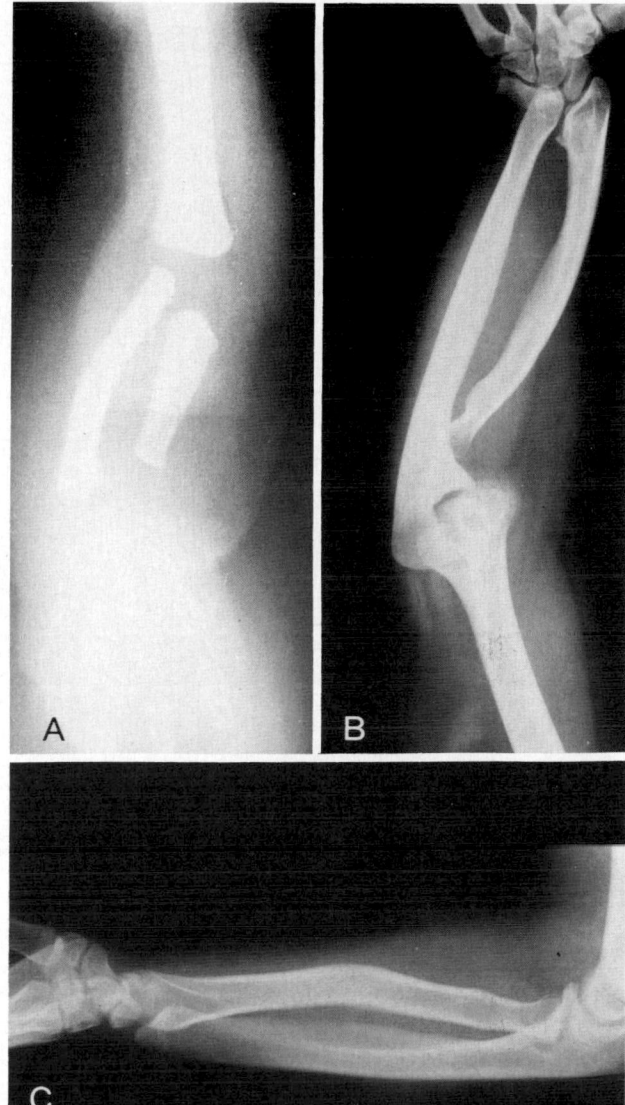

Fig. 4.5.   Middle segment shortening. A. Markedly shortened bowed bone in middle segment dwarfism. B. Typical short radius and ulna in Madelung's deformity of osteochondrosteosis. Also note increased carpal angle, and typical dislocation of the ulna in C.

Ballooned Bones

Ballooned bones are characterized by very wide shafts, thin cortices, and widely spaced trabeculae (Fig. 4.6). Conditions producing ballooned bones are listed in Table 4.4, but generally include familial hyperphosphatemia (10), mastocytosis (early stages) (23), the otopalitodigital syndrome (ballooning of metaphyses primarily), neurofibromatosis (focal involvement usually), Gaucher's disease (ballooning of metaphyses primarily), and the severe anemias (especially Cooley's anemia). With the anemias and mastocytosis (11, 23), ballooning results from marrow hypercellularity, while in Gaucher's disease, marrow infiltration with an abnormal cholesterol lipid is the cause. In the other conditions, ballooning is inherently part of the bony dysplasia, and in hyperphosphatemia it is the result of altered tubulation secondary to bone hypermetabolism and overgrowth.

Focal, or very localized ballooning can occur with fibrous dysplasia, multiple or solitary aneurysmal bone cysts (Fig. 4.6D), giant cell tumors, fibrous or cartilaginous bone tumors, and hemangiomas or lymphangiomas of bones. Apparent ballooning of bones

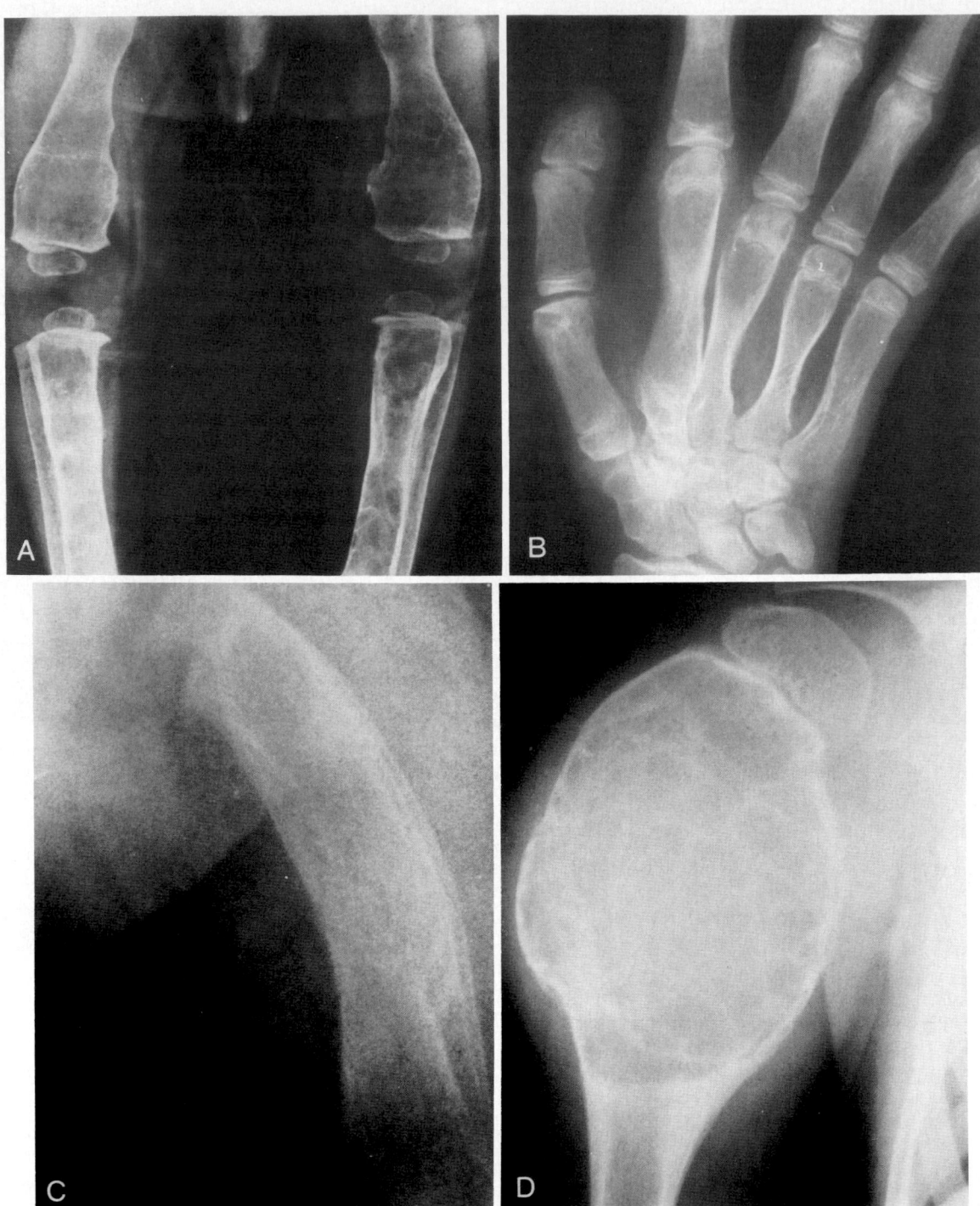

Fig. 4.6. Balloned bones. A. Typical expansion and ballooning due to bone marrow infiltration. This patient had mastocytosis. B. Generalized ballooning of the metaphyses, especially of the small bones in the hands in otopalatodigital syndrome. C. Marked ballooning of the femur in hyperphosphatemia. D. Focal ballooning due to aneurysmal bone cyst. ("A" reproduced with permission from Wooten WB, DeSantos LA, Finkelstein JB: *Skeletal Radiol* 3:53–55, 1978. "C" reproduced with permission from Dunn V, Condon VR, Rallison ML: *Am J Roentgenol* 132:541–545, 1979.)

Table 4.4 Ballooned Bones (Osteoectasia)

Generalized
  Severe anemia } Commonest

  Familial hyperphosphatemia
  Mastocytosis
  Otopalatodigital syndrome
  Gaucher's disease (metaphyseal
    regions)
  Pyle's metaphyseal dysplasia
    (metaphyseal regions)
} Relatively rare

Asymmetric or localized
  Healing fracture (ordinary or
    pathologic including battered
    child syndrome)
} Commonest

  Fibrous dysplasia
  Bone cysts
  Fibrous or cartilagaginus bone
    tumors
} Moderately common

  Hemangiomatous bone tumors
  Lymphangiomatous bone tumors
  Scurvy (healing-subperiosteal
    bleeding)
  Neurofibromatosis
} Relatively rare

occurs in the healing stages of massive subperiosteal bleeding such as occurs with pathologic fractures in patients with scurvy or neurogenic disease, neurofibromatosis (loose periosteal attachment), and hemo-

philia. It also can occur after severe ordinary fracturing, especially in the battered child syndrome (see Fig. 4.129).

Overtubulation: Long, Thin Bones (Table 4.5)

The major causes of long, thin bones are atrophy and congenital bony dysplasia. The commonest, of course, is atrophy and most often is secondary to the chronic disuse seen in a large number of neurogenic or neuromuscular diseases (Fig. 4.7A) including the heterogeneous arthrogryposis multiplex congenita group. However, it also can be seen with longstanding debilitating arthritic disease (usually rheumatoid arthritis) and in the debilitating storage disease known as Winchester's syndrome (22). In this latter condition, rheumatoid-like findings are seen.

Bony dysplasias leading to long, thin bones include osteogenesis imperfecta (Fig. 4.7B), Cockayne's syndrome, progeria, Marfan's syndrome (1), Marfan's contractural arachnodactyly (5, 7, 9, 13) (Fig. 4.7C), homocystinuria (1, 12, 14), Seckel's bird-headed dwarfism, the Kenny-Caffey or medullary stenosis syndrome (2, 3) (often associated with hypocalcemia and seizures), the Stickler syndrome, the Hallermann-Streiff and Werdnig-Hoffman syndromes, and a few instances of neurofibromatosis (focal thinning). Osteogenesis imperfecta, of course, is the most common and is characterized by impaired diaphyseal bone formation. In the Kenny-Caffey syndrome, in addition

Table 4.5 Overtubulation: Thin, Gracile Bones

Neurogenic-neuromuscular disease } Commonest

Osteogenesis imperfecta
Chronic illness with hypotonia or
  immobilization
Severe arthritic disease (rheuma-
  toid arthritis)
Arthrogryposis syndromes
} Moderately common

Marfan's syndrome
Homocystinuria
} Relatively rare

Cockayne's syndrome
Winchester's syndrome
Progeria
Kenny-Caffey (medullary stenosis
  syndrome)[a]
Marfan's contractural arachnodac-
  tyly
Stickler syndrome
Hallermann-Streiff syndrome
Seckel's bird-headed dwarf
} Rare

[a] Thin bones but thick, sclerotic cortex.

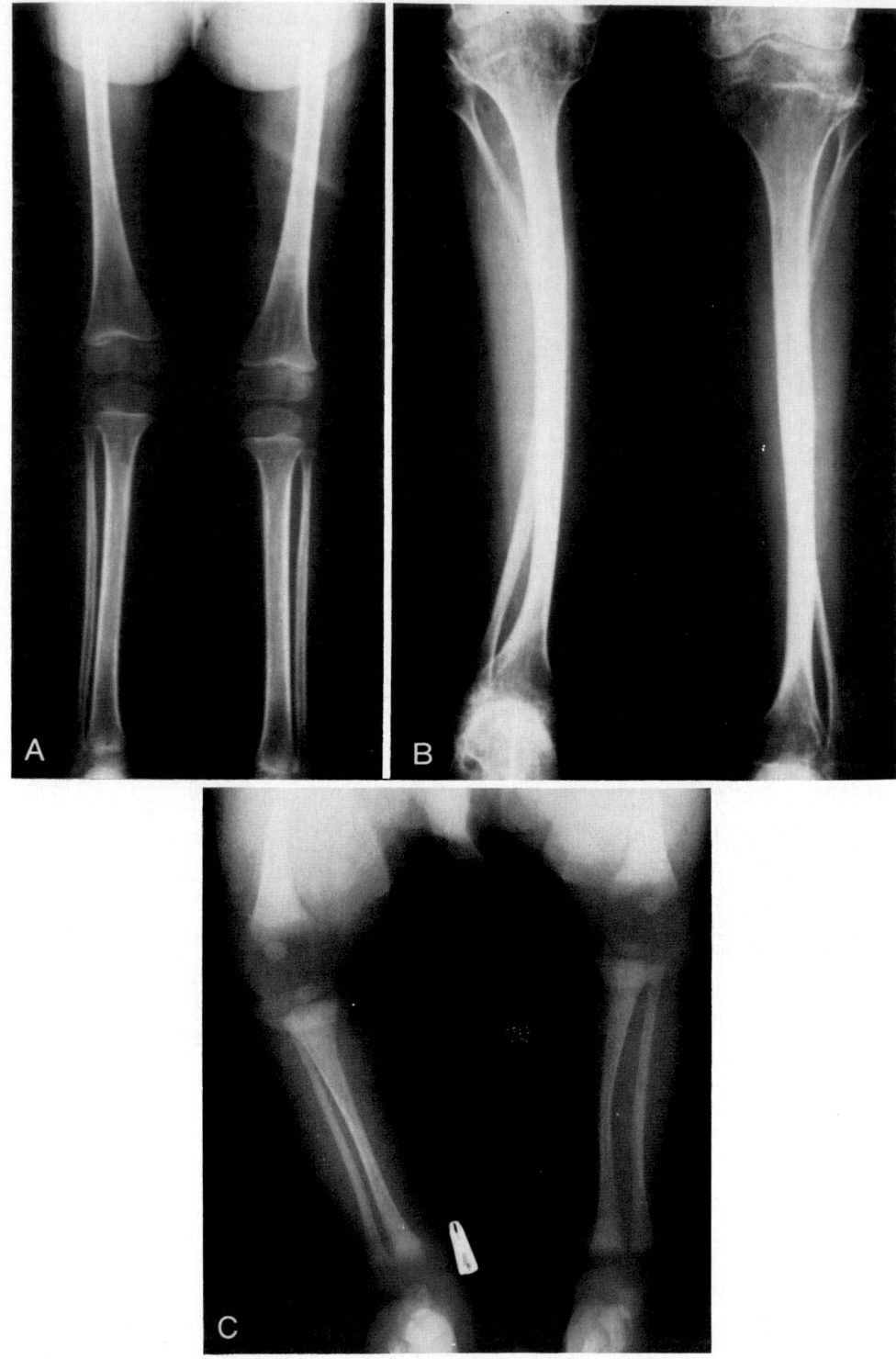

Fig. 4.7. Long, thin bones (overtubulation). A. Typical long thin bones in patient with long-standing neurogenic disease. B. Long, thin, somewhat bent bones in osteogenesis imperfecta. C. Long, thin bones in infant with Marfan's contractual arachnodactyly.

to the bones being thin, the cortices are very thick and sclerotic. Although in all of these conditions the long bones are thin and appear long, when they are truly long the best possibilities are Marfan's syndrome, Marfan's contractural arachnodactyly, and homocystinuria.

References

1. Brenton DP, Dow CJ, James JIP, Hay RL, Wynne-Davies R: Homocystinuria and Marfan's syndrome. A comparison. *J Bone Joint Surg* 54:277–298, 1972.
2. Caffey J: Congenital stenosis of medullary spaces in tubular bones and calvaria in two proportionate dwarfs—mother and son; coupled with transitory hypocalcemic tetany. *Am J Roentgenol Radium Ther Nucl Med* 100:1–11, 1967.
3. Frech RS, McAlister WH: Medullary steosis of the tubular bones associated with hypocalcemic convulsions and short stature. *Radiology* 91:457–461, 1968.
4. Glasgow JFT, Nevin NC, Thomas PS: Hypochondroplasia. *Arch Dis Child* 53:868–872, 1978.
5. Gruber MA, Graham TP Jr, Engle E, Smith C: Marfan's syndrome with contractural arachnodactyly and severe mitral regurgitation in a premature infant. *J Pediatr* 93:80–82, 1978.
6. Hall BD, Spranger J: Hypochondroplasia: clinical and radiological aspects in 39 cases. *Radiology* 133:95–100, 1979.
7. Hecht F, Beals RK: "New" syndrome of congenital contractural arachnodactyly originally described by Marfan in 1896. *Pediatrics* 49:574–579, 1972.
8. Heselson NG, Cremin BJ, Beighton P: The radiographic manifestations of hypochondroplasia. *Clin Radiol* 30:79–85, 1979.
9. Ho N, Khoo T: Congenital contractural arachnodactyly. *Am J Dis Child* 133:639–640, 1979.
10. Iancu TC, Almagor G, Friedman E, Hardoff R, Front D: Chronic familial hyperphosphatasemia. *Radiology* 129:669–676, 1978.
11. Lucaya J, Perez-Candela V, Aso C, Calvo J: Mastocytosis with skeletal and gastrointestinal involvement in infancy: two case reports and review of the literature. *Radiology* 131:363–366, 1979.
12. McCarthy JMI, Carey MC: Bone changs in homocystinuria. *Clin Radiol* 19:128, 1968.
13. MacLeod PM, Fraser FC: Congenital contractural arachnodactyly; a heritable disorder of connective tissue distinct from Marfan's syndrome. *Am J Dis Child* 126:810–812, 1973.
14. Morreels CL Jr, Fletcher BD, Weilbaecher RG, Forst JP: The roentgenographic featues of homocystinuria. *Radiology* 90:1150–1158, 1968.
15. Pease CN: Focal retardation and arrestment of growth of bones due to vitamin A intoxication. *JAMA* 182:980–985, 1962.
16. Robinow M, Silverman FN, Smith HD: A newly recognized dwarfing syndrome. *Am J Dis Child* 117:645–649, 1969.
17. Schedewie H, Willich E, Grobe H, Schmidt H, Muller KM: Skeletal findings in homocystinuria, a collaborative study. *Pediatr Radiol* 1:12–23, 1973.
18. Schultz G, Lang EK: Disseminated lipogranulomatosis: early roentgenographic changes. *Radiology* 82:675–678, 1964.
19. Stokes NJ, Sheat JH: Chondroectodermal dysplasia (Ellis-van Creveld syndrome). Case report. *Australas Radiol.* 15:259 263, 1971.
20. Swischuk LE: *Radiology of the Newborn and Young Infant,* ed 2. Baltimore, Williams & Wilkins, 1980, pp 680–701.
21. Swischuk LE, Hayden CK Jr: Rickets: a roentgenographic scheme for diagnosis. *Pediatr Radiol* 8:203–208, 1979.
22. Winchester P, Grossman H, Lim WN, Danes BS: A new acid mucopolysaccharidosis with skeletal deformities simulating rheumatoid arthritis. *Am J Roentgenol* 106:128–136, 1969.
23. Wooten WB, de Santos LA, Finkelstein JB: Case report 61, diagnosis: systemic mastocytosis. *Skeletal Radiol* 3:53–55, 1978.

BOWED BONES

Bowed bones can occur on a generalized or focal basis (Table 4.6). Focally bowed bones usually result from injury or infection while generalized bowing usually occurs with (*a*) bony dysplasias or syndromes where inherent disturbances of bone growth result in bowing, and (*b*) metabolic diseases where bones bow because they are osteomalacic and soft.

Table 4.6 Bowed Bones

A. Generalized bowing

Rickets	}	Commonest
Achondroplasia		

Osteogenesis imperfecta (congenita form with fractures)	}	Moderately common
Metaphyseal dysostosis		
Madelung's deformity (dyschondrosteosis)[a]		
Neonatal bowing		

Diastrophic dwarfism	}	Relatively rare
Hypochondroplasia		
Thanatophoric dwarfism		
Campomelic dwarfism		
Larsen's syndrome		
Pseudoachondroplasia		
Asphyxiating thoracic dystrophy		
Mucopolysaccharidoses		
Mucolipidoses		

Melnick-Needles syndrome	}	Rare
Neonatal Ellis-van Creveld syndrome		
Hypophosphatasia		
Hyperphosphatemia		
Parastremmatic dwarfism		
Marfan's contractural arachnodactyly		
Achondrogenesis		
Short-rib polydactyly syndromes		
Mesomelic dwarfism syndromes[a]		
Robinow-Silverman syndrome[a]		

B. Localized bowing

Plastic bending fracture (normal bone)	}	Commonest
Normal (radius, ulna, fibula, tibia)		
Bowed legs-knock knees (see Table 4.7)		

Post trauma or osteomyelitis	}	Moderately common
Neurofibromatosis (tibia-fibula)		
Prenatal bowing or bending		
Fractures in softened bones		
Focal fractures in osteomalacia		

Bowed tibia with or without absent fibula	}	Relatively rare

[a] Symmetric middle segment dwarfism predominates.

Generalized Bowing

Generalized bowing resulting from metabolic disease leading to soft, osteomalacic bones occurs in rickets, hyperparathyroidism, hypophosphatasia, and hyperphosphatemia. Rickets, of course, is most common, and in all of these conditions, because of weight bearing, bowing is most pronounced in the lower extremities (Fig. 4.8A). This is not so true of the bony dysplasias which include achondroplasia, hypochondroplasia, a large variety of neonatal dwarfs (8, 10, 12, 13), the Ellis-van Creveld syndrome, campomelic dwarfism, Larsen's syndrome, pseudoachondroplasia (multiple epiphyseal dysplasia and spondyloepiphyseal dysplasia types), diastrophic dwarfism, the mucopolysaccharidoses, the mucolipidoses, the metaphyseal dysostoses, Melnick-Needles syndrome (see Fig. 4.15), and parastemmatic dwarfism. In campomelic dwarfism and Larsen's syndrome, in addition to bowing, the long bones usually are underdeveloped and varying degrees of hypoplasia frequently are seen around the elbow. Larsen's syndrome also is characterized by multiple joint dislocations, and while in any of these conditions bowing is rather nonspecific, it still is an important part of their diagnosis (Fig. 4.8B).

Bowing also occurs in osteogenesis imperfecta, especially in the congenita form (Fig. 4.8C).

In some conditions, although bowing is generalized it is most noticeable in the middle segments of the upper or lower extremities (i.e., radius and ulna and the tibia and fibula). Classically, in the upper extremities such bowing occurs with Madelung's deformity, or so-called dyschondrosteosis (6). The typical distal, ulnar, subluxation, increased carpal angle, tilting of the radial epiphysis, and bowing of the radius and ulna make the diagnosis (see Fig. 4.5, B and C). Middle segment bowing also occurs in mesomelic dwarfism, the ulnofibular dysplasia syndromes of Reinhardt and Pfeiffer, and the Robinow-Silverman syndrome (11) (see Fig. 4.5A).

All of the foregoing abnormalities must be differentiated from normal curvatures of bones. For the most part, these involve the radius, ulna, fibula, and tibia. The typical normal curved shapes of these bones are illustrated in Figure 4.9, but variations can occur. Clearly, comparative views are important in the evaluation of both these and abnormal long bone curvatures.

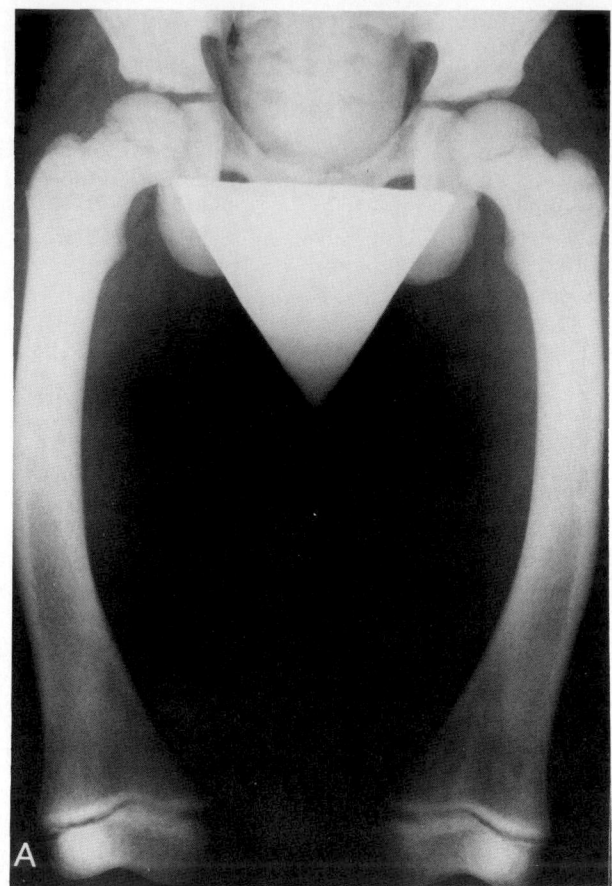

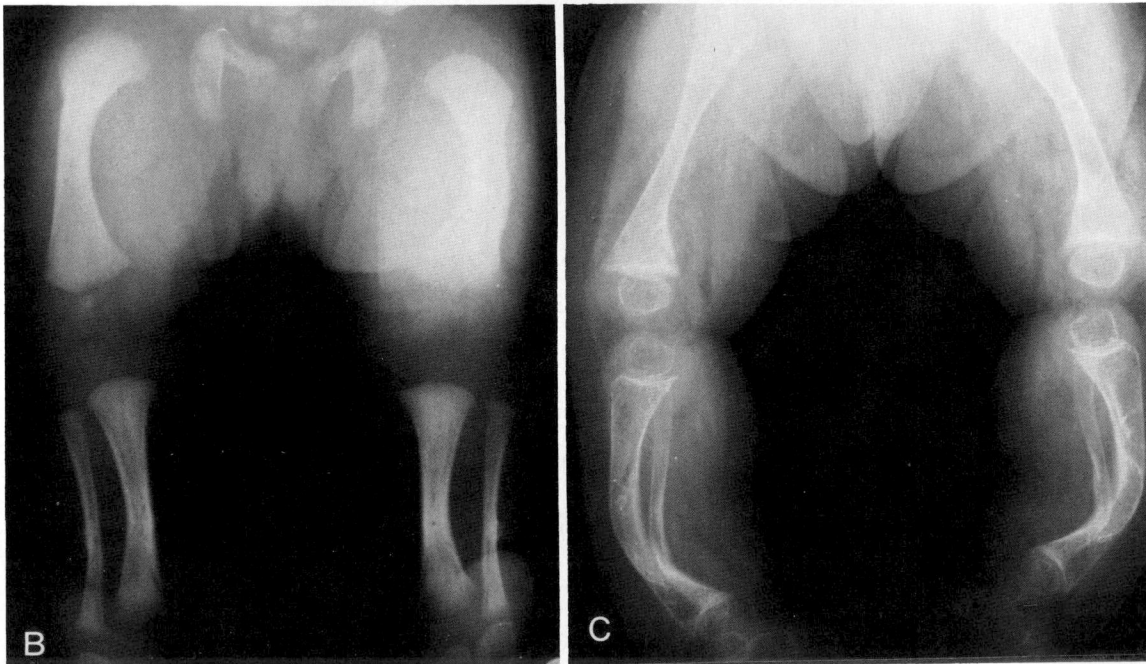

Fig. 4.8. Bowed bones. A. Typical bowing of the femurs in rickets. This is an example of bowing secondary to bone softening and weight bearing. B. Bowing of the shortened bones of the lower extremity in comptomelic dwarfism. Also note extostoses on the fibula. C. Bowing of the bones in osteogenesis imperfecta.

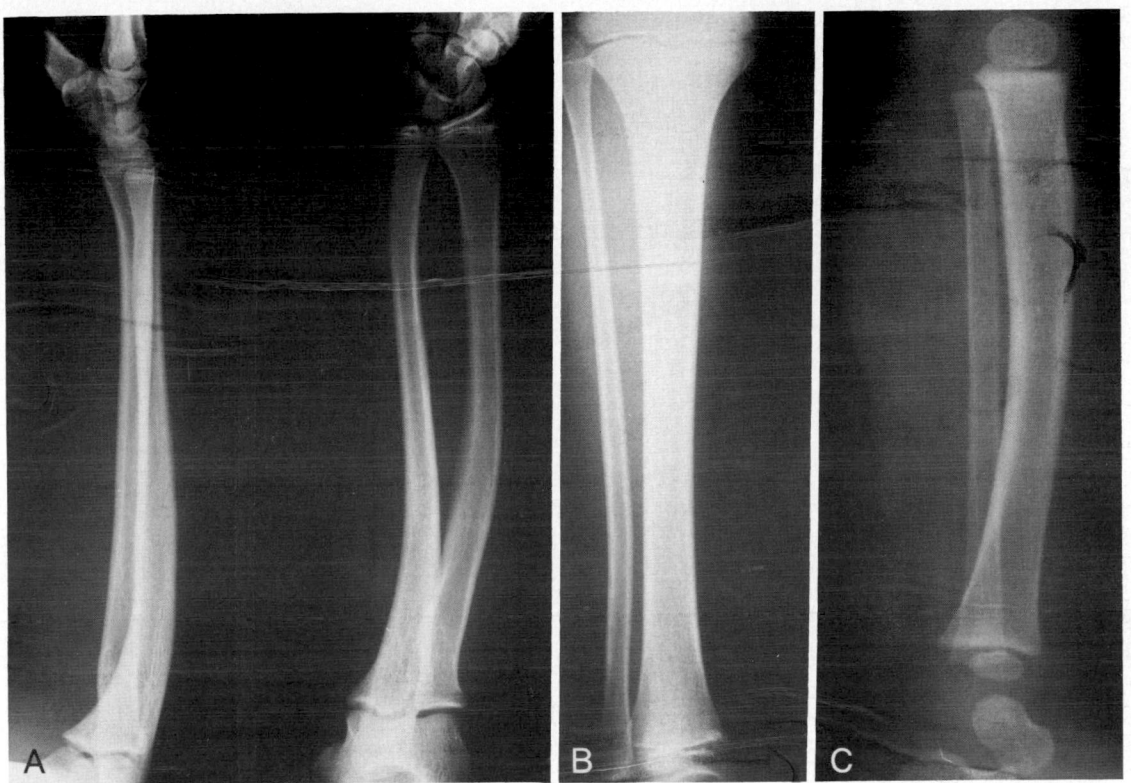

Fig. 4.9. Normal bowing of bones. A. Typical bowing of the radius and ulna on both frontal and lateral views. B. Typical inward bowing of the fibula on frontal view. C. Typical bowing of the tibia on lateral view.

Focal Bowing

Focal, asymmetric bowing of one or two bones most commonly is due to trauma and is seen with the so-called plastic bending or bowing fractures of childhood (1, 2, 5). With minimal injuries the bowing deformity will be missed unless the other extremity is examined at the same time (Fig. 4.10). Actually, these fractures are a variation of the well known greenstick fracture and can be considered the **"greenest of greenstick fractures."** Virtually unheard of just a few years ago, they now are known to be quite common in children. Most often they occur in the bones of the forearm, but they also can be seen in the fibula and clavicle. Rarely they are seen in the other long bones (3).

Bending or plastic fractures usually heal with persistent deformity and many years are required for any remodeling to occur. Indeed, complete remodeling may never occur and in addition, periosteal new bone deposition, in the healing phase, rarely is seen. Isotope bone scans, however, will be positive, but once the fracture is appreciated on plain films, there is little reason to obtain them. Perhaps the most important points regarding these fractures are that one (a) know of their existence, and (b) obtain views of the normal extremity for comparison. Otherwise, even the more obvious of these fractures can be overlooked.

Focal, unilateral or bilateral, bowing of the extremities also is seen with faulty intrauterine positioning of the fetus. In the broadest sense, such bowing also is due to trauma, and actually, is a form of the plastic bending fracture. Of course, these bent bones, as opposed to those seen with bending fracture in the older infant and child, tend to correct with time. Other instances where plastic bowing fractures occur include osteogenesis imperfecta and in bones softened by metabolic disease such as rickets, hypophosphatasia, and hyperphosphatemia.

Localized bowing, more pronounced at one end of a long bone, can be seen after epiphyseal injury secondary to trauma, infection, or irradiation (Fig. 4.11). Most often the problem is trauma and, indeed such bowing is common in the battered child syndrome. Similar epiphyseal-metaphyseal injuries are seen in metabolically weakened bones such as those occurring in rickets and scurvy. Indeed, any time the epiphyseal-metaphyseal junction is weakened, epiphyseal-metaphyseal fractures are more prone to occur, and then, bowing deformities can result.

Congenital pseudoarthroses are another cause of focal bowing and, although these can occur in almost any long bone, most commonly they occur in the lower extremity, in the tibia and fibula. In most of these cases, the problem is believed to be just another manifestation of the generalized mesenchymal defect seen in neurofibromatosis (Fig. 4.12, A and B) and, at first,

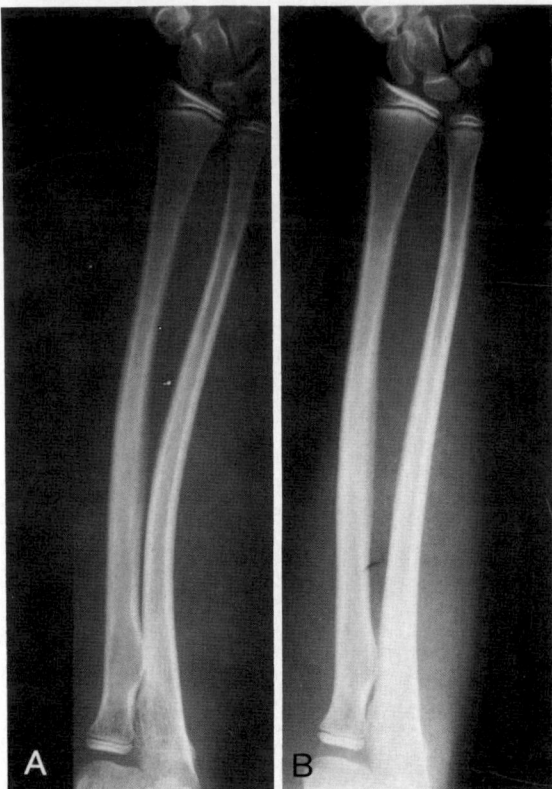

Fig. 4.10.   Focal bone bowing. A. Note exaggerated, abnormal bowing of the radius and ulna due to a plastic bending fracture. Alone, these findings could be missed, but when compared to the normal side, bowing is more apparent. B. Normal side for comparison.

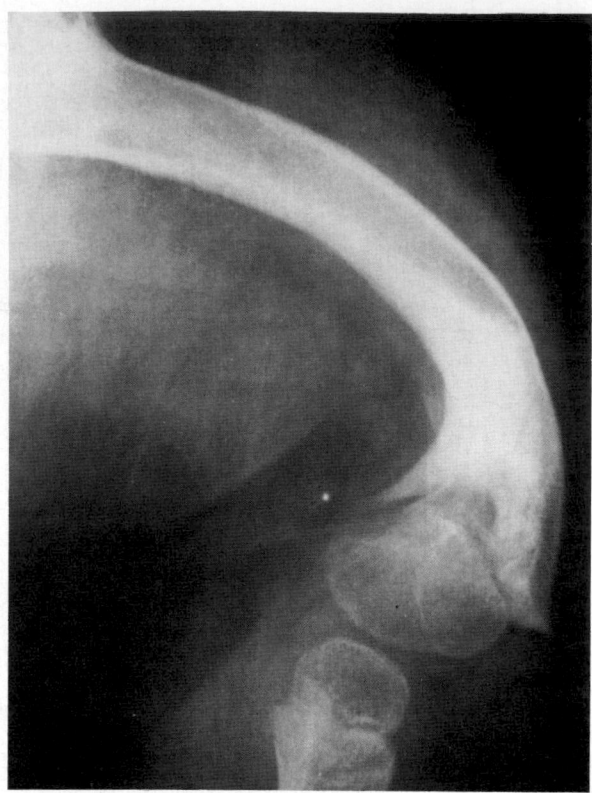

Fig. 4.11.   Severe bowing after epiphyseal insult. Note marked bowing of this femur secondary to osteomyelitis in the past.

only bowing and dysplasia are seen, but later frank pseudoarthrosis develops (see Fig. 4.25B). Recently, stabilization of the bony fragments with intramedullary nails has proven somewhat successful, but in the past, even with bone grafting, true healing seldom occurred; very often the end result was amputation of the extremity. For this reason it is important to differentiate this form of tibiofibular bowing from the rather benign form which occurs with abnormal fetal positioning (Fig. 4.13). For the most part, this differentiation is accomplished on the fact that, in the latter, curvature of the bones occurs in the opposite direction to that seen with the congenital pseudoarthrosis or neurofibromatosis. In addition, with positional bowing there is no evidence of bony dysplasia, while with the bowing of neurofibromatosis, the bone in the area of maximal bending is narrower than normal, dysplastic appearing, and associated with virtual obliteration of the medullary canal.

Bowing of the tibia, on an isolated basis (4, 7), usually occurs with congenital absence or hypoplasia of the fibula, but also can occur with an intact fibula (9). When the fibula is absent, the tibia is quite

kyphotic (Fig. 4.14), and the opposite, that is, absence of the tibia, also can occur (Fig. 4.14B). Other causes of localized bowing of long bones include fibrous dysplasia and juvenile (tertiary) syphilis. Fibrous dysplasia, of course, can involve any bone, but bending tends to involve the weight-bearing bones of the lower extremity. Juvenile syphilis usually involves the tibia, resulting in the so-called sabre-shin tibia. However, it is quite rare.

References

1. Borden S: Roentgen recognition of acute plastic bowing of the forearm in children. *Am J Roentgenol* 125:524–530, 1975.
2. Borden S: Traumatic bowing of the forearm in children. *J Bone Joint Surg* 56A:611–616, 1974.
3. Cail WS, Keats TE, Sussman MD: Plastic bowing fracture of the femur in a child.*Am J Roentgenol* 130:780–782, 1978.
4. Coventry MB, Johnson EW Jr: Congenital absence of the fibula. *J Bone Joint Surg* 34:646, 1952.
5. Crowe JW, Swischuk LE: Acute bowing fractures of the forearm in children. A frequently missed injury. *Am J Roentgenol* 128:981–984, 1977.
6. Felman AH, Kirkpatrick JA: Madelung's deformity: observations in 17 patients. *Radiology* 93:1037–1042, 1969.
7. Hootnick D, Boyd NA, Fixsen JA, Lloyd-Roberts GC:

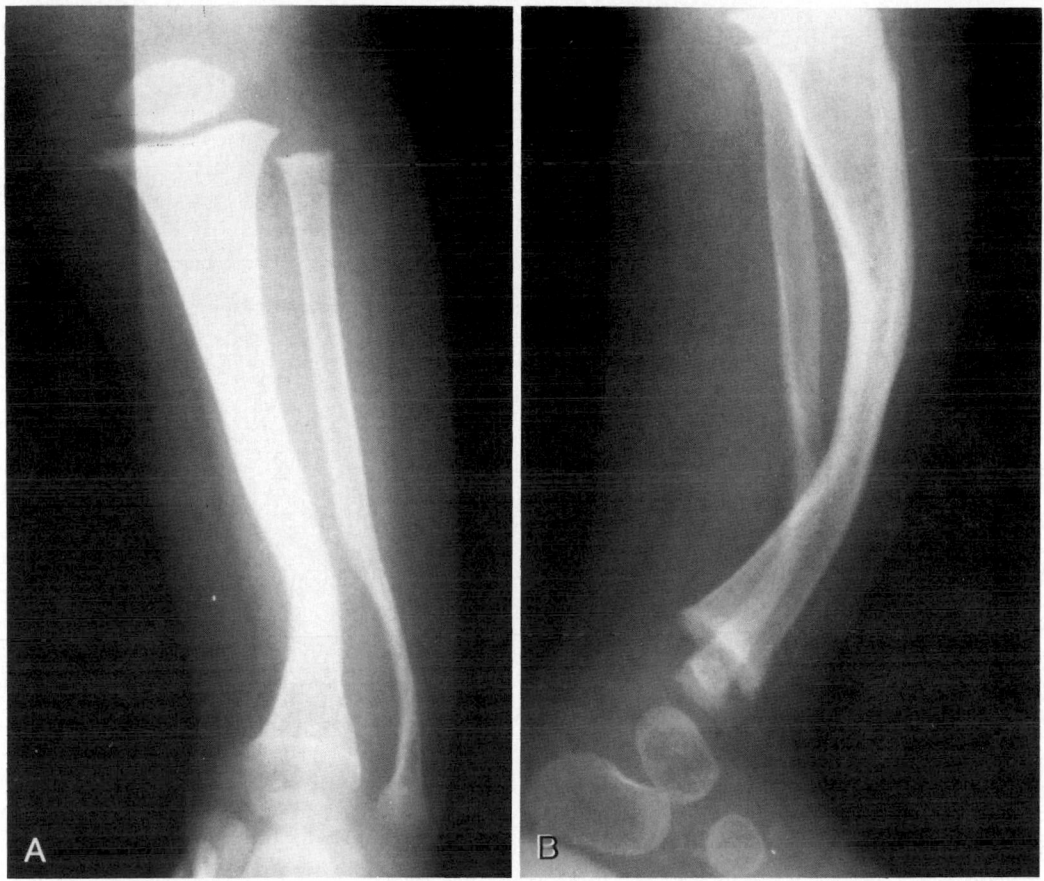

Fig. 4.12. Focal bowing; congenital pseudoarthrosis of lower extremity. A. Typical bowing and dysplasia of the tibia and fibula in congenital pseudoarthrosis, a common feature of neurofibromatosis. B. Typical findings on lateral view. Note especially, the dysplastic appearance of the thinned bones. Corticomedullary distinction is poor and eventually a pseudoarthrosis will develop through the area (see Fig. 4.25B).

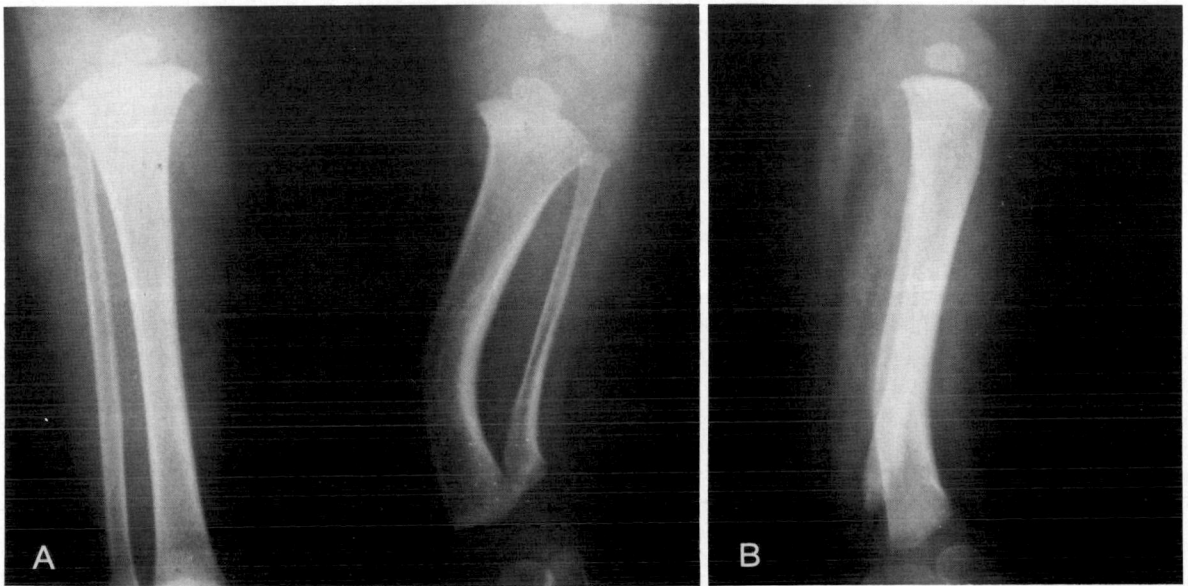

Fig. 4.13. Focal bowing; intrauterine bending. A. Typical frontal view of bowing due to intrauterine bending. Note the difference in appearance from the bending seen in Figure 4.12. B. Lateral view demonstrating typical findings, which again are quite different from those seen in Figure 4.12. Shortening, however, is present and may persist.

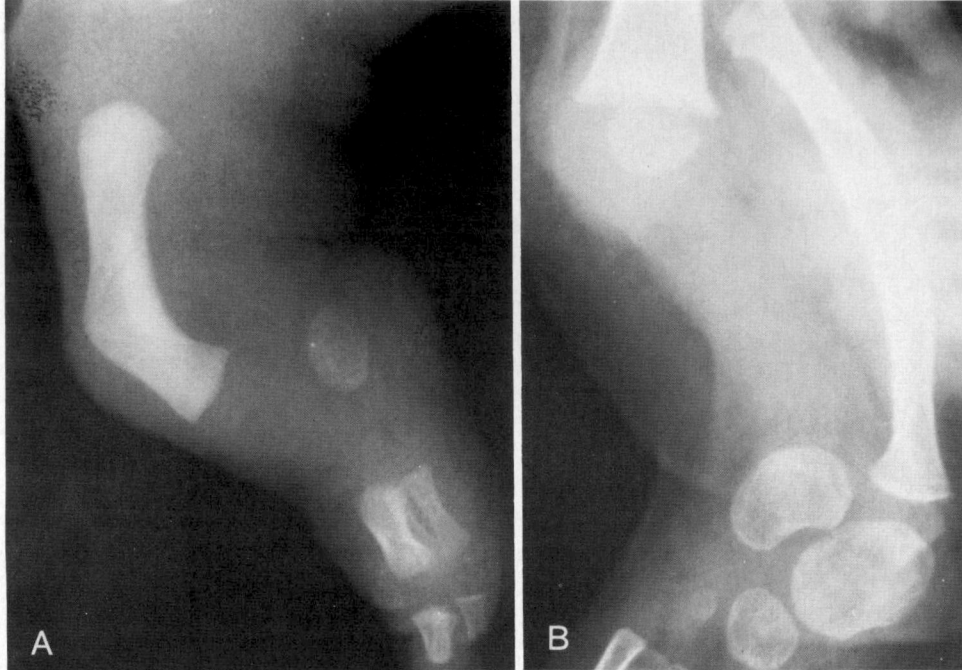

Fig. 4.14. Congenital bowing with absent bones. A. Tibial kyphosis, with absence of fibula. B. Fibular bowing with absence of tibia.

The natural history and management of congenital short tibia with dysplasia or absence of the fibula. *J Bone Joint Surg* 59:267–271, 1977.

8. Houston CS, Awen CF, Kent HP: Fetal neonatal dwarfism. *J Can Assoc Radiol* 23:45–61, 1972.

9. Jones D, Barnes J, Lloyd-Roberts GC: Congenital aplasia and dysplasia of the tibia with intact fibula. *J Bone Joint Surg* 60:31–39, 1978.

10. Kozlowski K, Butzler HO, Galatius-Jensen F, Tulloch A: Syndromes of congenital bowing of the long bones.

Pediatr Radiol 7:48, 1978.

11. Robinow M, Silverman FN, Smith HD: A newly recognized dwarfing syndrome. *Am J Dis Child* 117:645–649, 1969.

12. Swischuk LE: *Radiology of the Newborn and Young Infant,* ed 2. Baltimore, Williams & Wilkins, pp 681–704, 1980.

13. Thompson W, Oliphant M, Grossman H: Bowed limbs in the neonate; significance and approach to diagnosis. *Pediatr Ann* 5:50–62, 1976.

TWISTED OR CURVED BONES

Twisted bones are not common and, in the ribs, are referred to as "ribbon-like" bones. This type of rib deformity is seen most often in neurofibromatosis and the basal cell nevus syndrome (see Fig. 4.109). In both instances, the deformity represents a dysplastic aberration of bone growth, and in the basal cell nevus syndrome, vertebral anomalies, a large head, dentigerous cysts in the mandible and maxilla, and cyst-like lesions of the phalanges also are seen (1–4). Occasionally isolated congenital rib maldevelopment or post-surgical deformity of a rib or clavicle also can produce a "ribbon-like" deformity of these bones.

Generalized deformity of the skeleton, resulting in tortuous, twisted appearing bones occurs in the rather rare Needles-Melnick syndrome (5, 6). This generalized progressive bony dysplasia can lead to very bizarre appearing bones (Fig. 4.15A). Curved, somewhat swayed long bones can be seen in the otopalatodigital syndrome (Fig. 4.15B), and in Pyle's metaphyseal dysostosis. On an isolated basis, a long bone can appear twisted or curved after trauma, surgery, or

infection and also in osteogenesis imperfecta (Fig. 4.15C).

References

1. Becker MH, Kopf AW, Lande A: Basal cell nevus syndrome. Its roentgenologic significance. Review of the literature and report of four cases. *Am J Roentgenol* 99:817, 1967.

2. Dunnick NR, Head GL, Peck GL, Yoder FW: Nevoid basal cell carcinoma syndrome: radiographic manifestations including cystlike lesions of the phanges. *Radiology* 127:331–334, 1978.

3. Gorlin RJ, Golz R: Multiple nevoid basalcell epithelioma, jaw cysts and bifid rib syndrome. *New Engl J Med* 262:908, 1960.

4. Lile HA, Rogers JF, Gerard B: The basal cell nevus syndrome. *Am J Roentgenol* 103:214, 1968.

5. Melnick JC, Needles CF: An undiagnosed bone dysplasia; a 2 family study of 4 generations and 3 generations. *Am J Roentgenol* 97:39–48, 1966.

6. Moadel E, Byrk D: Melnick-Needles syndrome (osteodysplasia). *Radiology* 123:154, 1977.

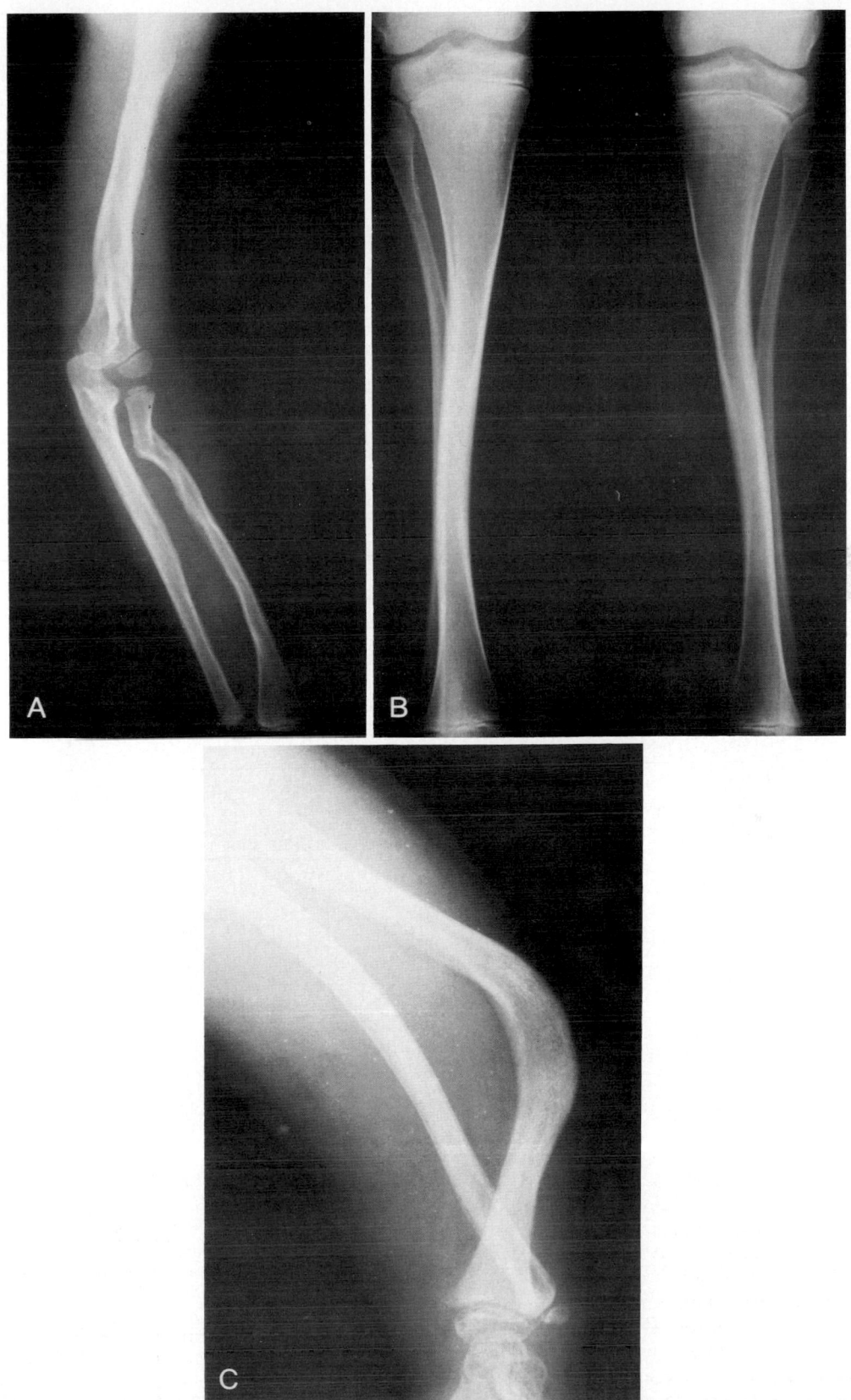

Fig. 4.15. Twisted or curved bones. A. Typical twisted undulating appearance of long bones in Needles-Melnick syndrome. B. Swayed, somewhat "S"-shaped bones of the lower extremity in the otopalatodigital syndrome. C. Curved bones in osteogenesis imperfecta. Patient had numerous episodes of fracturing.

BOWED LEGS AND KNOCK-KNEES

Both bowed legs and knock-knees are common in childhood, and actually, in either case most often the problem is physiologic (1, 4, 6, 7). This is especially true of bow legs. However, physiologic or not, the deformity in either case is due to increased vertical stresses being applied to one or other side of the lower extremities (5). With medial stresses bowed legs result, while with lateral stresses knock-knees occur (5). The effects of these stresses on the metaphyses of the growing bones are illustrated in Fig. 4.16. Bowed legs and knock-knees also occur in certain bony dysplasias and syndromes, and less commonly with any number of epiphyseal plate insults.

The many causes of bowed legs and knock-knees are summarized in Table 4.7, but the commonest cause of bowed legs is the condition known as tibial torsion. In these infants the lower tibiae are twisted forward and medially so that there is intoeing and accommodative bowing of the legs. Most often the problem is self-limiting and corrects itself by the age of 3 or 4 yr

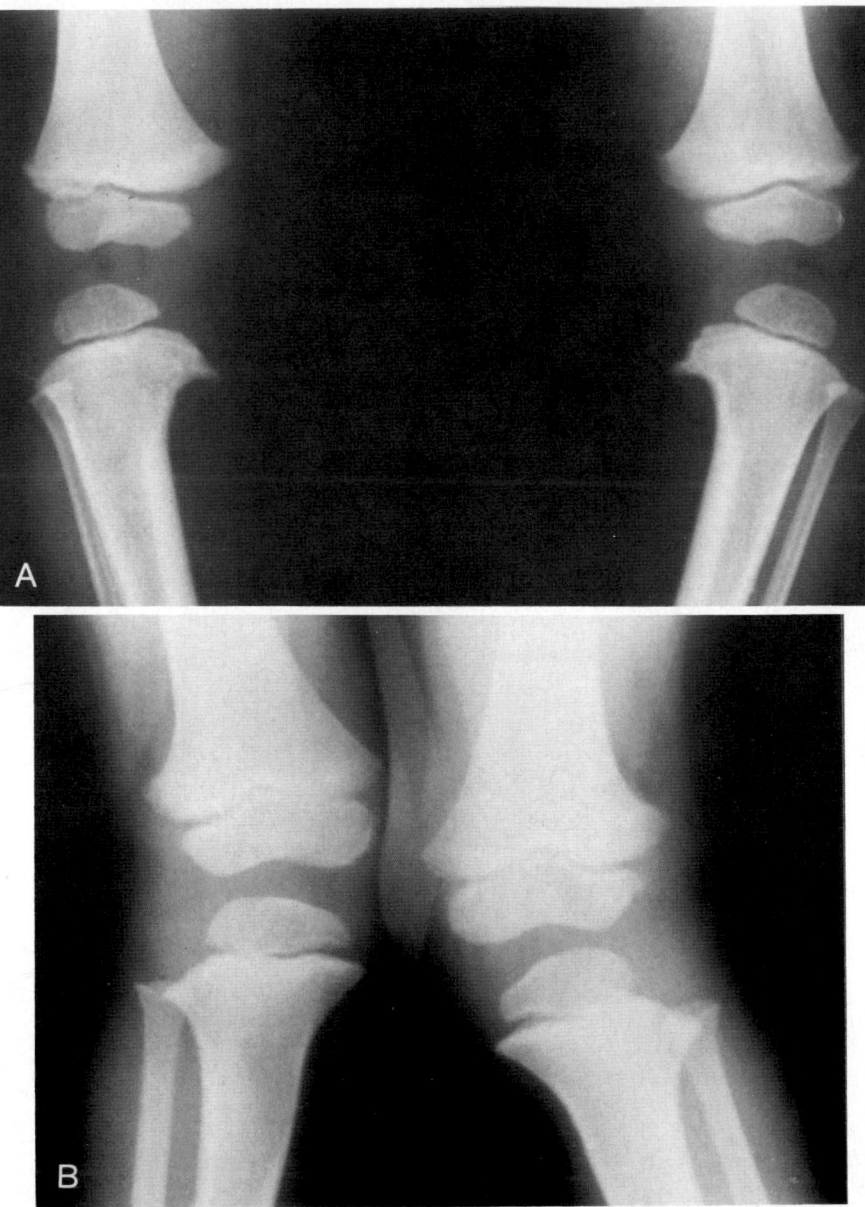

Fig. 4.16. Bowlegs and knock-knees; evidence of abnormal stresses. A. With bowlegs, bony stresses are more pronounced medially and, thus, there is flattening and impaction of the upper medial tibial metaphyses. Lesser changes are present in the lower medial femoral metaphyses. B. With knock-knees, changes are reversed. Note that there is flattening and impaction of the lateral aspects of the long bones, and that in addition there is cupping of the ulna.

(4, 6, 7). For this reason it is considered "physiologic", and hasty "corrective" osteotomies should be avoided (6). In terms of etiology, it is curious that the muscles in these patients almost always are well developed (Fig. 4.17A), and that the infants themselves are early walkers. It is likely that these factors lead to extra medial stress which then causes bending of the normal, but yet quite plastic, infantile bones.

In those patients where tibial torsion does not re-

solve, medial stresses lead to impaction fracturing and breaking of the medial tibial metaphysis. This leads to increased bowing (especially through the upper tibia) and so-called Blount's disease (2). As opposed to physiologic bowing, bowing due to Blount's disease (Fig. 4.17B) often requires corrective osteotomy. The condition can be unilateral or bilateral, and in some cases there is diastasis of the contralateral aspect (lateral) of the epiphyseal-metaphyseal junction (3). In other words, while there are compressive, fragmenting forces medially, distracting forces act laterally (i.e., see-saw like effect).

A less common cause of bowed legs is so-called femoral anteversion, or forward and internal rotation of the femur on its neck. This also is a physiologic or normal state in the neonate, but as the patient grows older it tends to correct itself. In those cases where correction is incomplete, femoral anteversion results. This also occurs in patients with cerebral palsy, presumably because of lack of normal weight bearing. Clinically, intoeing similar to that seen with tibial torsion occurs but, roentgenographically, the bow legs are less striking. Actually the problem is more clinical than radiologic and the bowing posture can be obliterated if the patient stands with the toes pointing out. However, to permanently correct the problem, derotational osteotomies, through the bent femurs, are required. Roentgenographically, the key finding is a coxa valga deformity of the upper femur, but it should be noted that this constitutes indirect evidence only. To determine whether anteversion is present or not, one must obtain true lateral views of the femur and then measure the femoral neck to femoral shaft angle.

Table 4.7   Bowed Legs and Knock Knees

Bowed legs		
Physiologic (tibial torsion)	}	Commonest
Rickets		
Femoral anteversion		
Bony dysplasias (see bony dysplasias with bowing, Table 4.6)	}	Moderately common
Blount's disease		
Epiphyseal injuries		
Hypophosphatasia		
Hyperphosphatemia	}	Relatively rare
Hyperparathyroidism		
Metaphyseal dysostoses		
Knock knees		
Physiologic	}	Commonest
Muscular weakness (see text)		
Bony dysplasias with hypotonia	}	Moderately common
Epiphyseal-metaphyseal injuries	}	Relatively rare
Trevor's disease		

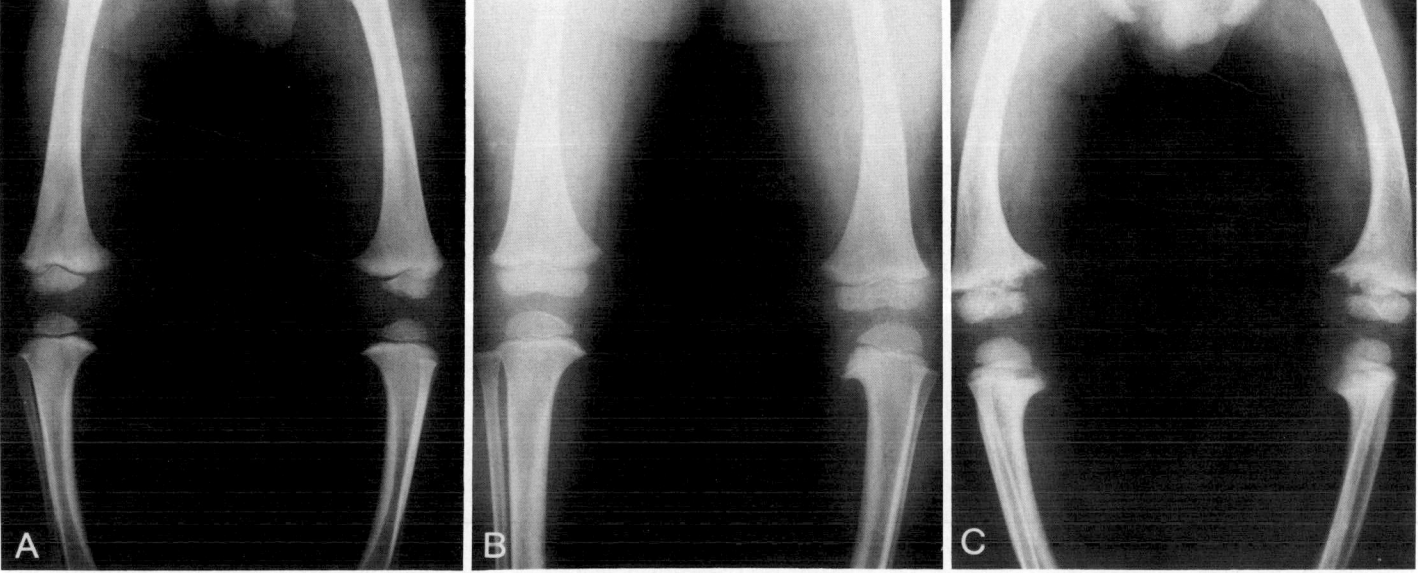

Fig. 4.17.   Bowed legs. A. Typical **physiologic bowing;** except for bowing the bones are normal. B. **Blount's disease.** On the left, note impaction and fragmentation of the upper medial metaphysis. This is the typical deformity of early Blount's disease. In this patient, the deformity corrected spontaneously. C. **Rickets.** Note bowing and characteristic metaphyseal changes of rickets.

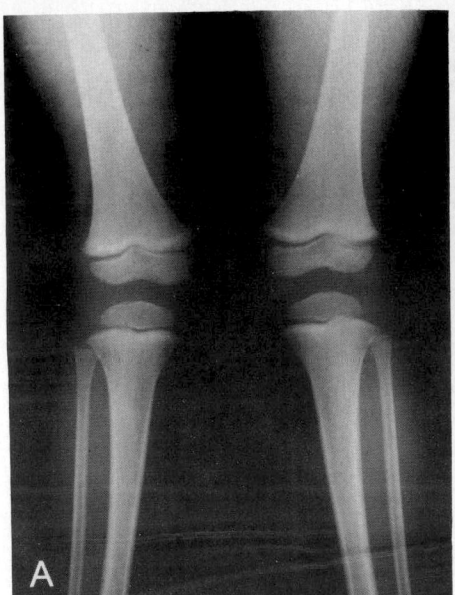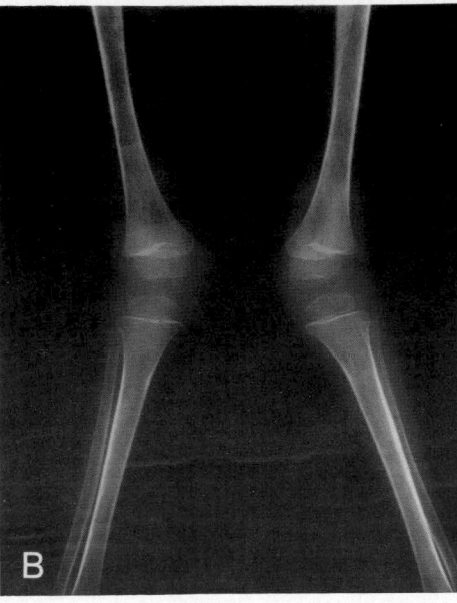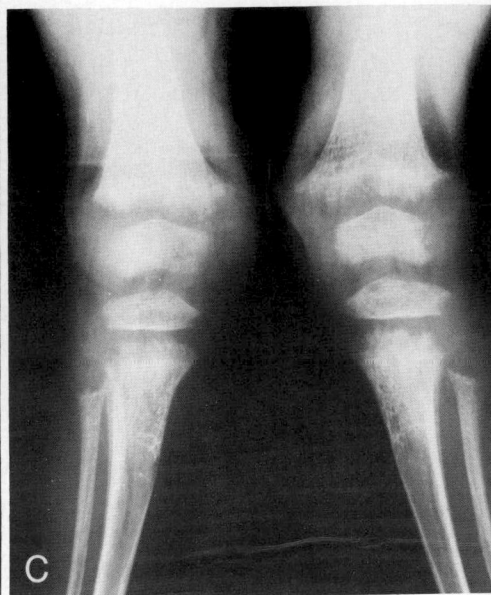

Fig. 4.18. Knock-knees. A. Normal knock-knees in 4-yr-old girl. B. Severe knock-knees in patient with neurogenic disease. Also note marked loss of soft tissues. C. Knock-knees in advanced rickets. This patient had dependent rickets and was bedridden. If the patient were ambulant, bowing would result.

The raw measurement thus obtained then must be applied to conversion tables available in most standard orthopedic textbooks or articles on the subject. However, more recently CT cross-sectional views of the femoral neck and its relation to the femoral shift have become available, and this has simplified measuring the angle of anteversion. Most likely, this will be the procedure of choice in the future.

Bowed legs, occurring in soft bones, most often are seen in rickets (8) (Fig. 4.17C), but also occur in hyperparathyroidism, hypophosphatasia, and hyperphosphatemia. Inherent bowing of the lower extremities occurs in a variety of bony dysplasias and dwarfing syndromes where there is bowing of the long bones in general (see Table 4.6). Unilateral, and occasionally, bilateral bow legs can result from epiphyseal-metaphyseal injury of any type (i.e., infection, trauma, radiation, and vitamin A intoxication). In such cases the involved extremity also usually is shortened and very often there is marked cupping of the associated metaphysis (see Fig. 4.11).

As far as knock-knees are concerned, once again the commonest cause is physiologic growth variation, occurring at about 3 to 6 yr of age (Fig. 4.18A) and more commonly in girls (4, 7). As with physiologic bowing, spontaneous correction is the rule. With pathologic knock knee deformity, the most common underlying problem is muscular weakness due either to neurologic or neuromuscular disease (Fig. 4.18B). Indeed, even in rickets, where bowing is characteristic, if associated

hypotonia exists, knock-knee deformity results (8) (Fig. 4.18C). For the same reason (i.e., associated muscle weakness), one can see knock-knees in conditions such as Pyle's disease, the various storage diseases, the nail-patella syndrome, Engelmann's diaphyseal dysostosis, and severe rheumatoid arthritis. Unilateral knock-knee deformity can be seen with any type of epiphyseal-metaphyseal injury, and Trevor's disease or dysplasia epiphysealis hemimelica.

References

1. Bateson EM: Non-rachitis bow leg and knock-knee deformities in young Jamaican children. *Br J Radiol* 39:92–101, 1966.
2. Bateson EM: The relationship between Blount's and bow legs. *Br J Radiol* 41:107–114, 1968.
3. Currarino G, Kirks DR: Lateral widening of epiphyseal plates in knees of children with bowed legs. *Am J Roentgenol* 129:208–312, 1977.
4. Greenberg LE, Swartz AA: Genu varum and genu valgum: another look. *Am J Dis Child* 121:219–221, 1971.
5. Kettelkamp DB, Chao EY: A method for quantitative analysis of medial and lateral compression forces at the knee during standing. *Clin Orthop* 83:202–213, 1972.
6. Shopfner CE, Cramer R, Cramer R: Growth remodelling of long bone osteotomies. *Br J Radiol* 46:512–519, 1973.
7. Shopner CE, Coin CG: Genu varus and valgus in children. *Radiology* 92:723–732, 1969.
8. Swischuk LE, Hayden CK Jr: Rickets: a roentgenographic scheme for diagnosis. *Pediat Radiol* 8:203–208, 1979.

COXA VARA AND COXA VALGA

Normally, with the legs internally rotated, and the toes pointing inward, the femoral neck to femoral shaft angle measures about 130° to 140°. However, if the roentgenogram is obtained with the toes pointing upward or outward, the angle is increased and an erroneous impression of coxa valga deformity results. Consequently, it is most important that correct positioning of the hips be present, and then, if the angle between the neck and shaft is increased, true coxa valga is present, and if it is decreased, coxa vara is present (Table 4.8).

Coxa vara deformities most frequently result from downward bending of the femoral neck in bones which are softer than normal or downward slipping of the femoral capital epiphysis because of a weakened epiphyseal-metaphyseal junction. In other cases, the deformity is due to a growth disturbance as part of a generalized bony dysplasia, and occasionally, coxa vara occurs because of an actual bony defect in the femoral neck. Such defects usually are congenital (i.e., congenital coxa vara) but occasionally can be acquired after severe infections or epiphyseal-metaphyseal fractures. The latter often occurs in the battered child syndrome.

In those cases where coxa vara is due to bending of soft bones, the problem usually is some metabolic disease such as rickets, hyperparathyroidism, or hypophosphatasia. Coxa vara deformities secondary to actual downward slipping of the femoral capital epiphysis usually occur on an idiopathic, chronic basis (Fig. 4.19). With acute slips the displaced head is surgically replaced into a normal position within hours of the injury and deformity does not result. With chronic slippage, however, femoral neck bone growth is altered and a coxa vara deformity slowly results. The most common cause of such chronic slipping is the so-called slipped capital epiphysis syndrome of adolescence. The etiology of this condition is unknown, but it does tend to occur in more obese adolescents, and a little more commonly in boys (5, 6). There also seems to be a genetically inheritable predisposition and, in this regard, it has been noted that often there is skeletal (bone age) immaturity in these patients. This may well be an important factor for it is quite possible that a combination of skeletal immaturity and increased vertical stress (i.e., overweight individual) leads to the problem. The disease usually is unilateral, but bilateral disease occurs in approximately 10% of patients. In these cases, one side tends to slip earlier than the other, and it is uncommon to have simultaneous slipping of both sides.

The coxa vara deformity in these cases is a late manifestation and, thus, before any significant degree of slippage occurs, the findings consist only of (a) demineralization of the bones of the hip, (b) some soft tissue muscle atrophy, and (c) widening and hyperlucency of the epiphyseal line (see Fig. 4.68C). This latter sign is the most important and the one to look for in the early detection of this condition.

Chronic, and indeed, occasionally acute superimposed, slippage of the femoral epiphysis also can occur with severe rickets, hyperparathyroidism, and hypothyroidism (3). In terms of rickets, renal osteodystrophy usually is the underlying cause (3, 7, 8, 10), but of

Table 4.8   Coxa Vara and Coxa Valga

Coxa vara	
Idiopathic slipped epiphysis Legg-Perthes disease (healing)	Commonest
Rickets (slipped epiphysis or simple bending) Fracture or infection of femoral neck Sickle cell disease (femoral head necrosis) Steroid therapy (femoral head necrosis)	Moderately common
Hyperparathyroidism (slipped epiphysis) Hypothyroidism (slipped epiphysis) Radiation therapy (ischemic necrosis) Osteogenesis imperfecta (fxs. in cong. form) Metatropic dwarfism Storage diseases	Relatively rare
Gaucher's disease (ischemic necrosis) Congenital coxa vara (femoral neck defect) Diastrophic dwarfism Kniest's syndrome Metaphyseal dysostosis Multiple epiphyseal dysplasia Spondyloepiphyseal dysplasia Cleidocranial dysostosis (defect) Pseudo or pseudopseudohypoparathyroidism (slipped epiphysis)	Rare
Coxa valga	
Underlying neurologic or neuromuscular disease Chronic muscle hypotonia (other)	Commonest
Turner's syndrome Mucopolysaccharidoses Mucolipidoses	Moderately common
Melnick-Needle's syndrome Prader-Willi syndrome Progeria Pyle's metaphyseal dysplasia	Rare

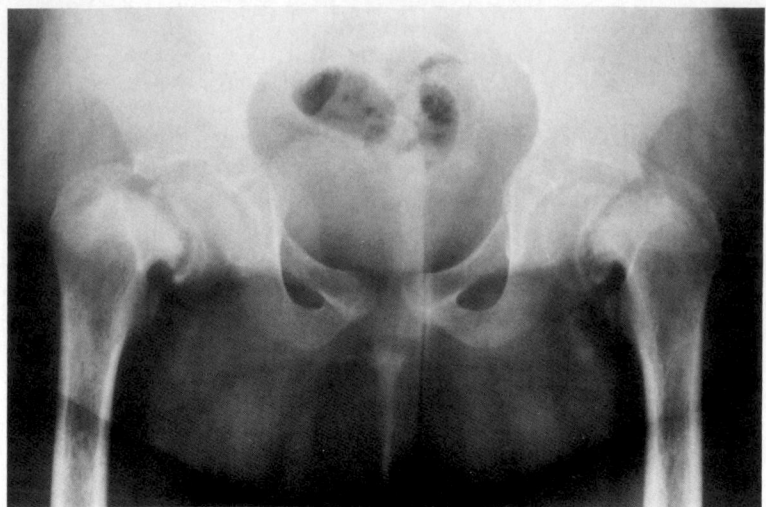

Fig. 4.19. Coxa vara. Bilateral coxa vara deformity secondary to markedly slipped femoral capital epiphyses.

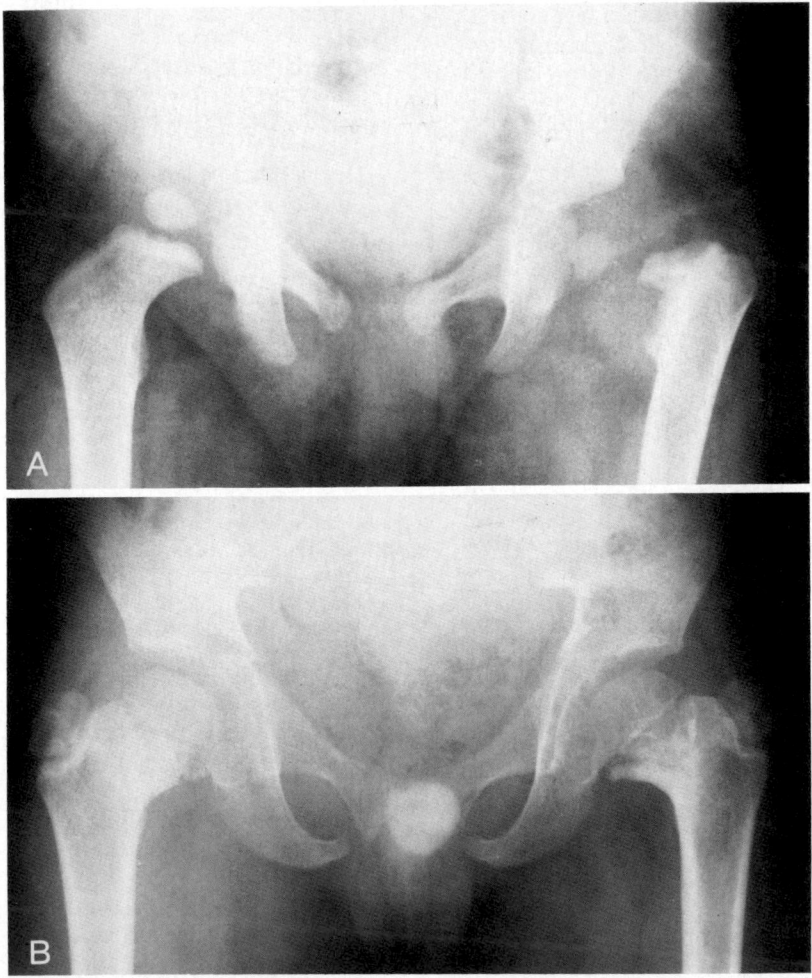

Fig. 4.20. Coxa vara. A. Congenital coxa vara on the left. Note that there is deficiency of ossification of the femoral neck. The femoral head remains relatively normal. B. Bilateral coxa vara deformities in older adolescent with metaphyseal dysostosis.

course, slippage can occur with any form of rickets. In rickets and hyperparathyroidism, the problem probably is related to weakened and softened bones, but in hypothyroidism the problem may be similar to that postulated in idiopathic slippage of the femoral capital epiphysis (i.e., delayed skeletal maturity and some degree of overweightness predispose to slippage).

Downward displacement of the femoral capital epiphysis also can be seen in the late, healing stages of ischemic necrosis of the femoral head (i.e., Legg-Perthes disease), steroid-induced infarction, infarction with the various collagen vascular diseases, Gaucher's disease, infarction after radiation therapy around the hip region (2, 13), and occasionally, with congenital dislocation of the hip. In these latter cases,

infarction of the femoral head is a complication of prolonged immobilization of the hips in a plaster splint. It does not occur very often.

So-called congenital coxa vara is not particularly common and often is considered to be the most minimal manifestation of the proximal focal femoral deficiency syndrome (1, 11). In these cases, when abnormality is severe, the upper end of the femur is phocomelic (see Fig. 4.22B) and the coxa vara deformity so gross that often it escapes observation. In milder cases, variable degrees of bony deficiency of the femoral neck lead to shortening, a more horizontal orientation with weight bearing, and thus, a coxa vara deformity (Fig. 4.20A). Similar femoral neck defects leading to coxa vara deformity also can be seen with cleidocranial

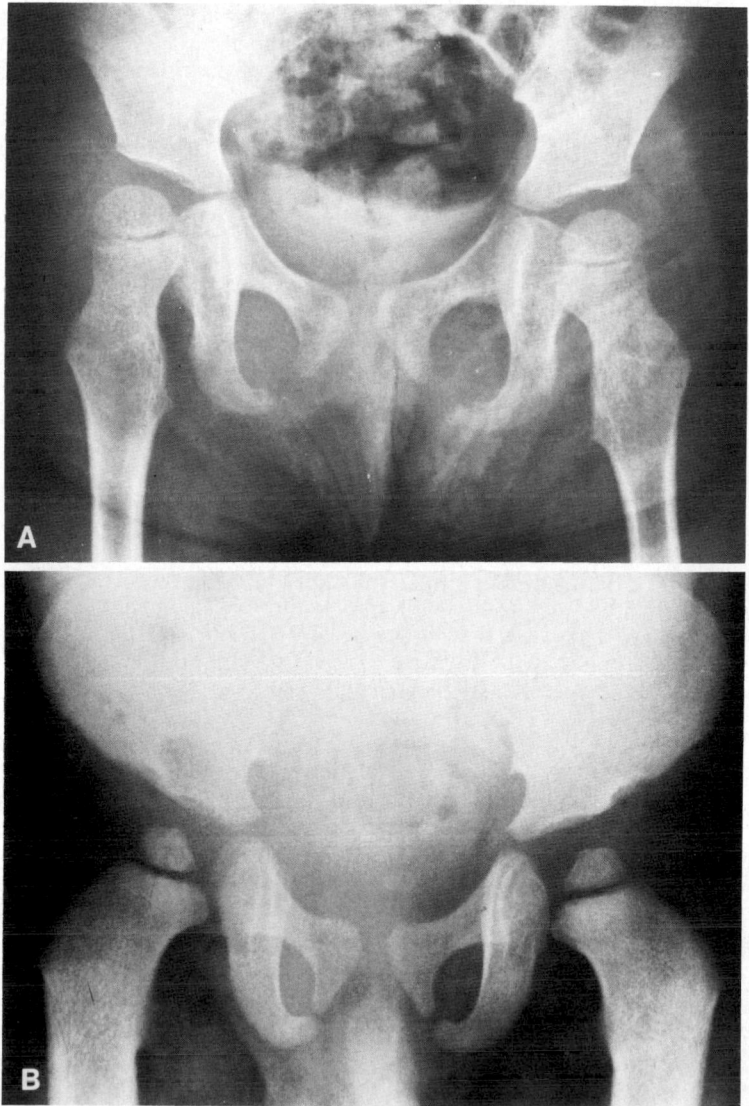

Fig. 4.21. Coxa valga. A. Typical coxa valga deformity of the hips in neurogenic disease. The hips are slightly subluxated. B. Coxa valga deformity in Hurler's disease. Also note that the bones are broad, and that the waist of the iliac wings is underdeveloped and narrow.

dysostosis and, on an acquired basis, with trauma or infection. Usually these latter problems occur in infancy, and as far as trauma is concerned, the battered child syndrome probably accounts for most cases. In addition, a few similar cases can be seen with osteogenesis imperfecta.

Other causes of coxa vara include a variety of dysplasias and dwarfing syndromes where intrinsic growth patterns of the upper femur lead to its prescence; i.e., achondroplasia, diastrophic dwarfism, metatrophic dwarfism, the Kniest syndrome, metaphyseal dysostosis (Fig. 4.20B), multiple epiphyseal dysplasia, Morquio's disease, spondyloepiphyseal dysplasia, and pseudo or pseudo-pseudohypoparathyroidism (12).

As far as **coxa valga** deformities of the upper femur are concerned, the commonest cause is underlying neurologic or neuromuscular disease (9). In these patients, lack of upright posture reduces vertical stresses on the femur and allows the femoral neck to grow in a more vertical direction (Fig. 4.21A). In many of these patients, the hips also are subluxated or frankly dislocated. The same problem occurs in a number of syndromes and dysplasias where hypotonia is inherently present (i.e., Turner's syndrome, Stickler's syndrome, the mucopolysaccharidoses, the mucolipidoses, Melnick-Needles syndrome, Prader-Willie syndrome, progeria, pycnodysostosis, and Pyle's metaphyseal dysplasia) (Fig. 4.21B).

References

1. Calhoun JD, Pierret G: Infantile coxa vara. *Am J Roentgenol* 115:561–568, 1972.
2. Chapman JA, Deakin DP, Green JH: Slipped upper femoral epiphysis after radiotherapy. *J Bone Joint Surg* 62B:337–339, 1980.
3. Goldman AG, Lane JM, Salvati E: Slipped capital femoral epiphyses complicating renal osteodystrophy: a report of three cases. *Radiology* 126:333–339, 1978.
4. Hirano T, Stamelos S, Harris V, Dumbovic N: Association of primary hypothyroidism and slipped capital femoral epiphysis. *J Pediatr* 93:262–264, 1978.
5. Kelsey JL: Epidemiology of slipped capital femoral epiphysis. *J Pediatr* 93:262–264, 1978.
6. Kelsey JL, Acheson RM, Keggi KJ: The body build of patients with slipped capital femoral epiphysis. *Am J Dis Child* 124:276–281, 1972.
7. Kirkwood JR, Ozonoff MB, Steinbach HL: Epiphyseal displacement after metaphyseal fracture in renal osteodystrophy. *Am J Roentgenol Radium Ther Nucl Med* 115:647–654, 1972.
8. Mehls O, Ritz E, Krempien B, Gilli G, Link K, Willich E, Scharer K: Slipped epiphyses in renal osteodystrophy. *Arch Dis Child* 50:545–554, 1975.
9. Griffiths GJ, Evans KT, Roberts GM, Lloyd KN: The radiology of the hip joints and pelvis in cerebral palsy. *Clin Radiol* 28:187–192, 1977.
10. Nixon JR, Douglas JF: Bilateral slipping of the upper femoral epiphysis in end-stage renal failure. *J Bone Joint Surg* 62B:18–21, 1980.
11. Pavlov H, Goldman AG, Freiberger RH: Infantile coxa vera. *Radiology* 125:631–640, 1980.
12. Steinback HL, Young DA: The roentgen appearance of pseudohypoparathyroidism (PH) and pseudo-pseudo-hypoparathyroidism (PPH), differentiation from other syndromes associated with short metacarpals, metatarsals, and phalanges. *Am J Roentgenol* 97:49–66, 1966.
13. Wolf EL, Berdon WE, Cassady JR, Baker DH, Freiberger R, Pavlov H: Slipped femoral capital epiphysis as sequela to childhood irradiation for malignant tumors. *Radiology* 125:781–784, 1977.

CUBITUS VALGUS (INCREASED CARRYING ANGLE)

Most commonly, this deformity of the elbow results from improperly reduced fractures or growth plate damage to the distal humerus. It also occurs, as a basic growth disturbance, in Turner's syndrome, Noonan's syndrome, and the cerebrohepatorenal syndrome.

CLUBFEET

There are so many syndromes in which the typical clubfoot deformity occurs that it is of questionable value to list all of them, and actually, these lists can be obtained from a number of currently available syndrome textbooks (see p 159). Indeed, seldom does one make the diagnosis of any one of these conditions on the basis of clubfeet alone; the only exception might be diastrophic dwarfism where clubbing is so pronounced that it becomes quite characteristic.

Overall, the commonest causes of clubfoot deformity are (a) faulty intrauterine positioning and (b) underlying neurologic or neuromuscular disease. It also occurs in feti developing in an amniotic fluid-deficient uterus, a phenomenon which occurs most commonly with Potter's syndrome (renal agenesis) or premature and prolonged leakage of amniotic fluid from the uterus (2, 3). It also can occur when the fetus develops in an abnormal saccule or portion of a bifed uterus (4). In all of these cases, direct compression of the fetus by the uterus results in a number of physical deformities, and clubfoot is one of these. The thorax in these patients also is chronically compressed in utero, and this is believed to inhibit lung growth and result in pulmonary hypoplasia (4).

References

1. Blanc WW, Apperson JW, McNally J: Pathology of newborn and of placenta in oligohydramnios. *Bull*

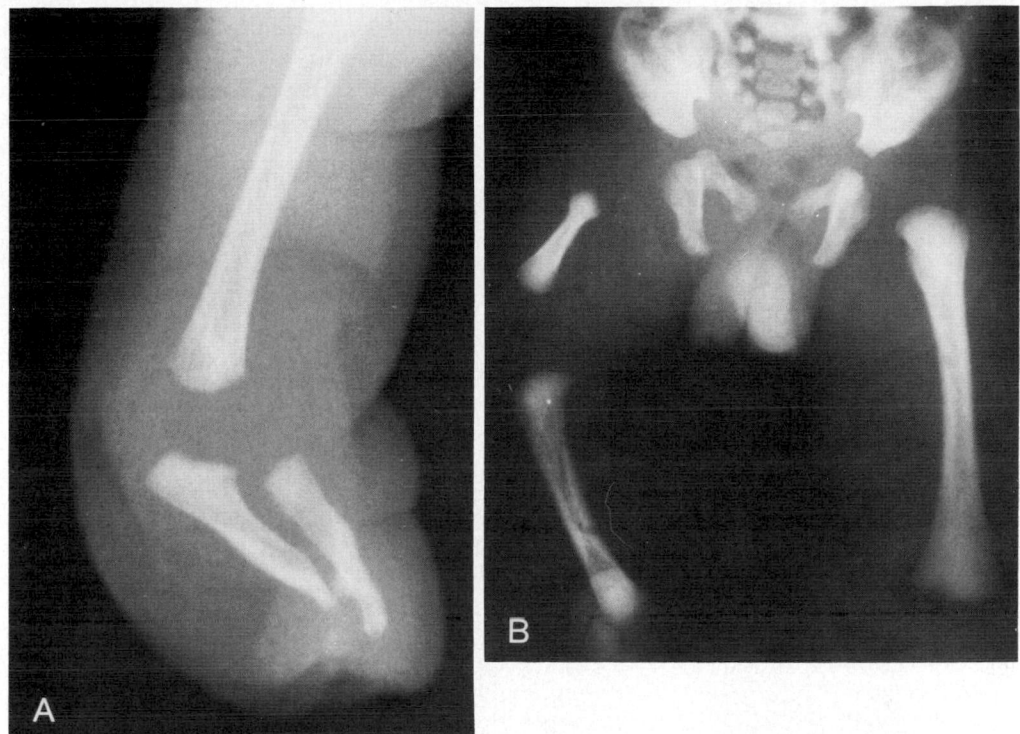

Fig. 4.22. Phocomelias and hypoplasias. A. Typical phocomelic abnormality of the forearm. B. Focal femoral deficiency causing underdevelopment of the right femur and absence of the upper femur and femoral neck. The clubbed end is typical of focal femoral deficiency. In other cases, the end is more pencil sharpened.

Sloane Hosp Women 8:51–64, 1962.
2. Potter EL: Facial characteristics of infants with bilateral renalagenesis. *Am J Obstet Gynecol* 51:885–888, 1946.
3. Sern L, Fletcher BD, Dunbar JS, Levant MN, Fawcett JS: Pneumothorax and pneumomediastinum associated

with renal malformations in newborn infants. *Am J Roentgenol* 116:785–791, 1972.
4. Swischuk LE: *Radiology of the Newborn and Young Infant,* ed 2. Baltimore, Williams & Wilkins, 1980, p 90.

PHOCOMELIAS, HYPOPLASIAS, AND APLASIAS

In terms of phocomelia, that is, peripheral underdevelopment or aplasia of the extremities, thalidomide embryonopathy usually first comes to mind. Indeed, for a time it was a common cause of this problem (3) and, both in these infants and those with other phocomelic deformities, the problem is believed to lie with an embryonic peripheral neuropathy (8). The neuropathy probably results from a drug or infection (virus?) causing damage to a primitive sclerotome. In turn, this leads to undergrowth of the extremity originating from the sclerotome, and finally phocomelia. Such deformities often are generalized and widespread, but focal hypoplasia of one or more of the long bones also can occur (Fig. 4.22A).

Of the focal hypoplasias, perhaps one of the best known examples is the so-called radial ray syndrome (Table 4.9). In this condition, the radius and first and second digits of the hand are variably underdeveloped (Fig. 4.23) and, for the most part, these changes occur in the Holt-Oram syndrome, Poland's syndrome, Fan-

Table 4.9 Focal Bony Hypoplasias

Radial ray syndrome
  Holt-Oram syndrome
  Poland's syndrome
  Fanconi's anemia
  TAR syndrome
	Commonest

Hypoplastic radial head with congenital dislocation Nonspecific focal hypoplasias (cause unknown)	Moderately common
Proximal focal femoral deficiency Absent fibula	Relatively rare
Absent tibia Mermaid deformity Thalidamide embryonopathy[a]	Rare

[a] Currently rare.

coni's anemia, and the related thrombocytopenia-hypoplastic radius (TAR) syndrome. In the TAR syndrome, the thumb often is not as hypoplastic as in Fanconi's anemia. Poland's syndrome is associated with ipsilateral underdevelopment of the pectoralis muscle and chest cage, and in the Holt-Oram syndrome, abnormally curved or hooked (handlebar) clavicles (see Fig. 4.92B), other congenital bone deformities, and cardiac disease (atrial septal defect, ventricular septal defect, or pulmonary stenosis) coexist.

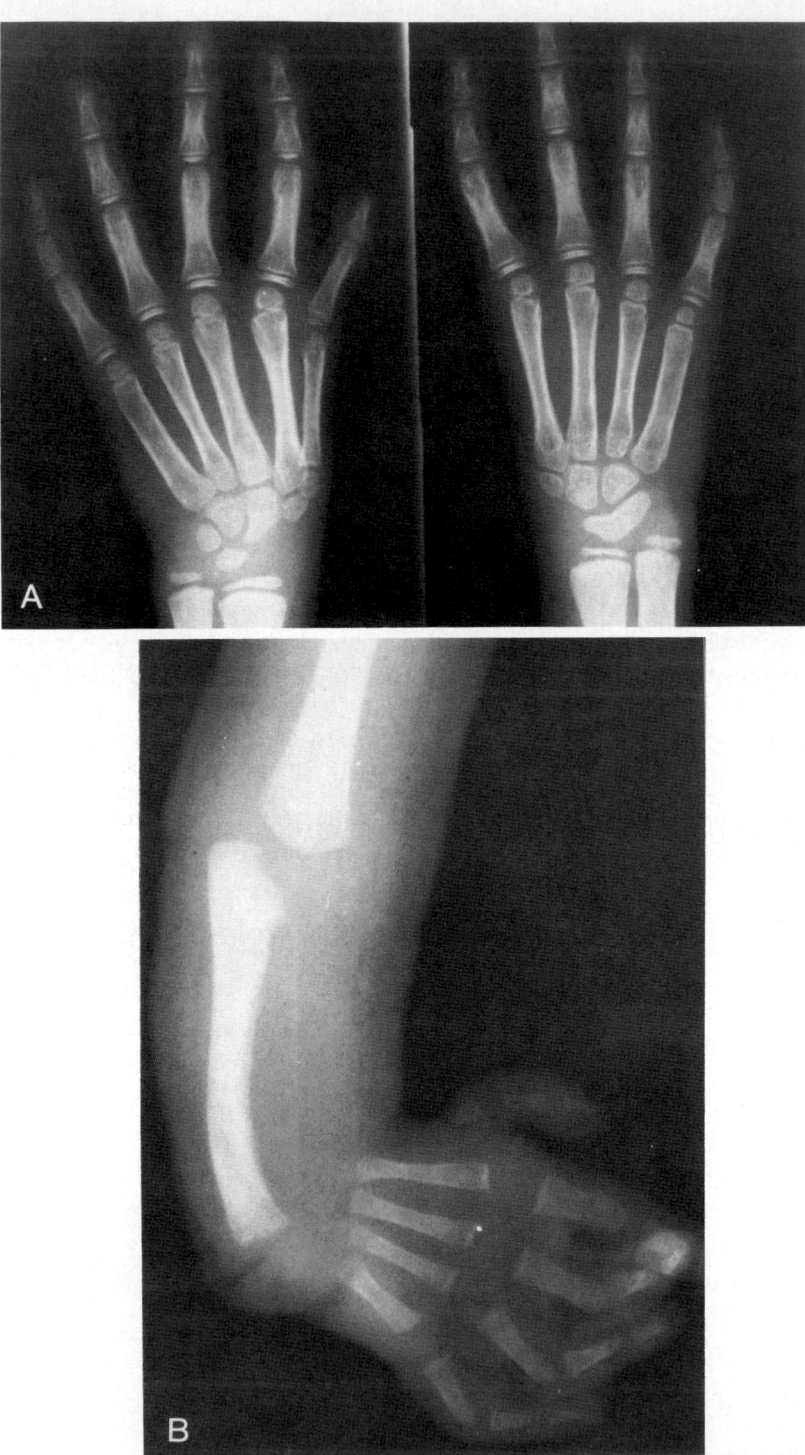

Fig. 4.23.   Radial ray syndrome. A. Patient with Holt Oram syndrome demonstrating absence of the thumb on one side, and severe hypoplasia of the thumb on the other. Also note corresponding carpal bone abnormalities. B. Another patient with the radial ray syndrome showing absence of the radius and a small, underdeveloped thumb.

Hypoplasia of the radial head commonly occurs with congenital dislocation of the head and this can occur either on a sporadic basis or in certain syndromes (see p 288).

Hypoplasia of the proximal femur, on a congenital basis, is referred to as the proximal focal femoral deficiency syndrome (5, 7, 10), and in severe cases results in a very short femur with a "pencil-sharpened" or "clubbed" upper end (Fig. 4.22B). In these more severe cases, the femoral head usually also does not develop properly, and all in all, the deformity is a major therapeutic problem. With lesser degrees of abnormality, the femoral head may develop to near normal size, but the upper femur remains hypoplastic and a femoral neck pseudoarthrosis (bony defect in the neck) may prevent normal ambulation. In the mildest form of this abnormality, the femoral neck is short and wide, the epiphyseal line wide and irregular, and although a major neck defect does not exist, a congenital coxa vara deformity is present (see Fig. 4.20A).

Isolated hypoplasia of either the tibia or fibula also can occur, and when the fibula is absent, a marked bowing deformity of the tibia results (see Fig. 4.14). Absence or hypoplasia of the tibia, on the other hand, usually is associated with a less bowed fibula. Extensive underdevelopment of the lower extremities and sacrum occurs in the so-called mermaid or caudal regression syndrome. Imperforate anus commonly is associated and the condition is more common in infants of diabetic mothers. It is believed that the entire deformity results from intrauterine vascular insufficiency of the lower segment of the body (1, 2, 4, 9).

Focal hypoplasia or underdevelopment of a bone also can result when severe infection or injury causes impaired epiphyseal-metaphyseal growth and, finally, generalized hypoplasia of the bones occurs in many dwarfing syndromes. These, for the most part, have been dealt with in the section dealing with tubulation abnormalities of the long bones (see p 165).

References

1. Assemany SR, Muzzo S, Gardner LI: Syndrome of phocomelic diabetic embryopathy (caudal dysplasia). *Am J Dis Child* 123:489–491, 1972.
2. Becker MH, Szatkowski JA, Bant EE: Case report 75, diagnosis; caudal regression syndrome. *Skeletal Radiol* 3:191–192, 1978.
3. Cuthbert R, Spiers AL: Thalidomide induced malformations. A radiological survey. *Clin Radiol* 14:163, 1963.
4. Duhamel, B: From mermaid to anal imperforation, syndrome of caudal regression. *Arch Dis Child* 36:152–155, 1961.
5. Goldman, AB, Schneider R, Wilson PD: Proximal focal femoral deficiency. *J Can Assoc Radiol* 29:101–107, 1978.
6. Jones D, Barnes J, Lloyd-Roberts GC: Congenital aplasia and dysplasia of the tibia with intact fibula. *J Bone Joint Surg* 60:31–39, 1978.
7. Levinson ED, Ozonoff MB, Royen PM: Proximal femoral focal deficiency (PFFD). *Radiology* 125:197–204, 1977.
8. McCredie J: Segmental embryonic peripheral neuropathy. *Pediatr Radiol* 3:163–168, 1975.
9. Passarge E, Lenz W: Syndrome of caudal regression in infants of diabetic mothers; observations of further cases. *Pediatrics* 37:672–675, 1966.
10. Schatz SL, Kopits SE: Proximal femoral focal deficiency. *Am J Roentgenol* 131:289–295, 1978.
11. Swischuk LE: *Radiology of the Newborn and Young Infant,* ed 2. Baltimore, Williams & Wilkins, 1980, pp 618–620.

ANKYLOSES

Acquired ankylosis is more common than congenital ankylosis and most often the problem is prior joint infection or inflammation as in septic or rheumatoid arthritis (Fig. 4.24A). Ankylosis after trauma is not as common. On a congenital basis, ankyloses can occur in isolated form, and often involve the elbow (1) (Fig. 4.24B). Ankylosis should not be confused with joint contracture (2, 3). Joint contractures may or may not demonstrate bony ankylosis, but most often they do not.

References

1. Card RY, Strachman J: Congenital ankylosis of the elbow. *J Pediatr* 46:81–85, 1955.
2. Pena SDJ, Shokeri MHK: Syndrome of camptodactyly, multiple ankylosis, facial anomalies, and pulmonary hypoplasia: a lethal condition. *J Pediatr* 85:373–375, 1974.
3. Punnett HH, Kistenmacher ML, Valdes-Dapena M, Ellison RT Jr: Syndrome of ankylosis, facial anomalies, and pulmonary hypoplasia. *J Pediatr* 85:375–377, 1974.

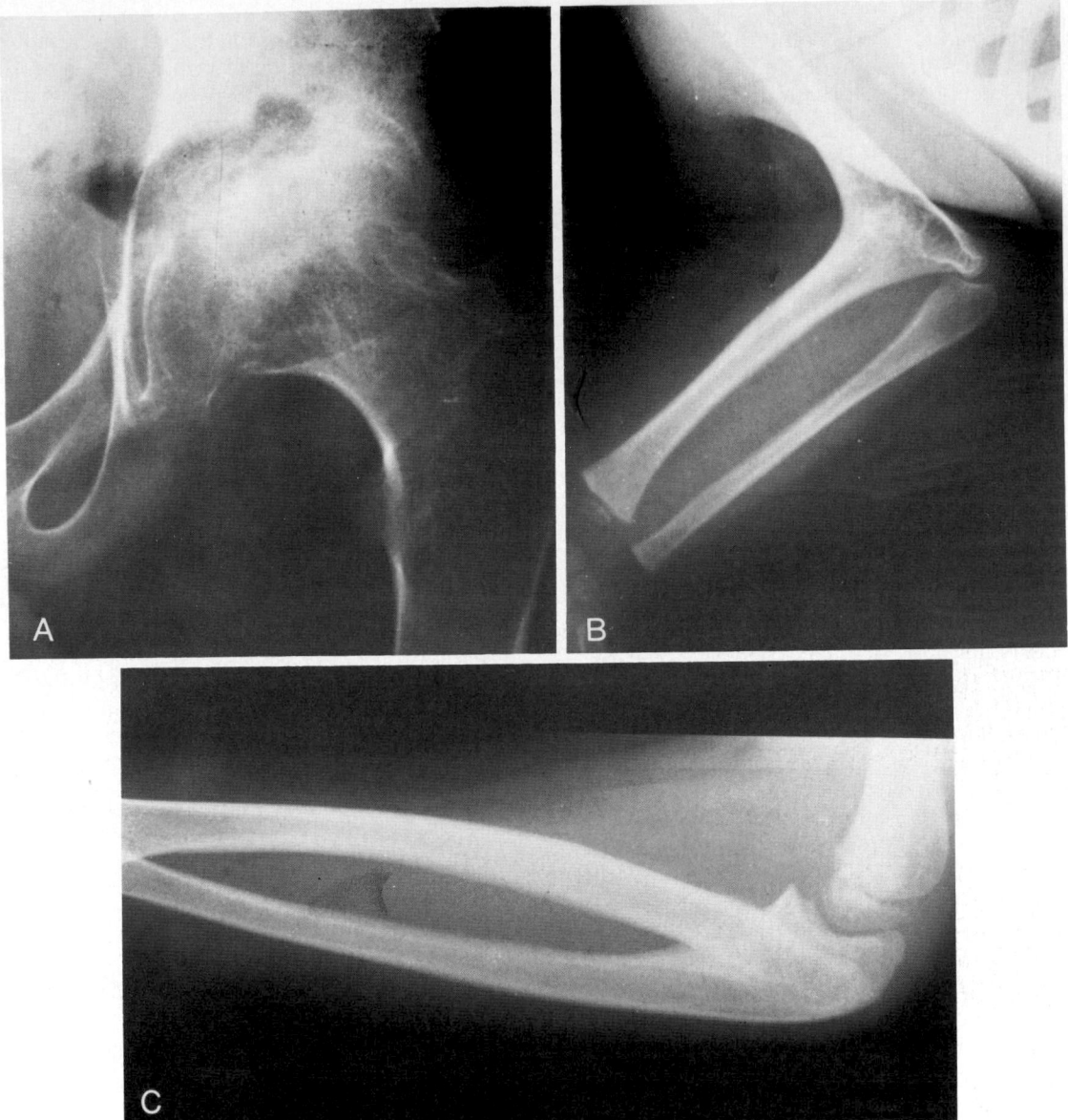

Fig. 4.24. Ankyloses and synostoses. A. Ankylosis of hip joint in rheumatoid arthritis. B. Congenital ankylosis of the elbow. C. Typical appearance of radioulnar synostosis. Note associated radial head dislocation.

SYNOSTOSES

Synostosis of bones can occur after severe inflammatory periostitis and the best known example of this is Caffey's infantile cortical hyperostosis. Similar synostoses can occur after extensive bleeding secondary to trauma, but overall congenital synostoses are more common and tend to occur in a variety of sex chromatin abnormalities. For the most part, these include Klinefelter's syndrome and the XXXY syndrome (1). In many of these cases, the synostoses involve the proximal radioulnar area and are associated with congenital radial head dislocation (Fig. 4.24C). Of course,

similar synostoses can occur in patients without these syndromes and synostoses also can be seen with the clover-leaf skull syndrome (Kleeblatschädel), Ehlers-Danlos syndrome, Holt-Oram's syndrome, and the mesomelic dwarfism syndrome.

Reference

1. Jancu J: Radioulnar synostosis: a common occurrence in sex chromosomal abnormalities. *Am J Dis Child* 122:10–11, 1971.

PSEUDOARTHROSES

Pseudoarthroses most commonly occur after nonunion of fractures, either in normal bones or bones with structural weakness secondary to osteomyelitis, tumor, or cysts (Fig. 4.25A) (Table 4.10). Pseudoarthroses also are encountered in conditions where bone fragility is increased (i.e., osteogenesis imperfecta, osteoporosis, and osteomalacia). On a congenital basis pseudoarthroses most commonly occur in the clavicle (1, 6) and lower extremity. In the clavicle, most often they are isolated findings but also can be seen with cleidocranial dysostosis. In the lower extremity, the tibia and fibula usually are involved, and the finding most commonly is associated with neurofibromatosis (Fig. 4.25B). These cases must be differentiated from those with somewhat similar, but innocuous, bowing resulting from faulty intrauterine positioning (9). In these latter cases, bowing of the tibia and fibula occurs in a direction opposite to that which occurs with congenital pseudoarthroses associated with neurofibromatosis (see Fig. 4.13). In addition, there is no evidence of dysplasia in these cases, only bending. With neurofibromatosis, the bent area is thinned, the cortex irregularity thickened, and the overall appearance dysplastic.

Congenital pseudoarthroses of the clavicle must be differentiated from nonunited clavicular fractures, and this usually is accomplished by noting absence of callous formation, shortening of both remaining portions of the clavicle, and smoothness of their inner ends (Fig. 4.25C). Congenital pseudoarthroses of other bones occurs rarely but can be seen in the radius (2), fibula (3, 8), and upper femur. In the femur, the problem occurs as part of the proximal focal femoral deficiency syndrome (4, 5, 7) (see Fig. 4.22B).

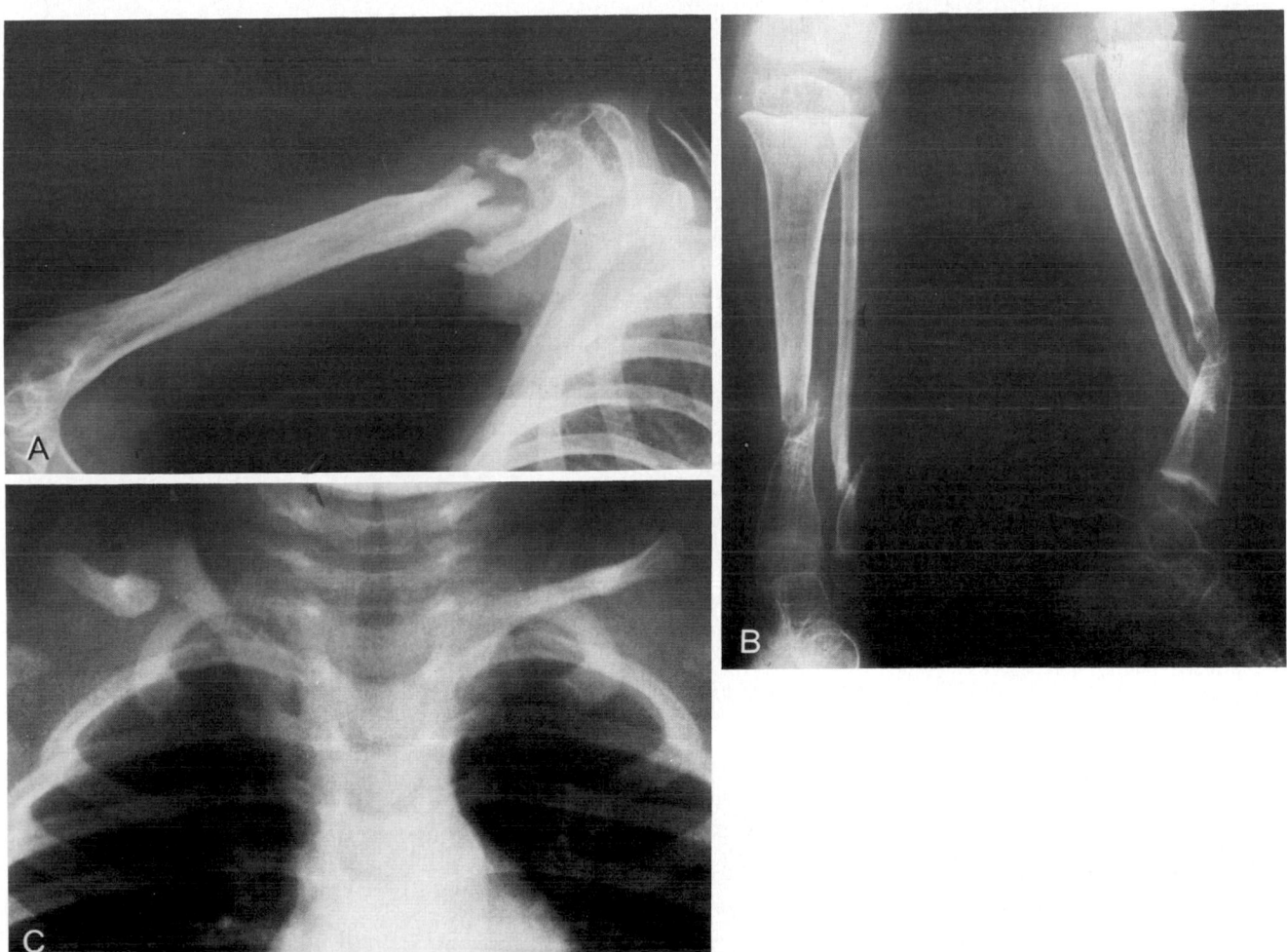

Fig. 4.25. Pseudoarthroses. A. Acquired pseudoarthrosis of humerus after pathologic fracture and severe osteomyelitis. B. Typical pseudoarthrosis of tibia and fibula in neurofibromatosis. C. Typical congenital pseudoarthrosis of the right clavicle. There are no signs of an old, healing, ununited fracture. The bone ends are smooth and rounded.

Table 4.10   Pseudoarthroses

Post fracture long bones or clavicle	Commonest
Congenital: clavicle Neurofibromatosis: tibia-fibula Postinfection (osteomyelitis) Osteogenesis imperfecta (fracture)	Moderately common
Congenital: radius, ulna, fibula Proximal focal femoral deficiency (upper femur) Postirradiation (path. fx)	Rare

References

1. Behringer BR, Wilson FC: Congenital pseudoarthrosis of the clavicle. *Am J Dis Child* 123:511–517, 1972.
2. Cleveland RH, Gilsanz V, Wilkinson RH: Congenital pseudoarthrosis of the radius. *Am J Roentgenol* 130:955–957, 1978.
3. Dooley BJ, Menelaus MB, Paterson DC: Congenital pseudoarthrosis and bowing of the fibula. *J Bone Joint Surg* 56:739–743, 1974.
4. Goldman, AB, Schneider R, Wilson, PD: Proximal focal femoral deficiency. *J Can Assoc Radiol* 29:101–107, 1978.
5. Levinson ED, Ozonoff MB, Royen PM: Proximal femoral focal deficiency (PFFD). *Radiology* 125:197–204, 1977.
6. Manashil G, Laufer S: Congenital pseudoarthrosis of the clavicle; report of three cases. *Am J Roentgenol* 132:678–679, 1979.
7. Schatz SL, Kopits SE: Proximal femoral focal deficiency. *Am J Roentgenol* 131:289–295, 1978.
8. Sprague BL, Brown GA: Congenital pseudoarthrosis of the radius. *J Bone Joint Surg* 56:191–194, 1974.
9. Swischuk LE: *Radiology of the Newborn and Young Infant,* ed 2. Baltimore, Williams & Wilkins Co., 1980, p 624.

SUBPERIOSTEAL BONE RESORPTION

Subperiosteal bone resorption (Table 4.11) can occur at multiple sites, and on a practical basis is almost synonymous with hyperparathyroidism. In children, as in adults, such bone resorption occurs at sites of musculotendinous attachment, but in children, certain areas tend to be more involved. These include the upper proximal tibia, femoral neck (especially the inner curvature), inner proximal humerus, and distal radius and ulna (Fig. 4.26). Of course, resorption also occurs at other sites and, as in the adult, can be seen at either end of the clavicle (12), the middle phalanges of the hand (lateral aspects), terminal tufts of the phalanges (9), and the lamina dura of the teeth. In more severe cases, almost all these sites are positive, but in early cases one of the best places to look for subperiosteal bone resorption in children is along the inner upper tibia (Fig. 4.26A). In addition, in all cases both endosteal and trabecular bone resorption coexist (1), but subperiosteal bone resorption receives most attention. Nonetheless, the other finding should be appreciated because the combination of endosteal, subperiosteal, and trabecular bone resorption produces a rather characteristic picture of an indistinct, fuzzy cortex and coarse trabeculae (Fig. 4.26).

Both primary and secondary forms of hyperparathyroidism can be encountered in children, but the secondary form is much more common. Most often it is seen with chronic renal disease, and then it is referred to as renal osteodystrophy (1, 2). In these cases, both rickets and hyperparathyroidism coexist, but eventually, the findings of hyperparathyroidism predominate. Rickets in these patients results from tubular dysfunction, and hyperparathyroidism from glomerular dysfunction (i.e., the latter leads to phosphorus retention, overstimulation of the parathyroid glands, and secondary hyperparathyroidism). In kidney disease where only tubular impairment occurs, secondary hyperparathyroidism does not arise. Conditions in which renal osteodystropy is seen include chronic glomerulonephritis, chronic pyelonephritis, hypoplastic kidneys, kidneys destroyed by hydronephrosis, and bilateral cystic disease of the kidneys.

Secondary hyperparathyroidism also can occur with severe nonrenal rickets, and in these cases it is believed that profound, chronic hypocalcemia leads to rebound, or secondary, hyperparathyroidism (11). Early or mild cases of rickets do not demonstrate this phenomenon, and actually only those forms of rickets capable of producing severe bony change show changes of hyperparathyroidism. For the most part, these in-

Table 4.11   Subperiosteal Bone Resorption

Hyperparathyroidism: secondary (renal osteodystrophy)	Commonest
Hyperparathyroidism: secondary severe rickets Focal, with tendon avulsion	Moderately common
Hyperparathyroidism: primary Hyperparathyroidism: secondary in pancreatitis Hyperparathyroidism in neonate Focal, with subperiosteal hematoma	Relatively rare
Jansen's metaphyseal dysostosis[a] Generalized gangliosidosis[a] Mucolipidoses[a] Lipogranulomatosis[a] Pseudohypohyperparathyroidism	Rare

[a] Present in infancy.

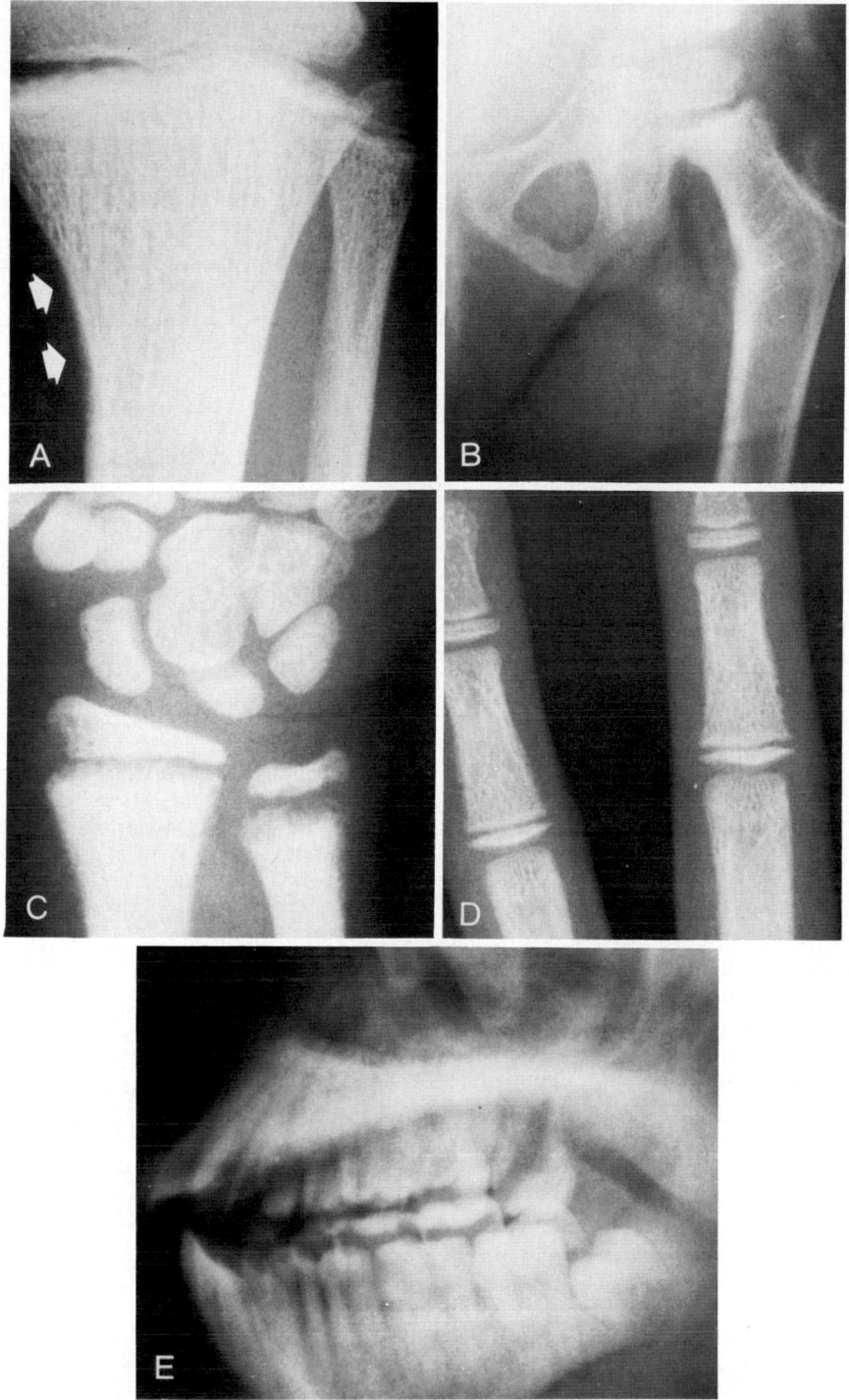

Fig. 4.26.   Subperiosteal bone resorption. A. Hyperparathyroidism. Typical subperiosteal resorption along the upper medial tibia (arrows). B. Same patient demonstrating subperiosteal bone resorption around the femoral neck. C. Another patient demonstrating subperiosteal bone resorption around the radius and ulna. D. Subperiosteal and endosteal bone resorption in the phalanges. E. Absence of lamina dura. (For normal lamina dura, see Fig. 2.14A).

clude deficiency, dependent, and dilantin-phenobarb rickets (11). Another uncommon cause of secondary hyperparathyroidism is pancreatitis. The problem here should not be confused with pancreatitis occurring in patients with primary hyperparathyroidism.

There is an increased incidence of pancreatitis in these patients, but pancreatitis-induced hyperparathyroidism can occur in any patient, with any type of pancreatitis. We have seen the findings in one patient with viral pancreatitis where features of hyperpara-

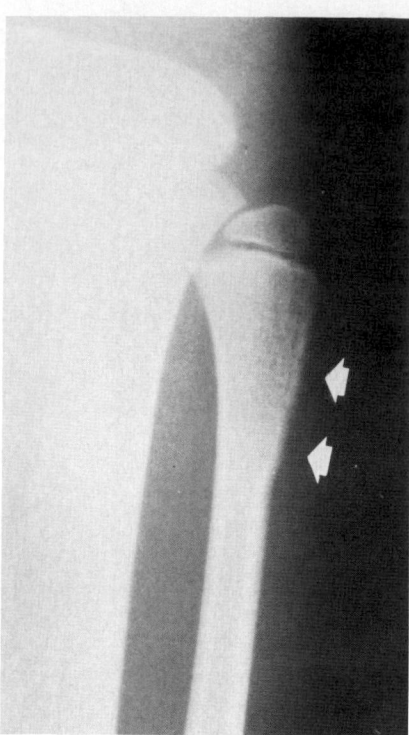

Fig. 4.27. Focal subperiosteal bone resorption. Note area of subperiosteal bone resorption from a chronic avulsion injury in a patient with cerebral palsy (arrows).

thyroidism developed 3 to 4 weeks after the onset of pancreatitis and all disappeared as the patient recovered. It is presumed that liberation of lipase in this patient caused binding of calcium, hypocalcemia, and rebound hyperparathyroidism.

Rarely, secondary hyperparathyroidism is seen in association with pseudo or pseudopseudohypoparathyroidism (8). In these cases, hyperparathyroidism also is believed to result from hypocalcemia, and when the findings of both of these aberrations of bone metabolism are seen together, the term pseudohypohyperparathyroidism is applied.

Primary hyperparathyroidism in the pediatric age group is quite uncommon but both sporadic and familial forms exist (5). Neonates also can be hyperparathyroid as a result of their mothers being hypoparathyroid (10), and finally, subperiosteal bone resorption, very similar to that seen with hyperparathyroidism, can occur in a few nonrelated conditions. It is not known exactly why this should occur, but the findings can mimic those of hyperparathyroidism ex-

actly. For the most part, this occurs in infants with the following conditions; Jansen's metaphyseal dysostosis (4), generalized gangliosidosis (3), mucolipidoses (6), and lipogranulomatosis (7).

Focal, or isolated subperiosteal resorption occurs with adjacent soft tissue inflammations, or tendon avulsions (see Fig. 4.27). The latter is more common, and can occur at any tendon insertion site. Subperiosteal resorption, eventually leading to a frank cortical defect, also is seen with posttraumatic subperiosteal hematomas, or so-called subperiosteal giant cell tumors (see Fig. 4.30).

References

1. Jensen PS, Klinger AS: Early radiographic manifestations of secondary hyperparathyroidism associated with chronic renal disease. *Radiology* 125:645–652, 1977.
2. Mehls O, Ritz E, Krempien B, Willich E, Bommer J, Scharer K: Roentgenological signs of the skeleton of uremic children. An analysis of the anatomical principles underlying the roentgenological changes. *Pediatr Radiol* 1:183–190, 1973.
3. O'Brien JS, Stern BB, Landing BH, O'Brien JK, Donnell GN: Generalized gangliosidosis. Another inborn error of ganglioside metabolism. *Am J Dis Child* 109:338–346, 1965.
4. Ozonoff MB: Metaphyseal dysostosis of Jansen. *Radiology* 93:1047–1050, 1969.
5. Sandler LM, Moncrieff MW: Familial hyperparathyroidism. *Arch Dis Child* 55:146–147, 1980.
6. Scott CR, Langunoff D, Trump BF: Familial neurovisceral lipidosis. *J Pediatr* 71:357–366, 1967.
7. Schultz G, Lang EK: Disseminated lipogranulomatosis: early roentgenographic changes. *Radiology* 82:675–678, 1964.
8. Steinback HL, Young DA: The roentgen appearance of hyperparathyroidism (PH) and pseudo-pseudo-hypoparathyroidism (PPH), differentiation from other syndromes associated with short metacarpals, metatarsals, and phalanges. *Am J Roentgenol* 97:49–66, 1966.
9. Sundaram M, Joyce PF, Shields JB, Riaz MA, Sagar S: Terminal phalangeal tufts: earlies site of renal osteodystrophy findings in hemodialysis patients. *Am J Roentgenol* 133:25–29, July, 1979.
10. Swischuk LE: *Radiology of the Newborn and Young Infant*, ed 2. Baltimore, Williams & Wilkins, 1980, pp 660–661.
11. Swischuk LE, Hayden CK Jr: Rickets: a roentgenographic scheme for diagnosis. *Pediatr Radiol.* 8:203–208, 1979.
12. Teplick JG, Eftekhari F, Haskin ME: Erosion of the sternal ends of the clavicles. A new sign of primary and secondary hyperparathyroidism. *Radiology* 113:323–326, 1974.

CORTICAL DEFECTS AND EROSIONS

Cortical defects and erosions can result from (*a*) intrinsic cortical lesions and (*b*) extrinsic focal erosions or areas of demineralization (Table 4.12).

Table 4.12 Cortical Defects and Erosions

Benign cortical defect Tendon avulsion injuries	Commonest

Focal subperiosteal bone resorption
  (see Table 4.11)
Metaphyseal bone destruction with:
  Lymphoma, leukemia
  Metastatic disease
  Infection, infarction
Juxtaarticular erosion with rheuma-
  toid arthritis
	Moderately common

Posttraumatic subperiosteal giant cell tumor Adjacent soft tissue tumors	Relatively rare

Intrinsic Cortical Lesions

The commonest intrinsic cortical lesion, producing a localized cortical defect is the so-called benign cortical, fibrous defect (4). These growth disturbances, primarily of long bones, are identified by their very eccentric and completely intracortical location. They occur in the metaphyses, and while some appear as small cortical cysts, others are just thin, flat defects (Fig. 4.28). Often they are more readily demonstrable on one view than another and, of course, the tangential view is the one which best demonstrates their cortical location. When seen en face, a more serious lesion often is erroneously suggested (i.e., osteomyelitis, primary or secondary bone tumor, and bone cysts) (Fig. 4.29).

Benign cortical defects usually are multiple and tend to be most common in the lower extremities. For the most part, they seem to cluster around the knees and ankles, but they can be seen in other long bones and, occasionally, even in a flat bone. Eventually they become filled with bone and disappear, (Fig. 4.29C) but in their early stages they are a problem for the unwary. In this regard, it should be noted that benign cortical defects, for the most part, are silent lesions. Usually they are noted when the extremity is being examined for some other reason. It is most important not to misinterpret these benign cortical defects for some more serious lesion, and the major step in avoiding such a misinterpretation is knowing what they look like and where they are likely to be seen. They are related to the more cystic, but still generally eccentric, cortical lesion known as the nonossifying fibroma (see Fig. 4.130A).

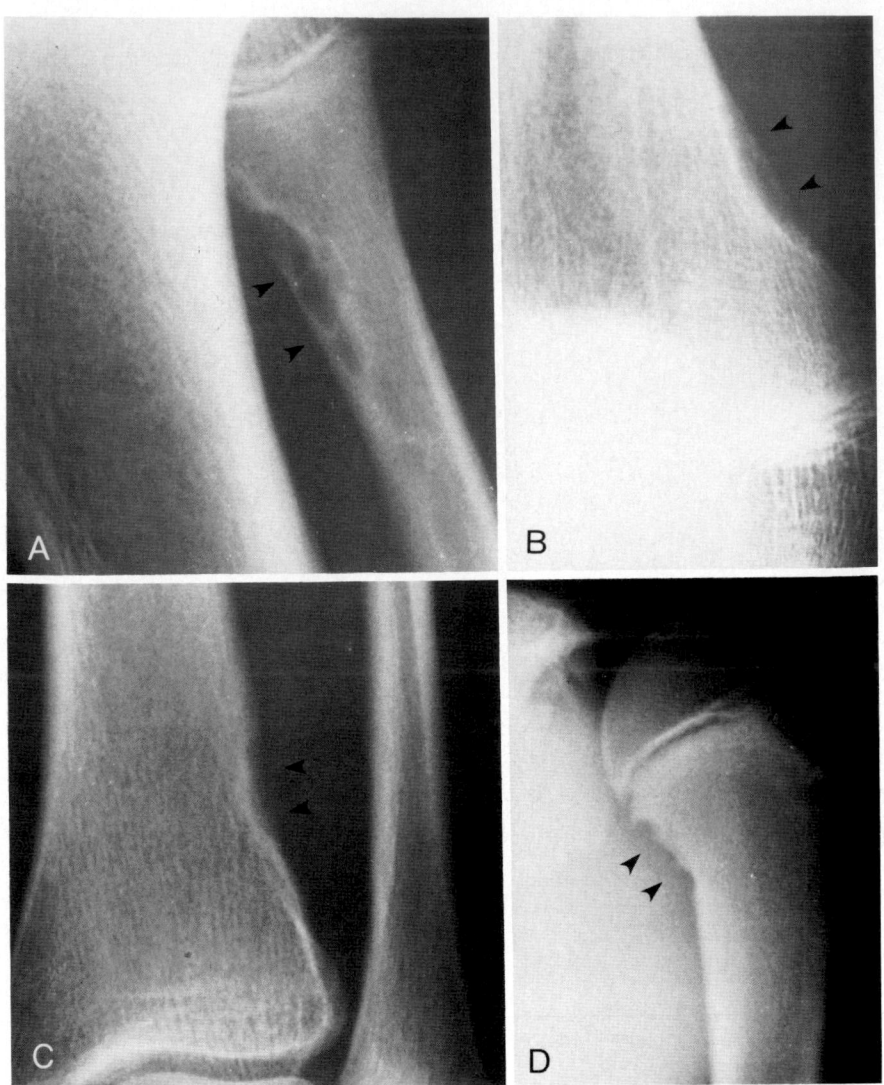

Fig. 4.28. Benign cortical defects. A. Rather large, multiloculated benign cortical defect (arrows). This type of defect could qualify for the related lesion, a nonossifying fibroma. B. Smaller, somewhat cystic appearing benign cortical defect (arrow). C. Small, almost invisible benign cortical defect (arrow). D. Lobulated benign cortical defect in upper humerus (arrows).

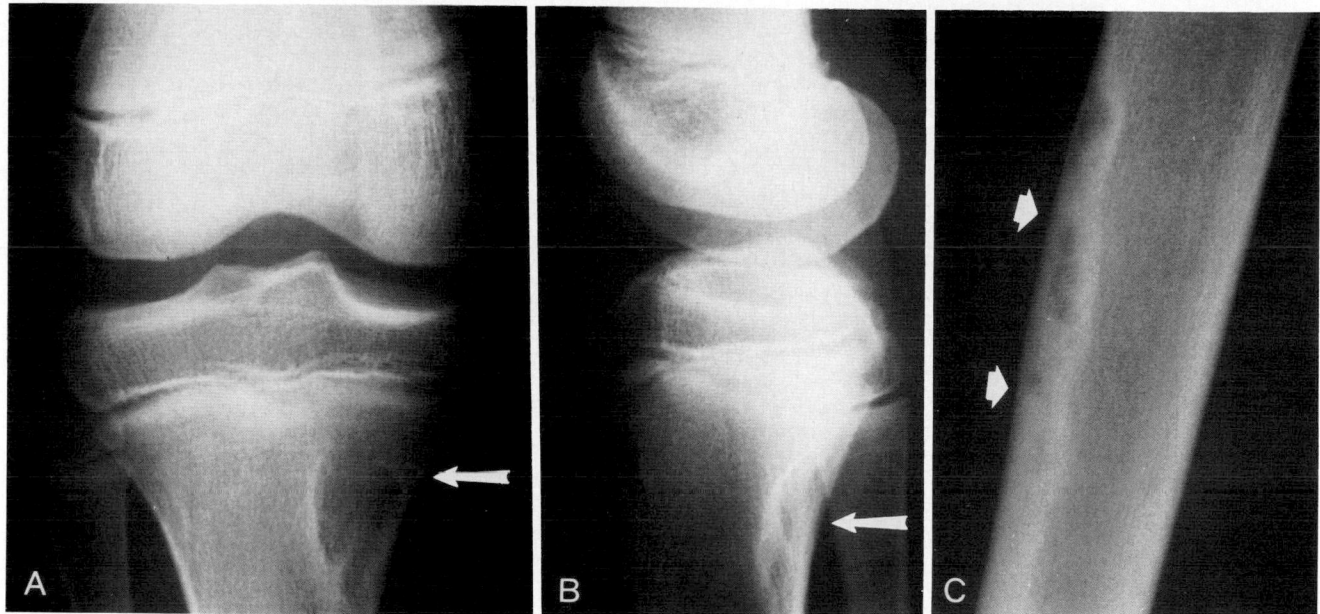

Fig. 4.29. Benign cortical defects. A. Typical appearance on frontal view (arrow). B. On lateral view, note eccentric cortical location (arrow). C. Another patient demonstrating a sclerotic, healing benign cortical defect (arrow).

Extrinsic Focal Cortical Erosions

Such erosions can result from pressure caused by adjacent soft tissue masses, tendon avulsion injuries, or focal, subperiosteal bone resorption. Erosions from **adjacent soft tissue masses** usually are smooth edged, but are least common. For the most part, the masses are visible but palpable clinically, and include tumors such as neurofibroma, fibroma, lipoma, and hemangioma. The malignant counterparts of these tumors (generally quite rare) may render the edge of the defect moth-eaten and irregular. A rare cause of an extrinsic "tumor" producing a focal cortical erosion is the so-called posttraumatic subperiosteal giant cell tumor. This lesion is not really a tumor, but rather a hematoma which causes focal bone resorption as it heals. The clue to its diagnosis is the history of preceding trauma, and its recognition is important, for histologically there is a tendency to misinterpret these lesions from a malignant bone tumor. Usually, they occur in the diaphysis of a long bone (Fig. 4.30).

Focal cortical erosions produced by **tendon avulsion injuries** are the most common cause of an extrinsic cortical defect or erosion. Of course, if the avulsed piece of bone is visible there is no problem with the diagnosis, but unfortunately in some cases no such avulsed fragment of bone is seen (see Fig. 4.27). Rather there is soft tissue change only, but then, with bleeding and inflammation, subsequent bone resorption at the site of avulsion occurs. These injuries can occur anywhere a tendon inserts onto a bone, but they are most common in the lower extremity, around the hip and knee. In the hip they tend to occur over

the superior crest of the iliac wing, just above the edge of the acetabulum, around either trochanter, and along the lower edge of the ischium (6, 10, 11). At most of these sites, in most cases, an avulsed piece of bone is visible from the onset, but along the lower edge of the ischium the reverse usually is true (Fig. 4.31). Indeed, all that usually is present in the early stages is slight fuzziness of the cortex. To be sure, the finding is so subtle that most often it is missed. On the other hand, when it is seen it tends to be misinterpreted for a more serious lesion such as a malignant bone tumor or area of osteomyelitis. This pitfall can be avoided if the characteristic site of this avulsion injury is remembered.

In the healing phase of an avulsion injury, as new bone is deposited, the findings may mimic a bone tumor even more (Fig. 4.32). Indeed, it is at this stage of the evolution of the lesion that one must maintain confidence in one's original diagnosis. Bone biopsy must be avoided because there is a tendency to misinterpret the findings for those of a malignant bone tumor. In addition, there is no point in obtaining an isotope bone scan, for while it is positive it does not differentiate between trauma, tumor, or infection. Realistically, then, once one identifies the lesion on plain films, the diagnosis must be made from the plain films.

In the knee, the best known avulsion injury is the one involving the cruciate ligaments and tibial spines, but this is not the injury causing most difficulty with diagnosis. Rather it is the avulsion injury involving

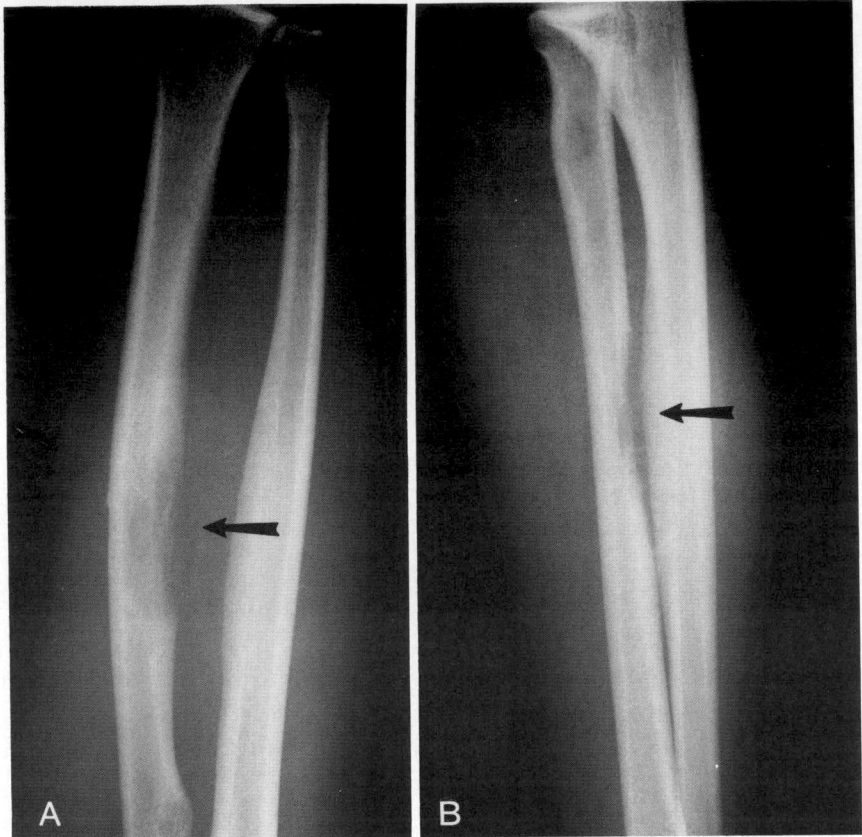

Fig. 4.30. Cortical defect—subperiosteal giant cell tumor. A. Note the extensive area of eccentric bone erosion (arrow) in this 18-yr-old patient with a subperiosteal hematoma producing bone resorption (arrow). B. Lateral view demonstrates same findings (biopsy proven).

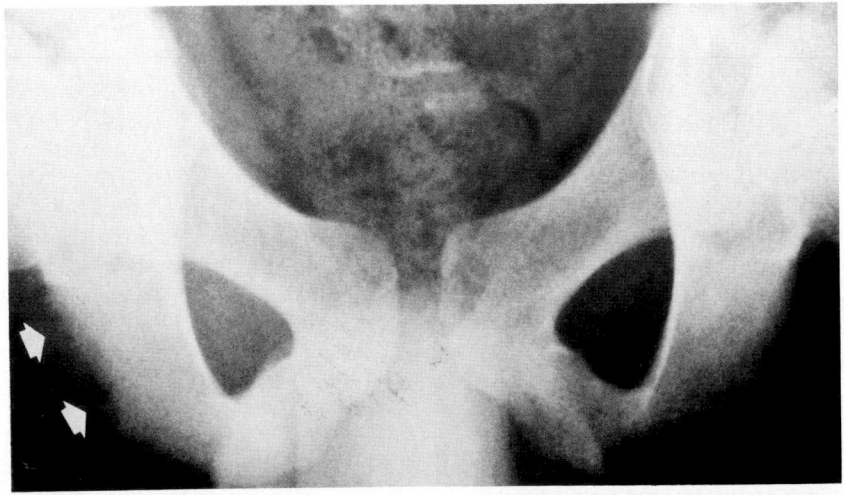

Fig. 4.31. Cortical defects—tendon avulsion. Indistinct but typical cortical defect due to tendon avulsion along the ischium (arrow). This patient had hip pain.

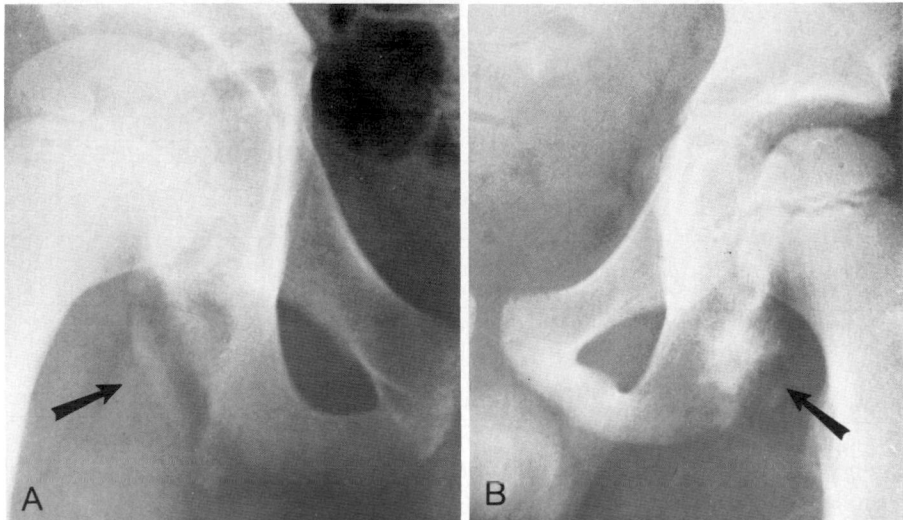

Fig. 4.32.   Healed ischial avulsions. A. Note new bone deposition during healing of an ischial avulsion (arrow). Same patient as in Figure 4.31. B. Another patient with tumor-like healing ischial avulsion (arrow).

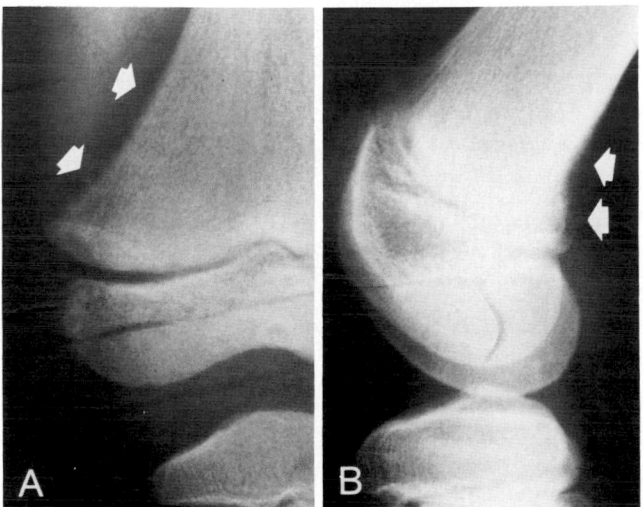

Fig. 4.33.   Cortical defect—distal femoral irregularity. A. Typical appearance of medial condylar irregularity due to tendon avulsion (arrows). B. Lateral view demonstrating similar findings in another patient (arrows). Oblique views often demonstrate these findings to better advantage.

the medial supracondylar ridge of the femur (Fig. 4.33). This injury is very similar to the one occurring along the lower ischium, but as opposed to the ischial lesion, the one around the femur usually is asymptomatic. To be sure, most cases are discovered incidentally when the knee is being investigated for some other reason. In spite of this fact, and that numerous documentations of this avulsion injury are available (1, 3, 5, 8, 9, 12), it still is commonly misdiagnosed for a bone tumor. In the past these lesions have been referred to as cortical desmoids or desmoblastic fibro-

mas, but most likely they represent nothing more than healing cortical avulsions (2, 5). All of these points notwithstanding, however, when the lesion is encountered it is difficult not to entertain such thoughts as parosteal sarcoma. Clinically, of course, some help should be present in that pain usually is not present over the area and that radiographically, there is no evidence of an associated soft tissue mass.

Occasionally, as has been mentioned earlier, erosions similar to those described in the pelvis and knee are seen in other bones. In this regard, such injuries can occur around the upper inner tibial metaphysis, or at the deltoid insertion on the humerus. None of these sites, however, are as common as those outlined around the hip and knee.

Focal cortical bone loss secondary to subperiosteal bone resorption is seen with hyperparathyroidism and conditions mimicking hyperparathyroidism. For the most part, these have been discussed in the preceding section and are noted in Table 4.11. In addition, however, juxtacortical erosions occur with rheumatoid arthritis (7) and can be mimicked by a number of metaphyseal destructive lesions when these lesions are very aggressive. In such cases, the cortex is destroyed from within, but the x-ray picture may suggest that an extrinsic cortical erosion is present. Conditions in which this can occur include leukemia, lymphoma, metastatic disease (Fig. 4.34), and the trophic (destructive) bone changes produced by congenital lues, and bone infarction.

References

1. Barnes GR Jr, Gwinn JL: Distal irregularities of the femur stimulating malignancy. *Am J Roentgenol* 122:180–185, 1974.
2. Barower AC, Culver JE Jr, Keats TE: Histologic nature

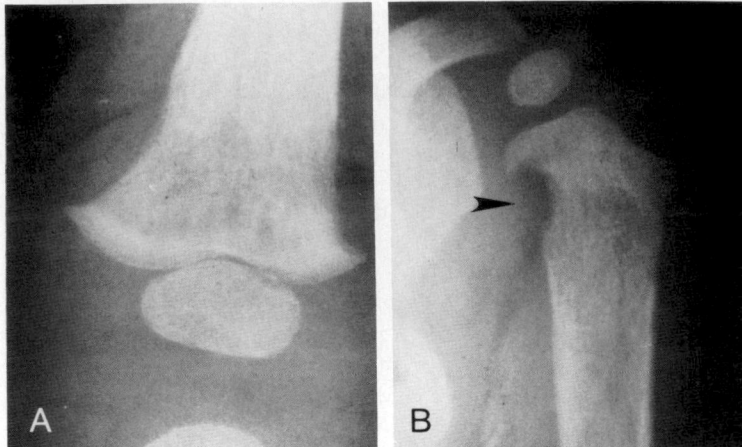

Fig. 4.34. **Cortical erosions—leukemia.** A. Note cortical erosions in the upper tibiae and lower femurs. Although destruction is occurring from within, the cortical erosions suggest an extrinsic process. B. Similar changes in the humerus (arrows).

of cortical irregularity of medial posterior distal femoral metaphysis in children. *Radiology* 99:389, 1971.

3. Bufkin WJ: The avulsion cortical irregularity. *Am J Roentgenol* 112:477–492, 1971.

4. Caffey J: *Pediatric X-Ray Diagnosis*, ed 6. Chicago, Year Book Medical Publishers, 1972, vol 2, pp 948–955.

5. Dunham, WK, Marcus NW, Enneking WF, Haun C: Developmental defects of the distal femoral metaphysis. *J Bone Joint Surg* 62(A):801–806, 1980.

6. Ellis RE, Green AG: Ischial apophyseolysis. *Radiology* 87:646–648, 1966.

7. Goel KM, Rawson SP, Shanks RA: Radiological assessment of fifty patients with juvenile rheumatoid arthritis: correlation with clinical and laboratory abnormalities.

Pediatr Radiol 2:51–60, 1974.

8. Prentice ID: Variations on the fibrous cortical defect. *Clin Radiol* 25:531–533, 1974.

9. Simon H: Medial distal metaphyseal femoral irregularity in children. *Radiology* 90:258–260, 1968.

10. Slayton CA: Ischial epiphysiolysis. *Am J Roentgenol* 76:11161–1162, 1956.

11. Swischuk LE: Avulsion and stress fractures in childhood. In Margulis A, Gooding CA (eds): *Diagnostic Radiology.* St. Louis, C.V. Mosby, 1981, pp 257–264.

12. Young, DW, Nogrady MB, Dunbar JS, Wiglesworth FW: Benign cortical irregularities in the distal femur of children. *J Can Assoc Radiol* 23:107–115, 1972.

CORTICAL BUMPS

Local cortical bumps are most commonly encountered with so-called buckle or torus fractures of the long bones. These bumps occur in the metaphyses where the cortex is weakest. Generally, the normal metaphyseal margins are smoothly curving and when one sees any type of buckle, kink, or bump, one should suspect a fracture (Fig. 4.35A). In the more subtle cases, these bumps will be missed unless comparative views of the other extremity are obtained. Other causes of cortical bumps include old healed fractures (Fig. 4.35B) and small sessile osteochondromas and enchondromas (Fig. 4.35C).

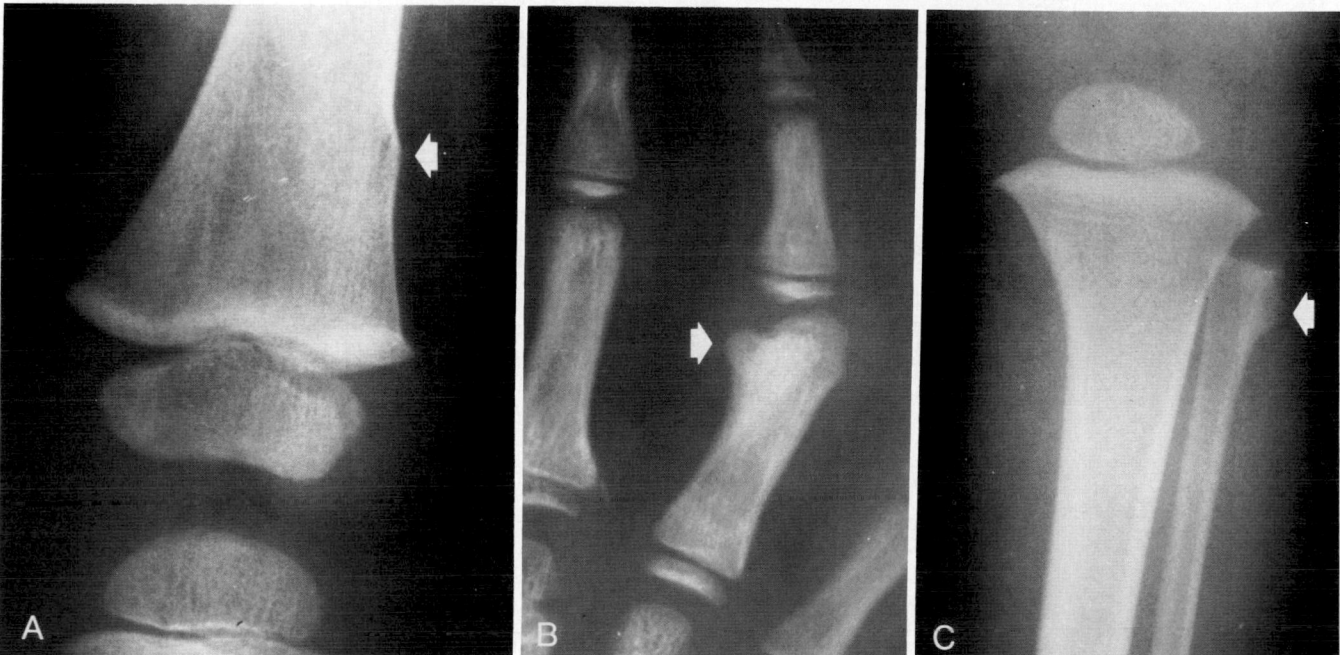

Fig. 4.35. Cortical bumps. A. Typical cortical bump due to buckle or torus fracture of the distal femur (arrow). Compare with the curved smoothness of the normal cortex on the other side. B. Cortical bump due to old epiphyseal-metaphyseal fracture (arrow). C. Cortical bump due to sessile osteochondroma (arrow) in 1-yr-old child. This patient came from a family with multiple osteochondromas and this is about as early as these lesions are seen.

CORTICAL THICKENING

The commonest cause of localized cortical thickening is a healed fracture or osteomyelitis. However, it can also be seen after healing of any type of bone lesion which first destroys or expands the cortex. Localized cortical thickening also is seen in osteoid osteoma and with prolonged periosteal new bone deposition for any reason. Thickening of the cortex also occurs in hyperphosphatemia, a condition where hypermetabolism of the bone leads to thick, coarsely trabeculated cortices. Thick, dense cortices also are seen in the Kenny-Caffey syndrome.

OSTEOLYSIS

Osteolysis, in general, is an uncommon problem, but three basic types have been identified: (a) massive osteolysis (Gorham's disease); (b) essential (carpal-tarsal) osteolysis; and (c) acro-osteolysis. None are particularly common in childhood, and of the three, acro-osteolysis probably is most common. Massive osteolysis is quite rare and also is known as vanishing or disappearing bone disease (1, 7). The basic problem in this condition is an underlying hemangioma or, more often, lymphangioma leading to virtual dissolution of bone. The process can cross joint spaces, generally is progressive, and usually involves the flat bones, including the ribs (Fig. 4.36). Essential, carpal-tarsal osteolysis is a progressive, slow, bone resorbing disease which affects the carpal and tarsal bones primarily. However, it also can involve the metacarpals, metatarsals, and bones around the elbow (4). Basically two types have been identified, a hereditary autosomal dominant form and a nonfamilial type associated with a fatal nephropathy (2–4, 6, 8, 10–14). The most likely underlying problem is a vasculitis leading to both bone and cartilage destruction. Similar destruction can be seen with rheumatoid arthritis and the mucopolysaccharidosis known as the Winchester syndrome (15). Bone lysis also occurs with neuropathic joints such as seen with lues, leprosy, syringomyelia, and scleroderma (4).

Acro-osteolysis refers to resorption of the terminal phalanges of the hands and feet, but often the finding is more pronounced in the hands. It is likely that in many cases a vasculitis leads to progressive bone resorption and the condition, along with other causes of phalangeal resorption, are dealt with at a later point (see p 245).

References

1. Abrahams J, Ganick D, Gilbert E, Wolfson J: Massive osteolysis in an infant. *Am J Roentgenol* 135:1084–1086, 1980.
2. Counahan R, Simmons MJ, Charlwood GJ: Multifocal

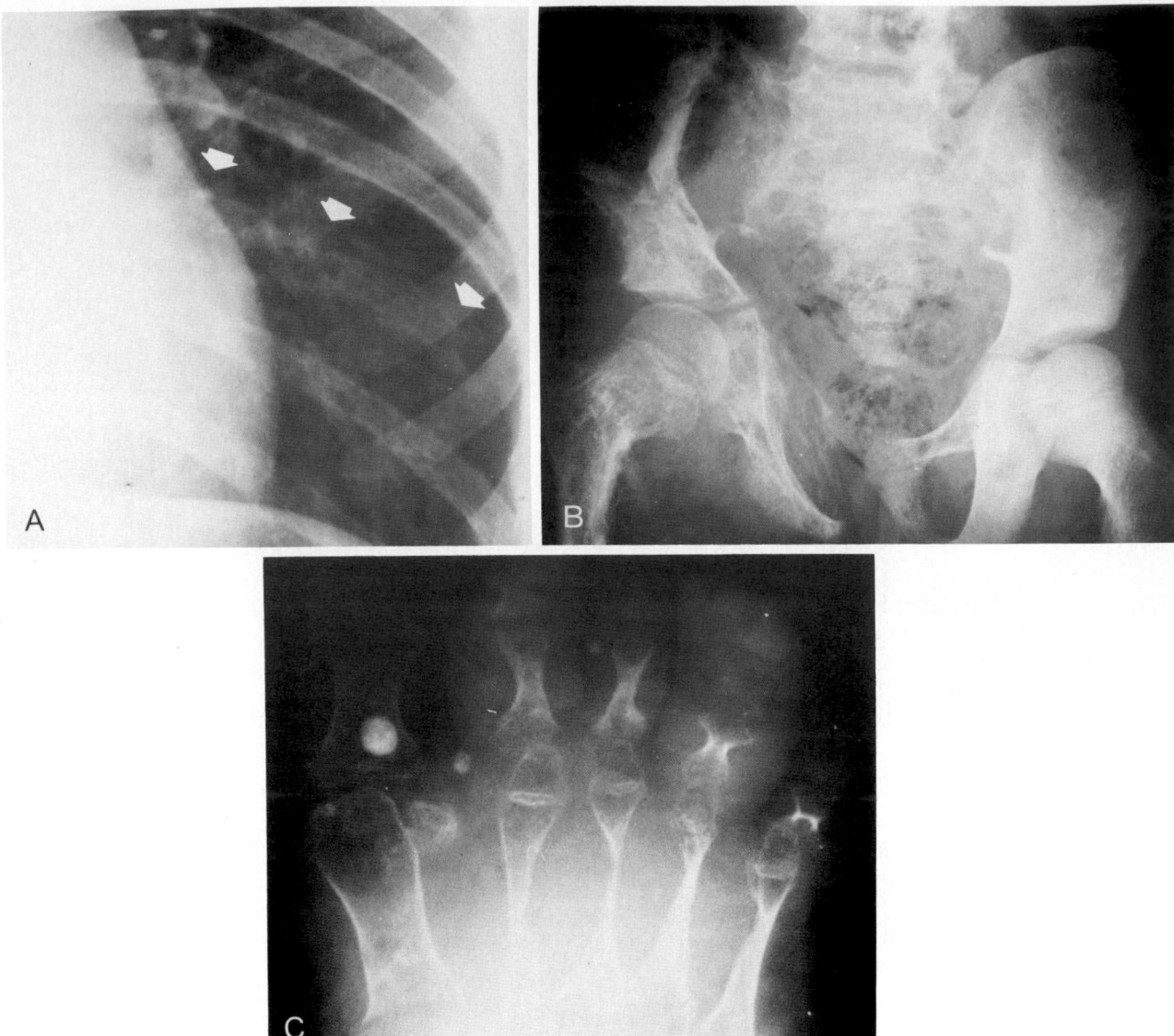

Fig. 4.36. Osteolysis. A. Note complete absence of the rib on the left (arrows) in this patient with disappearing bone disease secondary to lymphangioma of the bone. B. Extensive lysis of the pelvic bones and right femur in a patient with extensive soft tissue hemangiomas. C. Another patient with extensive lysis due to hemangioma. Note characteristic phleboliths.

osteolysis with nephropathy. *Arch Dis Child* 51:717–719, 1976.

3. Edeiken J, Hodes PJ: *Roentgen Diagnosis of Diseases of Bone*, ed 2. Baltimore, Williams & Wilkins, 1973, pp 58, 214, 928

4. Erickson CM, Hirschberger M, Sticker GB: Carpaltarsal osteolysis. *J Pediatr* 93:779–782, 1978.

5. Gilula LA, Bliznak J, Staple TW: Idiopathic nonfamilial acro-osteolysis with cortical defects and mandibular ramus osteolysis. *Radiology* 121:63–68, 1976.

6. Gluck J, Millier JJ III: Familial osteolysis of the carpal and tarsal bones. *J Pediatr* 81:506–510, 1972.

7. Heyden G, Kinblom LG, Nielsen JM: Disappearing bone disease: a clinical and histological study. *J Bone Joint Surg* 59:57–61, 1977.

8. Kohler E, Babbitt D, Huizenga B, Good TA: Hereditary osteolysis: A clinical, radiological and chemical study. *Radiology* 108:99–105, 1973.

9. Kozlowski K, Barylak A, Eftekhari F, Pasyk K: Acro-osteolysis. Problems of diagnosis—report of four cases. *Pediatr Radiol* 8:79–86, 1979.

10. Lemaitre L, Remy J, Smith M, Nuyts JP, Cousin J, Farine MO, Debeugny P: Carpal and tarsal osteolysis. *Pediatr Radiol* 13:219–226, 1983.

11. MacPherson RI, Walker RD, Kowall MH: Essential osteolysis with nephropathy. *J Can Assoc Radiol* 24:98–100, 1973.

12. Tyler T, Rosenbaum H: Idiopathic multicentric osteolysis. *Am J Roentgenol* 126:23–32, 1976.

13. Torg JS, Steel HH: Essential osteolysis with nephrop-

athy: a review of the literature and case report of an unusual syndrome. *J Bone Joint Surg* 50A:1629–1634, 1968.

14. Torg JS, DiGeorge AM, Kirkpatrick JA, Trujillo MM: Hereditary multicentric osteolysis with recessive trans-

mission. A new syndrome. *J Pediatr* 75:243–246, 1969.
15. Winchester P, Grossman H, Lim WN, Danes BS: A new acid mucopolysaccharidosis with skeletal deformities simulating rheumatoid arthritis. *Am J Roentgenol* 106:121–128, 1969.

FOCAL BONY SCLEROSIS

The commonest cause of focal bony sclerosis in childhood is a healing stress fracture (Table 4.13). Most commonly these fractures occur in the upper tibia, and the sclerosis is seen as they heal. At this stage, usually, there also is associated periosteal new bone deposition (Fig. 4.37A), and both the sclerosis and periosteal new bone are best demonstrated with laminography. The presence of these fractures also can be verified with isotope bone scans, but the roentgenographic findings are so characteristic that seldom is this required. In addition to the upper tibia, these fractures occur in the femoral neck, in the fibula, and in the second metatarsal as "march" fractures. Stress fractures in the upper extremities, or through the chest cage are uncommon except in very active children or those with underlying metabolic bone disease.

Other causes of focal bony sclerosis are not particularly common but perhaps the next group of conditions to be considered would include idiopathic focal sclerosis, bone infarction, healed benign cortical defect or nonossifying fibroma, and healed histiocytosis X. Idiopathic sclerosis occasionally is identified in entirely asymptomatic individuals (Fig. 4.37B). The cause of such areas of sclerosis is not known, but they may represent quiescent osteoid osteomas. Once an osteoid osteoma has burned itself out, sclerosis may

remain and yet no symptoms are present. Small, so-called bone islands (2, 5) are not particularly common in children (Fig. 4.37C) and are of no particular consequence.

Bone infarcts causing sclerosis occur, for the most part, in older children with sickle cell disease (Fig. 4.37D), and the findings are no different from those seen in adulthood. They consist of irregular areas of medullary sclerosis which, eventually, becomes more generalized, and at the same time, associated with irregular endosteal thickening. Healing in osteomyelitis (Fig. 4.38A), benign cortical defects (Fig. 4.38D), nonossifying fibromas, and histiocytosis X also can produce nonspecific sclerotic areas in the bone. With nonossifying fibromas and benign cortical defects (these most probably are related lesions), the eccentric, cortical location of the healed, sclerotic area is a clue to their etiology (Fig. 4.38D).

Osteoid osteoma, a benign bone tumor with an aberrant, radiolucent nidus of osteoid tissue in the center (Fig. 4.38B) and reactive bony sclerosis around it (Fig. 4.38, B and C), is moderately common in childhood (1, 7). It is associated with pain, worse at night, and characteristically relieved by aspirin. However, the clinical findings are not always so characteristic, and as noted earlier some osteoid osteomas seem to "burn-out" and become quiescent (Fig. 4.37B). In addition, when osteoid osteomas are located in the spine or pelvis, they may be difficult to detect. In this regard, isotope bone scans are quite useful in detecting the more occult of these tumors (6, 10). In any case, often there is difficulty differentiating an osteoid osteoma from a stress fracture, but when the central radiolucent nidus is demonstrated (Fig. 4.38B), the diagnosis is more or less assured. The radiolucent nidus often is more readily demonstrable with conventional laminography or CT scanning. Other, less common causes of focal bony sclerosis include Ewing's sarcoma (single or multiple), osteogenic sarcoma, fibrous dysplasia (usually skull), meningioma (skull), foreign body reaction, osteoma, healing mastocytosis, tuberous sclerosis, and osteoblastic metastases. The latter, of course, are quite uncommon in childhood, as far as osteogenic sarcoma is concerned, when it is multicentric (3, 9), multiple areas of focal sclerosis can be seen throughout the skeleton. This form of the tumor, however, is quite rare. In tuberous sclerosis, patches of dense bone frequently are seen in the flat bones and skull.

Table 4.13 Focal Bony Sclerosis

Stress fracture (healing)	}	Commonest
Fibrous dysplasia Bone infarct Healed cortical defect, nonossifying fibroma Healed histiocytosis X Osteoid osteoma	}	Moderately common
Idiopathic, bone island Ewing's sarcoma Osteogenic sarcoma (solitary) Meningioma (skull) Foreign body reaction Osteoma	}	Relatively rare
Osteogenic sarcoma (multiple) Tuberous sclerosis Healing mastocytosis Osteoblastic metastases	}	Rare

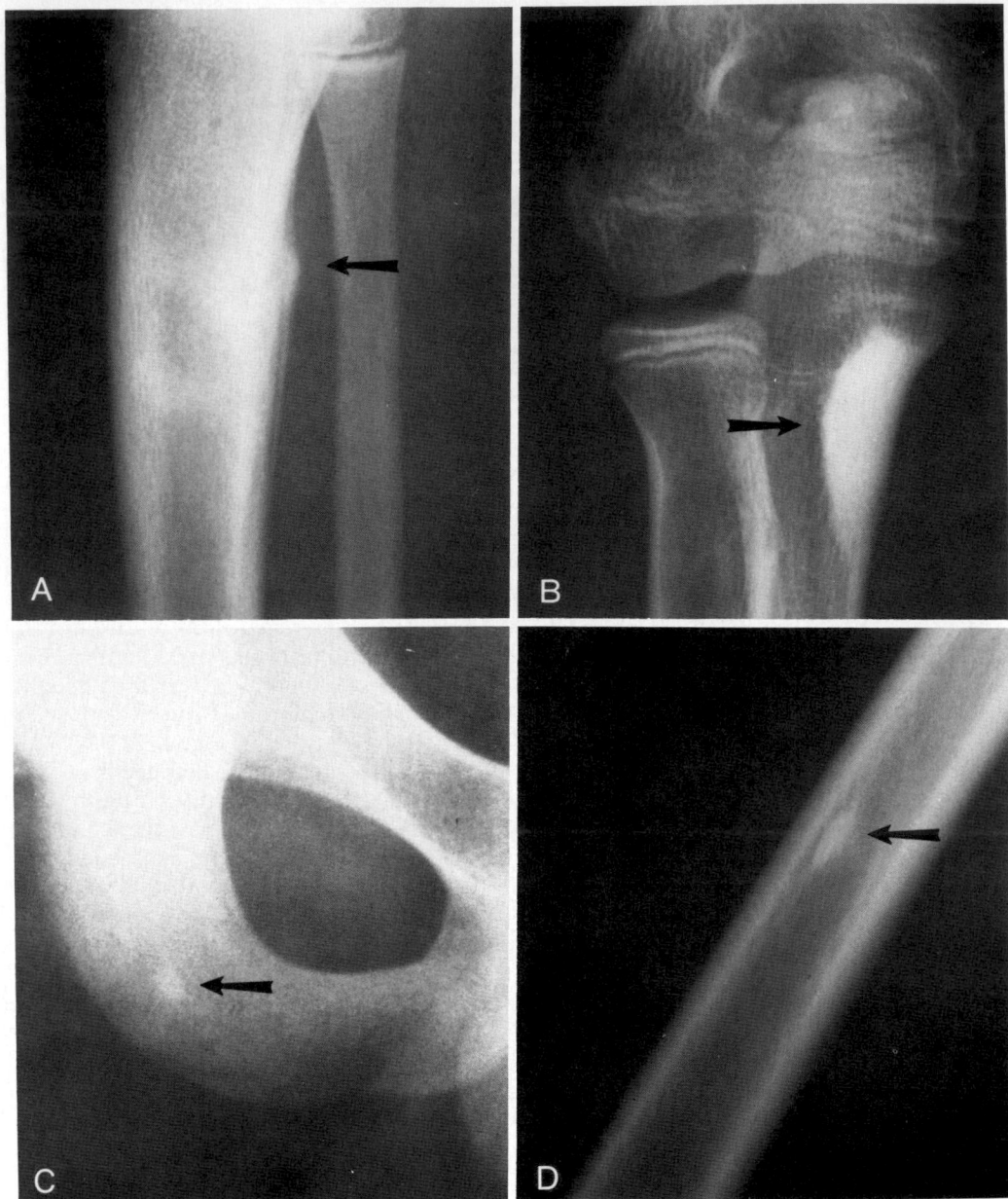

Fig. 4.37. **Focal bony sclerosis.** A. Typical sclerosis due to upper tibial stress fracture (arrow). Also note periosteal new bone. B. Idiopathic sclerosis in ulna (arrow). Possible quiescent osteoid osteoma. C. Bone island (arrow) in pubic bone. D. Small bone infarct (arrow) in older child with sickle cell disease.

References

1. Black JA, Levick RK, Sharrard WJW: Osteoid osteoma and benign osteoblastoma in childhood. *Arch Dis Child* 54:459–465, 1979.
2. Blank N, Lieber A: The significance of growing bone islands. *Radiology* 85:508–511, 1965.
3. Cremin BJ, Heselson NG, Webber BL: The multiple sclerotic osteogenic sarcoma of early childhood. *Br J Radiol* 49:416–419, 1976.
4. Freedman S, Taber P, Alter A: Benign osteoblastic lesion in the scapula of a child. *Am J Dis Child* 123:236–237, 1972.
5. Kim SK, Barry WF: Bone islands. *Radiology* 90:77–78, 1968.
6. Omojola MF, Cockshott WP, Beatty EG: Osteoid osteoma: an evaluation of diagnostic modalities. *Clin Radiol.* 32:199–204, 1981.
7. Orlowski JP, Mercer RD: Osteoid osteoma in children and young adults. *Pediatrics* 59:526–532, 1977.
8. Rowe CW, Haggard ME: Bone infarcts in sickle cell anemia. *Radiology* 68:661–667, 1957.
9. Singleton EB, Rosenberg HS, Dodd GD, Dolan PA: Sclerosing osteogenic sarcomatosis. *Am J Reoengenol Ther Nucl Med* 88:483–490, 1962.
10. Winter PF, Johnson PM, Hilal SK, Feldman F: Scintigraphic detection of osteoid osteoma. *Radiology* 122:177–178, 1977.

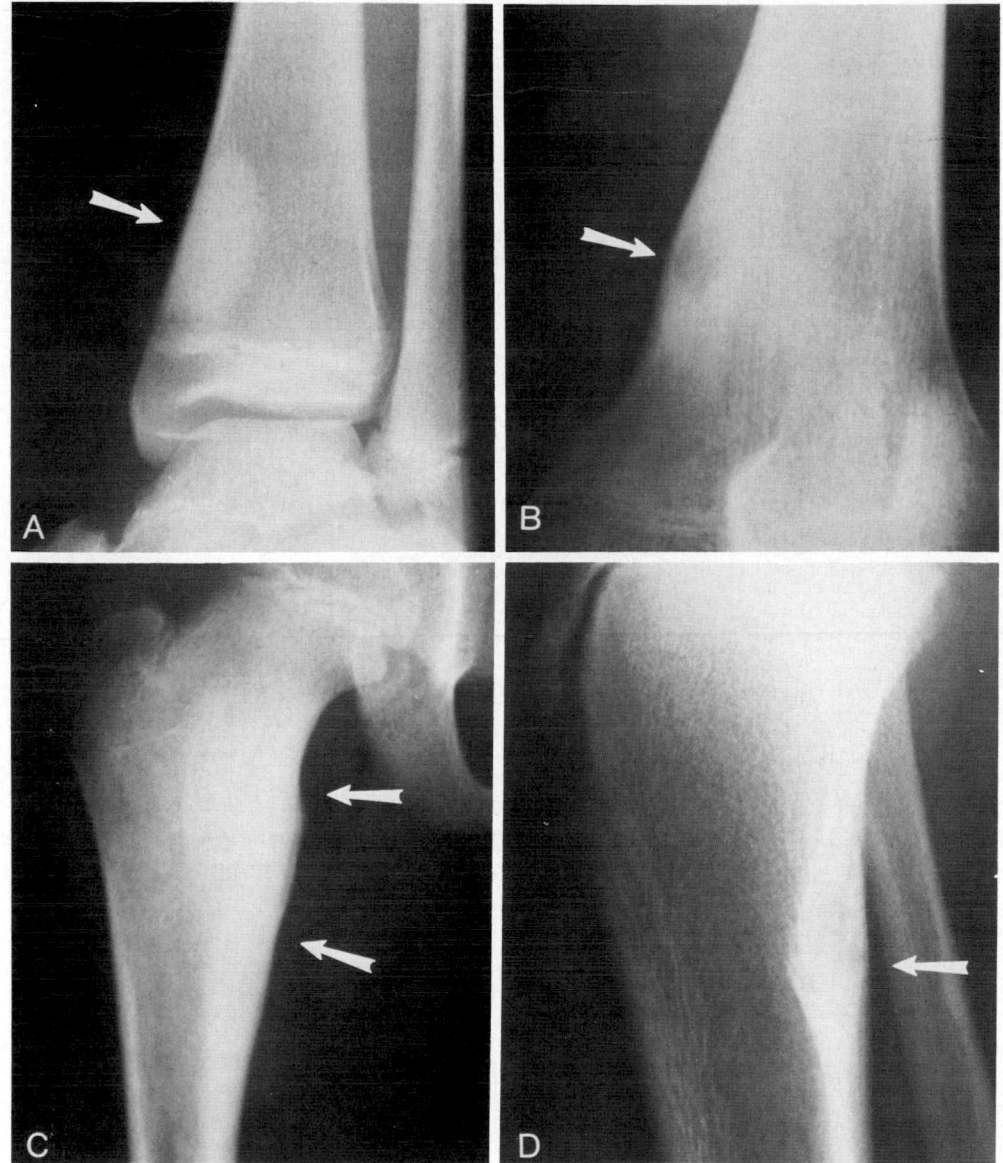

Fig. 4.38. **Focal bony sclerosis.** A. Focal bony sclerosis in healing, low grade osteomyelitis (arrow). B. Osteoid osteoma. Note characteristic focal sclerosis and central radiolucent nidus (arrow). C. Another osteoid osteoma along inner aspect of upper femur (arrow). D. Eccentric location identifies this healing, sclerotic nonossifying fibroma or benign cortical defect (arrow).

BONE SEQUESTRUM

For the most part when a bone sequestrum is seen, the problem is osteomyelitis and the sequestrum may be small or large. Typically it appears sclerotic (Fig. 4.39), and occasionally a similar finding can be seen with bone infarction in sickle cell disease or Gaucher's disease (the latter usually occurs in older children). A bone sequestrum also has been noted in cases of fibrous dysplasia (1). Bone sequestra in the calvarium also can be caused by histiocytosis X.

Reference

1. Pratt AD, Felson B, Wiot JF, Paige M: Sequestrum formation in fribrous dysplasia. *Am J Roentgenol Radium Ther Nucl Med* 106:162–165, 1969.

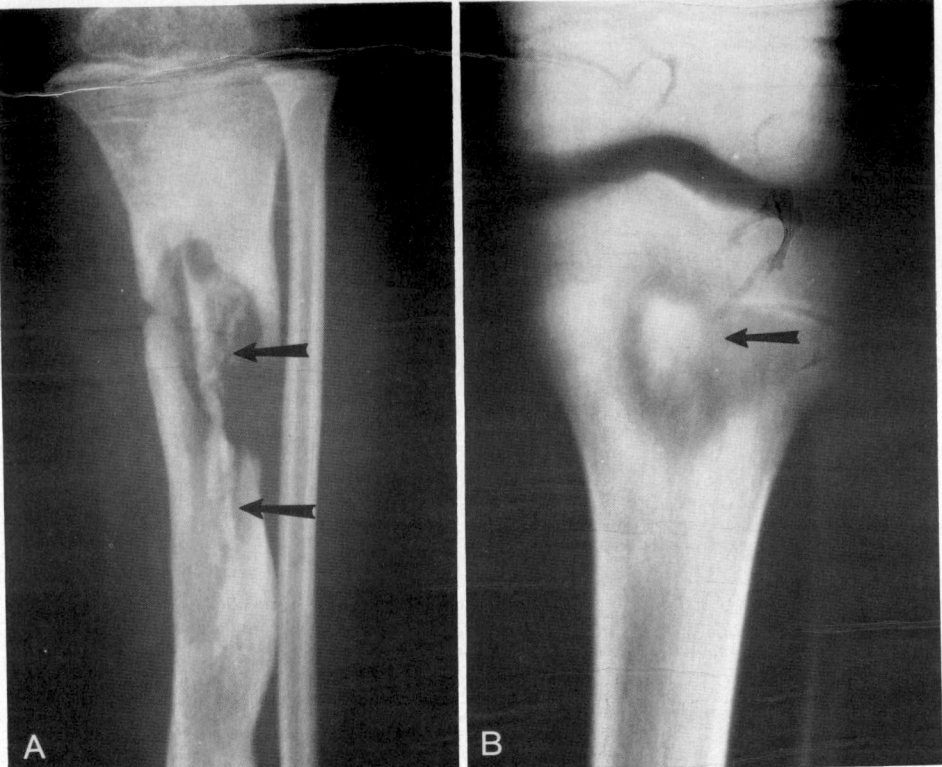

Fig. 4.39. **Bone sequestrum.** A. Note the dense, bone sequestrum (arrow) in this patient with treated osteomyelitis. B. Another patient with a dense, sclerotic sequestrum (arrow), secondary to osteomyelitis.

BONE-WITHIN-BONE APPEARANCE

With this finding, a miniature (more or less) of the involved bone seems to be present within the bone itself. Most commonly, this is seen in the spine, as a normal variation in newborn infants. It is especially common in premature infants and is believed to result from retarded enchondral bone formation secondary to nonspecific perinatal insults to the infant. Within a few days or weeks, normal bone growth resumes and the old ghosts of the bone are buried into the substance of the newly grown bone (Fig. 4.40A). This phenomenon can be exaggerated in infants with greater stresses than birth (i.e., sepsis, hyaline membrane disease, gastrointestinal problems, etc.), and occasionally can be seen in other bones (Fig. 4.40B). Apart from this, the bone-within-bone appearance in children is not very common at all, but when seen under other circumstances almost always occurs in osteopetrosis (Fig. 4.40C).

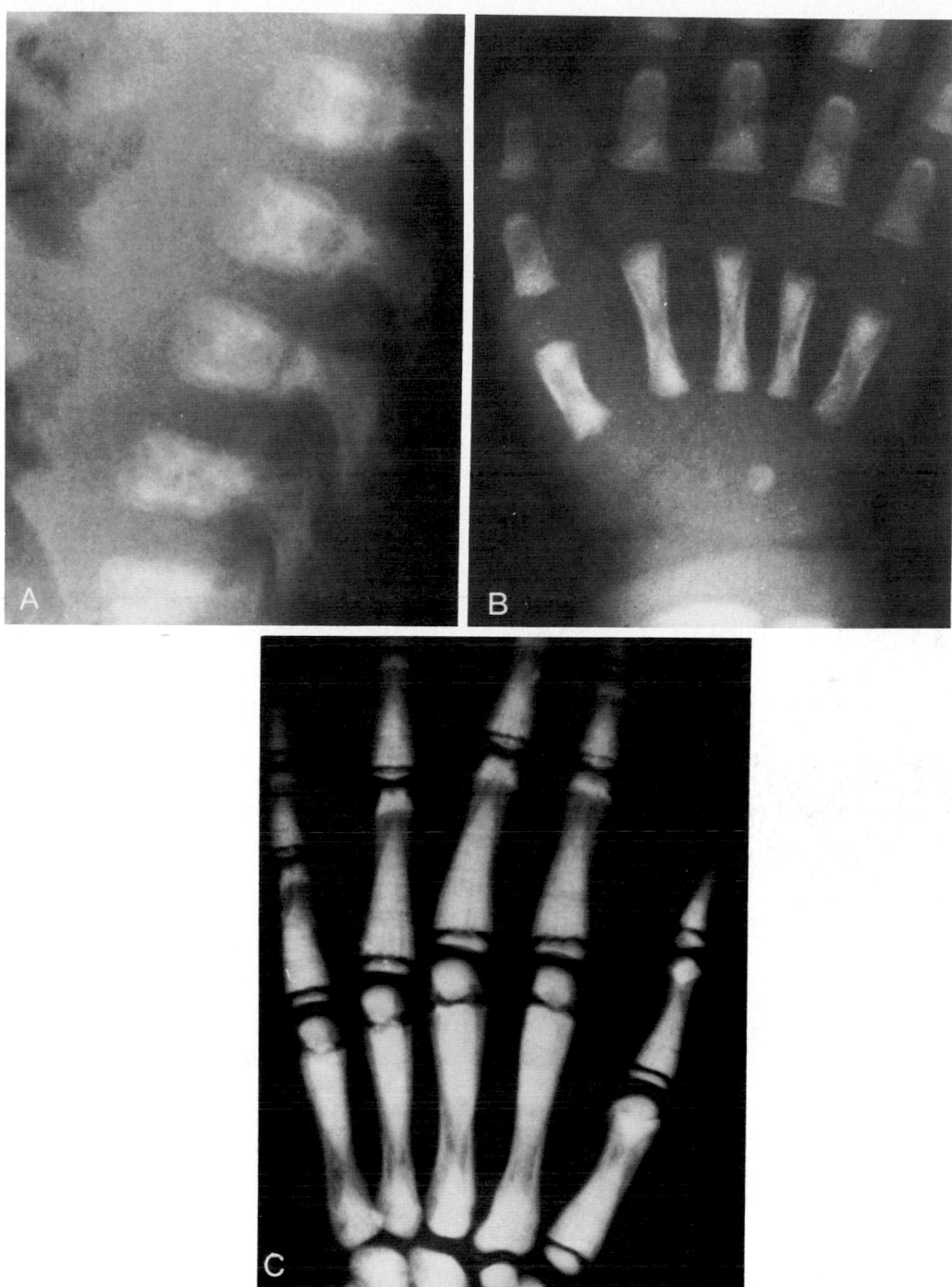

Fig. 4.40.   Bone in bone appearance. A. Typical bone in bone appearance in vertebra due to trophic disturbances in premature infant. The radiolucent rings correspond to the radiolucent trophic or stress lines seen in long bones (see Fig. 4.57). B. Same infant with bone in bone appearance of the small bones of the hands. C. Bone in bone appearance in osteopetrosis. A and B courtesy of Marvin Kogut, M.D., New Orleans.

EXOSTOSES

Exostoses are bony or cartilaginous outgrowths from long or flat bones, and while most are primary tumors others occur secondary to traumatic avulsions or myositis ossificans (Table 4.14). As far as the primary tumoral outgrowths are concerned, the commonest is the osteochondroma, a benign bone tumor with a cartilaginous cap which acts about the same as the epiphyseal plate of a growing long bone. Because

Table 4.14   Exostoses

Osteochondroma (single)	Commonest
Healed avulsion injuries Pronounced medial tibial metaphy- seal beaks in conditions with bowed legs Costoclavicular ligament exos- toses—midclavicle	Moderately common
Tuberous sclerosis Myositis ossificans progressiva Ellis-van Creveld syndrome Multiple osteochondromatosis Multiple enchondromatosis or Ol- lier's disease	Relatively rare
Supracondylar spur (humerus) Fong's lesion (iliac horn) Epiphyseal osteochondroma (Tre- vor's disease) Calcaneal spurs Hypertrophic (degenerative) spurs Iliac spur with tethered cord—li- poma syndrome Campomelic dwarfism Hemophilia	Rare

of this latter feature, osteochondromas grow until the patient's epiphyses fuse, and then growth stops. Morphologically, osteochondromas can be sessile or pedunculated and, when the latter, point away from the joint (Fig. 4.41A). Sessile osteochondromas do not demonstrate this phenomenon and, because of their flat appearance, are a greater problem in terms of diagnosis (Fig. 4.41B). To be sure, there is a distinct tendency for the uninitiated to assign them a more serious diagnosis; i.e., malignant bone tumor.

Osteochondromas can be single or multiple, and the multiple form is familial (11). Single osteochondromas, however, are much more common and although they can occur almost anywhere, most occur in the long bones of the lower extremities. Often they lie in close proximity to the joints, and thus can interfere with joint function. This problem is especially acute in the multiple exostoses syndrome, for the ends of the involved bones usually also are quite hypoplastic and deformed (see Fig. 4.86C).

Clinically, osteochondromas produce a variety of palpable lumps and bumps, joint deformity if para-articular, and when traumatized, pain. They also may interfere with tendon function and result in an actual tendonitis. When growth is complete, the edge of the exostosis is relatively smooth, but when inflammatory or trumatic changes supervene, raggedness of the periphery may erroneously suggest malignant degeneration (Fig. 4.41C). In actual fact, however, malignant degeneration is extremely uncommon in solitary osteochondromas, and overall probably occurs in less

than 1% of cases. With multiple familial exostoses, the incidence of malignancy often is quoted as being as high as 5 to 10%, but most likely also is considerably lower. When exostoses occur in the ribs, they can produce local bulges of the chest wall, and when posterior, can erode into the vertebral column and cause cord compression (4, 10). Laminography or CT scanning can demonstrate the precise location of these latter lesions.

Multiple osteochondromatosis should not be confused with multiple endochondromatosis or Ollier's disease. In Ollier's disease, the cartilaginous tumor is of central origin, but in some cases some of the lesions may resemble a sessile osteochondroma (see Fig. 4.138). Usually, however, the central origin of the radiolucent, cartilaginous tumor is readily apparent somewhere in the skeleton and this aids in diagnosis. Another point used to differentiate the two conditions is that, while in Ollier's disease the tumors tend to be unilateral, in multiple osteochondromatosis symmetry is the rule. A peculiar form of osteochondroma is that which occurs with **epiphyseal dysplasia hemimelica or Trevor's disease.** This condition tends to occur in the lower extremities (knee, ankle) but also can be seen in the arms (shoulder, wrist). Deformity and interference with joint motion are common and the whole problem arises because of a sessile epiphyseal osteochondroma (Fig. 4.41D). Other syndromes in which true exostoses can be seen include the Ellis-Van Creveld syndrome (humerus, tibia), Turner's syndrome, tuberous sclerosis, and dyschondrosteosis. In these latter conditions, except perhaps with tuberous sclerosis, the exostoses tend to occur in the upper medial tibia, and are associated with overgrowth of the ipsilateral femoral condyle. Exostoses also can be seen in association with camptomelic dwarfism (see Fig. 4.8B).

In the elbow one occasionally can encounter an exostosis referred to as a **supracondylar spur.** This vestigial structure is located anteromedially on the distal humerus and points toward the elbow (Fig. 4.42A). For the most part, the spur is of no consequence (1), but occasionally it can be fractured or cause traction on the median nerve. **Bony spurs off the iliac wings** (2, 6, 8, 12, 13), are seen in hereditary osteoonychodysplasia and are termed **Fong's lesion** (2) (Fig. 4.42B). This syndrome also is known as the nail-patella syndrome, for the nails are hypoplastic and the patellae absent. Another spine-like outgrowth from the iliac bone, just adjacent to the greater sciatic notch, also can occur. It is associated with sciatic nerve compression, a tethered cord, and a sacral lipoma (3, 5, 9). Calcaneal spurs are relatively uncommon in infants and children, either on a primary basis (7) or as acquired lesions secondary to diseases such as rheumatoid arthritis. Small **calcaneal spurs** have been seen in the neonate in campomelic dwarfism and also can occur normally (Fig. 4.42C). Another normal

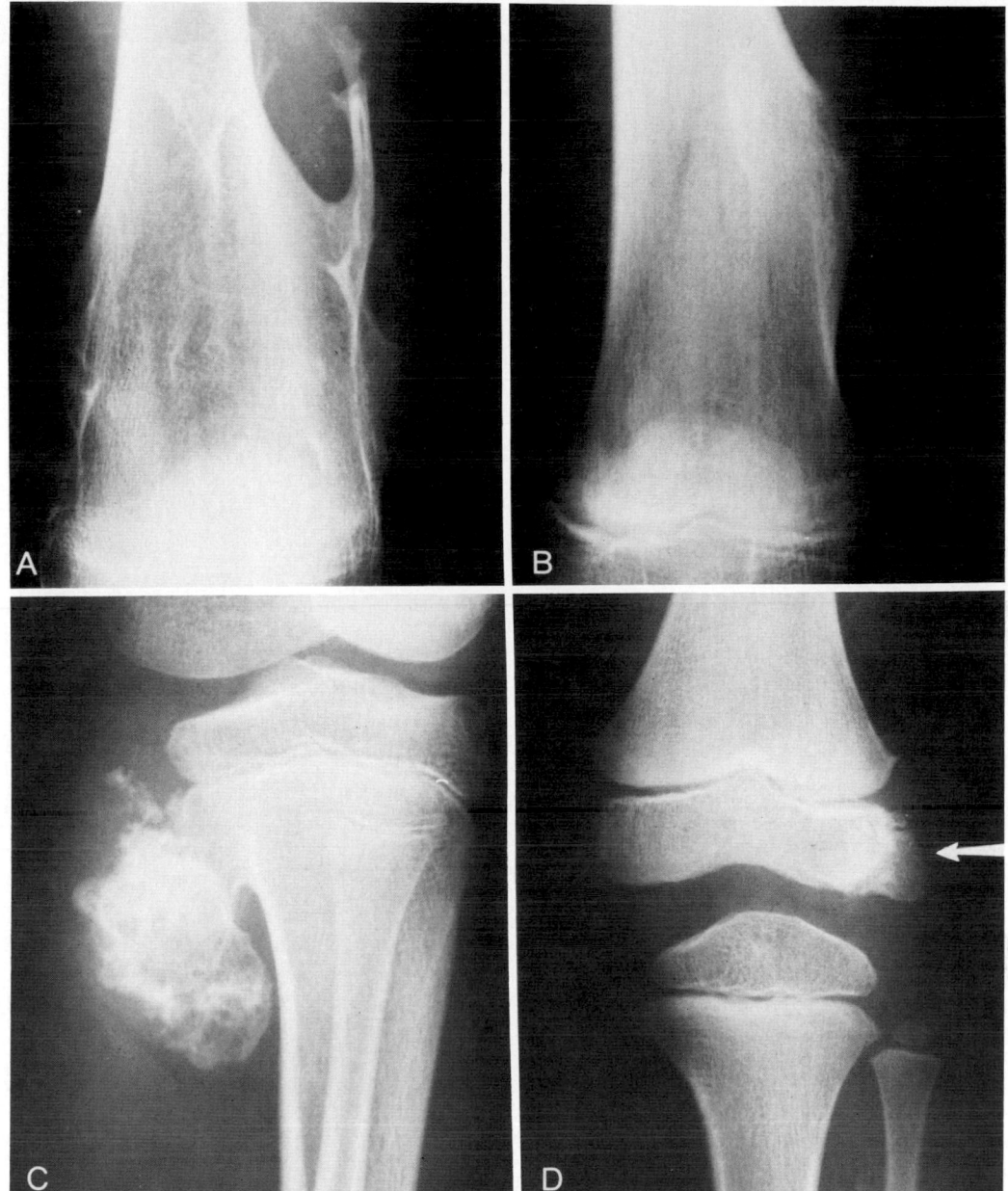

Fig. 4.41. Exostoses. A. Typical elongated osteochondroma. B. Sessile osteochondroma. C. Osteochondroma with irregular edge due to trauma. Note, however, that there is no associated soft tissue mass. D. Osteochondroma of epiphysis (arrow). This is a case of epiphyseal dysplasia hemimelica or Trevor's disease.

exostosis, occasionally seen in children, is that which occurs along the mid-clavicle just at the insertion of the costoclavicular ligament (Fig. 4.42D).

Bony exostoses also occur with healed avulsion injuries, degenerative joint disease, and myositis ossificans. The latter can be posttraumatic, posthemorrhagic in hemophilia, or part of the syndrome known as myositis ossificans progressiva (Fig. 4.42F). This latter condition is progressively debilitating, but not very common and of unknown etiology. It is characterized by generalized ligament calcification which

often is especially marked in the paraspinal ligaments. Hypertrophic, degenerative exostoses, or spurs, are rare in children but occasionally can be seen in the foot. At this site they occur most often on the superior aspects of the talus and navicular bone (at the joint) and result from chronic hyperflexion injuries to the joint. Elsewhere, degenerative spurs are less common, but can occur with long standing abnormalities of gait or extremity motion. For example, in little leaguer's elbow, exostosis can develop around the medial epicondyle, and in patients with a short leg and/or

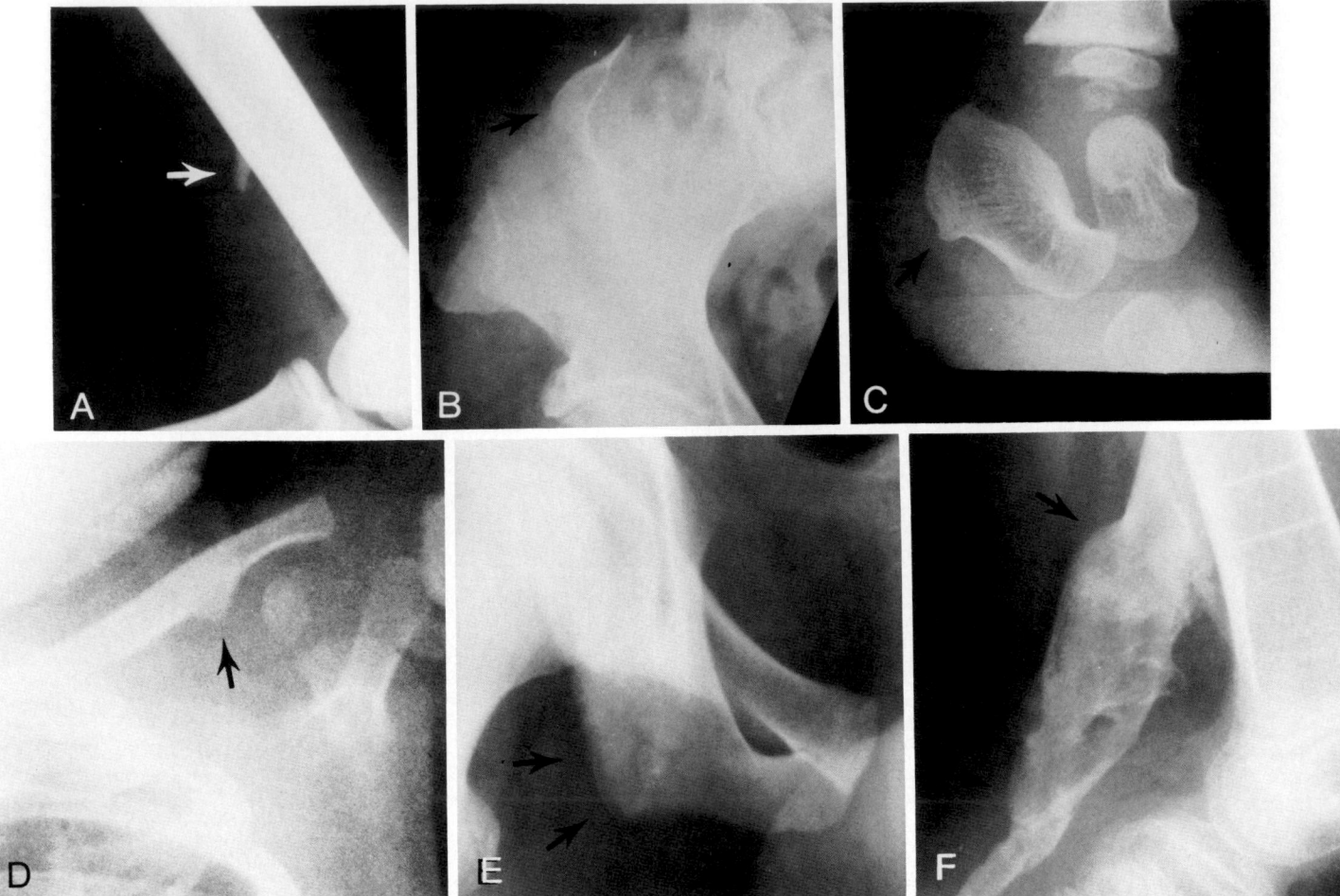

Fig. 4.42.   Exostoses and spurs. A. Typical supracondylar spur (arrow). B. Iliac wing spur in nail-patella syndrome. The spur (arrow) is referred to as Fong's lesion. C. Normal calcaneal spur in infant (arrow). D. Normal exostosis of clavicle at site of costoclavicular ligament insertion (arrow). E. Acquired exostosis due to ischial avulsion injury (arrows). F. Acquired exostosis in progressive myositis ossificans (arrows).

chronic limp, similar exostoses can be seen along the inferior aspect of the sacroiliac joints. Exostoses resulting from healed avulsion injuries can occur anywhere a muscle attaches onto a bone but most commonly are seen along the lower aspect of the ischium (Fig. 4.42E).

References

1. Barnard LB, McCoy SM: The suprocondyloid process of the humerus. *J Bone Joint Surg* 28:845–850, 1946.
2. Fong EE: Iliac horns (symmetrical bilateral central posterior iliac processes); case report. *Radiology* 47:517–518, 1946.
3. Lester PD, McAllister WH: Congenital iliac anomaly with sciatic palsy. *Radiology* 96:397–399, 1970.
4. Madigan R, Worrall T, McClain EJ: Cervical cord compression in hereditary multiple exostosis. *J Bone Joint Surg* 56A:401–404, 1974.
5. McAlister WH, Siegel MJ, Shackelford GD: A congenital iliac anomaly often associated with sacral lipoma and ipsilateral lower extremity weakness. *Skeletal Radiol* 3:161–166, 1978.
6. Palacios E: Hereditary osteo-onychodysplasia; the nail-patella syndrome. *Am J Roentgenol* 101:842–850, 1967.
7. Robinson HM: Symmetrical reversed plantar calcaneal spurs in children. *Radiology* 119:187–188, 1976.
8. Taybi H: *Radiology of Syndromes.* Chicago, Year Book Medical Publishers, 1975, p 199.
9. Theander G: Malformation of the iliac bone associated with intraspinal abnormalities. *Pediatr Radiol* 3:235–239, 1975.
10. Twersky J, Kassner EG, Tenner MS, Camera A: Vertebral and costal osteochondromas causing spinal cord compression. *Am J Roentgenol* 124:124–128, 1975.
11. Vinstein AL, Franken EA Jr: Hereditary multiple exostoses. *Am J Roentgenol* 112:405–407, 1971.
12. Williams HJ, Hoyer JR: Radiographic diagnosis of osteoonychodysostosis in infancy. *Radiology* 109:151–154, 1973.
13. Zimmerman C: Iliac horns; a pathognomonic roentgen sign of familial onchyo-osteodysplasia. *Am J Roentgenol* 86:478–483, 1961.

EPIPHYSEAL-METAPHYSEAL ABNORMALITIES

Stippled Epiphyses

Epiphyses which are stippled have a characteristic, dense, almost punctate pattern of fragmentation (Fig. 4.43). The commonest condition in which this occurs is punctate epiphyseal dysplasia, also known as chondrodystrophia calcificans congenita or Conradi's disease (4, 6, 7, 11). Similar findings can be seen in Zellweger's cerebrohepatorenal syndrome (1, 3, 9) and Warfarin embryonopathy (5, 8, 10). In all of these conditions, stippling also can be seen in the carpal and tarsal bones (actually quite common), the vertebral synchondroses, and at the cartilagenous junctions of the flat bones of the pelvis (i.e., Y cartilage). Indeed, in some cases the findings can be more striking at these sites than at the epiphyses. As far as punctate epiphyseal dysplasia is concerned, two forms exist, a recessive, rhizomelic form where neonatal death is common, and another milder, more common form which usually progresses to nothing more than deformed epiphyses in later life.

References

1. Bartoletti S, Armfield SL III, Lesema-Medina J: The cerebrohepatorenal (Zellweger's syndrome); report of four cases. *Radiology* 127:741–745, 1978.
2. Becker MH, Genieser NB, Finegold M, Miranda D, Spackman T: Chondrodysplasia punctata; is maternal Warfarin therapy a factor? *Am J Dis Child* 129:356–359, 1975.
3. Danks DM, Tippett P, Adams C, Campbell P: Cerebrohepatorenal syndrome of Zellweger. *J Pediatr* 86:382–387, 1975.
4. Heselson NG, Cremin BJ, Beighton P: Lethal chondrodysplasia punctata. *Clin Radiol* 29:679–684, 1978.
5. Johnson JF: Case report—Coumadin embryonopathy. *Skeletal Radiol.* 3:244–246, 1979.
6. LeMarec B, Passarge E, Dellenbach P, Kerisit J, Signargout J, Ferrang B, Senecal J: Lethal neonatal forms of chondroectodermal dysplasia with five case reports. *Ann Radiol* 16:19–26, 1973.
7. Mason RC, Kozlowski K: Chondrodysplasis punctata. A report of 10 cases. *Radiology* 109:145–150, 1973.
8. Pauli RM, Madden JD, Kranzler KJ, Culpepper W, Port R: Warfarin therapy initiated during pregnancy and phenotypic chondrodysplasis punctata. *J Pediatr* 88:506–508, 1976.
9. Poznanski AK, Nosanchuk J, Baublis J, Holt J: The cerebrohepatorenal syndrome (CHRS); Zellweger's syndrome. *Am J Roentgenol* 109:313–322, 1970.
10. Shaul WL, Emergy H, Hall JG: Chondrodysplasia punctata and maternal Warfarin use during pregnancy. *Am J Dis Child* 129:360–362, 1975.
11. Sheffield LJ, Danks DM, Mayne V, Hutchinson LA: Chondrodysplasia punctata—23 cases of a mild and relatively common variety. *J Pediatr* 89:916–923, 1976.

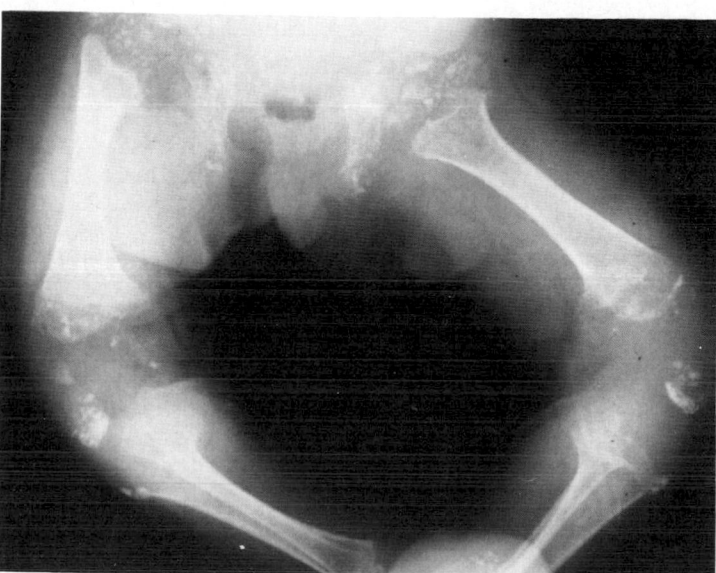

Fig. 4.43. Stippled epiphyses. Note characteristic stippling of the epiphyses in chondrodystrophia calcificans congenita (punctate epiphyseal dysplasia).

Fragmented or Irregular Epiphyses (Table 4.15)

Epiphyseal fragmentation, or extreme irregularity can occur because of (a) a primary epiphyseal growth disturbance or (b) some insult in the epiphysis. The former is more common and may be normal or pathologic. Normal, however, is commoner and most often is seen in the distal femoral epiphysis (Fig. 4.44A). To be sure, so common is this finding that one would expect to see it in other epiphyses on a regular basis, but this is not the case. Occasionally one can see normal fragmentation of the capitellum, and even rarer, the femoral head, but normal fragmentation of other epiphyses is uncommon. So called "normal" fragmentation of the femoral head constitutes Meyer's dysplasia (15), a condition which may be difficult to differentiate from aseptic necrosis (Fig. 4.44B). Isotope bone scans can aid in distinguishing the two because in aseptic necrosis decreased isotope activity in the femoral is seen, while in Meyer's dysplasia activity is normal. The changes in Meyer's dysplasia may be unilateral or bilateral, but most often are bilateral and may persist for years. Slowly, however, the fragments become larger and unite to form a single ossification center.

Table 4.15   Irregular—Fragmented Epiphyses

Normal (distal femur, capitellum) Legg-Perthes disease (hips)	Commonest
Aseptic necrosis, femoral head Sickle cell disease Steroid therapy	Moderately common

Multiple epiphyseal dysplasia
 Spondyloepiphyseal dysplasia
 Other aseptic necrosis (femoral head)
   Collagen vascular disease
   After congenital hip treatment
   With Gaucher's disease
   After hip surgery
 Epiphyseal dysgenesis (hypothyroidism)
 Frostbite hands and feet
 Osteomyelitis
 Rheumatoid arthritis
	Relatively rare

Morquio's disease Epiphyseal dysplasia hemimelica (Trevor's disease) Thiemann's disease (hand) Tricho-rhino-phalangeal syndrome (femoral head) Dyvvge-Melchior-Clausen syndrome Meyer's dysplasia hips Other arthritities Aseptic necrosis of epiphyses other than hips	Rare

Syndromes or diseases in which epiphyseal irregularity or fragmentation occur as a primary growth disturbance include multiple epiphyseal dysplasia (Fig. 4.44C), spondyloepiphyseal dysplasia, Morquio's disease (looks like spondyloepiphyseal dysplasia), Dyggve-Melchior-Clausen syndrome (resembles spondyloepiphyseal dysplasia and Morquio's disease), and the trichorhinophalangeal syndrome (primarily femoral head involvement). Fragmentation of the epiphyses also occurs in hypothyroidism and is referred to as epiphyseal dysgenesis (Fig. 4.44, D and E). The finding clears with therapy. When multiple epiphyseal dysplasia is seen in infancy, it usually takes the form of punctate epiphyseal dysplasia. In such cases there is premature and abnormal calcification of the epiphysis in characteristically stippled or punctate fashion (see Fig. 4.43).

As far as some insult leading to epiphyseal irregularity, the commonest problem is ischemic, aseptic necrosis, or Legg-Perthes disease of the femoral head (19, 20, 23). This condition, basically of unknown etiology, but generally believed to result from disruption of the blood supply to the growing femoral head, usually has onset with hip pain and limp. Roentgenographically, fluid accumulation in, and laxity of, the joint causes lateral displacement of the femoral head and widening of the joint space. In these early stages, the findings are difficult to differentiate from those of septic arthritis or more severe cases of transient (toxic) synovitis (see p 284). However, as opposed to these conditions the ossified nucleus of the femoral head in Legg-Perthes disease stops growing and soon becomes noticeably smaller than normal. Thereafter (usually within 3 or 4 months), the head becomes sclerotic (i.e., necrotic and impacted), and then fragmented (Fig. 4.45A). Fragmentation results from irregular resorption of the necrotic head, and eventually disappears. The ossified nucleus of the femoral head then reconstitutes and continues to grow. However, unless treated early, the new femoral head deforms and becomes large (coxa magna) and flat (coxa plana). At the same time, the femoral neck becomes shortened and a coxa vara deformity of the upper femur develops. Recently, osteotomies, either through the iliac wing or upper femur, have been utilized to prevent these deformities because they accomplish early repositioning of the femoral head under the acetabular roof. This offers the head a greater chance for regrowth into a normal, round, and smoothly articulating structure. Nonoperative treatment, in the form of various braces, can accomplish the same results and seems to be gaining in popularity again. Before leaving the discussion of Legg-Perthes disease, it should be noted that, during the active phase of the disease, associated irregularity of the epiphyseal metaphyseal junction and acetabular roof are common. These changes are believed to be secondary to the primary process in the

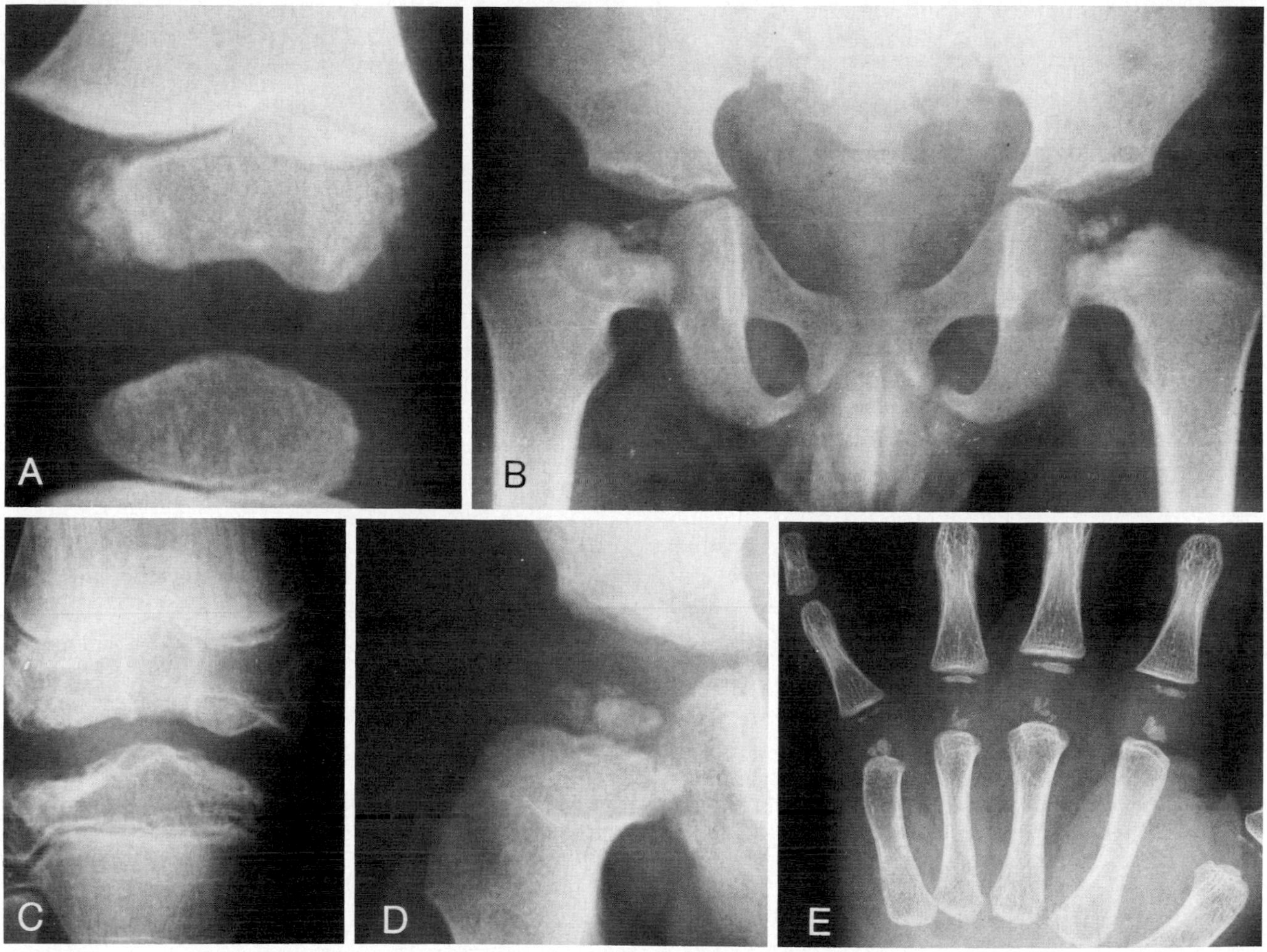

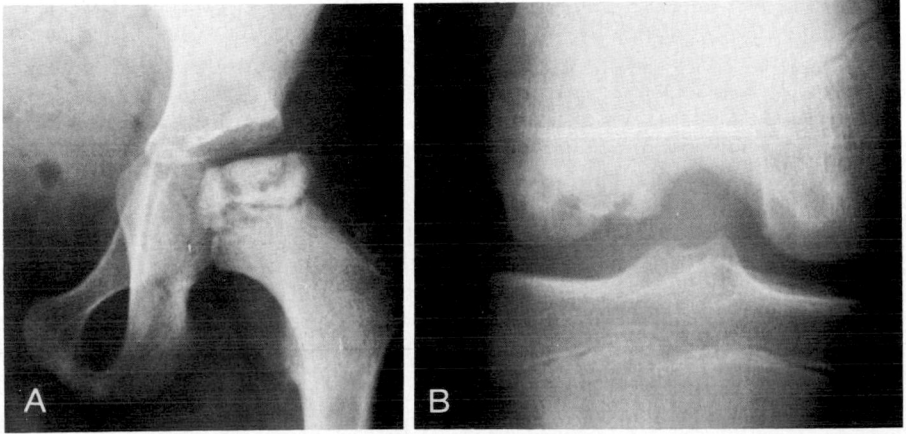

Fig. 4.44. Irregular epiphyses. A. Normal irregularity of distal femoral epiphysis in young child. B. Bilateral irregular, small, underdeveloped femoral capital epiphyses in asymptomatic patient with Meyer's dysplasia. Also note changes in metaphyses. C. Small irregular epiphyses in multiple epiphyseal dysplasia. D. Irregular femoral capital epiphysis in hypothyroidism. E. Numerous small, fragmented epiphyses and apophyses of the small bones of the hand in another patient with hypothyroidism.

Fig. 4.45. Irregular epiphyses. A. Typical, slightly small, sclerotic, and fragmented epiphysis of advanced Legg-Perthes disease. B. Irregular, distal femoral epiphyses due to ischemic necrosis in patient on steroid therapy for chronic renal disease.

femoral head and not the result of aseptic necrosis of these portions of the adjacent bones.

Aseptic necrosis of the femoral head also occurs with other conditions producing ischemia and, roentgenographically, the findings are indistinguishable from Legg-Perthes disease. These include steroid therapy (4), sickle cell disease (10, 13, 18), the collagen vascular diseases (1, 11), Gaucher's disease, a few cases of aseptic necrosis as a complication of closed reduction of congenital hip dislocation (8, 17), surgical hip nailing, hip fracture, some cases of osteomyelitis of the femoral neck with secondary epiphyseal damage (12), irradiation therapy to the hip area, and trauma (i.e., epiphyseal-metaphyseal fracture). Of all these, the most common are sickle cell disease and steroid therapy. Aseptic necrosis of the other epiphyses is rather uncommon, but occasionally can be seen after steroids (Fig. 4.45B), trauma, or frostbite (3, 22). The latter occurs mostly in the hands and feet. An unusual cause of a sclerotic, fragmented epiphysis in the hands is so-called Thiemann's disease (5), a condition presumed, but not universally accepted, as being a rare form of primary aseptic necrosis of the epiphysis of the small bones of the hand.

Rounding out the causes of epiphyseal irregularity are rheumatoid arthritis (9, 14), Winchester's syndrome, widespread infection (i.e., sepsis) (7), other joint inflammations, and epiphyseal dysplasia hemimelica. With epiphyseal dysplasia hemimelica, also known as Trevor's disease (2), the problem is an osteochondroma of the epiphysis and most often the changes are seen around knee or ankle (see Fig. 4.41D). However, the disease also occurs in the arm.

References

1. Bergstein JM, Wiens C, Fish AJ, Vernier RL, Michael A: Avascular necrosis of bone in systemic lupus erythematosus. *J Pediatr* 85:31–35, 1974.
2. Carlson DH, Wilkinson RH: Variability of unilateral epiphyseal dysplasia (Dysplasia Epiphysealis Hemimelic). *Radiology* 133:369–373, 1979.
3. Carrera GF, Kozin F, Flaherty L, McCarty DJ: Radiographic changes in the hands following childhood frostbite injury. *Skeletal Radiol* 16:33–37, 1971.
4. Cole WG, Neal BW: Corticosteroids and avascular necrosis of the femoral head in childhood. *Aust Paediatr J* 11:243–246, 1975.
5. Cullen JC: Thiemann's disease. *J Bone Joint Surg* 52B:532–534, 1970.
6. Danigelis JA, Fisher RL, Ozonoff MB, Sziklas JJ: ^{99m}Tc-polyphosphate bone imaging in Legg-Perthes disease. *Radiology* 115:407–413, 1975.
7. Fernandez F, Peuyo I, Jimenez JR, Vigil E, Guzman A: Epiphysiometaphyseal changes in children after severe meningococcic sepsis. *Am J Roentgenol* 136:1236–1238, 1981.
8. Gage JR, Winter RB: Avascular necrosis of the capital femoral epiphysis as a complication of closed reduction of congenital dislocation of the hip: a critical review of 20 years' experience at Gillette Children's Hospital. *J Bone Joint Surg* 54A:373–388, 1972.
9. Goel KM, Rawson SP, Shanks RA: Rdiological assessment of fifty patients with juvenile rheumatoid arthritis: correlation with clinical and laboratory abnormalities. *Pediatr Radiol* 2:51–60, 1974.
10. Hill MC, Oh KS, Bowerman JW, Siegelman SS, James AE Jr: Abnormal epiphyses in the sickling disorders. *Am J Roentgenol* 124:34–43, 1975.
11. Hurley RM, Steinberg RH, Patriquin H, Drummond KN: Avascular necrosis of the femoral head in childhood systemic lupus erythematosus. *Can Med Assoc J* 111:781–784, 1974.
12. Kemp HBS, Lloyd-Roberts CC: Avascular necrosis of the capital epiphysis following osteomyelitis of the proximal femoral metaphysis. *J Bone Joint Surg* 56:688–697, 1974.
13. Lee REJ, Golding JSR, Sergeant GR: The radiologic features of avascular necrosis of the femoral head in homozygous sickle cell disease. *Clin Radiol* 32:205–214, 1981.
14. Martel W, Holt JF, Cassidy JT: Roentgenologic manifestations of juvenile rheumatoid arthritis. *Am J Roentgenol* 88:400–423, 1962.
15. Meyer J: Dysplasia epiphysealis capitis femoris. *Acta Orthop Scand* 34:183–197, 1964.
16. Norman LE, Pischnotte WO: Morquio's disease. *Am J Dis Child* 124:719–722, 1972.
17. Salter RB, Kostuik J, Dallas S: Avascular necrosis of femoral head as a complication of treatment for congenital dislocation of hip in young children: a clinical and experimental investigation. *Can J Surg* 12:44–61, 1969.
18. Slovis TL, Haller JO, Berdon WE, Baker DH: Aseptic necrosis of the femoral head in a white boy with S-D hemoglobinopathy. *Pediatr Radiol* 1:250–252, 1973.
19. Spragge JW: Legg-Clave-Perthes disease. *Curr Probl Radiol* 3:30, 1973.
20. Suramo I, Puranem J, Keikkinen E, Vuorinen P: Disturbed patterns of venous drainage of the femoral neck in Perthes disease. *J Bone Joint Surg* 56:448–453, 1974.
21. Sutherland AD, Savage JP, Foster BK: The nuclide bone-scan in the diagnosis and management of Perthes' disease. *J Bone Joint Surg* 62B:300–306, 1980.
22. Wensl JE, Burke EC, Bianco AJ Jr: Epiphyseal destruction from frostbite of the hands. *Am J Dis Child* 114:668–670, 1967.
23. Wynne-Davies R, Gormley J: The etiology of Perthes Disease. *J Bone Joint Surg* 60B:6–14, 1978.

Irregular or Fragmented Apophyses (Table 4.16)

Apophyses are not true epiphyses, but in many regards function in the same fashion. They are growth centers which allow continued growth of a child's bones, but as opposed to epiphyses, they do not have articular surfaces. Overall, they normally tend to be more fragmented and irregular than epiphyses and most commonly this occurs in the feet, shoulder, and elbow. The findings should not be misinterpreted for those of aseptic necrosis or comminuted fracture (Fig. 4.46), but anytime the question arises, it is helpful to obtain isotope bone scans; they will be normal unless aseptic necrosis is the cause of irregularity. The most common source of such misinterpretation is the normally sclerotic, and often, markedly fragmented calcaneal apophysis. Usually it is considered aseptically necrotic and erroneously referred to as Siever's disease (Fig. 4.46D). In actual fact, Siever's disease probably

does not exist, and indeed, with normal weighbearing the calcaneal apophysis should be dense and sclerotic (2). Irregular, dense apophyses also occur in the scapula, primarily over the coracoid and acrominal processes (Fig. 4.46B).

The tibial tubercle, that is, the apophysis of the upper tibia, normally is not fragmented or particularly irregular, but with chronic avulsion of the inserting infrapatellar tendon, irregularity and sclerosis frequently develop. The condition then is known as Osgood-Schlatter's disease (1, 3, 4) and is quite common in the active youngster. In the acute phase, it is associated with soft tissue swelling and focal pain over the tibial tubercle, but fragmentation may be minimal. With healing and repeated avulsions, however, fragmentation and hypertrophic bone formation can become quite profound (Fig. 4.46E). Irregularity of the apophyses, in general, also occurs in hypothyroidism and trisomy 21, and once again, in both conditions the changes are most pronounced in the hands and feet (see Fig. 4.44E).

Table 4.16   Irregular—Fragmented Apophyses

Normal
    Hands, feet
    Distal humerus
    Calcaneal apophysis
    Scapula
	Commonest

Tibial tubercle (Osgood-Schlatter's disease)	Moderately common
Hypothyroidism (hands, feet) Trisomy 21 (hands, feet)	Relatively rare

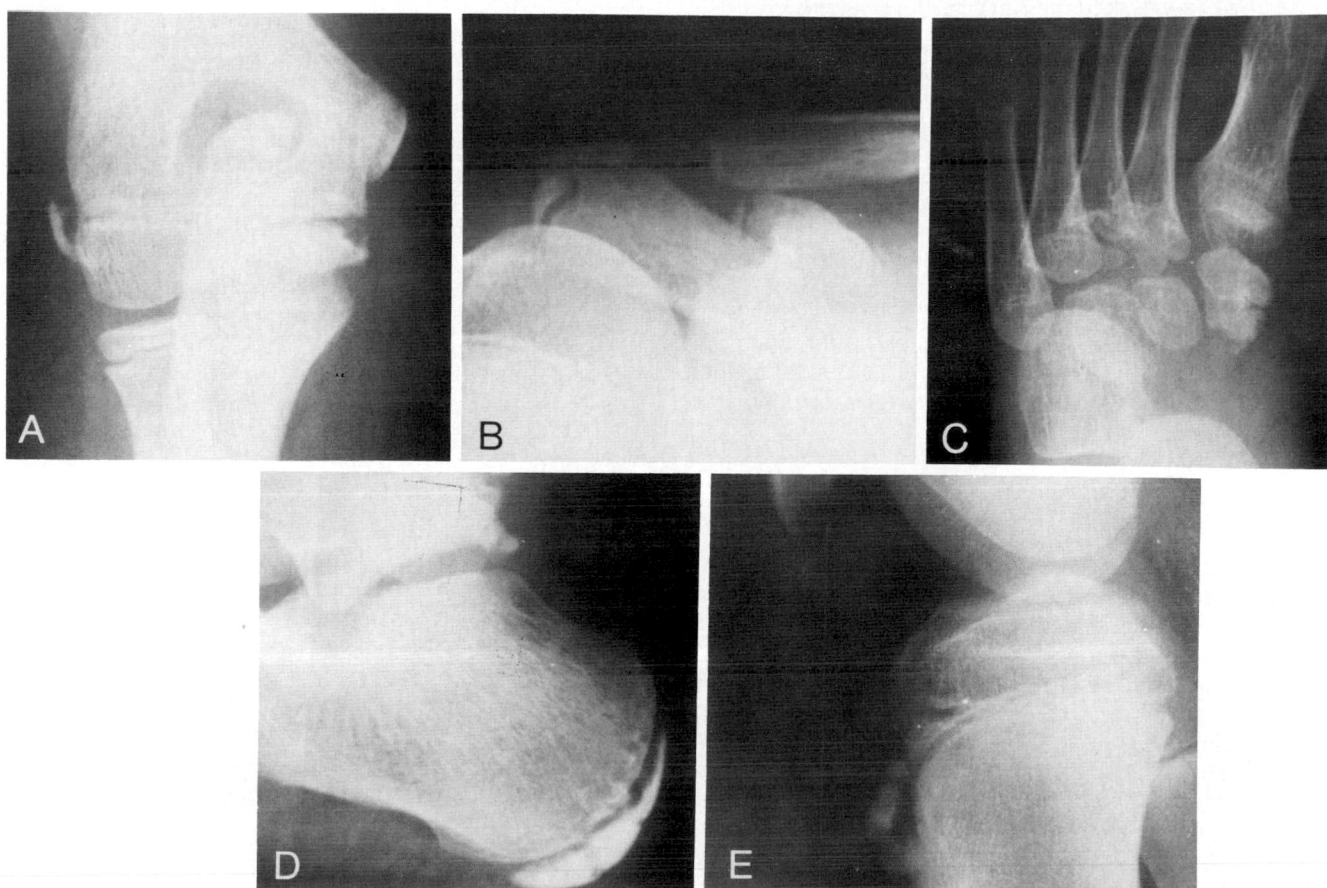

Fig. 4.46.   Irregular and sclerotic apophyses. A. Normal irregular apophyses around the elbow. B. Normal irregular apophyses around the shoulder. C. Normal irregular apophyses of metatarsals. D. Normal sclerotic, irregular calcaneal apophysis. E. Markedly irregular tibial tubercle in Osgood-Schlatter's disease (arrow). See Figure 4.44E for fragmented apophyses in hypothyroidism.

References

1. Cohen B, Wilkinson RW: The Osgood-Schlatter lesion: a radiological and histological study. *Am J Surg* 95:731, 1958.
2. Shopfner CE, Coin CG: Effect of weight-bearing on the appearance and development of the secondary clacaneal epiphysis. *Radiology* 86:201–206, 1966.
3. Willner P: Osgood-Schlatter's disease: etiology and treatment. *Clin Orthop* 62:178–179, 1969.
4. Woolfrey BF, Chandler EF: Manifestations of Osgood-Schlatter's disease in later teen age and early adulthood. *J Bone Joint Surg* 42A:327–332, 1960.

Ivory Epiphyses

Ivory epiphyses usually are of normal size and shape, but very dense (Fig. 4.47). Most often they occur in the hands and feet, and of the two, occurrence in the hands is more common. In this regard, the distal phalanges most often are involved, and the individuals in whom this is seen usually are normal (1). It might be noted, however, that many of these children are examined for short stature, and even though a cause for this problem is not always determined, it is debatable whether these individuals are completely normal. In this regard, ivory epiphyses do occur in patients with hypopituitarism and on a practical basis, then, one probably sees more ivory epiphyses in a child of short stature than in one perfectly normal. It may be that the ivory epiphysis simply reflects slow bone growth.

When multiple ivory epiphyses are seen in the proximal phalanges, there is a better chance that some syndrome is present and then one might consider conditions such as multiple epiphyseal dysplasia, Cockayne's syndrome (bone age also usually advanced), the tricho-rhino-phalangeal syndrome, Seckel's bird-headed dwarf, and rarely, Thiemann's disease (2). In the latter condition, aseptic necrosis of the epiphysis of the small bones of the hands is believed to be the problem. Dense epiphyses also can occur in any conditions where the bones generally are dense.

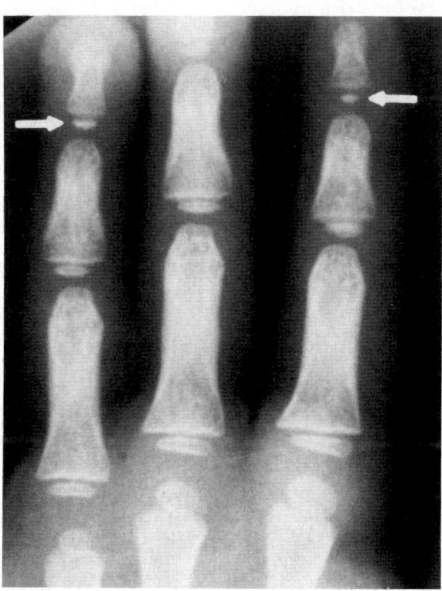

Fig. 4.47. Ivory epiphysis. Typical appearance of ivory epiphyses of a number of the small bones of the hands (arrows). This patient had growth retardation of undetermined etiology.

Reference

1. Kuhns LR, Poznanski AK, Harper HAS, Garn SM: Ivory epiphyses and the hands. *Radiology* 109:643–648, 1973.

Large Epiphyses (Table 4.17)

Generalized enlargement of all of the epiphyses occurs with many dwarfing syndromes where the long bones are short and squat, and the epiphyses relatively enlarged. By the same token, epiphyses become disproportionately large in conditions leading to thin bony shafts (i.e., osteogenesis imperfecta, neurologic-neurogenic disease, etc.), but in neither case are the large epiphyses used as a specific diagnostic feature of the conditions. When a large epiphysis is used for diagnostic purposes, it is focal, and most often secondary to chronic joint infection or inflammation. The hyperemia so produced results in epiphyseal overgrowth and osteoporosis and because of this the epiphysis becomes large, glassy, and coarsely trabeculated (Fig. 4.48). The most common causes of such epiphyseal enlargement are rheumatoid arthritis (2) and

Table 4.17 Large—Overgrown Epiphyses[a]

Rheumatoid arthritis[b] Hemophiliac arthritis[b] Healed Legg-Perthes disease (coxa plana-magna)	Commonest
Tuberculous arthritis[b]	Moderately common
Pyogenic arthritis (chronic) Fungal arthritis[b] Winchester's syndrome[b] Epiphyseal dysplasia hemimelica Fibrous dysplasia of epiphysis	Rare

[a] Does not include various bone dysplasias where long bones are short or thin and the epiphyses relatively large.
[b] Epiphysis often large and glassy.

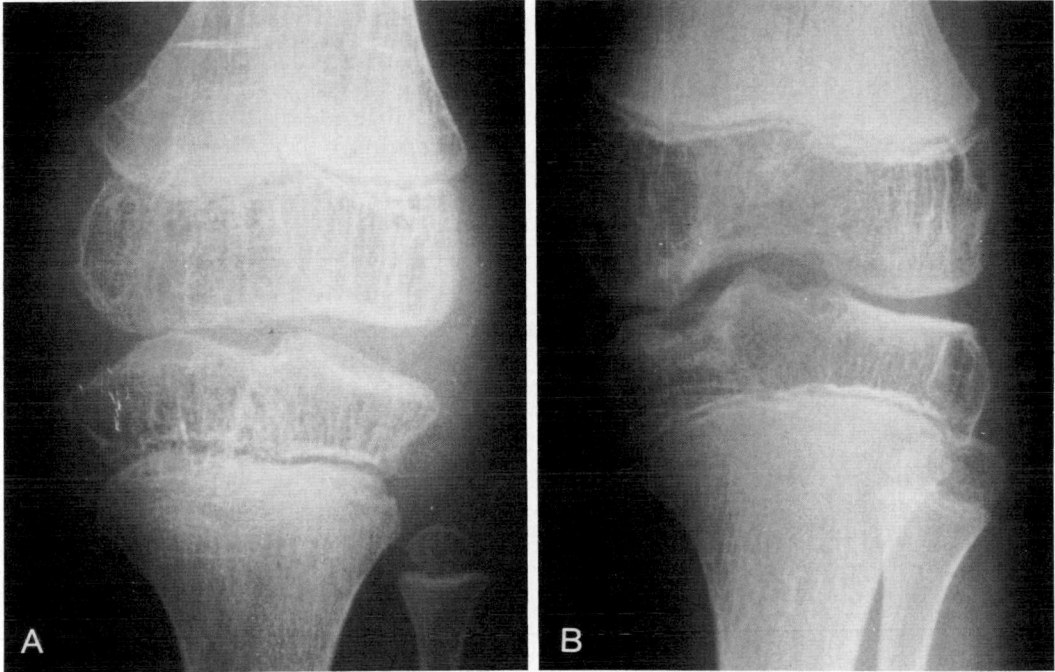

Fig. 4.48. Large, glassy epiphyses. A. Large glassy epiphyses in chronic infection; tuberculosis. B. Large glassy epiphyses in patient with hemophilia. Also note characteristic widening of the intercondylar notch.

hemophiliac arthropathy, but it also occurs in tuberculous arthritis, fungal arthritis, and the rheumatoid arthritis mimicking storage disease known as Winchester's syndrome (3, 6). In hemophiliac arthropathy, there also is widening of the intercondylar notch of the distal femur (Fig. 4.48B), and although this configuration is near pathognomonic of the condition, it also has been documented with tuberculous arthritis (4). It does not occur with rheumatoid arthritis.

Enlargement of an epiphysis also can occur with lingering, low grade pyogenic arthritis, but generally this is uncommon. Most often, with pyogenic arthritis, the infection is of short duration and rapid onset, and the epiphysis is more likely to be destroyed than overgrown. In those few, chronic cases where enlargement occurs, it is slight only, and the glassy effect does not develop. An enlarged, but flattened, epiphysis is seen in healed Legg-Perthes disease (i.e., coxa plana, coxa magna), and irregular enlargement of an epiphysis, especially of the lower extremity, can be seen with epiphyseal dysplasia hemimelica (1). In this condition, the problem actually is an osteochondroma of the epiphysis, and epiphyseal enlargement usually is eccentric (see Fig. 4.41D). Fibrous dysplasia leading to a large epiphysis also has been recorded (5), but is very rare.

References

1. Carlson DH, Wilkinson RH: Variability of unilateral epiphyseal dysplasia (dysplasia epiphysealis hemimelica). *Radiology* 133:369–373, 1979.
2. Goel KM, Rawson SP, Shanks RA: Radiological assessment of fifty patients with juvenile rheumatoid arthritis: correlation with clinical and laboratory abnormalities. *Pediatr Radiol* 2:51–60, 1974.
3. Hollister DW, Rimoin DL, Lachman RS, Cohen AH, Reed WB, Estin GW: The Winchester syndrome: a nonlysosomal connective tissue disease. *J Pediatr* 84: 701–709, 1974.
4. Nixon SP: Tuberculosis synovitis with widening of the intercondylar notch of the distal femur. *Br J Radiol* 42:703–704, 1969.
5. Nixon GW, Condon VR: Epiphyseal involvement in polyostotic fibrous dysplasia: a report of two cases. *Radiology* 106:167–170, 1973.
6. Winchester P, Grossman H, Lim WN, Danes BS: A new acid mucopoly-saccharidosis with skeletal deformities simulating rheumatoid arthritis. *Am J Roentgenol* 106:128–136, 1969.

Large Medial Femoral Condyle

There are some conditions where the distal femoral epiphysis becomes prominent, but mostly by way of the medial condyle. Often there is associated depression of the ipsilateral upper medial tibial plateau (Fig. 4.49), and for the most part the phenomenon occurs in the following conditions: Turner's syndrome, Prader-Willi syndrome, Cornelia de Lange syndrome, dychondrosteosis, vitamin D-resistant rickets, and Blount's disease (see Fig. 4.17B). Prominence of the medial femoral condyle also occurs in most of the chondrodystrophic dwarfs producing short, bowed bones, but in these conditions it is not of that much value for specific diagnosis.

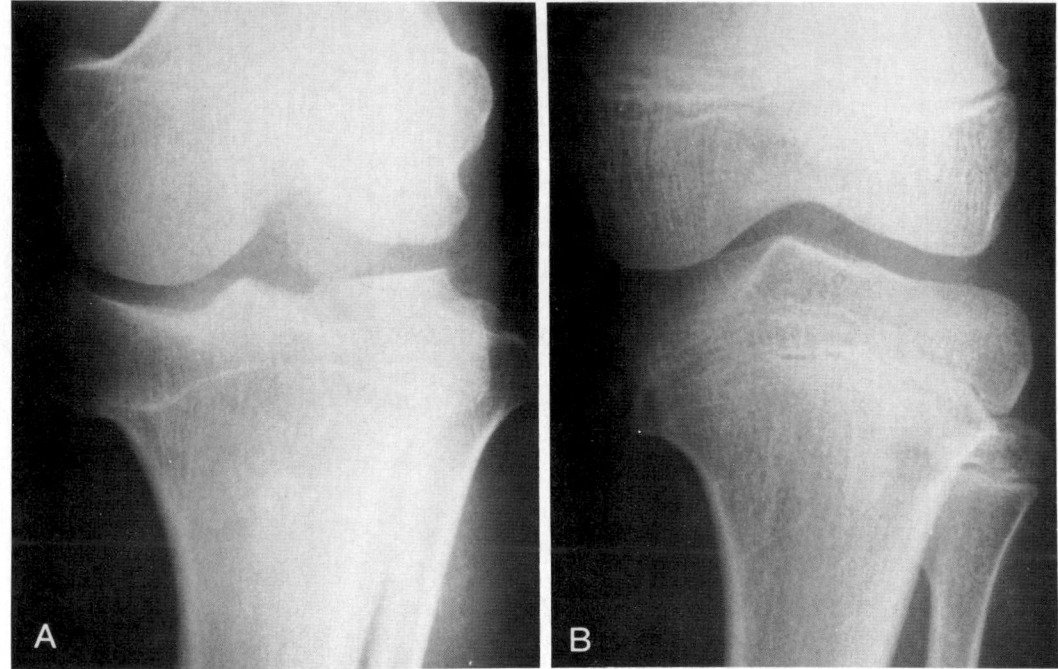

Fig. 4.49.   Prominent medial femoral condyles. A. Typical prominence of the medial femoral condyles in Turner's syndrome. B. Similar prominence of the medial femoral condyles in dyschondrosteosis. Also note associated flattening of the upper medial, tibial metaphysis and the small exostosis.

Small Epiphyses (Table 4.18)

Small epiphyses can occur on a generalized or focal basis. On a generalized basis, small epiphyses can be seen with any condition where bone age is delayed, but smallness of the epiphysis is not that important in the diagnosis of these conditions. On the other hand, there are certain diseases where the small epiphyses are used for specific diagnosis and these include multiple epiphyseal dysplasia, spondyloepiphyseal dysplasia, Morquio's disease (a storage disease which looks like spondyloepiphyseal dysplasia), and hypothyroidism. In both hypothyroidism and the epiphyseal dysplasias, in addition to the epiphyses being small, they are fragmented and irregular (see Fig. 4.44, C–E) and, with the epiphyseal dysplasias, frequently sclerotic.

Generalized smallness of the epiphyses, on an acquired basis, almost always occurs with widespread

Table 4.18   Small Epiphyses

A. Generalized	
Delayed bone age—any cause	Commonest
Hypothyroidism Multiple epiphyseal dysplasia	Moderately common
Spondyloepiphyseal dysplasia Morquio's disease	Relatively rare
B. Unilateral	
Early Legg-Perthes disease Congenital dislocating hip	Commonest
After infection, injury, etc. Normal (minimal asymmetry)	Moderately common

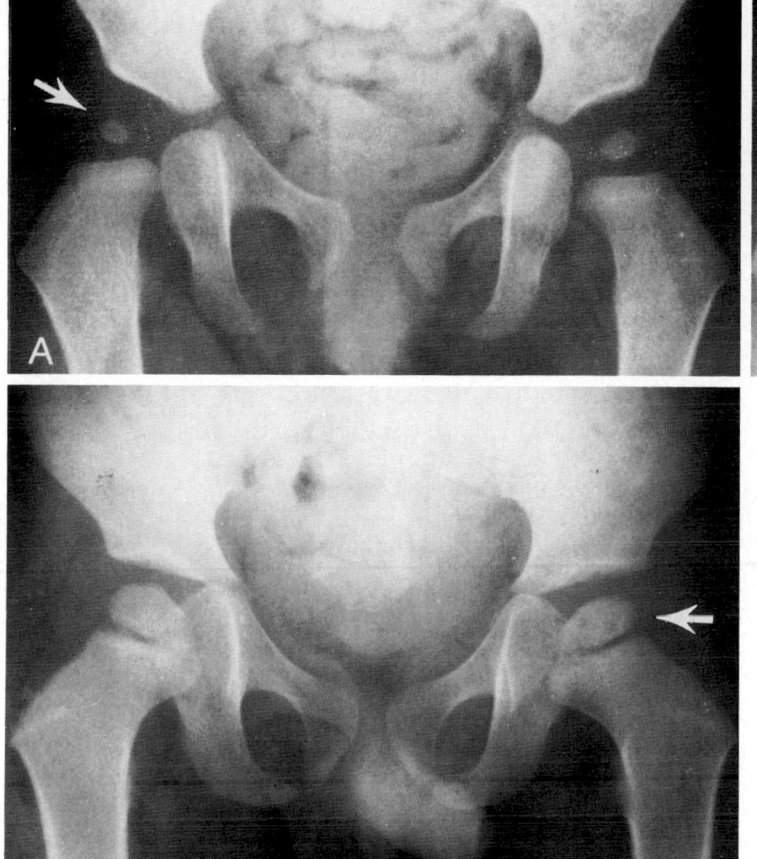

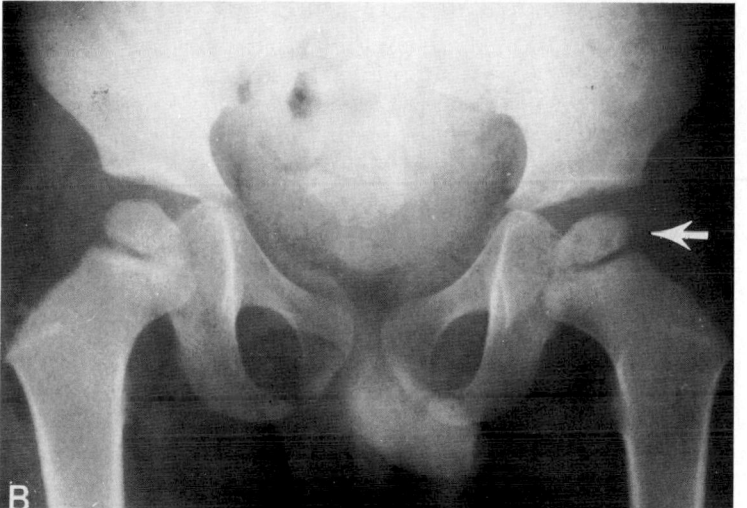

Fig. 4.50. **Small, nonfragmented epiphyses.** A. Congenital hip dislocation. Note small proximal femoral epiphysis on the right (arrow). Also note that the acetabular roof is more slanted and less cupped than normal, and that the hip is laterally displaced. B. Small epiphysis on the left (arrow) in patient with early Legg-Perthes disease. C. Another patient with later stage Legg-Perthes disease demonstrating more smallness, and sclerosis, of the femoral head on the left (arrow). Also note slight lateral luxation of the hip. Later on, the femoral head undergoes fragmentation (see Fig. 4.45A).

arthritic disease such as rheumatoid arthritis or the rheumatoid arthritis mimicking storage disease known as Winchester's syndrome (3, 4). The latter, of course, is quite rare, and so are other chronic arthropathies, such as pigmented villinodular synovitis. In many of these acquired conditions, not only are the epiphyses small and irregular, but also scalloped and deformed.

On a focal basis, a small epiphysis results from some insult to the epiphysis or because its extremity is not being used. The latter can occur in any neurologic, neuromuscular, or arthritic disease leading to disuse of an extremity, and one of the best examples of this phenomenon is congenital dislocation of the hip. In this condition, the femoral head remains small as long as the hip is located out of the acetabulum (Fig. 4.50A). If, however, early therapy is instituted, and the femoral head relocated under the acetabular roof, head size catches up with the normal side. Smallness of an

epiphysis, secondary to its destruction or resorption by inflammation, infection, or infarction is self evident, and in terms of infarction, the most common situation is the ischemically necrotic femoral head of Legg-Perthes disease (Fig. 4.50, B and C). To be sure, smallness of the femoral capital epiphysis is one of the earliest findings of this condition (1) and reflects cessation of growth of the ossified nucleus of the femoral head. However, even though the ossified nucleus becomes small and then fragments, the cartilage cap remains relatively normal, and it is only later, in long standing cases, that the femoral head becomes flattened, large, and deformed (i.e., coxa magna and coxa plana). If, however, therapy is instituted early (braces, osteotomies) and the femoral head is relocated under the acetabular roof, it retains a more normal round configuration.

Occasionally, a solitary, normal epiphysis may be

small, but in such cases difference in size from the other side is minimal. In such cases, if there is question as to whether the epiphysis is small and normal, or small and ischemically necrotic, one can utilize isotope scans. If the problem is ischemia, decreased isotope activity is seen (2).

References

1. Caffey J: The early roentgenographic changes in essential coxa plana; their significance in pathogenesis. *Am J Roentgenol* 102:620–634, 1968.

2. Danigelis JA, Fisher RL, Ozonoff MB, Sziklas JJ: ^{99m}Tc-Polyphosphate bone imaging in Legg-Perthes disease. *Radiology* 115:407–413, 1975.
3. Hollister DW, Rimoin DL, Lachman RS, Cohen AH, Reed WB, Westin GW: The Winchester syndrome: a nonlysosomal connective tissue disease. *J Pediatr* 84:701–709, 1974.
4. Winchester P, Grossman H, Lim WN, Danes BS: A new acid mucopolysaccharidosis with skeletal deformities simulating rheumatoid arthritis. *Am J Roentgenol Radium Ther Nucl Med* 106:128–136, 1969.

Cone-Shaped Epiphyses (Table 4.19)

Cone-shaped epiphyses have a cone-like projection into the center of the metaphysis and most commonly occur in the hands and feet. They can be seen in normal individuals (1, 5), especially in the feet (Fig. 4.51A) and occasionally in the knee (Fig. 4.51B). On a pathologic basis, coned epiphyses occur in a number of syndromes and the best known such association is with the tricho-rhino-phalangeal syndrome of Giedion (2–4, 6) (4.51C). Similar coning occurs in the lesser known conorenal syndrome, a condition associated with chronic renal disease, in the form of familial nephronophthisis (3, 9). Other conditions in which such cone-shaped epiphyses are seen include achondroplasia (see Fig. 4.4A), acrodysostosis, the Ellis-van Creveld syndrome, cleidocranial dysostosis, the orodigitofacial syndromes, the otopalatodigital syndrome, the acrocephalosyndactyly syndromes, asphyxiating thoracic dystrophy, nonspecific brachydactyly (Fig. 4.51D), Marchesani's syndrome, osteopetrosis, multiple and spondyloepiphyseal dysplasia, metaphyseal dysostosis, Seckel's bird-headed dwarfism, pseudo or pseudopseudohypoparathyroidism (10), and multiple osteochondromatosis. In the latter condition, the cone deformity often occurs laterally, while in most of the other conditions the cone is central.

On an acquired basis, a cone-shaped epiphysis can be seen secondary to any type of epiphyseal-metaphyseal injury or insult. Furthermore, in addition to occurring in the small bones of the hands and feet, acquired cone-shaped epiphyses commonly occur in the long bones (see Fig. 4.11). The specific epiphyseal-metaphyseal injury may be simple trauma (very often the battered child syndrome), pathologic epiphyseal-metaphyseal fracture, osteomyelitis, bone infarction (i.e., sickle cell disease), radiation injury, frostbite, hypophosphatasia (knees), or chronic vitamin A intoxication (7). In some of these cases, the resulting cone-shaped deformity is quite pronounced and deep.

References

1. de Iturriza JR, Tanner JM: Cone-shaped epiphyses and other minor anomalies in the hands of normal British children. *J Pediatr* 75:265–272, 1969.
2. Giedion A: Cone-shaped epiphyses of the hands and their diagnostic value: the tricho-rhino-phalangeal syndrome. *Ann Radiol* 10:322–329, 1967.
3. Giedion A: Phalangeal cone shaped epiphysis of the hands (PhCSEH) and chronic renal disease—the Conorenal syndromes. *Pediatr Radiol* 8:32–28, 1979.
4. Gorlin RJ, Cohen MM Jr, Wolfson J: Trichorhinophalangeal syndrome. *Am J Dis Child* 118:595–599, 1969.
5. Hertzog KP, Garn SM, Church SF: Cone-shaped epiphyses in the hand: population frequencies, anatomic distribution and developmental stages. *Invest Radiol* 3:433–441, 1968.
6. Kozlowski K, Blaim A, Malolepsky E: Tricho-rhinophalangeal syndrome. *Australos Radiol* 16:411–416, 1972.
7. Pease CN: Focal retardation and arrestment of growth of bones due to vitamin A intoxication. *JAMA* 182:980–985, 1962.
8. Poznanski AK: Diagnostic clues in the growing ends of bones. *J Can Assoc Radiol* 29:7–21, 1978.
9. Saldino RM, Mainzer F: Cone-shaped epiphyses (CSE) in siblings with hereditary renal disease and retinitis pitmentosa. *Radiology* 98:39–46, 1971.
10. Steinback HL, Young DA: The roentgen appearance of pseudohypoparathyroidism (PH) and pseudo-pseudo-hypoparathyroidism (PPH), differentiation from other syndromes associated with short metacarpals, metatarsals, and phalanges. *Am J Roentgenol* 97:49–66, 1966.

Table 4.19　Cone-Shaped Epiphyses

Normal (especially feet)	}	Commonest
Trauma Infection	}	Moderately common
Bone infarction (sickle cell) Frostbite (hands, feet) Other syndromes and dysplasias[a]	}	Relatively rare
Tricho-rhino-phalangeal syndrome[b] Vitamin A intoxication (chronic)	}	Rare

[a] See text for list.
[b] Rare condition, but cone-shaped epiphyses important.

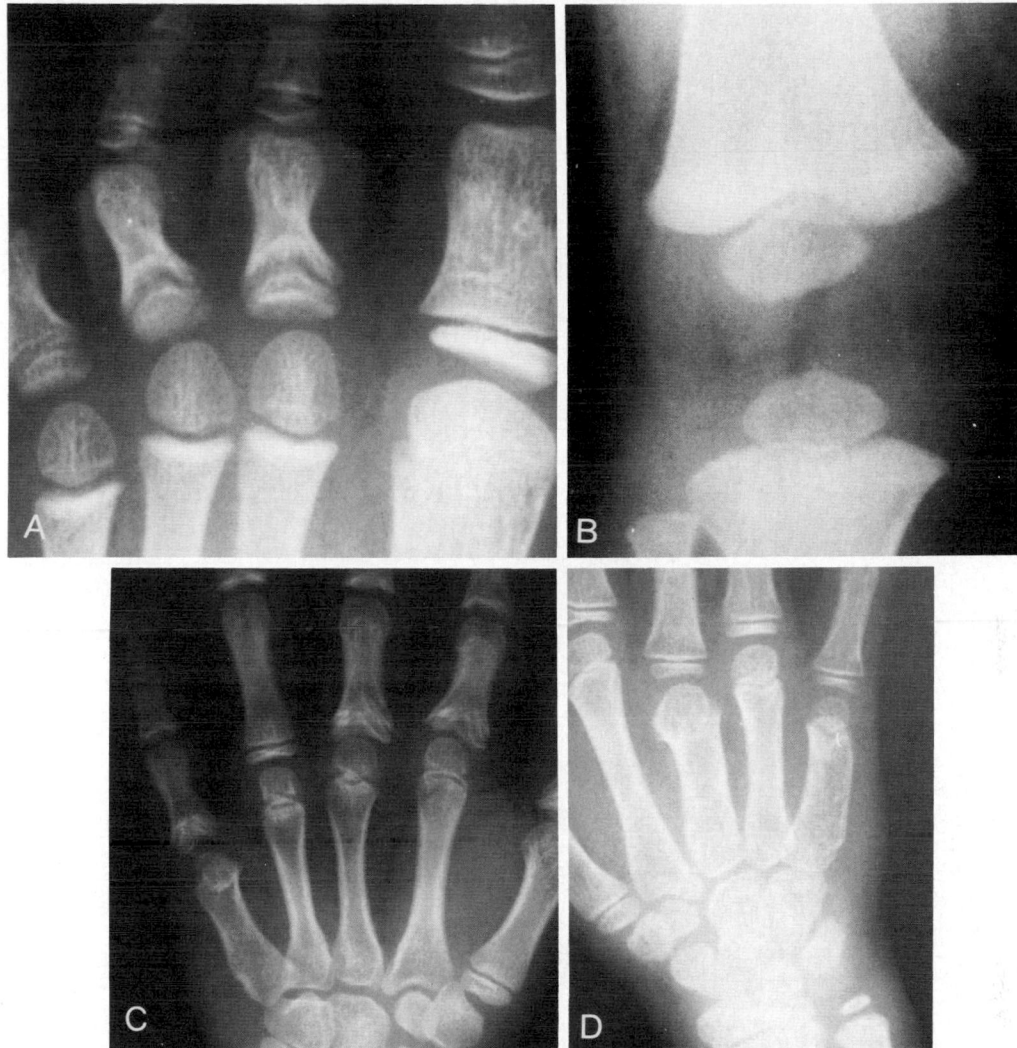

Fig. 4.51. Cone-shaped epiphyses. A. Normal cone-shaped epiphyses in feet. B. Normal cone-shaped epiphyses in knee of infant. C. Typical cone-shaped epiphyses in tricho-rhino-phalangeal syndrome. D. Cone-shaped epiphyses in nonspecific brachydactyly.

Indistinct Epiphyseal Margins (Table 4.20)

Normally the epiphysis has a readily visualized and intact margin around its periphery. However, when calcification is less than normal the edge of the epiphysis becomes indistinct. Most often this occurs with conditions producing osteomalacia, that is rickets and hyperparathyroidism (see Fig. 4.18C). However, it also occurs with hypophosphatasia, hypothyroidism and, in infancy, in conditions which mimic hyperparathyroidism (i.e., Jansen's metaphyseal dysostosis, generalized gangliosidosis, and mucolipidosis II).

Ringed Epiphyses (Table 4.20)

The commonest cause of a ringed epiphysis is severe, chronic osteoporosis because, while the center of the epiphysis becomes more and more radiolucent, the relatively less demineralized cortex remains thin and dense. This can be seen with any cause of osteoporosis but is most common in neurogenic or neuromuscular disease with disuse atrophy (Fig. 4.52A). The finding also is seen in osteogenesis imperfecta, and when seen in scurvy (rare these days), is referred to as Wimberger's ring (Fig. 4.52B).

Less delicate, and often very dense, rings are seen in the healing phase of any condition which first leads to an indistinct epiphyseal margin (see previous section). In these conditions, including rickets, hyper-

Table 4.20   Indistinct and Ringed Epiphyses

Indistinct epiphyseal margins	
Rickets	
Hyperparathyroidism (secondary) i.e., renal osteodystrophy	Commonest
Hypothyroidism	Moderately common
Hyperparathyroidism (primary)	
Jansen's metaphyseal dysostosis	Relatively rare
Mucolipidosis II	
Generalized gangliosidosis	
Ringed epiphysis	
Severe chronic osteoporosis (see Table 4.2 for causes)	Commonest
Healing rickets	Moderately common
Healing hypothyroidism	Relatively rare
Osteogenesis imperfecta	
Scurvy (Wimberger's ring)	Rare

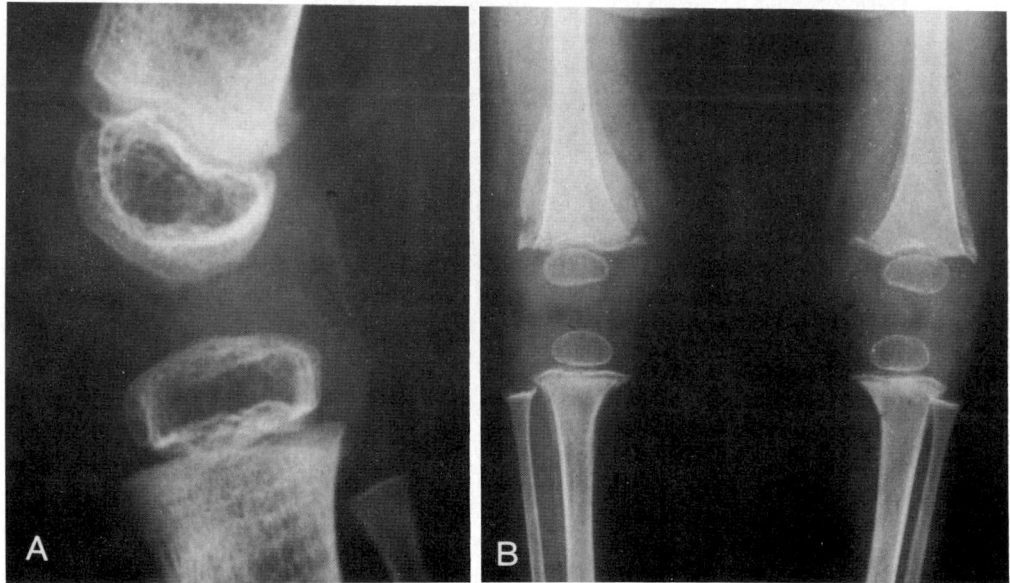

Fig. 4.52.   Ringed epiphyses. A. Marked disuse osteoporosis causing ringed epiphysis in patient with neurogenic disease. B. Ringed epiphyses in scurvy. Note other characteristic changes in the metaphyses including the white line of scurvy, the scurvy zone (radiolucent band), corner fracturing, and subperiosteal bleeding with new bone deposition.

parathyroidism, renal osteodystrophy, and hypothyroidism, the problem is similar to that seen with transverse metaphyseal bands (see p 226). In other words, when an insult to enchondral bone growth occurs, the edge of the epiphysis becomes indistinct, and then, with recovery, the cortex reconstitutes and a ring is formed.

Crenated (Crinkled) Epiphyses

This epiphyseal configuration resembles that of a crenated red blood cell. For the most part, it occurs in the distal femur and, while a certain degree of crenation can be seen in normal individuals, when it becomes more pronounced, one should think of rheumatoid arthritis (1) (Fig. 4.53).

Reference

1. Martel W, Holt J, Cassidy J: Roentgenographic manifestations of juvenile rheumatoid arthritis. *Am J Roentgenol* 88:400–423, 1962.

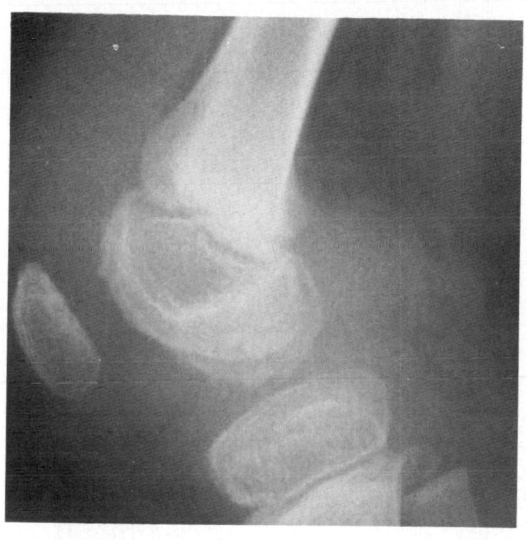

Fig. 4.53. Crinkled epiphysis. Note crinkled appearing distal femoral epiphysis in patient with rheumatoid arthritis. Slight crinkling also can occur in normal individuals. However, note that this patient has intra-articular fluid.

Defects of the Epiphyses (Table 4.21)

Perhaps the most important point to note about an epiphyseal defect is whether it is associated with joint fluid. The reason for this is that, when fluid is present, infection or trauma almost surely also are present. If the defect is due to an acute avulsion (i.e., cruciate ligament avulsion), the fluid is blood and since the avulsed fragment is seen, there is no problem with the diagnosis. When the problem is infection, chronic synovial hypertrophy is the cause of the defect. Almost invariably, in such cases, the problem is tuberculous (Fig. 4.54A) or rheumatoid arthritis (1–3, 6, 8, 9), but occasionally it is due to subacute pyogenic arthritis (4) (Fig. 4.54B). In the distal femoral epiphysis normal fibrous defects should not be confused with those due to infection (Fig. 4.54C) and in the hip, the normal defect of the fovea centralis can mimic a pathologic defect (Fig. 4.54D).

In the knee, another common epiphyseal defect is that seen with osteochondritis dissecans (5, 7). The condition may be asymptomatic and usually there is no significant joint fluid accumulation. Characteristically, the defect involves the medial femoral condyle, is somewhat anterior in position, and associated with an avulsed bone fragment (Fig. 4.55, A and B). Although osteochondritis dissecans can occur at other sites (i.e., patella, talus), it is by far most common in the distal femur. A normal defect, not to be confused with that of osteochondritis dissecans, can occur in either femoral condyle. In these cases, its posterior location is the clue to proper diagnosis (Fig. 4.55, C and D). Other causes of epiphyseal defects include histiocytosis X, rarely a synovial tumor, and occasionally a benign fibrous defect.

References

1. Cassidy JT, Brody GL, Martel W: Mono-articular juvenile rheumatoid arthritis. *J Pediatr* 70:867–875, 1967.

Table 4.21 Epiphyseal Defects

Fovea centralis (normal femoral head defect)	Commonest
Osteochondritis dissecans (distal femur) Normal femoral condyle defects Avulsion injuries (usually knee) Rheumatoid arthritis	Moderately common
Osteochondritis dissecans (other bones) Tuberculous arthritis Fungal arthritis Other chronic arthritities Osteomyelitis of epiphysis	Relatively rare
Histiocytosis X Synovial tumors Fibrous defects	Rare

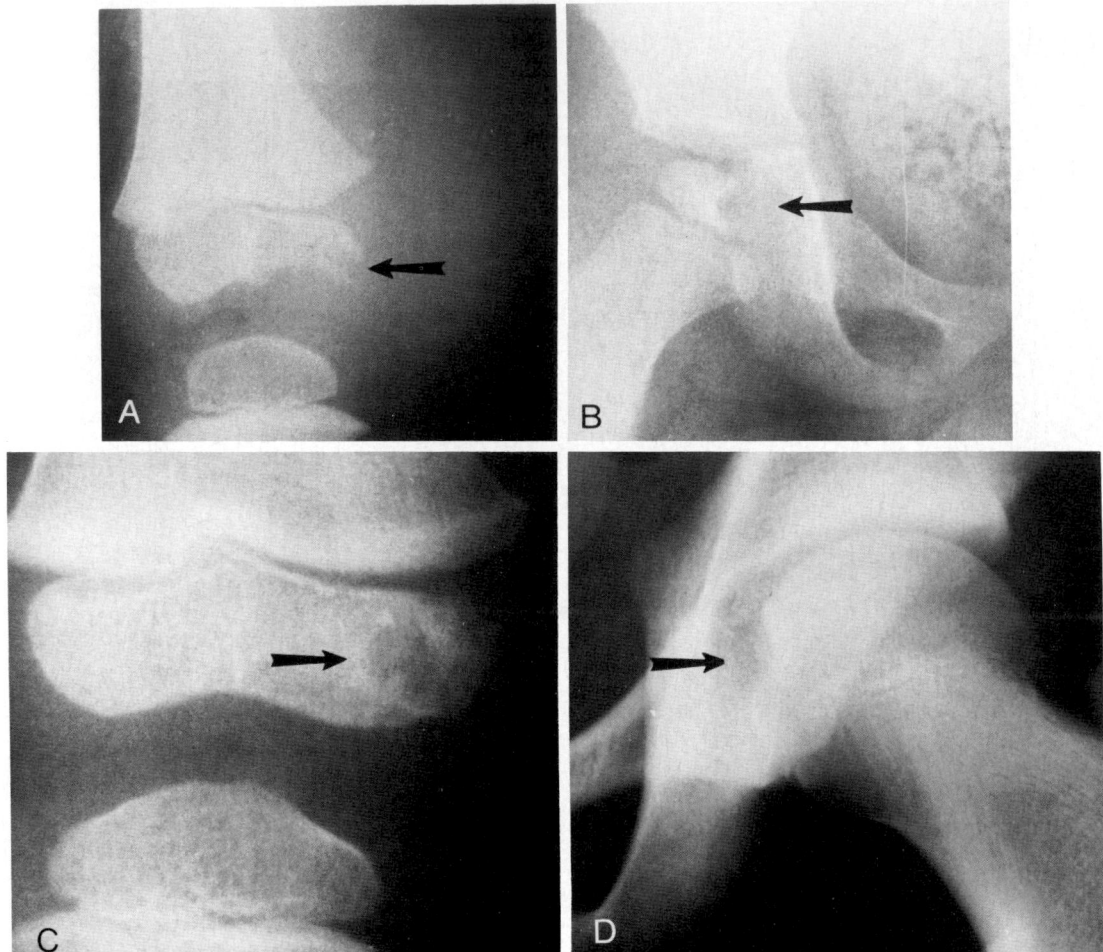

Fig. 4.54. **Epiphyseal defects.** A. Defect of distal femoral epiphysis due to tuberculous arthritis (arrow). Note extensive associated joint distention and swelling. B. Epiphyseal defect of proximal femoral epiphysis due to subacute pyogenic osteomyelitis (arrow). C. Normal, fibrous defect in distal femoral epiphysis (arrow). D. Normal defect in femoral capital epiphysis (arrow) due to fovea centralis.

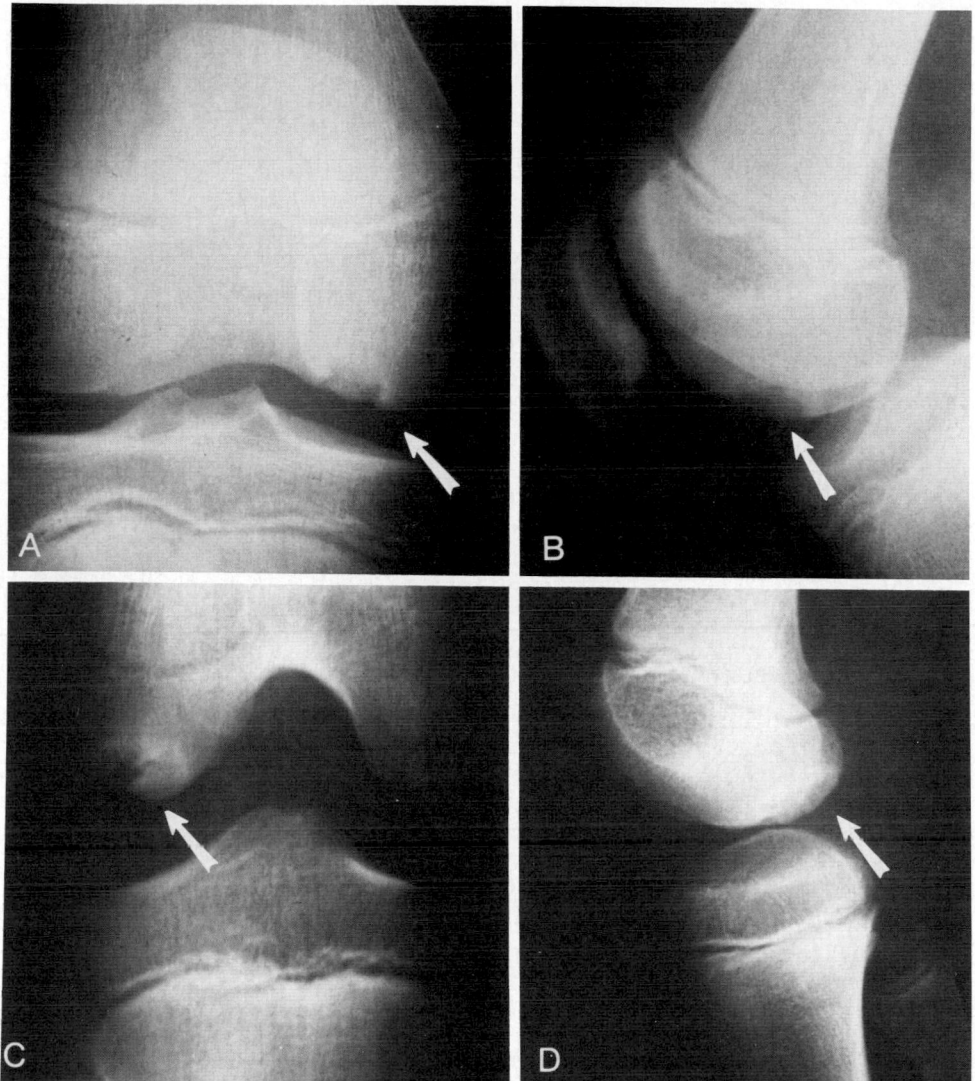

Fig. 4.55.   Epiphyseal defect—osteochondritis desicans. A. Note typical defect in medial femoral condyle (arrow). B. Lateral view demonstrating typical anterior location of defect (arrow). C. Normal irregularity mimicking osteochondritis desicans (arrow). This type of defect can occur on either condyle. D. Characteristically this defect is located posteriorly (arrow). Figures C and D courtesy Virgil Graves, M.D., Great Falls, Montana.

2. Cremin BJ, Fisher MB, Levinsohn MB: Multiple bone tuberculosis in the young. *Br J Radiol* 43:638–645, 1970.
3. Edeiken J, Hodes PJ: *Roentgen Diagnosis of Diseases of Bone,* ed 2. Baltimore, Williams & Wilkins, 1973, vol 2, pp 664–733.
4. Green NE, Beauchamp RD, Griffin PP: Primary subacute epiphyseal osteomyelitis. *J Bone Joint Surg* 63A: 107–114, 1981.
5. Green WT, Banks HII: Osteochondritis dissecans in children. *J Bone Joint Surg* 35-A:26–47, 1953.
6. Martel W, Holt J, Cassidy J: Roengenographic manifes- tations of juvenile rheumatoid arthritis. *Am J Roentgenol* 88:400–423, 1962.
7. Milgram JW: Radiological and pathological manifestations of osteochondritis dissecans of the distal femur. A study of 50 cases. *Radiology* 125:305–311, 1978.
8. Phemister DB: Changes in the articular surfaces in tuberculosis and in pyogenic infections of joints. *Am J Roentgenol* 12:1–14, 1924.
9. Phemister DB, Hatcher CH: Correlation of pathological and rorengenological findings in diagnosis of tuberculosis arthritis. *Am J Roentgenol* 29:736–752, 1933.

Epiphyseal Clefts

Epiphyseal clefts, are normal variations in the epiphysis and most commonly occur in the great toe (Fig. 4.56A). They can occur in other epiphyses (1), but are most problematic in the great toe, where often they are misinterpreted for similar clefts caused by fracturing of the epiphysis (Fig. 4.56B). This problem does not arise as often at other sites, for clefts then usually represent epiphyseal fractures.

Reference

1. Harrison RB, Keats TE: Epiphyseal clefts. *Skeletal Radiol* 5:23–27, 1980.

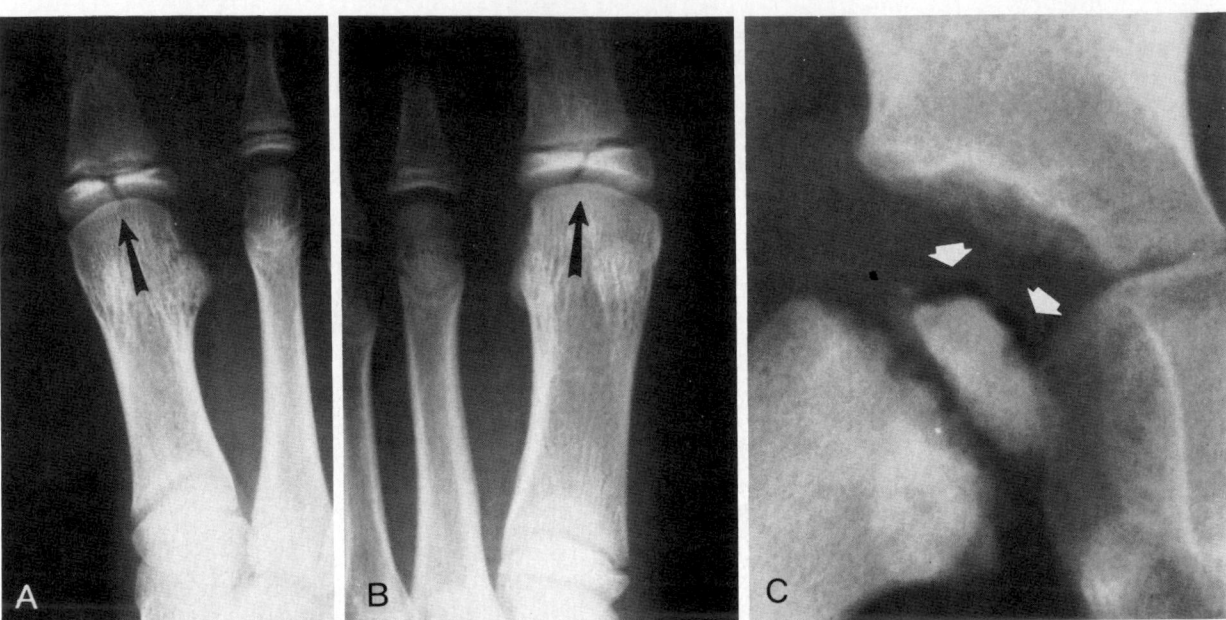

Fig. 4.56. Epiphyseal clefts. A. Normal epiphyseal cleft (bipartite epiphysis) of great toe (arrow). B. Defect of epiphysis due to fracture (arrow). C. **Intraepiphyseal gas.** Characteristic intraepiphyseal gas (arrows) in Legg-Perthes disease.

Intraepiphyseal Gas

Gas within the epiphysis almost exclusively occurs with aseptic necrosis of the proximal femoral epiphysis, that is Legg-Perthes disease (1). It has, however, been described with osteochondritis of the capitellum (2), and at either site is quite characteristic (Fig. 4.56C). The phenomenon of gas in the epiphysis is not unlike that which occurs with the so-called vacuum joint (see p 291). As a consequence, intraepiphyseal gas is seen only with traction on the joint, and perhaps this is why it is most commonly recorded in the hip. In the hip, standard roentgenographic examination consists of AP and frogleg views. On the frogleg view, there is a certain amount of traction applied to the joint, and it may be that this is why intraepiphyseal gas appears on this study so commonly. The reason the gas accumulates in the epiphysis is that there is a subchondral fracture present, and because of this the fractured fragment can separate from the main portion of the head. The negative pressures then are transmitted intraepiphyseally, and intraepiphyseal gas results. In the case of a joint, a vacuum joint is seen.

References

1. Caffey J: The early roentgenographic changes in essential coxa plana; their significance in pathogenesis. *Am J Roentgenol* 103:620–634, 1968.
2. Jacobs P: Intra-epiphyseal gas in osteochondritis of capitellum. *Clin Radiol* 21:318–319, 1970.

METAPHYSEAL ABNORMALITIES

Transverse Metaphyseal Bands (Table 4.22)

These bands can be radiolucent or radiodense, and actually, most times both coexist. Radiolucent bands generally reflect episodes of poor enchondral bone formation and dense bands the ensuing recovery phase. Often the dense bands are referred to as growth arrest or Parks's lines (1, 4, 5, 9), even though the term "arrest" is somewhat of a misnomer. More accurately the dense lines are recovery lines, for they

Table 4.22 Transverse Metaphyseal Bands

A.	Alternating radiolucent and radio-opaque	
	Trophic	
	Severe illness, trauma[a]	
	Battered child syndrome, deprivational dwarf[b]	Commonest
	Healing rickets[a]	
	Healing neonatal infections[a]	
	Chronic diseases[b]	Moderately common
	Chemotherapy, etc.[b]	
	Osteopetrosis[b]	Rare
B.	Solitary radiolucent band (no opaque band)	
	Severe illness, trauma	
	Leukemia, lymphoma[c]	Commonest
	Metastatic disease[c]	
	Neonatal infections (especially syphilis)[c]	Moderately common
	Scurvy[c]	Rare
C.	Solitary radiodense band	
	Normal, physiologic	Commonest
	Chronic lead intoxication	Moderately common
	Other heavy metal or chemical intoxication	
	Radiation injury by bone seeking isotopes	Relatively rare
	Idiopathic hypercalcemia	
	Hypervitaminosis D	

[a] Single line usually.
[b] Multiple lines.
[c] Fracture (pathologic) through line often associated.

result from the rapid deposition of new bone after the insult causing poor bone growth is gone.

The foregoing combination of radiolucent and radiodense transverse metaphyseal bands is rather nonspecific (Fig. 4.57), but at the same time, quite common. The reason is that these lines can result from almost any form of insult to the growing body; i.e., severe infections or fractures and chronic relapsing diseases such as asthma, diabetes, cystic fibrosis, osteopetrosis, treated malignancies (chemotherapy, radiation therapy), rheumatoid arthritis (8), and the battered child-deprivation dwarfism syndrome (6). These bands also occur in the neonate as a result of the "normal" insults sustained during birth and the immediate postnatal period (especially in premature infants), and pathologically, in perinatal infections such as rubella, CID, herpes, toxoplasmosis, and syphilis (2, 3, 11, 12). These lines even can develop before birth as a result of maternal infections or fetal insults

such as intestinal perforation. In addition the lines occur with healing rickets and treated hypothyroidism.

As noted earlier these transverse bands frequently are multiple and the radiolucent-opaque sequence clearly visible. However, if one obtains a roentgenogram during the first, or only, episode of impaired enchondral bone formation, then one will see only a single transverse radiolucent band. It will be located at the very distal end of the metaphysis, and to the uninitiated can appear quite worrisome (Fig. 4.57E). The reason for this is that similar bands can be seen with more serious problems such as leukemia (Fig. 4.57F), lymphoma, and metastatic disease, and uncommonly (these days) with scurvy (see Fig. 4.52B). In leukemia the transverse radiolucent line is referred to as the "leukemia line" while in scurvy it is termed the scurvy zone. The thin white line just distal to the radiolucent line in scurvy is called the scurvy line. In most of these pathologic states, the bone through the radiolucent zone also is weakened and pathologic fractures through the area are common. Indeed, grossly disorganized epiphyseal-metaphyseal areas often result (see Fig. 4.67, E and F).

Radiodense bands, in the absence of preceding radiolucent lines also occur in both normal and abnormal patients. Overall, however, the commonest cause of such a line is overexuberant calcification of the zone of provisional calcification in normal children. This commonly is seen in children exposed to extended periods of sunlight, especially after the winter months. Indeed, in some of these cases the line is so dense that chronic lead intoxication is suggested (Fig. 4.58). A similar phenomenon can occur with vitamin D intoxication and hypercalcemia, but certainly both are far less common and, of course, also are pathologic.

Other pathologic radiodense lines occur with chronic lead poisoning (Fig. 4.58B), and in some cases the lines are multiple. When so, they can be associated with a modeling error of the metaphysis leading to splaying or an Erlenmeyer flask deformity (10) (see Fig. 4.64C). The deformity and dense bands occur together only with chronic lead intoxication and although some lead is deposited in the region of the white lines, most of the increase in whiteness is due to excess deposition of calcium in thicker and more numerous trabeculae (10). Similar lines can be seen in bismuth, arsenic, phosphorus, fluoride, mercury, lithium, and radium poisoning. Radiodense bands also are seen in osteopetrosis (see Fig. 4.57C).

References

1. Caffey J: *Pediatric X-Ray Diagnosis,* ed 6. Chicago, Year Book Medical Publishers, 1972, vol 2, pp 969, 972, 973–976, 1237–1243, 1247–1248.
2. Coblentz DR, Cimini R, Mikity VG, Rosen R: Roent-

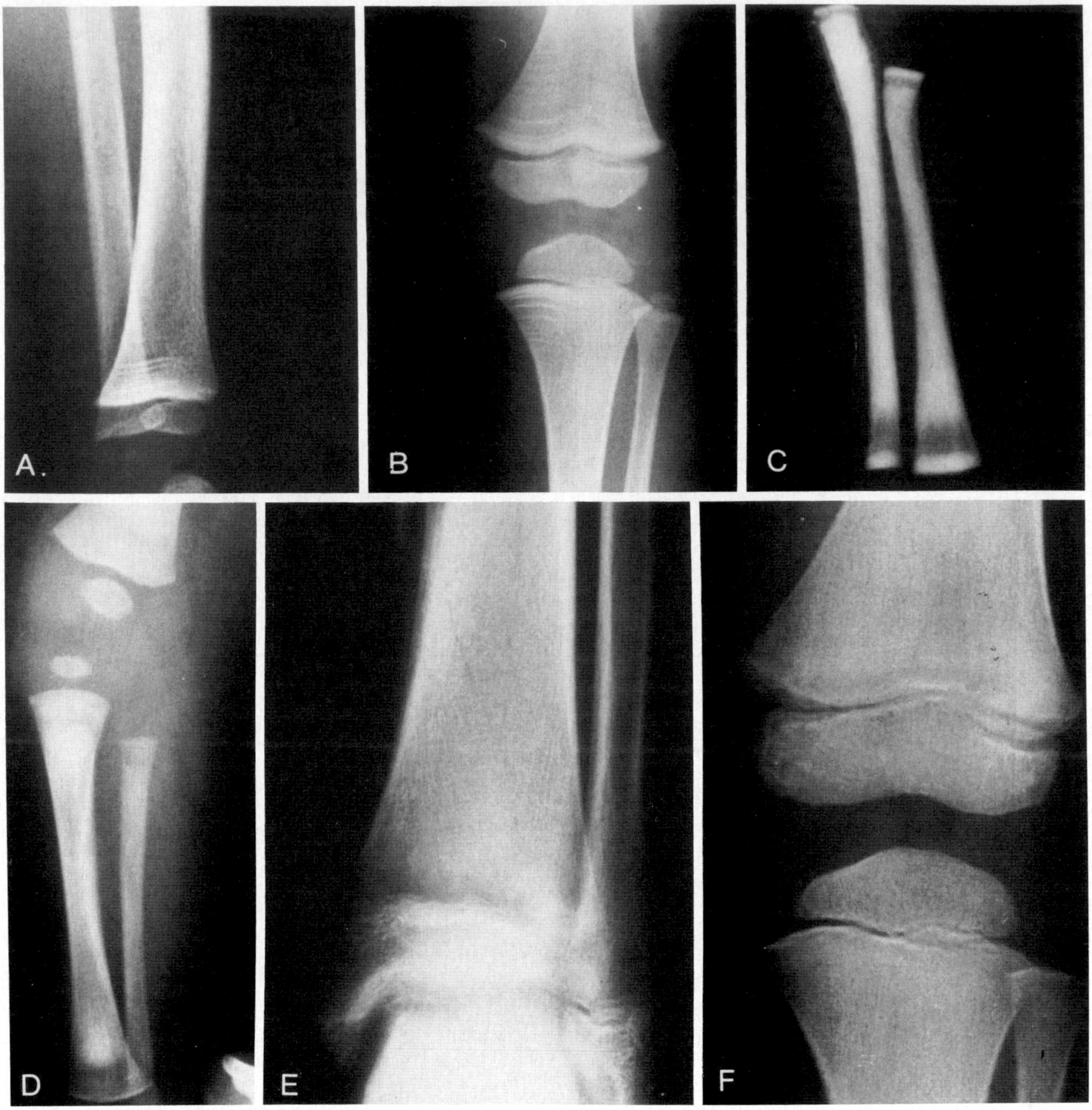

Fig. 4.57. Transverse lucent metaphyseal lines. A. Repeated alternating radiolucent and radio-opaque lines in patient with asthma. B. Numerous transverse lines in deprivational dwarfism. C. Broad radiolucent and dense bands in osteopetrosis. D. Broad, nonspecific radiolucent bands in patient with arthrogryposis. E. Broad radiolucent metaphyseal band in patient with fracture of tibia. F. Tranverse radiolucent band in distal femur and proximal tibia in leukemia.

genographic diagnosis of congenital syphilis in the newborn. *JAMA* 212:1061–1064, 1970.

3. Cremin BJ, Fisher RM: The lesions of congenital syphilis. *Br J Radiol* 43:333–341, 1970.

4. Follis RH Jr, Park EA: Some observations on bone growth, with particular respect to zones and transverse lines of increased density in the metaphysis. *Am J Roentgenol* 68:709–724, 1952.

5. Garn SM, Silverman FN, Hertzog KP, Robmann CG: Lines and bands of increased density; their implication to growth and development. *Med Radiogr Photogr* 44:58–88, 1968.

6. Hernandez RJ, Poznanski AK, Hopwood NJ, Kelch RP: Incidence of growth lines in psychosocial dwarfs and idiopathic hypopituitarism. *Am J Roentgenol* 131:477–479, 1978.

7. Leone AJ Jr: On lead lines. *Am J Roentgenol* 103:165–167, 1968.

8. Martel W, Holt JF, Cassidy JT: Roentgenologic manifestations of juvenile rheumatoid arthritis. *Am J Roent-*

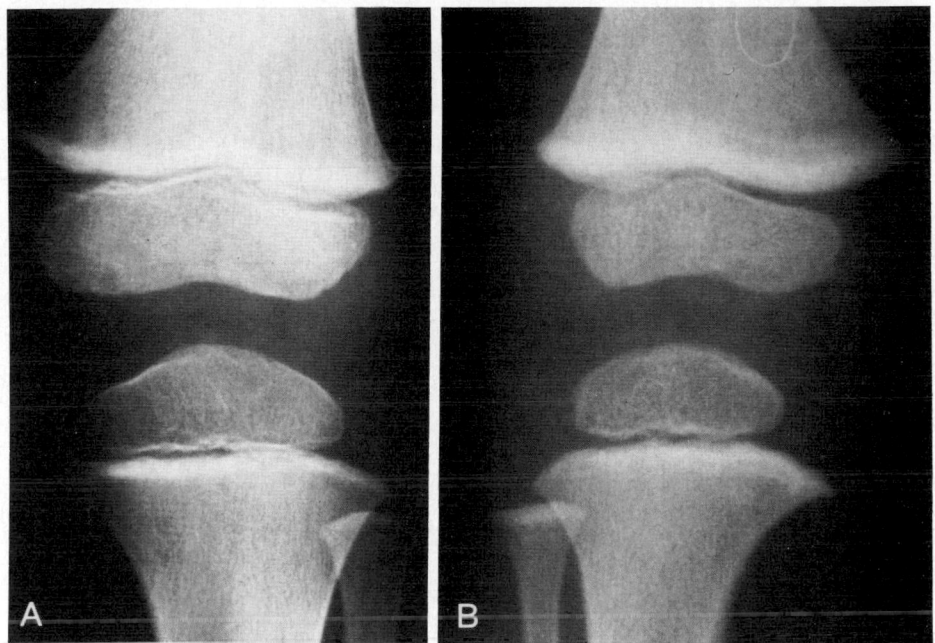

Fig. 4.58. Transverse white metaphyseal bands. A. Normal, dense zones of provisional calcification. B. Dense white lines in chronic lead intoxication.

genol 88:400–423, 1962.
9. Park EA: The imprinting of nutritional disturbances on growing bone. *Pediatrics* (Suppl, Part 2): 815, 1964.
10. Pease CN, Newton GB: Metaphyseal dysplasia due to lead poisoning. *Radiology* 79:233–240, 1962.
11. Rabinowitz JG, Wolf BS, Greenberg EI, Rausen AR: Osseous changes in rubella embryopathy (congenital

rubella syndrome). *Radiology* 85:494–499, 1965.
12. Rudolph AJ, Singleton EB, Rosenberg HS, Singer DB, Phillips CA: Osseous manifestations of congenital rubella syndrome. *Am J Dis Child* 110:428–433, 1965.
13. Wolfson JJ, Engel RR: Anticipating meconium peritonitis from metaphyseal bands. *Radiology* 92:1055–1060, 1969.

Dense Vertical Metaphyseal Lines

These lines are not particularly common in childhood, but on an isolated basis, can be seen after any type of epiphyseal injury. In such cases the finding probably results from a focally induced aberration of metaphyseal growth which causes a streak of thickened trabecular bone to extend into the metaphysis. Occasionally this also is seen on an entirely normal basis (Fig. 4.59A).

When numerous vertical lines are seen in the metaphyses one should think of the rare condition known as osteopathia striata (Fig. 4.59B). Usually an innocuous problem, in some instances it can be associated with hearing difficulties, cranial nerve dysfunction, frontal bossing, a depressed nasal bridge, apparent hypertelorism, and thickening and sclerosis of the skull and facial bones (1). Vertical lines also are seen in congenital infections such as rubella (Fig. 4.59C). The finding is much less common with cytomegalic inclusion disease and lues. The appearance of the vertical striations in the metaphyses of these latter conditions has led to the term **celery stalk metaphysis.** A less delicate form of celery stalk metaphysis can be seen with hypophosphatasia, and the occasional case of metaphyseal dysostosis.

Reference

1. Paling MR, Hyde I, Dennis NR: Osteopathia striata with sclerosis and thickening of the skull. *Br J Radiol* 54:344–348, 1981.

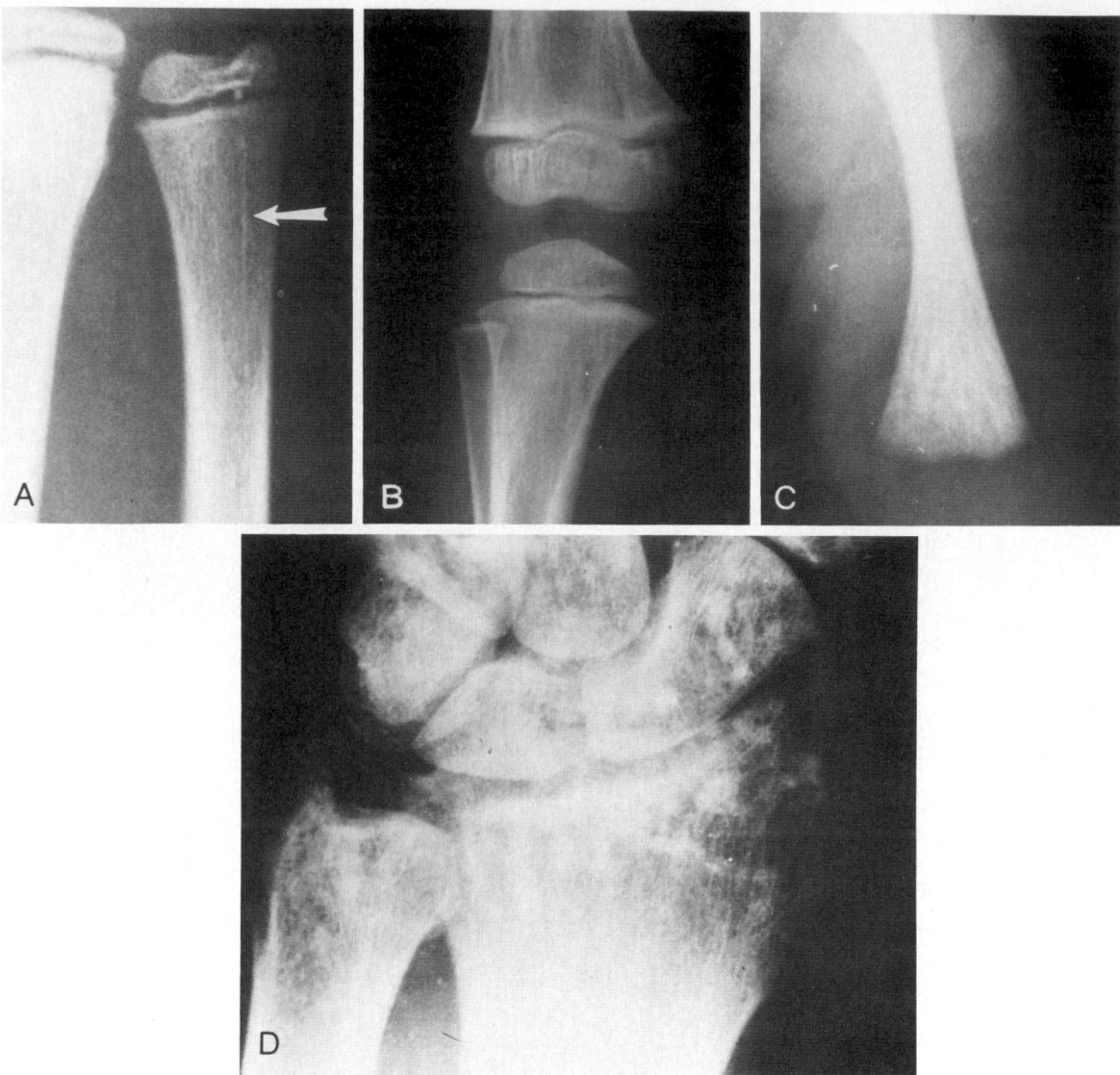

Fig. 4.59.   Vertical metaphyseal lines. A. Note normal, vertical metaphyseal line (arrow) associated with a normal epiphyseal line spicule. B. Vertical metaphyseal lines in osteopathia striata. C. Vertical, somewhat coarse, metaphyseal lines in congenital rubella. Note also that the bones are dense, a common feature of this infection. D. **Spotted metaphyses.** Note dense bone islands in the metaphyses and carpal bones of this young adult with osteopoikilosis.

Spotted Metaphyses

Basically there is only one condition which produces this finding, and in childhood it is not particularly common. It is termed osteopathia condensans disseminata or osteopoikilosis, and usually is asymptomatic (1–3). The dense areas in the metaphyses are small islands of compact bone and also can be seen in the epiphyses, the tarsal and carpal bones, and the flat bones of the pelvis (Fig. 4.59C). Osteopoikilosis also can be seen in association with melorheostosis and pachydermoperiostosis (2, 3).

References

1. Archer MC, Fox KW: Osteopoikilosis: Report of two new cases. *Radiology* 47:279–283, 1946.
2. Green AE, Ellswood WH, Collins JR: Melorheostosis and osteopoikilosis. *Am J Roentgenol* 87:1096–1111, 1962.
3. Holly LE: Osteopoikilosis: A five year study. *Am J Roentgenol* 36:512–517, 1936.

Indistinct-Frayed Metaphyses

Indistinctness, with fraying of the metaphysis is due to poor calcification of the zone of provisional calcification. For the most part, this occurs in conditions producing osteomalacia and certainly the most common of these is rickets (Fig. 4.60A). It also occurs in hypophosphatasia (Fig. 4.60B), in a few cases of metaphyseal dysostosis, and in severe hyperparathyroidism.

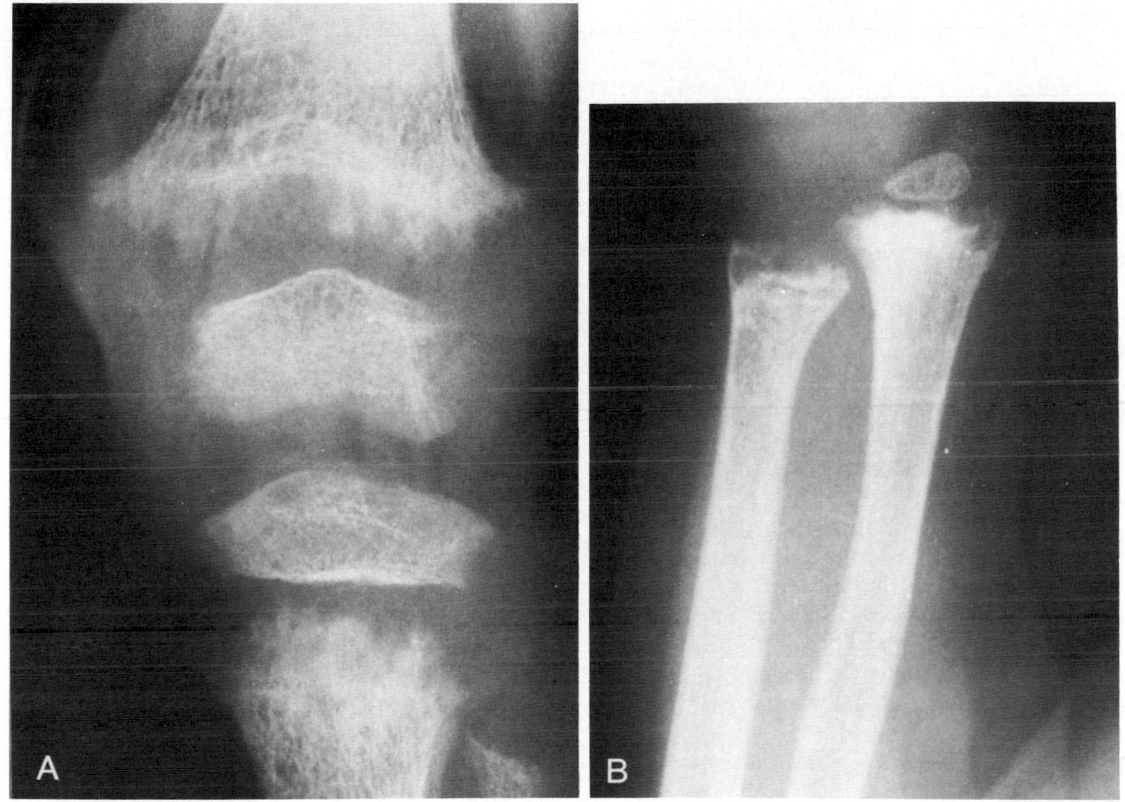

Fig. 4.60. Indistinct, frayed metaphyses. A. Typical indistinct frayed metaphyses of rickets. Also note severe osteomalacia and indistinctness of the epiphyseal margins. B. Indistinct, somewhat frayed metaphyses in hypophosphatasia.

Crinkled, Dense Metaphyseal Edge

Normally the edge of the metaphysis is smooth and demarcated by a variably sclerotic line, the zone of provisional calcification (see Fig. 4.58A). In some instances, however, metaphyseal growth is so disturbed that the edge of the metaphysis becomes very irregular or crinkled, and usually dense. Most commonly this occurs with healing epiphyseal metaphyseal fractures (Fig. 4.61A), but in more florid form occurs in conditions such as metaphyseal dysostosis (Fig. 4.61B), hypophosphatasia, pseudoachondroplasia (spondylo and multiple epiphyseal dysplasia types), and healing rubella infection in the neonate (Fig. 4.61C).

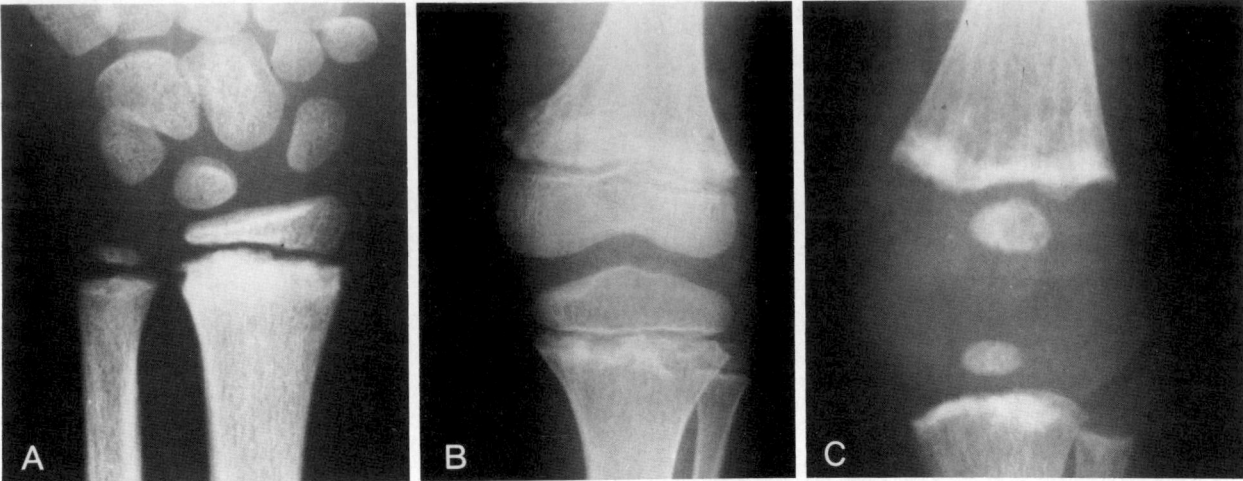

Fig. 4.61. Crinkled dense metaphyses. A. Typical, irregular and sclerotic (crinkled) metaphysis in healing epiphyseal-metaphyseal fracture. B. Crinkled metaphyses in metaphyseal dysostosis. C. Crinkled, dense metaphyses in rubella infection of infancy.

Metaphyseal Beaks (Table 4.23)

Metaphyseal beaks may be solid or fragmented, and most commonly occur as corner fractures in epiphyseal injuries where they become more pronounced as healing occurs (Fig. 4.62, A and B). Such beaking usually is focal and asymmetric, but when it occurs in the battered child syndrome may be more widespread, and even reasonably symmetric. Similar beaking resulting from trauma also is seen in the neonate delivered by breech and with pathologic fractures occurring in conditions such as neurogenic disease with bone atrophy, scurvy (beaks are termed Pelkan spurs; see

Fig. 4.52B) hyperparathyroidism, rickets, Menkes' kinky hair syndrome, leukemia, lymphoma, metastatic disease, osteomyelitis, and congenital infections such as lues, CID, and rubella.

The next most common cause of metaphyseal beaking is that which occurs as a normal variation along the upper medial tibia and distal femur (Fig. 4.62C). In most of these cases, tibial torsion, leading to so-called physiologic bowing of the legs usually also is present, and probably the two conditions are interrelated (i.e., beaking probably results from the abnormal, vertical stresses being placed on the medial aspect of the knee because of the bowlegs). There is a distinct tendency for this phenomenon to occur in more sturdy infants, with more ample muscle bulk and early ambulation. In more advanced cases beaking of the distal femur also is seen, and can be especially worrisome on oblique views (Fig. 4.62D). In older children, when the tibial beak is large and fragmented, the condition then is known as Blount's disease (see Fig. 4.17B). As opposed to physiologic bowing and beaking of the young infant, Blount's disease is a true pathologic state requiring treatment. Beaking around the knees also occurs with almost any other cause of bowed legs, and consequently is seen in conditions such as rickets, the various chondodystrophic dwarfs, metaphyseal dysostosis, etc. (Fig. 4.62E).

Table 4.23 Metaphyseal Beaking

Normal (knees; especially with bowing) Other causes of bowed legs (see Table 4.7) Epiphyseal metaphyseal fractures in normal bones	Commonest
Blount's disease Epiphyseal metaphyseal fractures in Battered child syndrome Breech delivery Rickets Hyperparathyroidism Neurogenic disease Leukemia, lymphoma Metastatic disease Osteomyelitis Trophic (ischemia) changes with congenital infections	Moderately common
Menkes' kinky hair syndrome Scurvy (Pelkan spurs)	Rare

References

1. Bateson EM: The relationship between Blount's disease and bowlegs. *Br J Radiol* 41:107, 1968.
2. Golding JSR, Bateson EM, McNeil-Smith JDG: Infantile tibia vara (Blount's disease or osteochondrosis deformans tibiae). In Rang M (ed): *The Growth Plate and Its Disorders.* Baltimore, Williams & Wilkins, 1969, pp 109–119.

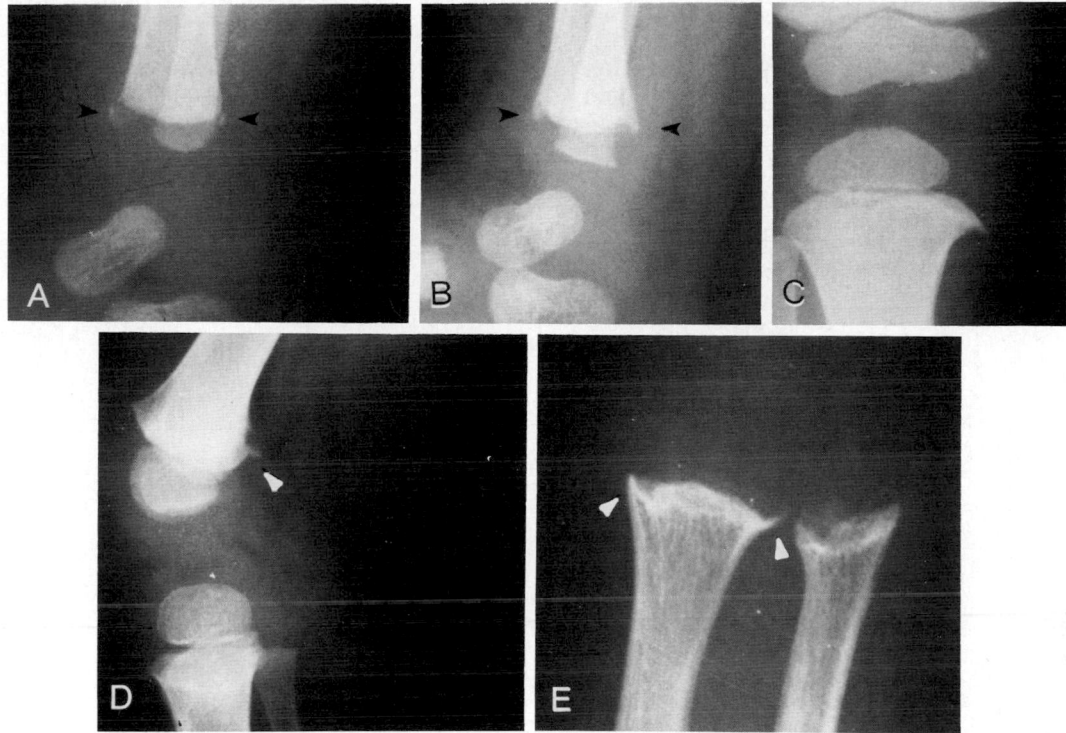

Fig. 4.62.   Metaphyseal beaking. A. Typical corner fractures with epiphyseal-metaphyseal injury (arrows). B. Later on with healing metaphyseal beaks are seen (arrows). C. Normal upper tibial metaphyseal beaking. D. Oblique view showing normal but rather worrisome distal femoral beaking (arrow). E. Beaking, associated with cupping in spondyloepiphyseal dysplasia (arrows).

Metaphyseal Flaring (Splaying) and Cupping (Table 4.24)

Very often both flaring and cupping are seen together, and indeed, it is difficult to have cupping without flaring. These changes occur as (a) inherent bone growth disturbances with some bony dysplasias or syndromes and (b) acquired growth disturbances associated with epiphyseal-metaphyseal injury or metabolic bone disease. With injury, the changes often are asymmetric and localized to one joint while with the other conditions they usually are generalized. In all instances the problem is failure of proper long bone tubulation causing failure of the metaphyses to decrease in diameter as they become incorporated into the diaphyses.

Inherent flaring and cupping of the metaphyses occurs in a large number of chondrodystrophies and bone dysplasias; i.e., achondroplasia (Fig. 4.63A), hypochondroplasia, pseudoachondroplasia (Fig. 4.63B), thanatophoric dwarfism, metatropic dwarfism, Kniest's syndrome, Ellis-van Creveld syndrome, mesomelic dwarfism, the short rib polydactyly syndromes, diastrophic dwarfism, punctate epiphyseal dysplasia congenita, the various metaphyseal dysostoses (Fig. 4.63C), hypophosphatasia (Fig. 4.63E), spondylometaphyseal dysplasia (Kozlowski), the Taybi-Lindner syndrome, osteodysplasia or the Mel-

nick-Needles syndrome, Weissenbacher-Zweymuller syndrome, phenylketonuria and a variety of immune deficiency syndromes such as the metaphyseal dysostosis-thymolymphopenia syndrome, the Schwachman-Diamond syndrome, and McKusick's metaphyseal dysostosis associated with neutropenia and pancreatic insufficiency (1, 4, 6, 7, 9, 11).

The best known cause of acquired metaphyseal flaring and cupping is rickets, and along with indistinctness of the metaphyseal margin (i.e., loss of zone of provisional calcification), is quite characteristic. Often cupping is more readily detectable when healing ensues (Fig. 4.63D). Acquired flaring and cupping also can be seen after epiphyseal-metaphyseal injury due to trauma (3), infection, radiation therapy, bone infarction (2), hypervitaminosis A, and scurvy (usually after pathologic fracturing). In many of these conditions, cupping is very deep so that the epiphysis becomes buried in the metaphysis and a **ball and socket metaphysis** results (Fig. 4.63E). In actual fact, the deformity also can be described as a cone-shaped epiphysis (see Fig. 4.11). The phenomenon probably is more common with acquired cupping but also can be seen in some of the chondrodystrophies leading to neonatal dwarfism, and in hypophosphatasia.

Before leaving the topic of metaphyseal cupping, it should be noted that a mild, or even moderate, degree of cupping occurs normally in certain bones. Most often this is seen in the distal ulna, proximal fibula, and the small bones of the hands and feet. Of course, such cupping is then exaggerated when any of the conditions producing pathologic cupping are present.

Table 4.24 Metaphyseal Flaring, Widening, and Cupping

Metaphyseal flaring and cupping (also affects anterior rib ends)	
Rickets[b]	
Normal[a]	
Ulna, fibula	Commonest
Small bones hands-feet	
Epiphyseal-metaphyseal injury[b, c]	
Achondroplasia[b, c]	Moderately common
Metaphyseal dysostosis[b]	
Hypochondroplasia[c]	
Pseudoachondroplasia[b]	
Thanatophoric dwarfism[b, c]	
Hypophosphatasia[b, c]	Relatively rare
Immunologic diseases[b]	
Bone infarctions[b, c]	
Metatrophic dwarfism[b, c]	
Kniest's syndrome[b, c]	
Ellis-van Creveld syndrome[b]	
Mesomelic dwarfism[b]	
Short rib polydactyly syndromes[b, c]	
Diastrophic dwarfism[b]	
Stippled epiphyses congenita[b]	
Hypophosphatasia[b, c]	
Spondylometaphyseal dysplasia[b]	Rare
Taybi-Lindner syndrome[b]	
Osteodysplasia (Melnick-Needles)[c]	
Hypervitaminosis A[b, c]	
Scurvy[b, c]	
Phenylketonuria[b]	
Weissenbucher-Zweymuller syndrome	
Metaphyseal widening (Erlenmeyer flask metaphyses)	
Chronic anemias	
Sickle cell	Commonest
Cooley's	
Pyle's disease	
Other craniometaphyseal dysostoses	Relatively rare
Gaucher's disease	
Chronic lead intoxication	
Mastocytosis	Rare

[a] Cupping predominantly.
[b] Cupping and flaring.
[c] Ball and socket metaphysis.

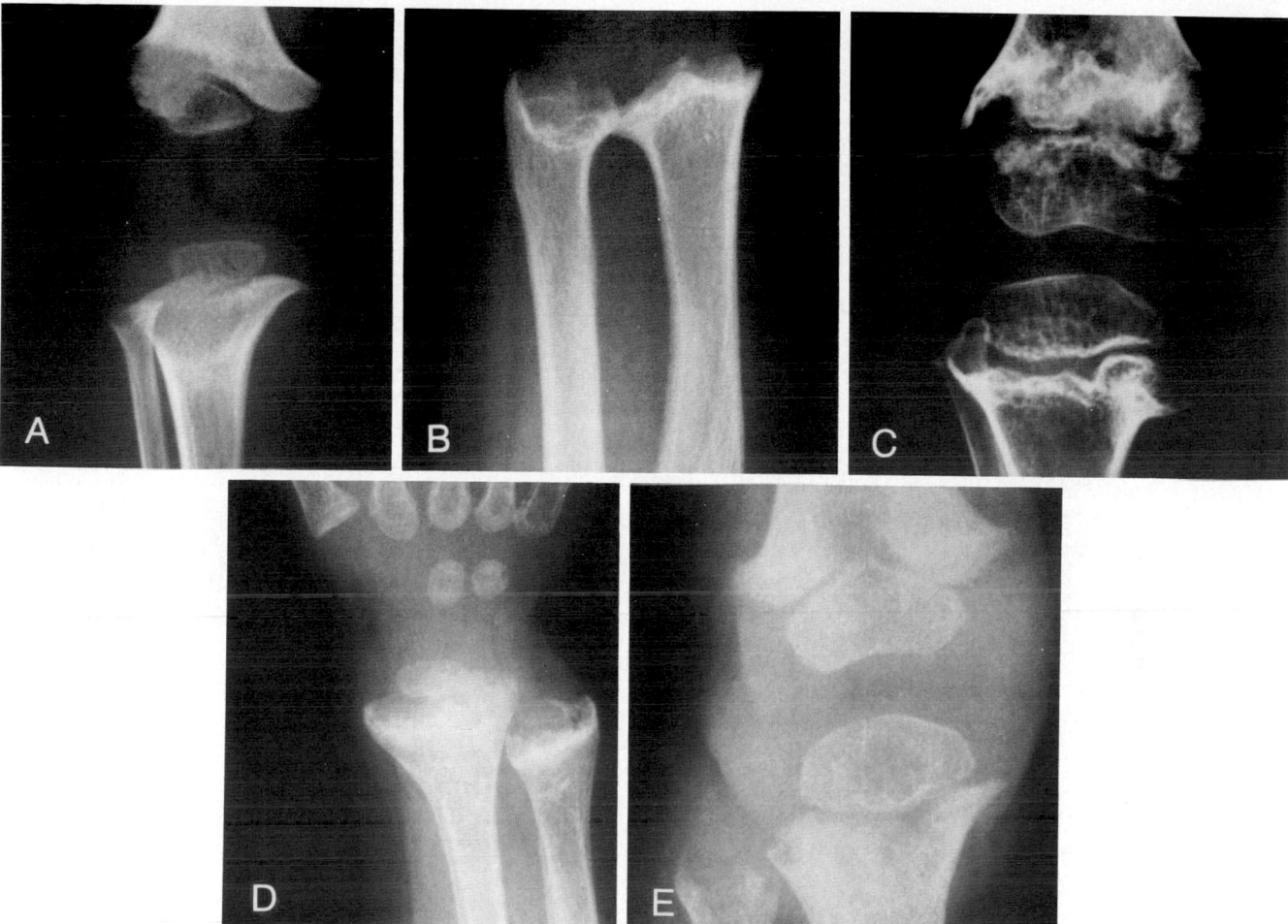

Fig. 4.63. Metaphyseal splaying and cupping. A. Metaphyseal splaying and slight cupping in achondroplasia. B. Rather marked cupping in pseudoachondroplasia. Note well defined zone of provisional calcification, but delayed epiphyseal and carpal bone development. C. Marked cupping in metaphyseal dysostosis. Also note severe irregularity of the epiphyseal-metaphyseal junction (dense, crinkled metaphyseal edge), but reasonably large epiphyses. This is typical of metaphyseal dysostosis. D. Marked cupping in healing rickets. Cupping in rickets often is more pronounced during the healing phase. Also note periosteal new bone formation. E. Hypophosphatasia. Note cupping of the fibula (arrow). Cupping was less marked in the other bones. Note, however, a deep ball and socket type epiphyseal-metaphyseal junction in the distal femur.

Metaphyseal Widening without Cupping

Metaphyseal widening without cupping occurs most commonly with bone marrow hypercellularity problems and the storage diseases. As far as bone marrow hypercellularity is concerned the problem arises almost exclusively in Cooley's anemia and mastocytosis. Occasionally it can be seen in sickle cell disease (Fig. 4.64A) and with the storage diseases the most common offender is Gaucher's disease (Fig. 4.64C). Occasionally, however, similar widening can be seen with Niemann-Pick disease and very rarely with histiocytosis X.

Metaphyseal widening also occurs in chronic lead intoxication (8) and here, multiple lead lines provide a clue to its etiology (Fig. 4.64B). Similar widening of the epiphysis, but without the lead lines, is seen in Pyle's cranial metaphyseal dysostosis, other cranial metaphyseal dysplasias, the otopalatodigital syndrome and in osteopetrosis (Fig. 4.64D). In most of these conditions, when widening is quite pronounced, the term **Erlenmeyer flask deformity** often is used.

References

1. Alexander WJ, Dunbar JS: Unusual bone changes in thymic alymphoplasia. *Ann Radiol* 11:389–394, 1968.
2. Bohrer SP: Growth disturbances of the distal femur following sickle cell bone infarcts and/or osteomyelitis. *Clin Radiol* 25:221–235, 1974.
3. Caffey J: Traumatic cupping of the metaphyses of grow-

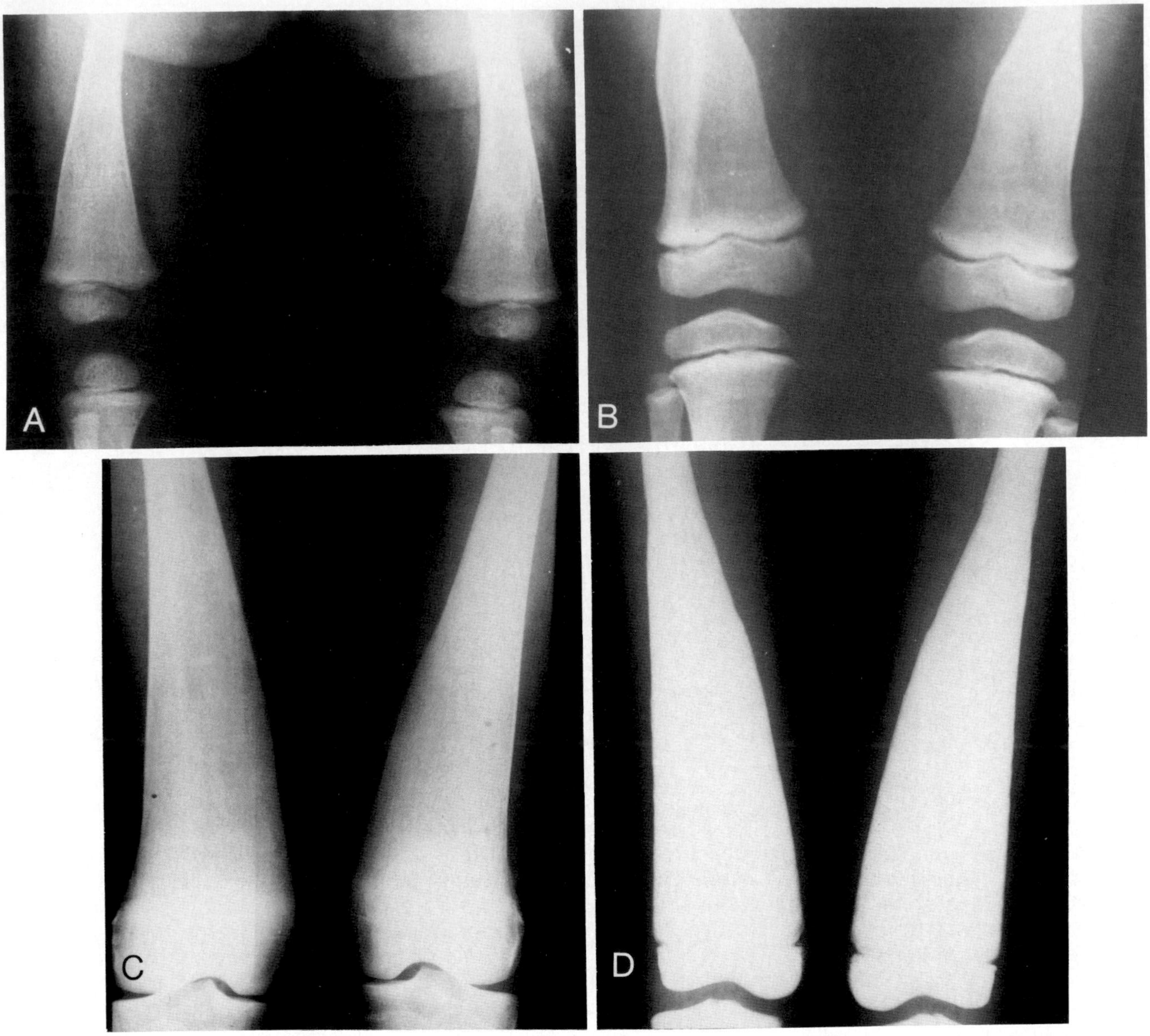

Fig. 4.64. Metaphyseal widening without cupping. A. Minimal widening of the metaphyses of the femurs in a young child with sickle cell disease. B. Marked widening in chronic lead intoxication. Note faint radio-opaque transverse lines. C. Marked metaphyseal widening in older patient with Gaucher's disease. D. Pronounced widening of the metaphyses and extreme increase in bone density in osteopetrosis.

ing bones. *Am J Roentgenol* 108:451–460, 1970.

4. Cederbaum SD, Kaitila I, Rimoin DL, Steihm ER: The chondro-osseous dysplasia of adenosine deaminase deficiency with severe combined immunodeficiency. *J Pediatr* 89:737–742, 1976.

5. Daeschner CW, Singleton EB, Hill LL, Dodge WF: Metaphyseal dysostosis. *J Pediatr* 57:844–854, 1960.

6. Fellman K, Kozlowski K, Senger A: Unusual bone changes in exocrine pancreas insufficiency with cyclic neutropenia. *Acta Radiol* 12:428–432, 1972.

7. McLennan TW, Steinbach HL: Schwachman's syndrome: the broad spectrum of bony abnormalities. *Radiology* 112:167–173, 1974.

8. Pease CN, Newton GG: Metaphyseal dysplasia due to lead poisoning in children. *Radiology* 79:233–240, 1962.

9. Say B, Tinaztepe B, Tinaztepe K, Kiran O: Thymic dysplasia associated with dyschondroplasia in an infant. *Am J Dis Child* 123:240–244, 1972.

10. Schwachman H, Diamond LK, Oski FA, Kwaw K: The syndrome of pancreatic insufficiency and bone marrow dysfunction. *J. Pediatr* 65:645–663, 1964.

11. Taybi H, Mitchell AD, Friedman GD: Metaphyseal dysostosis and the associated syndrome of pancreatic insufficiency and blood disorders. *Radiology* 93: 563–571, 1969.

Metaphyseal Destruction (Table 4.25)

Although bone destruction is the same no matter where it occurs, many times with generalized diseases, bone destruction localized to the metaphysis provides the first clue to the diagnosis. For this reason it is of some merit to consider metaphyseal destruction alone, and in this regard the patterns of destruction encountered include (*a*) mottled destruction, (*b*) homogeneous destruction, and (*c*) focal or cyst-like or scalloped destruction.

Table 4.25 Metaphyseal Destruction

A. Mottled destruction	
Leukemia, lymphoma Metastatic disease	Commonest

Primary bone sarcoma
    Ewing's sarcoma
    Osteomyelitis
	Relatively rare

B. Homogeneous destruction (no
     mottling)
    Osteomyelitis
	Commonest

Bone infarction (sickle cell) Histiocytosis X	Moderately common

Leukemia, lymphoma (advanced)
    Metastatic disease
    Primary bone sarcomas
    Ewing's sarcoma
	Relatively rare

C. Focal cyst-like destruction
    Osteomyelitis
    Histiocytosis X
    Benign cortical defect, en
      face
	Commonest

Small bone cysts
    Leukemia
    Lymphoma
    Metastatic disease
	Moderately common

Primary bone tumor	Relatively rare

Generalized Mottled Destruction

Generalized mottled destruction usually belies a serious problem, and indeed, underlying malignancy usually is the cause. Associated permeative destruction of the cortex commonly occurs and overall, one's first diagnostic considerations should be leukemia, lymphoma, or metastatic disease (Fig. 4.65A). In the early stages, the findings may be difficult to differentiate from simple coarse trabecular demineralization, but with advancing disease, the destructive pattern becomes more obvious. Mottled destruction usually does not occur with infection or infarction, but of course, can occur with primary malignant bone tumors such as fibrosarcoma, osteosarcoma, chondrosarcoma, and Ewing's tumor.

Metaphyseal destruction which is more homogeneous can occur with all the conditions producing mottled destruction, but usually does so when such destruction is very advanced (Fig. 4.65C). Otherwise the problem is more likely to be infection (osteomyelitis) (Fig. 4.65B), infarction (usually in sickle cell anemia), histiocytosis X, or bone necrosis secondary to trophic (ischemic) bone disturbances associated with intrauterine infections such as syphilis, CID, and rubella (2, 3, 7).

In some cases of homogeneous bone destruction **large scooped out areas** of the metaphysis are seen. This type of destruction is especially common in neonates and young infants with widespread osteomyelitis, infants with bone infarction (usually sickle cell disease), and with congenital lues. In congenital lues, when the finding occurs in the upper medial tibiae, the term **Wimberger's sign** is utilized (Fig. 4.65D).

Large scooped out areas of destruction also can occur with advanced lymphoma, leukemia, or meta-

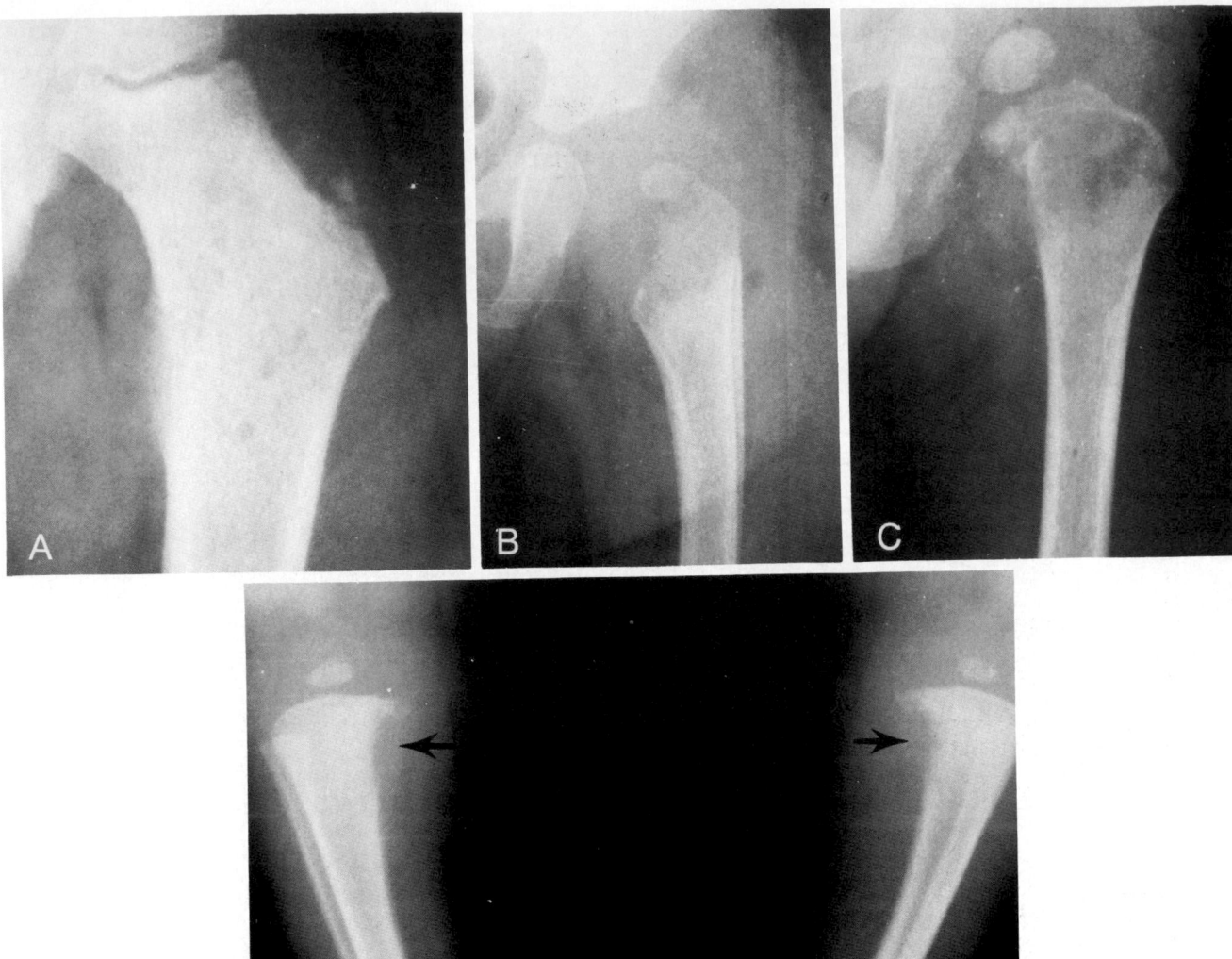

Fig. 4.65. **Metaphyseal destruction.** A. Typical, mottled destruction characteristic of malignancy. This patient had metastatic neuroblastoma. B. Diffuse, homogeneous destruction of upper femur, more characteristic of infection, infarction, etc. This patient had atypical tuberculosis of the bone and hip joint. Note periosteal new bone deposition. C. Homogeneous destruction, with pathologic fracture through upper femur (arrow) in patient with leukemia. D. **Scooped out** medial metaphyseal regions in the upper tibiae in patient with congenital lues (arrows). This constitutes Wimberger's sign.

static disease, and are common in the condition known as infantile fibromatosis (1, 7). Indeed, the lesions in this condition often are virtually indistinguishable from those of congenital syphilis. The cause of the condition is unknown but both bony and systemic varieties exist. If only bone involvement occurs, the prognosis is good, but if widespread visceral involvement is present, the prognosis is poor.

The commonest cause of **focal, cyst-like destruction** within a metaphysis is osteomyelitis (Fig. 4.66A). Many times, a moderately to markedly sclerotic margin of osteoblastic reaction is seen around the area of destruction (Fig. 4.66B). The degree of sclerosis de-

pends on the chronicity of the lesion, and the lesion itself is referred to as a Brodie's abscess. Focal, cyst-like destructive lesions, without any significant sclerosis can be seen with more active osteomyelitis but also are characteristic of histiocytosis X, leukemia, lymphoma, and metastatic disease. Occasionally a small hemangioma, fibroma, chondoma, chondromixoid fibroma, or even an early malignant bony sarcoma also can produce such destruction. More detailed descriptions of some of these lesions are available later (see p 308).

Small bone cysts usually pose no problem in diagnosis because their thin, well-corticated margin and

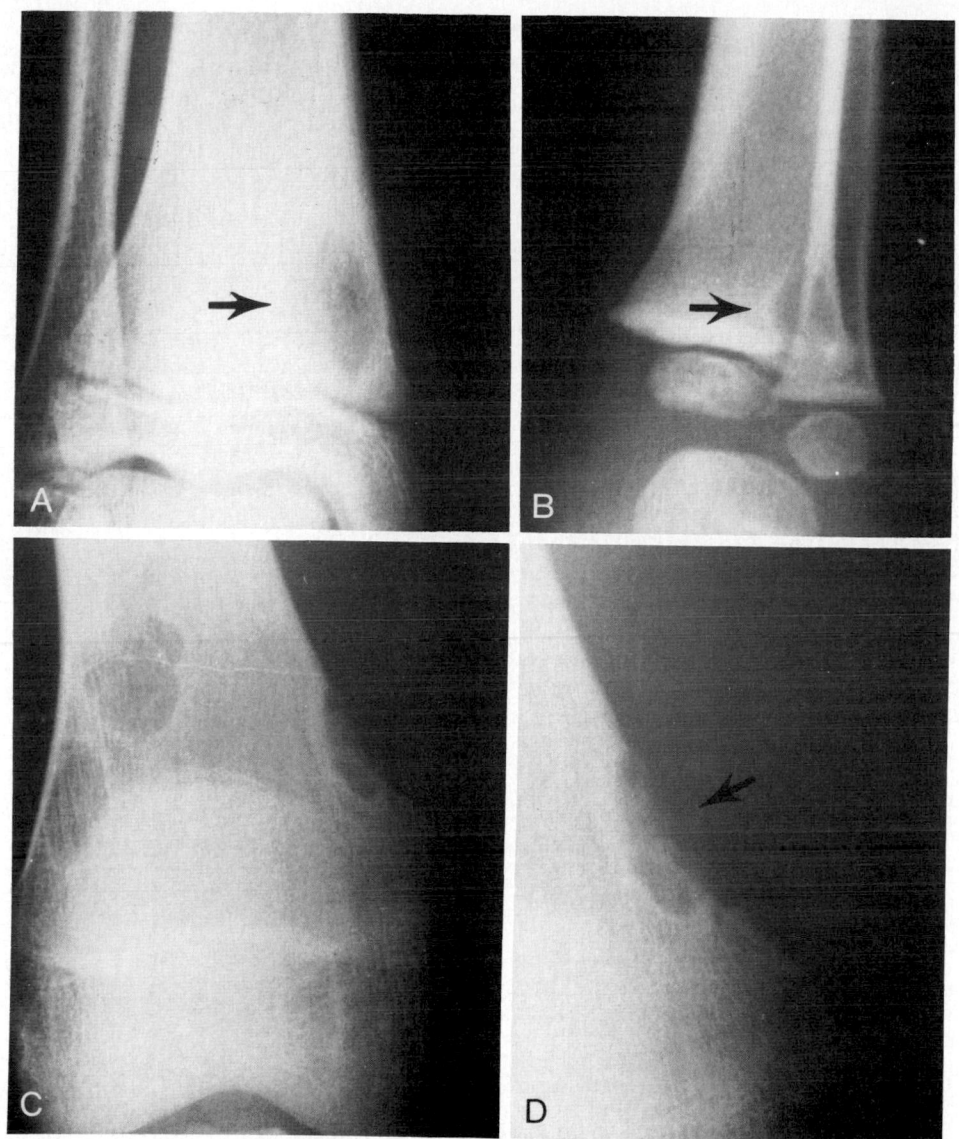

Fig. 4.66.   Metaphyseal destruction—focal. A. Note area of homogeneous destruction (arrow) in distal tibia. There is very little, if any sclerosis. This patient had osteomyelitis. B. Another patient with osteomyelitis showing slight sclerosis around an area of metaphyseal destruction (arrow). A cyst-like appearance is mimicked, but note that the lesion extends into the epiphyseal-metaphyseal plate. C. Typical benign cortical defects in distal femur. D. The eccentric cortical location of one of them (arrow) is diagnostic.

markedly radiolucent interior are characteristic. However, the benign cortical defect, when seen en face, can mimic a focal, cystic, intramedullary lytic lesion and cause problems in diagnosis. It is only when the eccentric nature of this lesion is appreciated that its true identity is established (Fig. 4.66, C and D).

References

1. Baer JW, Radkowski MA: Congenital multiple fibromatosis; a case report with review of the world literature. *Am J Roentgenol* 118:200–205, 1973.
2. Coblentz DR, Cimini R, Mikity VG, Rosen R: Roentgenographic diagnosis of congenital syphilis in the newborn. *JAMA* 212:1061–1064, 1970.
3. Cremin BJ, Fisher RM: The lesions of congenital syphilis. *Br J Radiol* 43:333–341, 1970.
4. Familusi JB, Nottidge VA, Anita AU, Attah EB: Congenital generalized fibromatosis. *Am J Dis Child* 130:1215–1217, 1976.
5. Morettin LB, Mueller E, Schreiber M: Generalized hamartosis (congenital generalized fibromatosis). *Am J Roentgenol* 114:722–734, 1972.
6. Plaschkes J: Congenital fibromatosis. Localized and generalized forms. *J Pediatr Surg* 9:95–101, 1074.
7. Swischuk LE: *Radiology of the Newborn and Young Infant,* ed 2. Baltimore, Williams & Wilkins, 1980, pp 641–650, 685–697.

Grossly Disorganized Epiphyseal-Metaphyseal Areas (Table 4.26)

When one encounters grossly disorganized epiphyseal-metaphyseal areas, almost always a fracture is present. In such cases, excessive motion and bleeding at the fracture site lead to fragmentation, hypercallosis, and marked periosteal new bone deposition. The phenomenon is common in the battered child syndrome and in patients with underlying neurologic or neuromuscular disease (3, 4) for, in either case, excess post-injury motion is common (Fig. 4.67). In neurogenic patients, even with passive flexion and extension, such fractures are commonly induced. Other grossly disorganized epiphyseal-metaphyseal fractures associated with sensory neuropathies, can be seen in chronic diabetes mellitus, syringomyelia, peripheral nerve injury (Fig. 4.67D), tertiary lues, amyotrophic lateral sclerosis, and congenital insensitivity to pain (1, 2, 5). All of these conditions are relatively rare in children.

Gross disorganization of the epiphyseal-metaphyseal regions secondary to fractures also occurs in pathologically diseased bones weakened by severe bone infection (especially osteomyelitis in neonates and infants), bone infarction (usually sickle cell disease in infancy), neonatal infections with trophic disturbances (i.e., lues, rubella, CID), widespread metastatic disease, scurvy, rickets and hyperparathyroidism (Fig. 4.67, E and F).

References

1. Dehen H, et al.: Congenital insensitivity to pain, and endogenous morphine-like substances. *Lancet* 2:293, 1977.
2. Drummond RP, et al.: A twenty-one-year review of a case of congenital indifference to pain. *J Bone Joint Surg* 57B:241, 1975.
3. Gyepes MT, Newbern DH, Neuhauser EBD: Metaphyseal and physeal injuries in children with spina bifida and meningo-myeloceles. *Am J Roentgenol* 95:168–177, 1965.
4. Siegelman SS, Heimann WG, Manin MC: Congenital indifference to pain. *Am J Roentgenol* 97:242, 1966.
5. Silverman FN, Gilden JJ: Congenital insensitivity to pain: A neurologic syndrome with bizzarre skeletal lesions. *Radiology* 72:176, 1959.
6. Vardy PA, Greenberg LW, Kachel C, Falewski de Leon G: Congenital insensitivity to pain with anhidrosis. *Am J Dis Child* 133:1153, 1979.

Table 4.26 Grossly Disorganized Epiphyseal Metaphyseal Junctions

Battered child syndrome Fractures in neurogenic or neuro- muscular disease	Commonest

Fractures in weakened bone
   Osteomyelitis
   Infarction
   Neonatal infections
   Metastatic disease
   Rickets
   Hyperparathyroidism
	Moderately common

Congenital insensitivity to pain
Other sensory neuropathies
   Diabetes mellitus
   Syringomyelia
   Lues
   Amyotrophic lateral sclerosis
Osteogenesis imperfecta
	Rare

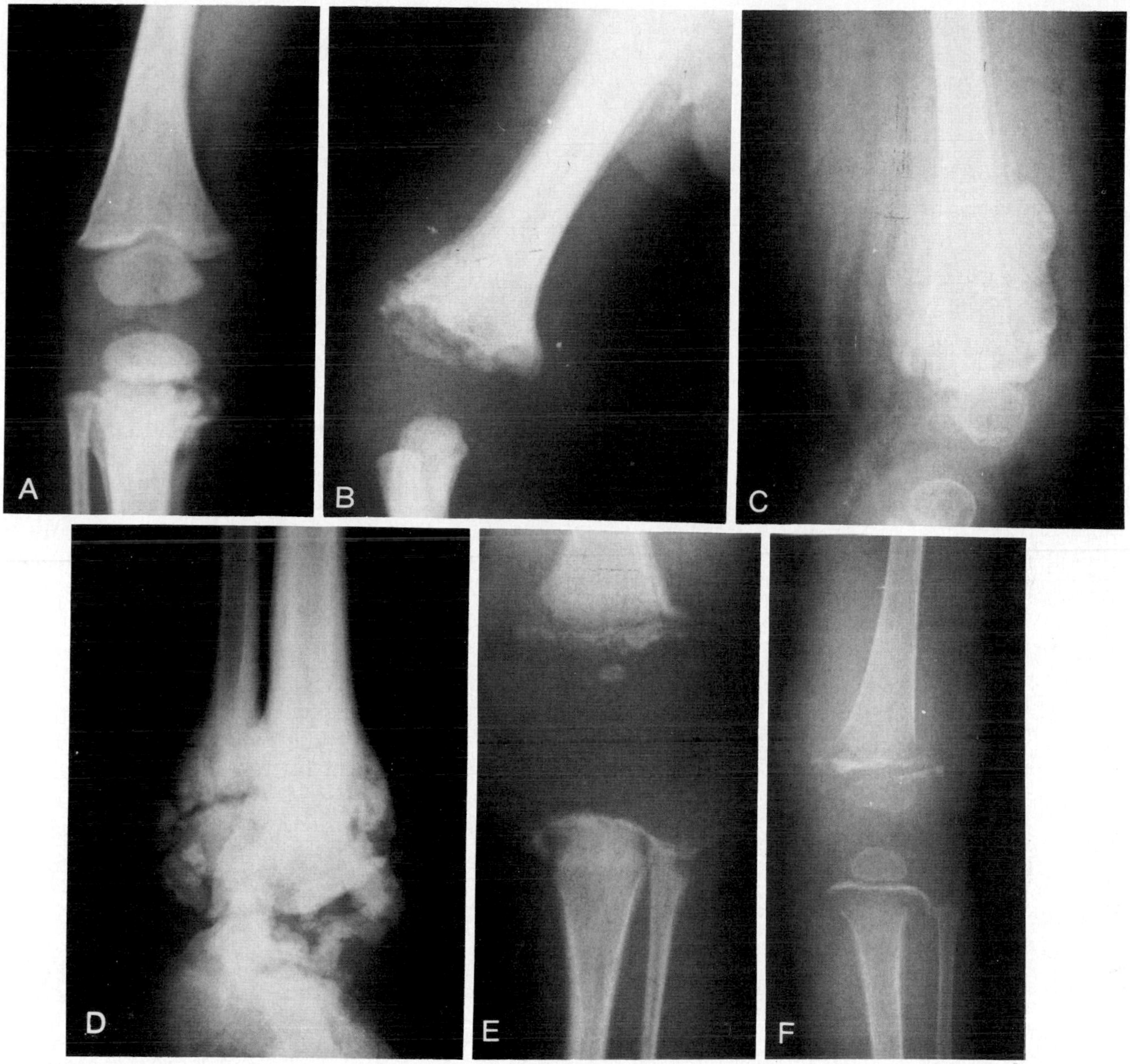

Fig. 4.67. Grossly disorganized epiphyseal-metaphyseal areas. A. Moderately disorganized upper tibial epiphyseal-metaphyseal area secondary to healing fracture in battered child syndrome. Note bending of distal femur from old injury. B. Extensive disorganization of both ends of the humerus in infant with fractures in the battered child syndrome. C. Hypercallosis in neurogenic fracture. Note atrophy of muscle and abundance of fat. Also note that the bones are osteoporotic and thin. D. Severe disorganization-Charcot joint secondary to peripheral nerve injury. E. Disorganized epiphyseal-metaphyseal region with pathologic fracture in congenital lues. F. Similar changes in infant with scurvy.

EPIPHYSEAL LINE ABNORMALITIES

Widened Epiphyseal Line (Table 4.27)

Abnormal widening of the epiphyscal line (physis) generally is due to (*a*) traumatic separation of the epiphysis from the metaphysis or (*b*) impaired enchondral bone formation at the epiphyseal-metaphyseal junction. With the latter the findings tend to be generalized, while with the former they are localized. As far as defective enchondral bone formation is concerned, the commonest cause is some form of rickets (Fig. 4.68A) including renal osteodystrophy. In addition to widening of the epiphyseal line in such cases, the edges of the metaphyses and epiphyses also are indistinct. Similar findings occur with severe hypothyroidism, hypophosphatasia, and conditions mimicking hyperparathyroidism in infancy (i.e., Jansen's meta-

Table 4.27 Widened Epiphyseal Line

Epiphyseal metaphyseal fractures (normal bones) }	Commonest
Epiphyseal metaphyseal fractures (pathologic bones) Rickets (any type) Hyperparathyroidism (secondary in renal osteodystrophy) }	Moderately common
Hyperparathyroidism (primary) Metaphyseal dysostosis }	Relatively rare
Hypophosphatasia Jansen's metaphyseal dysostosis[a] Gangliosidosis[a] Mucolipidosis II[a] }	Rare

[a] Mimic hyperparathyroidism in infancy.

physeal dysostosis, gangliosidosis, mucolipidosis II). In the more chronic forms of hypophosphatasia and in the other metaphyseal dysostoses, although the epiphyseal line may be widened, the edges of the epiphysis and metaphysis are less fuzzy or frayed. Indeed, in metaphyseal dysostosis, the edges may be white and undulating or crinkled (see Fig. 4.61B).

Separation of the epiphysis from the metaphysis, secondary to trauma, most commonly occurs in normal bones (Fig. 4.68B), but it also occurs in structurally weakened bones (i.e., in scurvy, rickets, leukemia, lymphoma, metastatic disease, hyperparathyroidism, etc.). In any of these cases, shearing forces applied across the epiphyseal-metaphyseal junction are the cause of the separations. In such cases, when the epiphysis is markedly displaced, or when there are associated corner fractures of the metaphysis, the fact that an epiphyseal fracture has occurred is not difficult to detect. However, when these associated findings are not present, widening of the epiphyseal line may be the only clue to the presence of the fracture (Fig. 4.68B). Indeed, this is a common situation in the pediatric age group, and it is under such circumstances

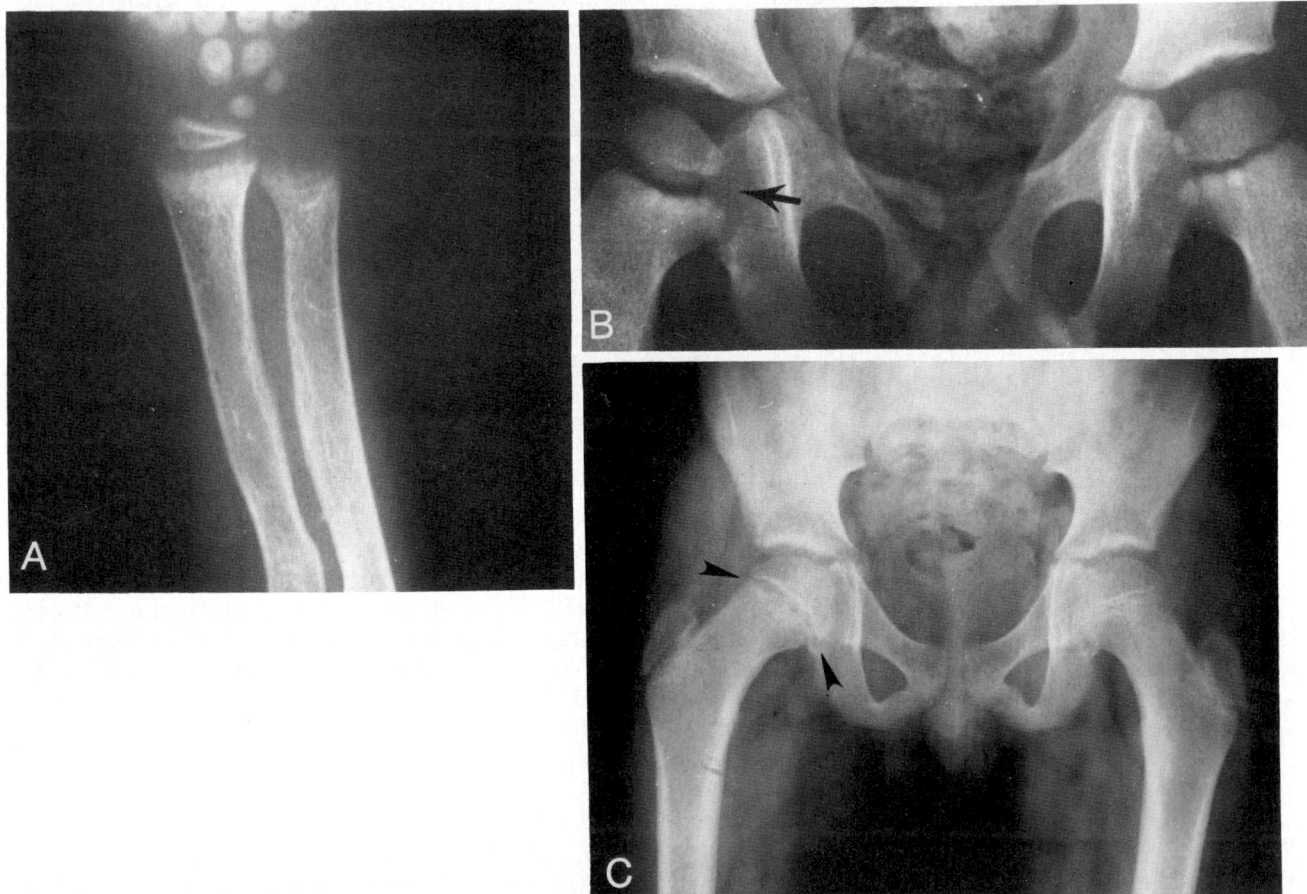

Fig. 4.68. Widened epiphyseal line. A. Widening of the epiphyseal line in rickets. Note also fraying of the metaphysis. B. Widened epiphyseal line (arrow) secondary to epiphyseal-metaphyseal fracture. C. Subtle widening of the epiphyseal line on the right (arrow) secondary to slipped capital femoral epiphysis; early changes.

that examination of the normal side for comparison is extremely important.

Chronic, posttraumatic widening of the epiphyseal line most commonly is seen as the earliest finding in the so-called slipped capital femoral epiphysis syndrome of adolescence. This condition, of unknown etiology, but common in overweight adolescents (especially boys) presents with insidious onset of pain, which then lasts for weeks or months. Often the first roentgenographic findings consist of little more than increased radiolucency and slight widening of the epiphyseal line (Fig. 4.68C).

Finally, before leaving the topic of the widened epiphyseal line, it should be noted that in many perfectly normal children the line may appear unduly wide to the uninitiated examiner. This is especially prone to occur in the wrist, and many times only comparative views finally convince one that the finding is normal.

Spicules in Epiphyseal Line

Most commonly these spicules are seen in perfectly normal children (Fig. 4.69). They probably represent

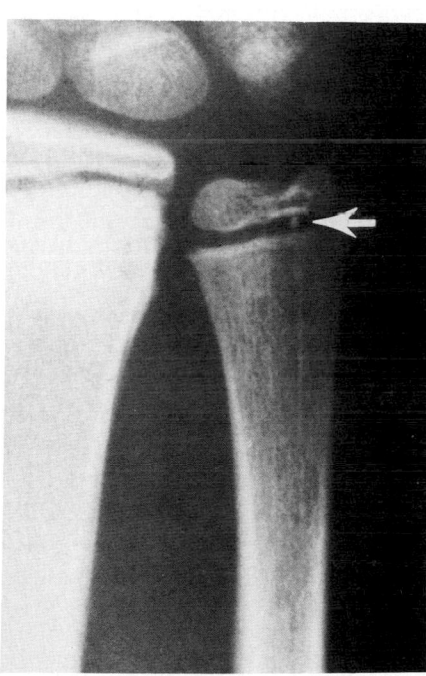

Fig. 4.69. Epiphyseal line spicules. Note spicule (arrow) in the epiphyseal line of the ulna. This patient was normal.

lingering fingers of calcified cartilage and have no particular significance. However, they also have been described with phenylketonuria, homocystinuria, other aminoacidurias (1–5), and also can be seen in some cases of healing rickets. In all cases, these spicules, as growth progresses, can be incorporated into the metaphysis as short, vertical dense lines (Figs. 4.59A and 4.69). Recently, in phenylketonuria it has been demonstrated that these spicules do not occur in adequately treated children (6).

References

1. Feinberg SB, Fisch RO: Roentgenologic findings in growing long bones in phenylketonuria. *Radiology* 78:394–397, 1962.
2. Feinberg SB, Fisch RO: Bone changes in untreated neonatal phenylketonuric patients, a new roentgenographic observation and interpretation. *J Pediatr* 81:540–543, 1972.
3. Fisch RO, Craven HJ, Feinberg SB: Growth and bone characteristics of phenylketonurics. Comparative analysis of treated and untreated phenylketonuric children. *Am J Dis Child* 112:3–10, 1966.
4. Holt JF, Allen RJ: Radiologic signs in the primary aminoacidurias. *Ann Radiol* 10:317–321, 1967.
5. Morreels CL: The roentgenographic features of homocystinuria. *Radiology* 90:1150–1153, 1968.
6. Woodring JH, Rosenbaum HD: Bone changes in phenylketonuria reassessed. *Am J Roentgenol* 137:241–243, 1981.

THE HANDS AND FEET

There are so many findings, both normal and abnormal, in the hands and feet that one can be overwhelmed with details. By the same token, not all are of equal importance, and thus, this section deals with those utilized most often in sorting out various diseases, syndromes, and dysplasias. Generally, changes in the hands are more important than those in the feet, and foot changes are alluded to only if they are diagnostically specific. If they are similar to those in the hands, no specific mention is made.

Terminal Phalanges

Before analyzing terminal phalangeal changes it should be noted that there is considerable difference in appearance of these bones from one normal person to another. Some terminal phalanges are tapered, while others are more clubbed (Fig. 4.70) and actually, differentiation between normal and abnormal may be difficult. However, some of the changes are specific enough to allow them to be utilized in the differential diagnosis of certain conditions.

CLUBBING OF TERMINAL PHALANGES

Clubbing is a soft tissue phenomenon and usually is more readily detectable clinically than roentgenographically. However, in some cases there is enough widening of the terminal tufts of the distal phalanges to allow roentgenographic identification. Clubbing occurs with chronic cyanotic congenital heart disease, chronic gastrointestinal disease, chronic respiratory disease, intrathoracic tumors such as mesothelioma, and in the condition known as pachydermoperiostitis. The latter condition is familial and associated with idiopathic periosteal new bone deposition and calvarial defects. Clubbing also occurs in acromegaly, but acromegaly is an adult diagnosis. In childhood gigantism is the counterpart, and clubbing is not a significant feature.

DRUMSTICK TERMINAL PHALANGES

Drumstick terminal phalanges result any time the shaft of the phalanx is disproportionately thinned in comparison to the tuft (Fig. 4.71). Clearly, the problem can be either in the tuft or in the shaft and, furthermore, some degree of drumsticking is present in some

normal individuals. However, true drumstick terminal phalanges have been identified in Turner's syndrome, trisomy 21, the Cri du Chat syndrome, Coffin's syndrome, and the cardiomelic or Holt-Oram syndrome (1-5). One must hasten to add, however, that not every case of these syndromes demonstrates drumstick terminal phalanges.

References

1. Coffin GS, Siris E, Wegienka LC: Mental retardation with osteocartilaginous anomalies. *Am J Dis Child* 112:205, 1066.
2. Kosowicz J: The roentgen appearance of the hand and wrist in gonadal dysgenesis. *Am J Roentgenol* 93:354–361, 1965.
3. Necic S, Grant DB: Diagnostic value of hand x-rays in Turner's syndrome. *Acta Paediatr Scand* 67:309–213, 1978.
4. Poznanski AK: *The Hand in Radiologic Diagnosis*. Philadelphia, W.B. Saunders, 1974, p 228.
5. Procopis PG, Turner B: Mental retardation, abnormal fingers and skeletal anomalies: Coffin's syndrome. *Am J Dis Child* 214:258–261, 1972.

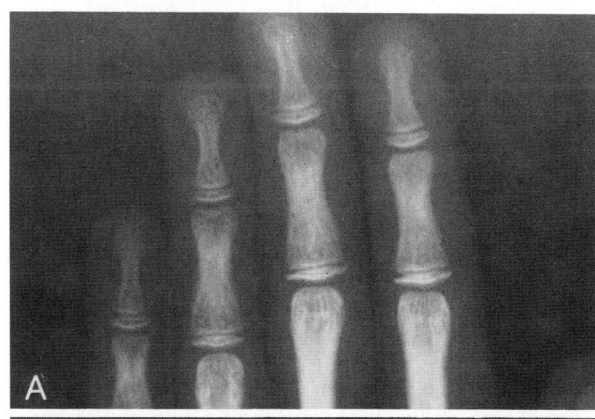

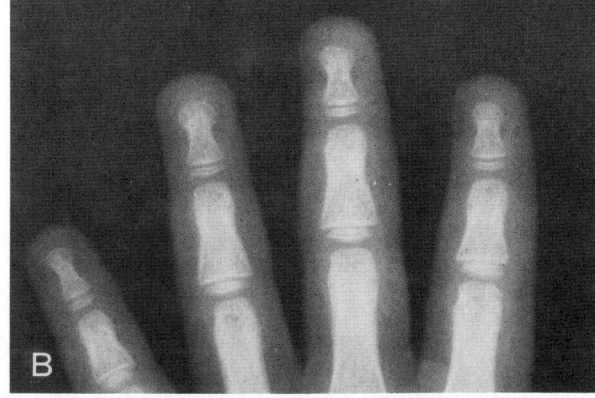

Fig. 4.71. Drumstick terminal phalanges. A. Typical drumstick-shaped terminal phalanges in Turner's syndrome. B. Another patient with suspected Turner's syndrome and squat, drumstick terminal phalanges.

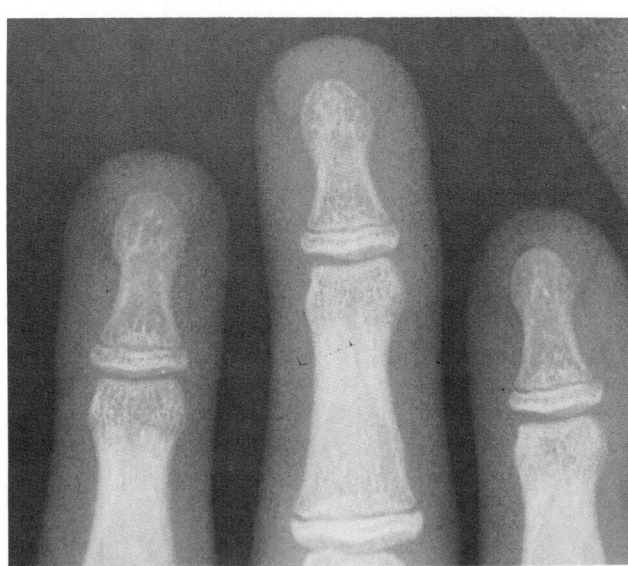

Fig. 4.70. Normal terminal phalanges. Note slightly club-shaped terminal phalanges in a normal child.

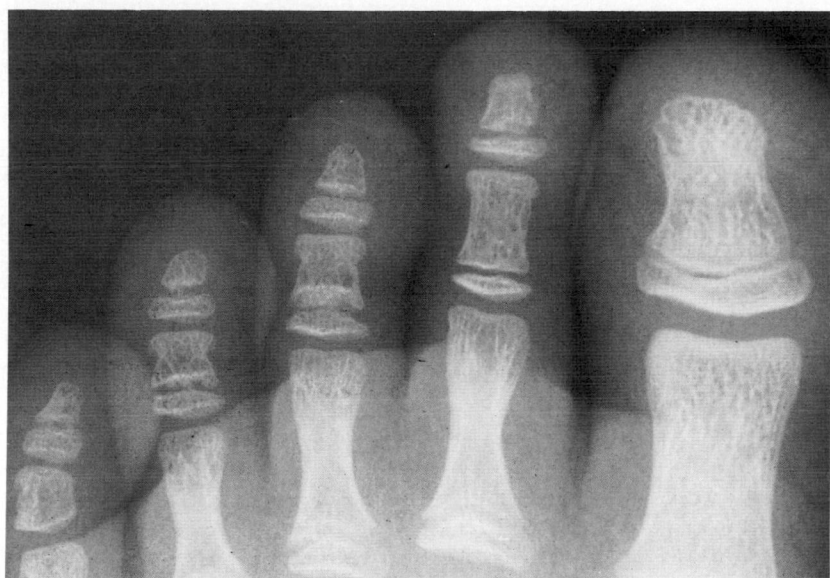

Fig. 4.72. **Hypoplastic terminal phalanges.** A. Normal, small terminal phalanges in foot.

HYPOPLASTIC TERMINAL PHALANGES

Hypoplastic terminal phalanges should be differentiated from destroyed or eroded terminal phalanges. The latter are dealt with in the next section, and in this section only those terminal phalanges which are inherently underdeveloped, or hypoplastic, are considered. Such phalanges may appear spindle-shaped or frankly stubbed-off, but once again variation is common. Stubbed-off phalanges are common in the normal foot (Fig. 4.72), but in the hand, when a hypoplastic terminal phalanx is encountered some pathologic condition should be considered. For the most part these include: any number of conditions associated with hypoplastic fingernails (7), trisomy 18, trisomy 13, Aarskog syndrome, cleidocranial dysostosis (Fig. 4.73, A and B), asphyxiating thoracic dystrophy, dilantin embryonopathy (2) (Fig. 4.73, C and D), Ellis-van Creveld syndrome, otopalatodigital syndrome, scalp defect and hand anomaly syndrome (1), pseudo and pseudopseudohypoparathyroidism, Larsen's syndrome, Coffin-Siris syndrome (1, 5), Turner's syndrome (2–4), and all of the conditions producing a spade hand (see Fig. 4.81). In some cases of terminal phalangeal underdevelopment, the epiphysis is overgrown and is of a size, near equal to that of the phalanx. In such cases, hyperphalangealism erroneously is suggested (Fig. 4.73D), and most recently this has been described in dilantin embryonopathy (2).

References

1. Barr M Jr, Poznanski AK, Schmickel RD: Digital hypoplasia and anticonvulsants during gestation; a teratogenic syndrome? *J Pediatr* 84:254–256, 1974.
2. Coffin GS, Siris E, Wegienka LC: Mental retardation with osteocartilaginous anomalies. *Am J Dis Child* 112:205, 1966.
3. Kosowicz J: The roentgen appearance of the hand and wrist in gonadal dysgenesis. *Am J Roentgenol* 93:354–361, 1965.
4. Necic S, Grand DB: Diagnostic value of hand x-rays in Turner's syndrome. *Acta Paediatr Scand* 67:309–313, 1978.
5. Poznanski AK: *The Hand in Radiologic Diagnosis.* Philadelphia, W. B. Saunders, 1974, p 228.
6. Procopis PG, Turner B: Mental retardation, abnormal fingers and skeletal anomalies: Coffin's syndrome. *Am J Dis Child* 214:258–261, 1972.
7. Taybi H: *Radiology of Syndromes.* Chicago, Year Book Medical Publishers, 1975, p 328.
8. Wood BP, Young LW: Pseudohyperphalangism in fetal dilantin. *Radiology* 131:371–372, 1979.

DISTAL PHALANGEAL RESORPTION OR DESTRUCTION

The most common cause of resorption of the terminal tufts of the distal phalanges is hyperparathyroidism in childhood and, in this regard, secondary hyperparathyroidism, or renal osteodystrophy, is much more common than primary hyperparathyroidism. Nonetheless, in either situation resorption of the terminal phalanges is rather characteristic (Fig. 4.74). Other acquired causes of terminal phalangeal resorption or destruction include frostbite, thermal injury, syringomyelia, trauma, infection, leprosy (6), psoriasis, the hyperuricemia (fingerbiting syndrome of Lesch-Nyhan) (1), and polyvinyl chloride toxicity (2). In almost all of these cases, except for hyperparathyroidism, the problem probably results from a vasculitis or vessel spasm leading to bone necrosis. Indeed, even in congenital causes of distal phalangeal resorption, the same problem likely is present, and as far as these

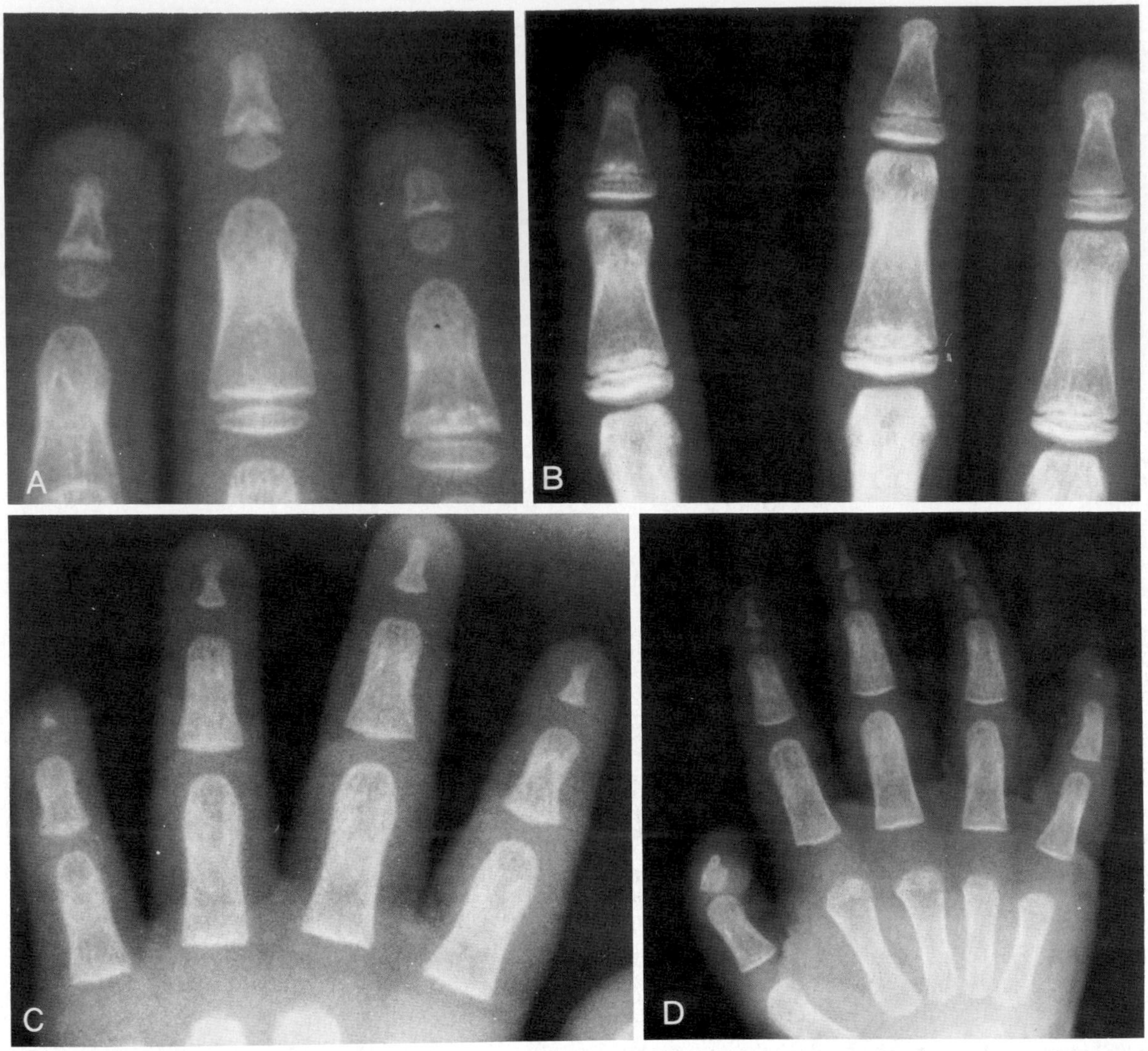

Fig. 4.73. Hypoplastic terminal phalanges. A. Small hypoplastic terminal phalanges in young child with cleido-cranial dysostosis. Also note slight cone-shaped epiphysis. B. Older child with cleidocranial dysostosis showing thin, tapered distal phalanges. C. Infant with Dilantin embryopathy and small spindle-shaped terminal phalanges. D. Another child with Dilantin embryopathy showing small, hypoplastic terminal phalanges and so-called **pseudohy-perphalangealism.**

syndromes are concerned, one should consider the following: idiopathic acro-osteolysis (2), progeria, pyc-nodysostosis, osteopetrosis (5), Ehler-Danlos syn-drome (3), pseudoxanthoma elasticum, Rothmund's syndrome (4), congenital insensitivity to pain (con-genital sensory neuropathy), and epidermolysis bul-losa. Distal phalangeal resorption also can occur, on an isolated basis, with osteomyelitis of the distal pha-lanx, and on a more generalized basis in patients with burn contractures (with or without associated osteo-myelitis).

References

1. Becker MH, Wallin JK: Congenital hyperuricosuria: associated radiologic features. *Radiol Clin North Am* 6:239–243, 1968.

2. Brown DM, Bradford DS, Gorlin RJ, Desnick RJ, Lan-ger LO Jr, Jowsey J, Sauk JJ Jr: The acroosteolysis syndrome: morphologic and biochemical studies. *J Pe-diatr* 88:573–575, 1976.
3. Mabille JP, Castera D, Chapuis JL, Lambert D, Cha-pelon M: A case of Ehlers-Danlos syndrome with ac-roosteolysis. *Ann Radiol* 15:781–786, 1972.
4. Maurer RM, Langford OL: Rothmund's syndrome. A cause of resorption of phalangeal tufts and dystorphic calcification. *Radiology* 89:706–708, 1967.
5. Moss A, Mainzer F: Osteopetrosis: an unusual cause of terminal-tuft erosion. *Radiology* 97:631–632, 1970.
6. Newman H, Casey B, DuBois JJ, Gallagher T: Roentgen features of leprosy in children. *Am J Roentgenol* 114:402–410, 1972.
7. Taybi H: Radiology of syndromes. Chicago, Year Book Medical Publishers, 1975, p 328.

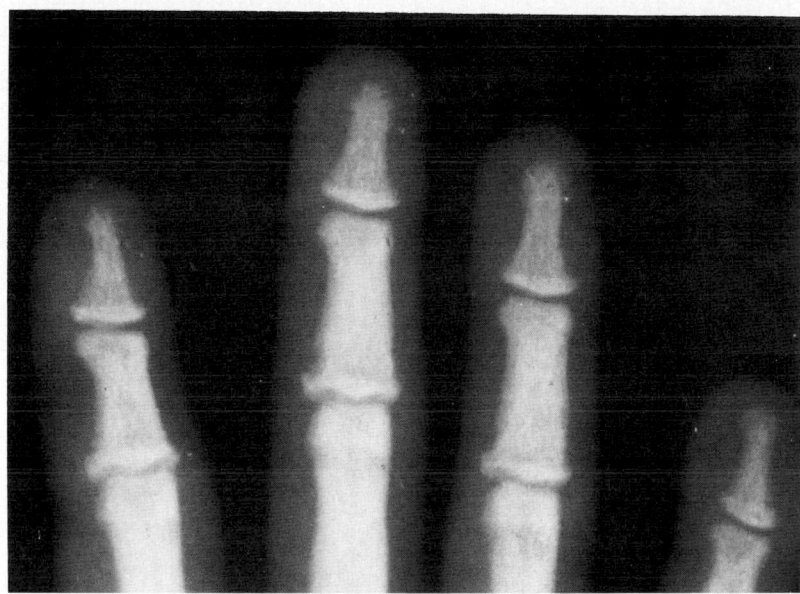

Fig. 4.74. Distal phalangeal resorption. Note resorption of terminal phalanges in advanced secondary hyperparathyroidism.

Middle and Proximal Phalanges

Except for the middle phalanx of the fifth digit, middle or proximal phalangeal hypoplasia is relatively uncommon. Hypoplasia of the middle phalanx of the fifth digit is dealt with later (see Fig. 4.80B). Middle or distal phalangeal underdevelopment can be acquired after osteomyelitis, bone infarction, trauma, or septic arthritis. On a congenital basis, generalized shortening of the middle phalanges, often is associated with hypoplasia of the distal phalanges and can be seen in the following syndromes: acrocephalosyndactyly (Apert's syndrome; see Fig. 4.77C), Poland's syndrome, and the tricho-rhino-phalangeal syndrome (see Fig. 4.51C). There are no specific syndromes where the proximal phalanges are shortened on an isolated basis.

Metacarpals and Metatarsals

For the most part, metacarpal and metatarsal problems center around shortening of one or more of these bones. Overly long metacarpals and metatarsals also can be seen but usually occur as part of an underlying syndrome such as Marfan's syndrome, homocystinuria, etc. In such cases, they are not used selectively for diagnosis.

Shortening of the first metacarpal and metatarsal are dealt with later along with other abnormalities of the thumb and great toe. In this section, shortening of the other metacarpals and metatarsals is considered, and generally what can be said for the metacarpals holds for the metatarsals.

SHORT METACARPALS AND METATARSALS

It is helpful to consider the third, fourth, and fifth metacarpals as a unit, even though only one of these may be shortened. The reason for this is that many syndromes cause shortening of these bones as a unit. However, when only the fourth and fifth metacarpals appear shortened, it is important to determine whether one's observations are true because often, perfectly normal metacarpals appear shortened to the inexperienced observer. To determine whether the fourth and fifth metacarpals are truly shortened one can apply the so-called metacarpal line. Originally developed for assessing metacarpal shortening in Turner's syndrome (2–5), the line is drawn along the heads of the fourth and fifth metacarpals and then it is noted where it intersects the third metacarpal. When the sign is positive, the line intersects the head of the third metacarpal, when borderline it just grazes the head, and when normal, it misses the head (Fig. 4.75).

Perhaps the two conditions best known for producing shortening of the third through fifth metacarpals are the just-mentioned Turner's syndrome and pseudo or pseudopseudohypoparathyroidism (5, 6) (Fig. 4.76, A and B). In addition to these conditions, the metacarpals or metatarsals can be shortened on an isolated basis (Fig. 4.76C), and with the following syndromes: basal cell nevus syndrome, Beckwith-Wiedemann syndrome, Biedmon syndrome, Larsen's syndrome, the multiple exostoses syndrome, the various epiphyseal

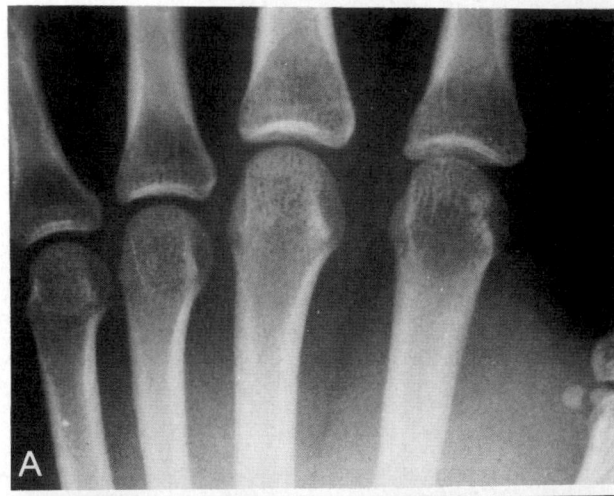

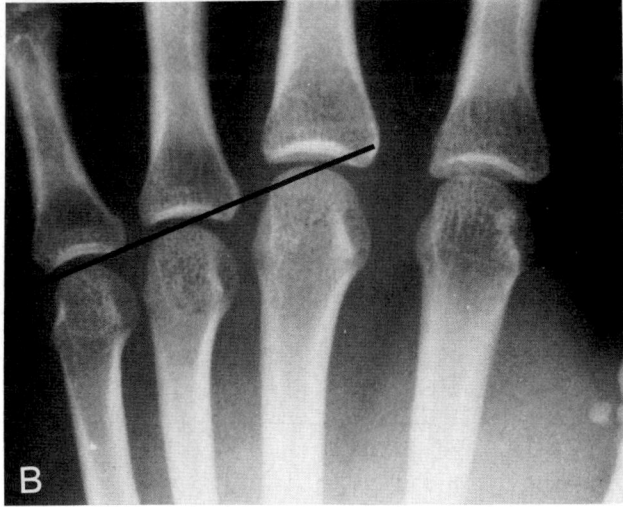

Fig. 4.75. Positive, metacarpal sign. A. Note shortening of the fourth and fifth metacarpals. B. Metacarpal line drawn across the heads of the fourth and fifth metacarpals intersects head of the third metacarpal.

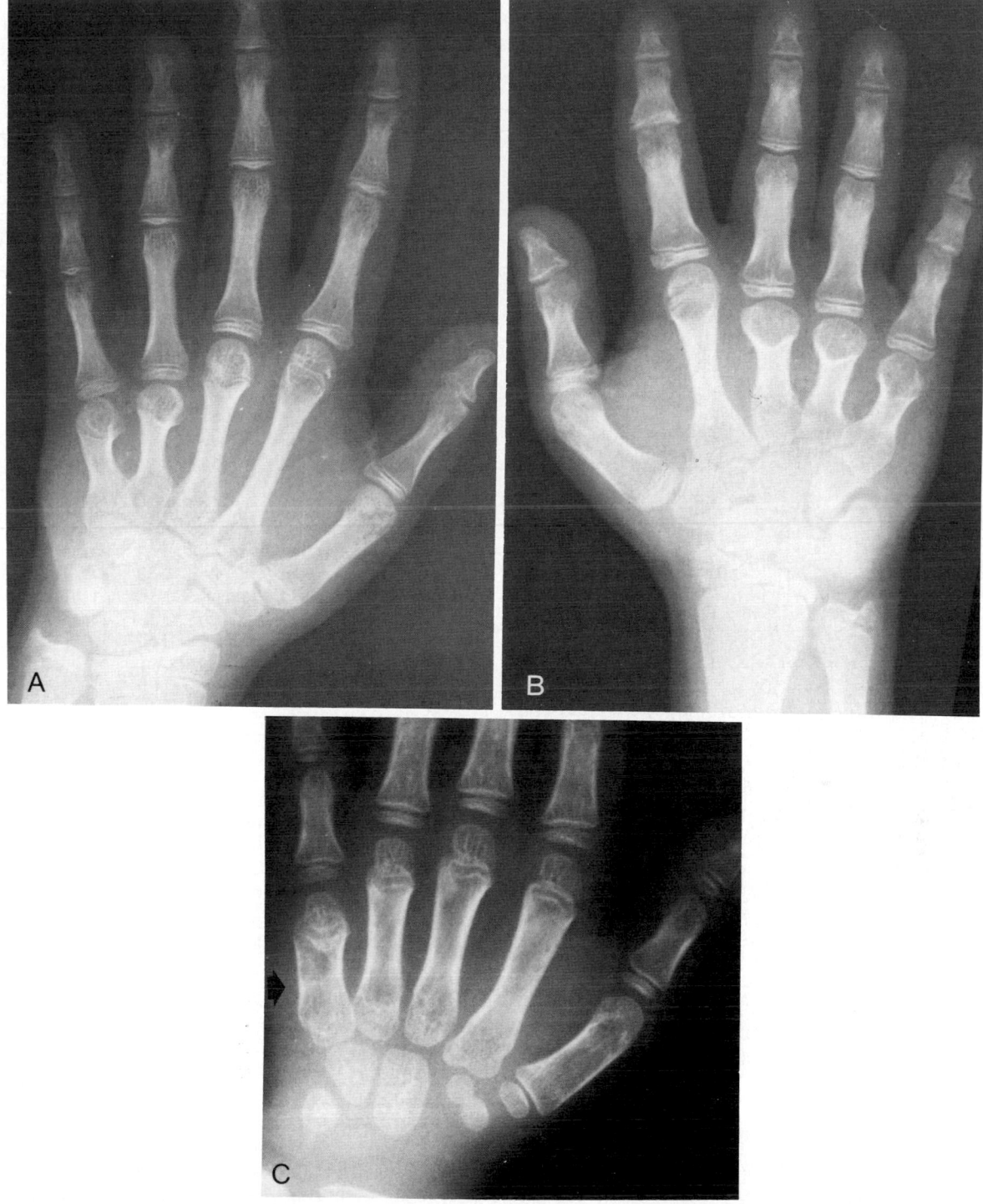

Fig. 4.76.   Short metacarpals. A. Typical short fourth and fifth metacarpals in Turner's syndrome. Also note carpal fusion and drumstick terminal phalanges. B. Similar shortening of the fourth, fifth, and sixth metacarpals in pseudohypoparathyroidism. Note that all of the small bones of the hands are shortened. C. Isolated, incidental shortening of the fifth metacarpal (arrow), in normal individual.

dysplasias, and the tricho-rhinophalangeal syndrome. In any of these conditions, only the fifth metacarpal may be shortened. Other conditions in which only the fifth metacarpal is shortened include the cat-cry (Cri-du-Chat) syndrome and Russell-Silver dwarfism (congenital hemiatrophy). Finally, it should be noted that short fourth and fifth metacarpals, of no consequence at all, occur in approximately ten percent of normal individuals (1).

References

1. Bloom RA: The metacarpal sign. *Br J Radiol* 43:133–135, 1970.
2. Finby N, Archibald RM: Skeletal abnormalities associated with gonadal dysgenesis. *Am J Roentgenol* 89:1222–1235, 1963.
3. Kosowicz J: The roentgen appearance of the hand and wrist in gonadal dysgenesis. *Am J Roentgenol* 93:354–

361, 1965.
4. Necic S, Grant DB: Diagnostic value of hand x-rays in Turner's syndrome. *Acta Paediatr Scand* 67:309–312, 1978.
5. Poznanski AK, Werder EA, Giedion A: The pattern of shortening of the bones of the hand in PHP and PPHP-A comparison with brachydactyly E, Turner syndrome, and acrodysostosis. *Radiology* 123:707–718, 1977.
6. Steinback HL, Young DA: The roentgen appearance of pseudohypoparathyroidism (PH) and pseudo-pseudo hypoparathyroidism (PPH), differentiation from other syndromes associated with short metacarpals, metatarsals and phalanges. *Am J Roentgenol* 97:49–66, 1966.

The Thumb and Great Toe

SHORT, BROAD THUMB OR GREAT TOE

Shortening of the first digit often is more evident clinically than radiographically, and perhaps the most striking radiologic findings are seen in the Rubenstein-Taybi (mental retardation and broad thumbs), and acrocephalosyndactyly syndromes (Fig. 4.77, A–C). In both of these conditions, the thumbs and great toes also may be double. Other conditions demonstrating broad thumbs and great toes, but not usually duplicated, include the otopalatodigital syndrome (Fig. 4.77D), the hand-foot-uterus syndrome, progressive myositis ossificans (Fig. 4.77E), diastrophic dwarfism, the frontodigital syndrome, and pleonosteosis. The thumb also is short and broad when there is isolated hypoplasia of the distal phalanx of the thumb. This particular deformity has no diagnostic specificity, and usually occurs as an isolated finding in otherwise normal individuals.

HYPOPLASTIC, THIN THUMB

Conditions producing a hypoplastic, but thin, thumb include the Holt-Oram syndrome (see Fig. 4.23), Fanconi's anemia, the thrombocytopenia absent radius syndrome (thumb only minimally hypoplastic or normal), trisomy 18, the Cornelia de Lange syndrome, and any of the conditions leading to a triphalangeal thumb (see next section).

TRIPHALANGEAL THUMB

In this deformity the thumb has an extra phalanx and appears more like the other digits. Rarely it can occur as a normal variation, and in any case may be associated with duplication of the thumb or absence of the contralateral thumb. As far as syndromes are concerned, triphalangeal thumbs can occur in the Blackfan-Diamond congenital anemia syndrome (2, 3), the Holt-Oran syndrome (Fig. 4.78) trisomy 13-15 (rarely), Poland's (absent pectoralis muscle) syndrome, Werner's mesomelic dysplasia (1), the Juberg-Hayward syndrome, and thalidomide embryonopathy (4).

References

1. Hall CM: Werner's mesomelic dysplasia and ventricular septal defect and Hirschsprung's disease. *Pediatr Radiol* 10:247–249, 1981.
2. Jones B, Thompson H: Triphalangeal thumbs associated with hypoplastic anemia. *Pediatrics* 52:609–612, 1973.
3. Murphy S, Lubin B: Triphalangeal thumbs and congenital erythroid hypoplasia: report of a case with unusual features. *J Pediatr* 81:987–989, 1972.
4. Poznanski AK, Garn SM, Holt JF: The thumb in the congenital malformation syndromes. *Radiology* 100:115–129, 1971.

HYPOPLASTIC FIRST METACARPAL OR METATARSAL

A hypoplastic first metacarpal, or metatarsal, can be seen as an isolated anomaly, but more often is seen in some syndrome (1). Perhaps the best known conditions resulting in shortening of the first metacarpal are those constituting the so-called radial ray syndrome (hypoplastic radius and thumb). For the most part, these include Fanconi's anemia, the Holt-Oram syndrome (see Fig. 4.23), and the thrombocytopenia absent radius (TAR) syndrome. In the latter, however, changes in the thumb usually are minimal or virtually nonexistent. Hypoplasia of the first metacarpal also occurs with syndromes exhibiting a triphalangeal thumb (see previous section). Other syndromes in which the first metacarpal, or metatarsal, are shortened or hypoplastic include the Juberg-Hayward syndrome, the Cornelia de Lange syndrome, progressive myositis ossificans (Fig. 4.79A), trisomy 18 (Fig. 4.79B), the hand-foot-uterus syndrome, diastrophic dwarfism, the VATER syndrome, and all of the conditions presenting with short broad thumbs and toes.

Reference

1. Poznanski AK, Garn SM, Hold JF: The thumb in the congenital malformation syndromes. *Radiology* 100:115–129, 1971.

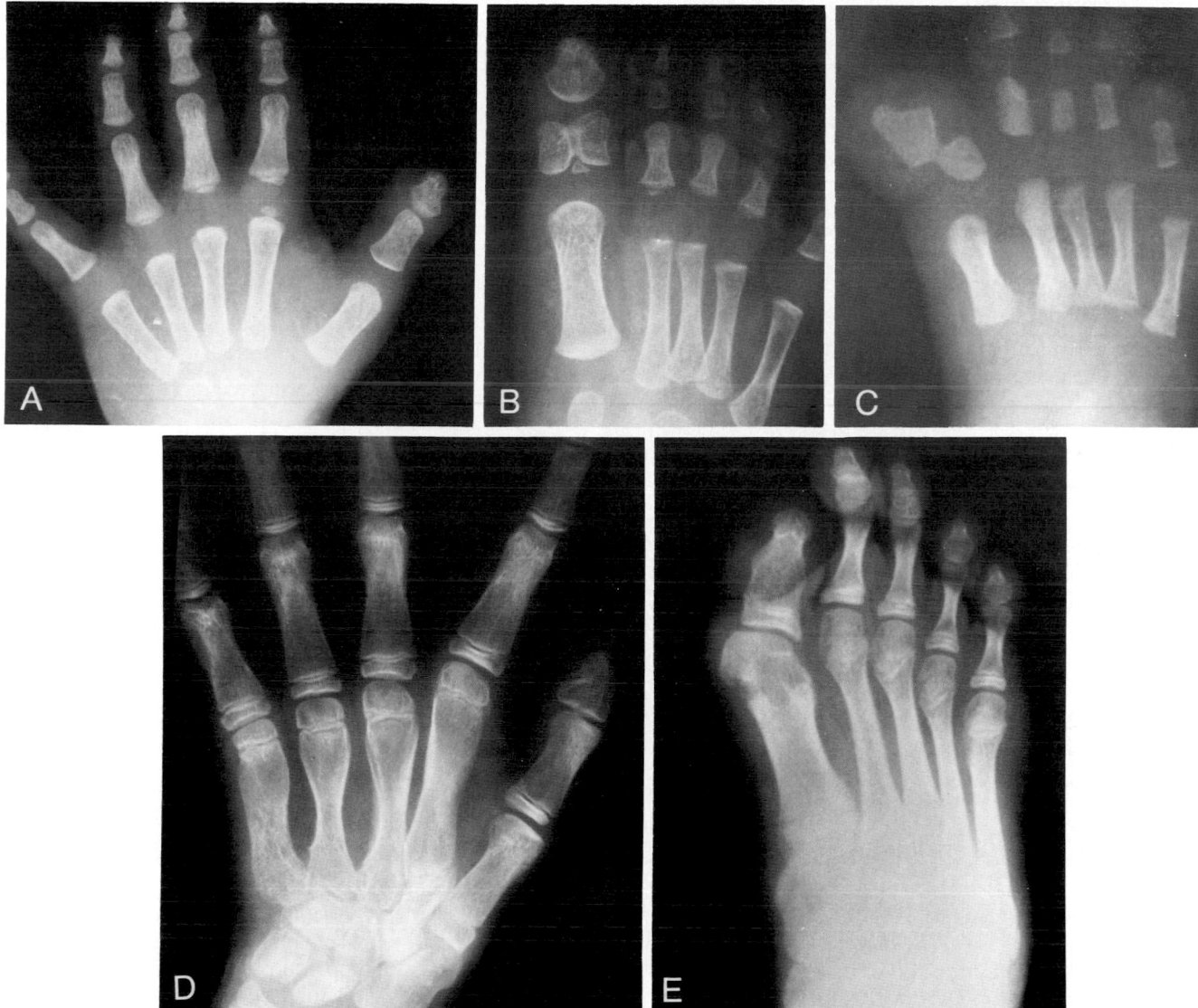

Fig. 4.77. Short broad thumbs and toes. A. Broad thumb in Rubenstein-Taybi syndrome. B. Broad, bifid great toe in same patient. C. Short broad toe in acrocephalosyndactyly. Note other anomalies including symphalangism and hypoplasia of the phalanges. D. Broad thumb in otopalatodigital syndrome. Note other characteristic changes. E. Short, somewhat broad great toe, with fusion of the phalanges, in progressive myositis ossificans.

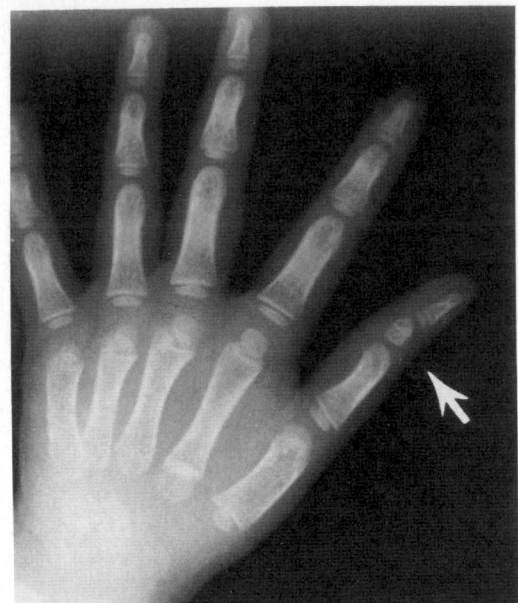

Fig. 4.78.   Triphalangeal thumb. Typical triphalangeal thumb (arrow) in Holt-Oram syndrome.

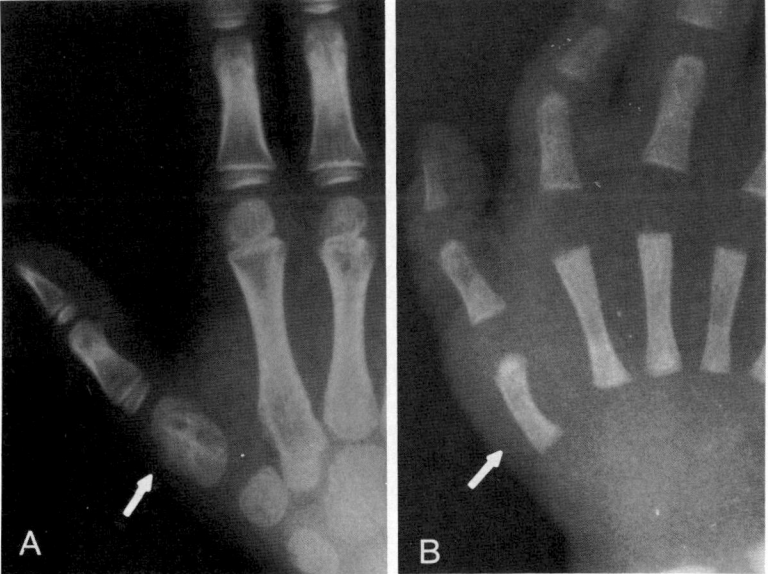

Fig. 4.79.   Short, hypoplastic first metacarpal or metatarsal. A. Note short metacarpal in progressive myositis ossificans (arrow). B. Short metacarpal (arrow) with slight shortening of the phalanges of the thumb in trisomy 18 (arrow). For a thin, hypoplastic metacarpal in Fanconi's anemia, see Figure 4.23.

Fifth Digit Abnormalities

For the most part, abnormalities of the **fifth digit involve the hand,** and are incurving deformities, i.e., clinodactyly and Kirner's deformity. Clinodactyly of the fifth digit is associated with hypoplasia of the middle phalanx while Kirner's deformity is isolated to the terminal phalanx. (Fig. 4.80). Some believe it to be a form of epiphyseal dysplasia (1, 3, 5). The condition usually is bilateral and occurs as an isolated finding (Fig. 4.79A). However, it can be seen, with some frequency, in the Cornelia de Lange and Russell-Silver syndromes. The findings are rather typical but often misinterpreted for posttraumatic or infectious changes.

Ordinary clinodactyly of the fifth digit is seen in so many conditions that its diagnostic value is diminished (Table 4.28). In addition, it can be seen, on an isolated basis, in some normal individuals (1, 2).

References

1. Blank E, Girdany BR: Symmetric bowling of the terminal phalanges of the fifth fingers in a family (Kirner's deformity). *Am J Roentgenol* 93:367–373, 1965.

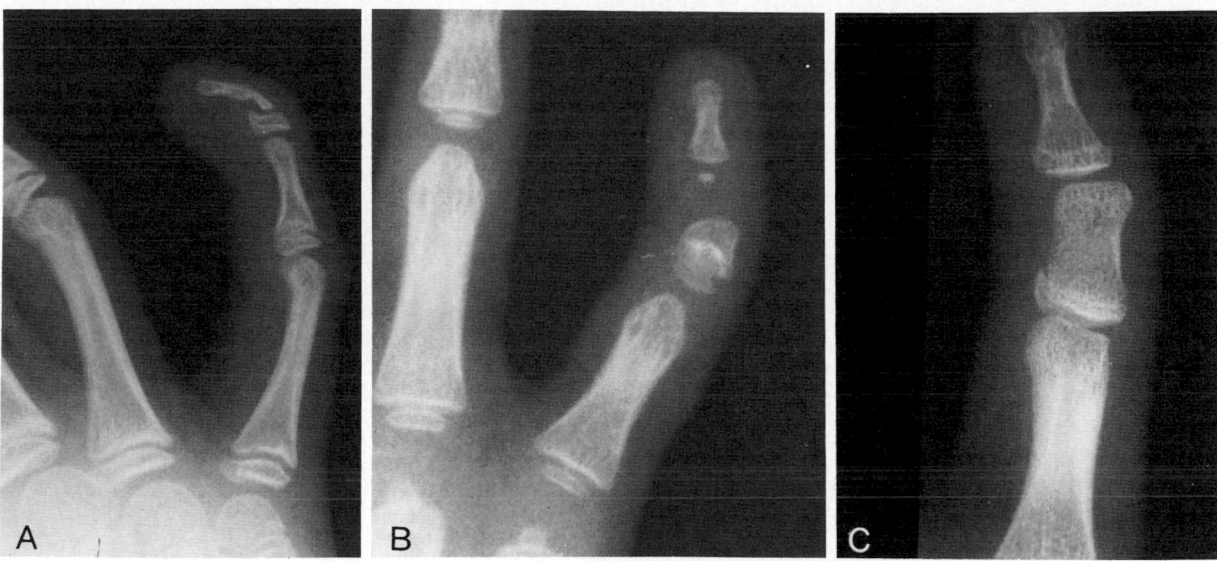

Fig. 4.80. Curved fingers. A. Typical configuration of Kiner's deformity. Note that the terminal phalanx of the fifth digit appears dysplastic. B. Curved fifth digit with hypoplastic middle phalanx in trisomy 21. C. Normal individual with curved fifth digit and hypoplastic middle phalanx.

Table 4.28   Clinodactyly Fifth Digit

More Common Conditions	Less Common Conditions
Normal	Syndromes
Sporadic	Aarskog syndrome
With other middle phalanx hypoplasia	Bloom's syndrome
Syndromes	Cerebrohepatorenal syndrome
Acrocephalosyndactyly	Cri-du-Chat (cat-cry) syndrome
Campomelic dwarfism	Holt-Oram syndrome
Cornelia de Lange syndrome	Nievergelt's syndrome
Fanconi's anemia	Osteo-onychodysplasia
Goltz's syndrome	Oro-digital-facio syndrome I, II
Hand-foot syndrome	Otopalatodigital syndrome
Klinefelter's syndrome	Popliteal pterygium syndrome
Laurence-Moon-Biedl-Bardet syndrome	Rieger's syndrome
Marfan's syndrome	Senior syndrome
Myositis ossificans progressiva	Seckel's bird-headed dwarf
Noonan's syndrome	Thrombocytopenia-absent radius (TAR) syndrome
Oculo-dento-osseous dysplasia	Tricho-rhino-phalangeal syndrome
Poland's syndrome	Penta X (XXXXX) syndrome
Russell-Silver syndrome	Wolf's syndrome (4p syndrome)
Trisomy 18	XXXY syndrome
Trisomy 21	Whistling face syndrome
Trisomy 13	Oculodentodigital syndrome

2. Greulich WW: A comparison of the dysplastic middle phalanx of the fifth finger in mentally normally Caucasions, Mongoloids, and Negroes with that of individuals of the racial groups who have Down's syndrome. *Am J Roentgenol* 118:259–281, 1973.

3. Kaufmann HJ, Taillard WF: Bilateral incurving of the terminal phalanges of the fifth fingers: an isolated lesion of the epiphyseal plate. *Am J Roentgenol* 86:490, 1961.

4. Laporte G: Clinodactyly. *Ann Radiol* 23:60–68, 1980.

5. Staheli LT, Clawson DK, Capps JH: Bilateral curving of terminal phalanges of little fingers: report of two cases. *J Bone Joint Surg* 48A:1171–1176, 1966.

Other Hand and Foot Deformities

SPADE HAND

The spade hand is quite square and results from shortening of all of the bones of the hand. There are a fair number of conditions in which such a hand occurs, but the largest group consists of the chondrodystrophies: i.e., achondroplasia (Fig. 4.81A), pseudoachondroplasia (multiple epiphyseal and spondyloepiphyseal types), hypochondroplasia (mild changes), thanatophoric dwarfism, achondrogenesis, the storage diseases, the short rib polydactyly syndromes, metatrophic dwarfism, Kniest's syndrome, diastrophic dwarfism, peripheral dysostosis or acrodysostosis (1, 2, 4) (Fig 4.81C), asphyxiating thoracic dystrophy (minimal changes), plenosteosis, and metaphyseal dysostosis (more severe in Jansen type). In the storage diseases, in addition to the hands being spade-like, the metacarpals are proximally tapered and bullet-shaped (Fig. 4.81B).

A spade hand also can occur in osteogenesis imperfecta (due to multiple fractures in congenita form), punctate epiphyseal dysplasia, Ruvalcaba syndrome (3), the Taybi-Lindner syndrome, and the otopalatodigital syndrome.

References

1. Arkless R, Graham CB: An unusual case of brachydactyly. Peripheral dysostosis? Pseudo-pseudo-hypoparathyroidism? Cone epiphyses? *Am J Roentgenol* 99:724–735, 1967.

2. Robinow M, Pfeiffer RA, Gorlin RJ, McKusick VA, Renuart AW, Johnson GF, Summitt RL: Acrodysostosis. *Am J Dis Child* 121:195–203, 1971.

3. Ruvalcaba RHA, Reichert A, Smith DE: A new familial syndrome with osseous dysplasia and mental deficiency. *J Pediatr* 79:450–455, 1971.

4. Singleton EB, Daeschner CW, Teng CT: Peripheral dysostosis. *Am J Roentgenol* 84:499–505, 1960.

CAMPTODACTYLY

The term camptodactyly designates a flexion deformity of one or more of the digits, and the findings usually are more striking in the hand than in the foot. Bending occurs primarily at the proximal interphalangeal joints, and one or more fingers may be involved. Clinical detection is easier than roentgenographic detection, for the findings may be difficult to differentiate from faulty positioning of the fingers. Camptodactyly occurs in a number of syndromes (Table 4.29), but the one usually coming to mind first is trisomy 18 (Fig. 4.82). Other syndromes in which camptodactyly occur are listed in Table 4.29, and it also should be noted that flexion deformities of the digits can be acquired secondary to old burns, infections, fractures, and contractures.

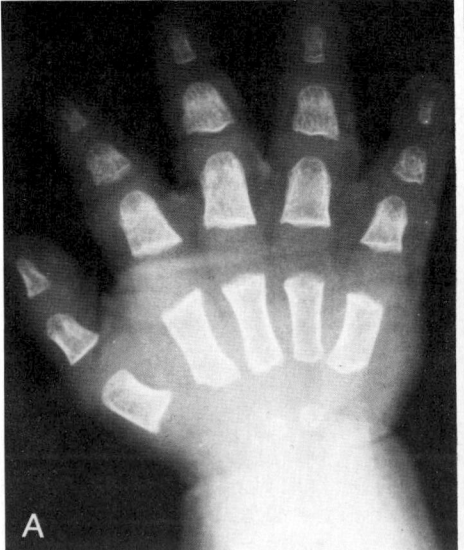
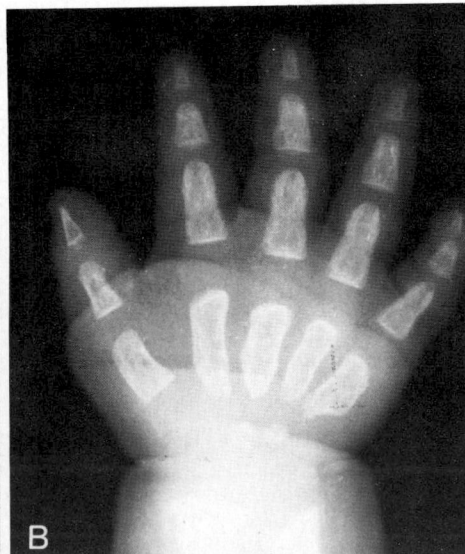
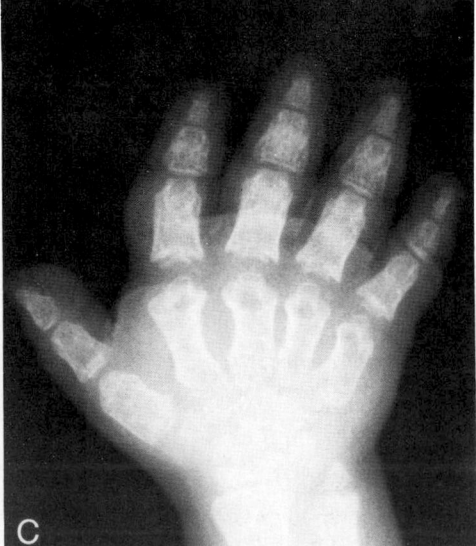

Fig. 4.81. Spade hand. A. Typical spade hand of achondroplasia. B. Spade hand in Hurler's disease. Note bullet shaped, proximally tapered metacarpals. C. Spade hand in acrodysostosis.

Table 4.29 Camptodactyly

More Common Conditions	Less Common Conditions
Holt-Oram syndrome	Isolated phalangeal hypoplasia or absence
Arthrogryposis congenita	Oro-facio-digital syndromes I, II
Poland's syndrome	
Trisomy 18	Aarskog's syndrome
Acquired	Cerebrohepatorenal or Zellweger's syndrome
Burns	
Infections	Goltz's syndrome
Fractures	Marfan's contractural arachnodactyly
Contractures	Osteo-onychodysplasia
	Popliteal pterygium syndrome
	Tricho-rhino-phalangeal syndrome
	Camptodactyly-ankylosis-pulmonary hypoplasia syndrome

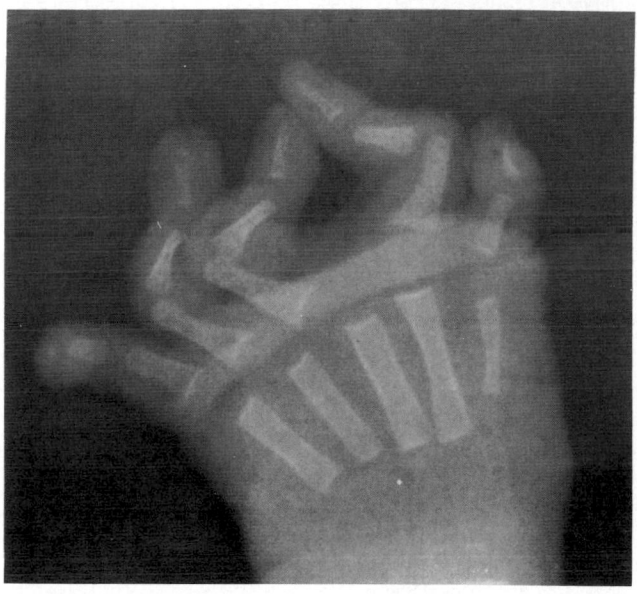

Fig. 4.82. Camptodactyly. Note bent fingers in trisomy 18. Also note hypoplastic thumb and first metacarpal.

SYNDACTYLY AND POLYDACTYLY

Syndactyly can involve either the soft tissues alone or both the bones and soft tissues (Fig. 4.83A). In addition, it can occur as an isolated finding or as a feature of certain syndromes (Table 4.30). In a few cases, the metacarpals also can be fused, while in others, polydactyly or duplication of the middle digits occurs.

Polydactyly can involve the outer or inner aspect of the hand (Fig. 4.83B). When it involves the ulnar side, it is termed postaxial, while on the radial side, it is called preaxial polydactyly (1). Polydactyly often is associated with syndactyly, and both can occur on an isolated sporadic basis. However, polydactyly also oc-

curs with a number of syndromes and is useful in defining these syndromes (Table 4.31).

Reference

1. Poznanski AK: *The Hand in Radiologic Diagnosis.* Philadelphia, W. B. Saunders, 1974, pp 197–204.

SYMPHALANGISM

In this condition there is fusion of the phalanges in the same digit. Most often the condition is seen as an isolated abnormality in the hands or feet and because the condition is believed to have existed in John Talbot, the first Earl of Shrewsbury, the finding often is referred to as the mark of Shrewsbury. It is inherited as a mendelian dominant trait and most often the

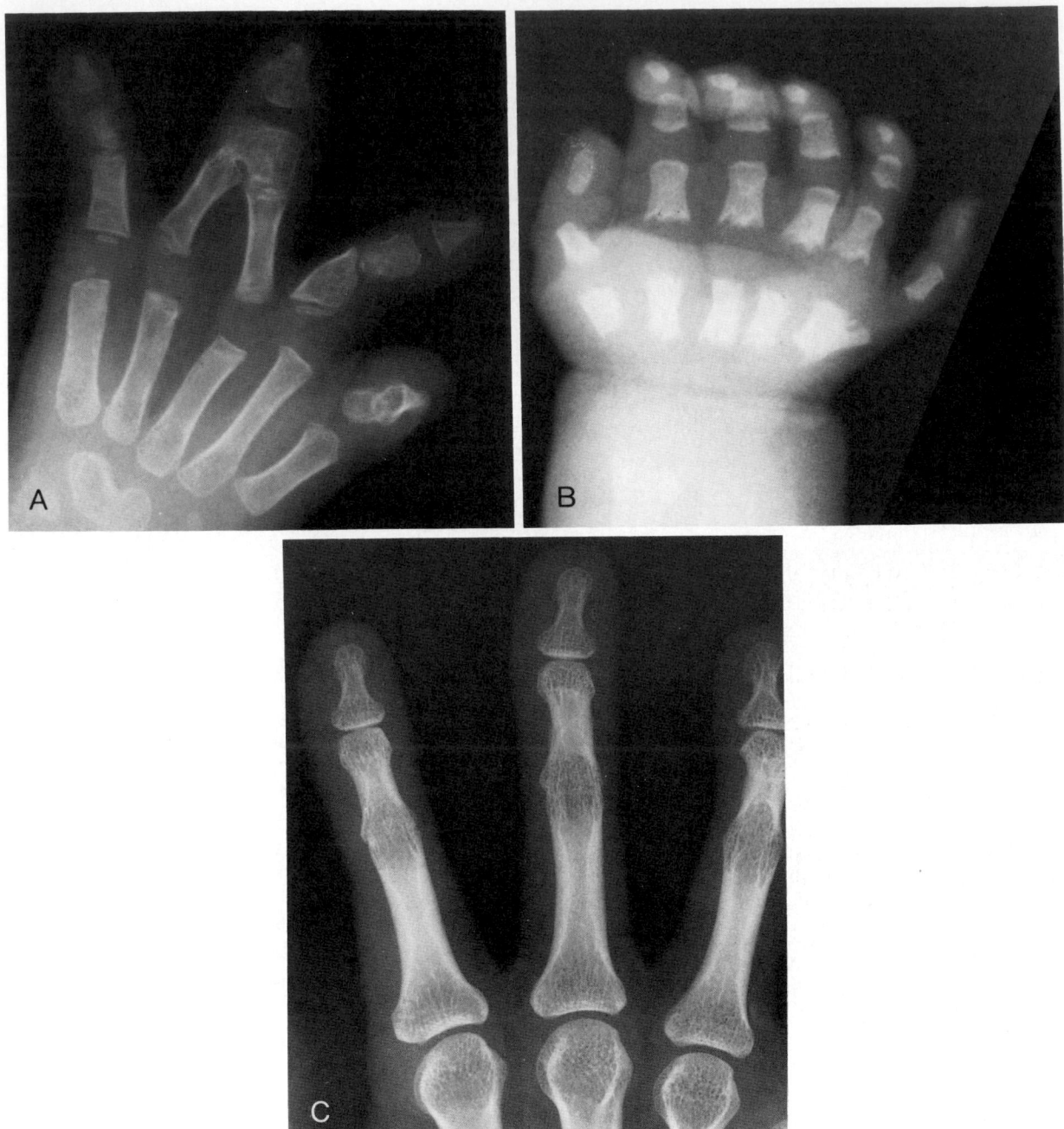

Fig. 4.83. Syndactyly and polydactyly. A. Note typical syndactyly and peripheral hypoplasia in Apert's syndrome. Also note carpal bone fusion. B. Short-rib polydactyly syndrome of Saldino-Noonan. C. **Symphalangism.** Note fusion of the distal intraphalangeal joints.

proximal interphalangeal joints of the fingers and distal interphalangeal joints of the toes are affected. However, involvement of the distal interphalangeal joints of the hands also can occur (Fig. 4.83C). Other anomalies can be seen in some patients and the condition has been reported in association with carpal and tarsal coalition (2, 3). It also occurs in diastrophic dwarfism, isolated brachydactyly, the popliteal pte-

rygium syndrome, and some cases of the acrocephalosyndactyly syndrome (4).

References

1. Daniel GH: A case of hereditary anarthrosis of the index finger, with associated abnormalities in the proportions of the fingers. *Ann Eugen* 7:281–296, 1936.
2. Elkington SG, Huntsman RG: The Talbot fingers: a

Table 4.30 Syndactyly

More Common Conditions	Less Common Conditions
Acrocephalosyndactyly (including Apert's)	Normal
Cornelia de Lange	Sporadic
Fanconi's anemia	Syndromes
Holt-Oram syndrome	Aarskog syndrome
Poland's syndrome	Aglossia-adactyly syndrome
Thrombocytopenia-absent radius (TAR)	Bloom's syndrome
Trisomy 13	Carpenter's syndrome
Trisomy 18	Punctate epiphyseal dysplasia (Conradi's)
Syndromes with polydactyly (Table 4.31)	Goltz's syndrome
	Laurence-Moon-Biedl
	Möbius's syndrome
	Popliteal pterygium syndrome
	Rothmund-Thomson's syndrome
	Rubinstein-Taybi syndrome
	Smith-Lemli-Opitz syndrome
	Robinow-Silverman syndrome

Table 4.31 Polydactyly

More Common Conditions	Less Common Conditions
Acrocephalosyndactyly[a]	Normal
Blackfan-Diamond anemia[a]	Sporadic
Fanconi's anemia[a]	Syndromes
Holt-Oram syndrome[a]	Acro-pectoro-vertebral dysplasia[a]
	Asphyxiating thoracic dystrophy[b]
	Biedmond syndrome[b]
	Bloom's syndrome
	Ellis-van Creveld syndrome[a]
	Goltz's syndrome[b]
	Hereditary hydrometrocolpos[b] (McKusick-Kaufman syndrome)
	Imperforate anus vertebral anomalies[a] (Vater syndrome)
	Mohr's syndrome[a, b]
	Möbius's syndrome
	Myositis ossificans progressiva
	Orodigitofacial syndrome
	Trisomy 13
	Short rib polydactyly syndrome[b]
	Werner's mesomelic dysplasia[a]

[a] Preaxial (radial side).
[b] Postaxial (ulnar side).

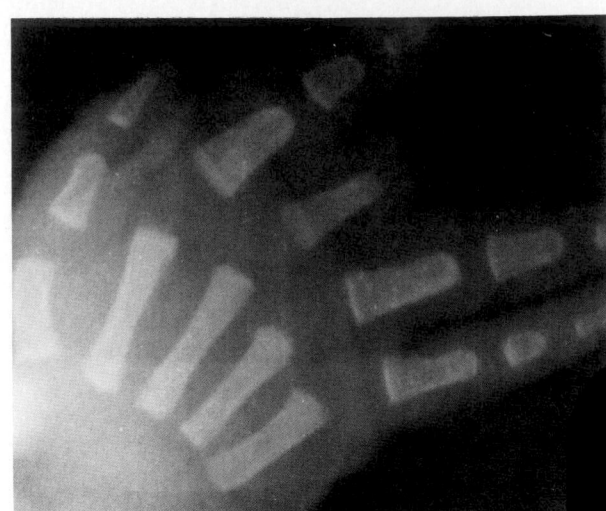

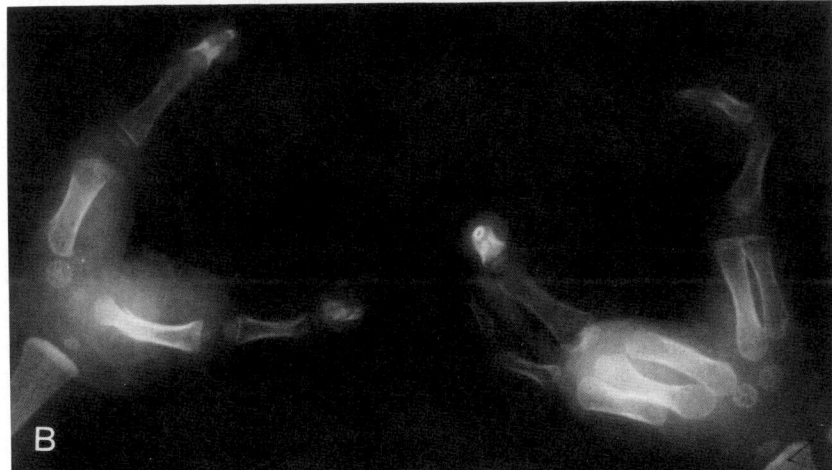

Fig. 4.84. **Amputated digits.** A. Note amputation of middle digit due to amniotic band. B. Absent middle digits in Claw Hand deformity.

study in symphalangism. *Br Med J* 1:407–411, 1967.

3. Geelhoed G, Neel JV, Davidson RT: Symphalangism and tarsal coalitions: a hereditary syndrome. A report on two families. *J Bone Joint Surg* 51B:278–298, 1969.
4. Harle TS, Stevenson JR: Hereditary symphalangism associated with carpal and tarsal fusions. *Radiology* 89:91–94, 1967.
5. Strasburger AK, Hawkins MR, Eldridge R, Hargrave RL, McKusick VA: Symphalangism: Genetic and clinical aspects. *Johns Hopkins Med J* 117:108–127, 1965.
6. Walker G: Remarkable cases of hereditary anchyloses, or absence of various phalangeal joints. *Johns Hopkins Med J* 12:129–133, 1901.
7. Wildervanck LS, Goedhard G, Meijer S: Proximal symphalangism of fingers associated with fusion of os tibiale externum) in an European-Indonesian-Chinese family. *Acta Genet* 17:166–177, 1967.

ABSENT OR AMPUTATED DIGITS

Acquired conditions such as trauma, burns, and infection most commonly cause amputation of the digits. Less common acquired causes include advanced psoriasis and frostbite (the latter is more common in colder climates). Congenital amputation also occurs and is seen in the aglossia-adactyly, Cornelia de Lange, Mobius's, and thalidomide embryonopathy syndromes. Amputation of the digits also can occur with amniotic or so-called Streeter's bands (Fig. 4.84A).

Absence of the middle digits of the hands can be seen with the so-called clawhand deformity (Fig. 4.84B). This deformity often is seen with anomalies of the face including cleft lip and palate, mandibulo-facial dysostoses, congenital deafness, etc. Absence of the digits on one or the other side of the hand is termed the **radial or ulnar ray syndrome.** The radial ray syndrome is more common, and often the thumb bears the brunt of the hypoplasia. Conditions demonstrating the radial ray syndrome include Klippel-Feil deformity, ectodermal dysplasia, Fanconi's anemia, Holt-Oram syndrome, thrombocytopenia ab-

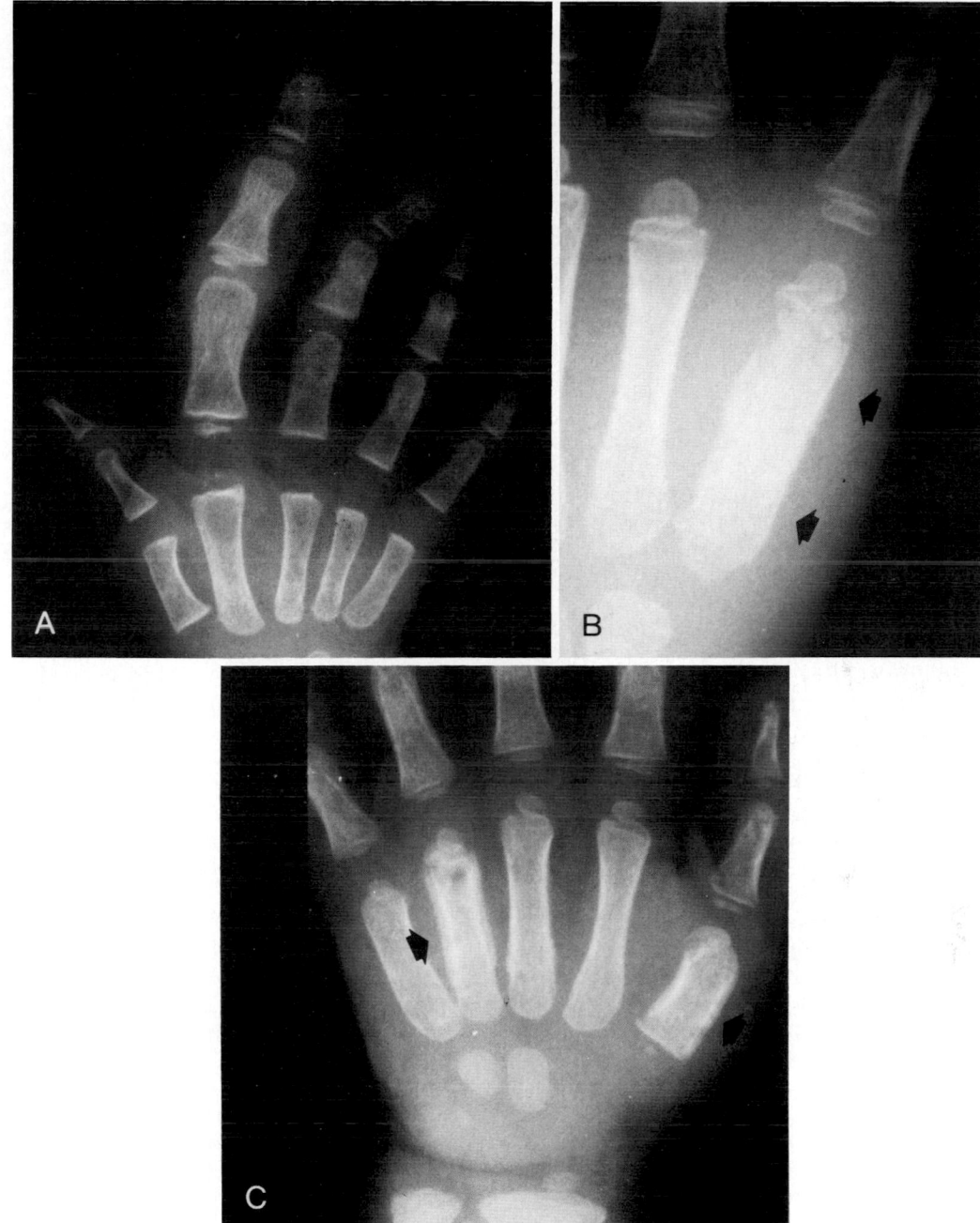

Fig. 4.85.   A. Gigantism. Note enlargement of the second and third digits in this patient with neurofibromatosis.
B. Dactylitis. Coccidiomycosis of metacarpal (arrows). **C. Dactylitis.** Hand-foot syndrome in sickle cell disease
(arrows).

sent radius (TAR) syndrome (thumb usually well developed but radius absent), thalidamide embryonopathy, Vater syndrome, and trisomy 18. Conditions associated with the ulnar ray syndrome (i.e., fourth and fifth digits) include the Cornelia de Lange syndrome, Nievergelt's and Pfeiffer's ulnofibular dysplasias, Wegner's syndrome, and Weyer's oligodactyly.

MACRODACTYLY

Enlargement of one or more of the digits is not common, and most often is associated with a heman-giomatous or lymphangiomatous tumor of the hand or foot, neurofibromatosis (Fig. 4.85A), or macrodystrophia lipomatosa congenita. Occasionally macrodactylia is seen in the absence of any of these conditions and the cause is unknown (1). In most cases the middle digits are more involved.

Reference

1. Poznanski AK: *The Hand in Radiologic Diagnosis.* Philadelphia, W.B. Saunders, 1974, pp 218–220.

Table 4.32 Dactylitis

Infection (osteomyelitis) Infarction (hand-foot syndrome) }	Commonest
Frostbite }	Relatively rare
Radiation injury Microgeodic syndrome Tumor (mimicking dactylitis) Ewing's sarcoma Hemangioma Metastatic neuroblastoma }	Rare

DACTYLITIS

Dactylitis infers an infection or inflammation of the fingers (Table 4.32). There are, however, other conditions in which the bony changes of infection can be mimicked. As far as infection is concerned, perhaps the most common cause of dactylitis is osteomyelitis in certain immune deficiency syndromes and tuberculosis (spina ventosa). Many times the findings in the bones consist of destruction, sclerosis with healing, and generalized expansion of the bone (Fig. 4.85B). Similar findings can be seen with bone infarction (i.e., hand-foot syndrome of sickle cell disease) (Fig. 4.85C), frostbite (2), radiation necrosis, and rarely tumors such as Ewing's sarcoma, hemangiomas, and metastatic neuroblastoma. With Ewing's sarcoma and metastatic neuroblastoma, spiculated new bone formation may accompany the changes. Changes resembling dactylitis are seen in the rare phalangeal microgeodic syndrome of infancy (1).

References

1. Maroteaux P: Cinq observations d'une affection microgeodique des phalanges du nourrisson d'etiologie inconnue. *Ann Radiol* 13:229, 1970.
2. Sweet EM, Smith MGH: Winter fingers. Bone infarction in Scottish children as a manifestation of cold injury. *Ann Radiol* 22:71–75, 1979.

Carpal and Tarsal Abnormalities

DECREASED (MORE ACUTE) CARPAL ANGLE

The carpal angle is the angle formed by the lines drawn tangent to the lunate, scaphoid, and triquetral bones. Normally the angle measures somewhere between 125° and 140° (1). When it is decreased (i.e., more acute), especially in more severe cases, there is associated slanting of the distal radial and ulnar articulating surfaces (Fig. 4.86). The most common condition associated with a decreased carpal angle is Turner's Syndrome (1–3) but other conditions where it can be decreased include dyschondrosteosis (Madelung's deformity), Morquio's disease, multiple osteochondromatosis, Hurler's syndrome (1), and other storage diseases with more severe bony changes. When angulation is profound, often there is an erosion of the upper medial aspect of the radius (see Fig. 4.86B). This erosion, we have determined, is due to herniation of the synovial lining of the wrist joint (4).

References

1. Harper HAS, Poznanski AK, Garn SM: The carpal angle in American populations. *Invest Radiology* 9:217–221, 1974.
2. Kosowicz J: The roentgen appearance of the hand and wrist in gonadal dysgenesis. *Am J Roentgenol* 93:354–361, 1965.
3. Necic S, Grant DB: Diagnostic value of hand x-rays in Turner's syndrome. *Acta Paediatr Scand* 67:309–312, 1978.
4. Swischuk LE, Hayden CK: The Radial Notch and Decreased Carpal Angle. In preparation.

CARPAL-TARSAL COALITION

The carpal bones probably undergo fusion more often than the tarsal bones, and the phenomenon can occur on an isolated basis in normal patients or as a part of certain syndromes. On an isolated basis (most common), carpal coalition is more common in the black race (1, 2, 4) and, in this regard, the most common fusion is between the triquetral and the lunate bones (Fig. 4.87A). However, numerous other combinations can occur both in the hand and foot (Fig. 4.87B). In the foot, isolated coalition between the talus and calcaneus is not uncommon, and may be associated with pes planus.

In syndromes, coalition patterns may be more bizarre, and in the foot they are likely to involve mostly the cuneiforms, and the metatarsals (3). Syndromes in which fusion occurs are outlined in Table 4.33, but perhaps the one that comes to mind first is the Ellis-van Creveld syndrome. Acquired carpal or tarsal fusion can be seen after trauma, inflammation, or infection. In terms of inflammation, the best known cause is rheumatoid arthritis (Fig. 4.87C).

References

1. Cockshott WP: Carpal fusions. *Am J Roentgenol* 89:1260–1271, 1963.
2. Cope JR: Carpal coalition. *Clin Radiol* 25:261–266, 1974.
3. Poznanski AK: Foot manifestations of the congenital malformation syndromes. *Semin Roentgenol* 5:354–366, 1970.
4. Poznanski AK, Holt FF: The carpals in congenital malformation syndromes. *Am J Roentgenol* 112:443–459, 1971.

SCALLOPED CARPAL-TARSAL BONES

Scalloping deformities of the carpal or tarsal bones most commonly occur with multiple epiphyseal dysplasia (Fig. 4.88A), but similar findings can be seen

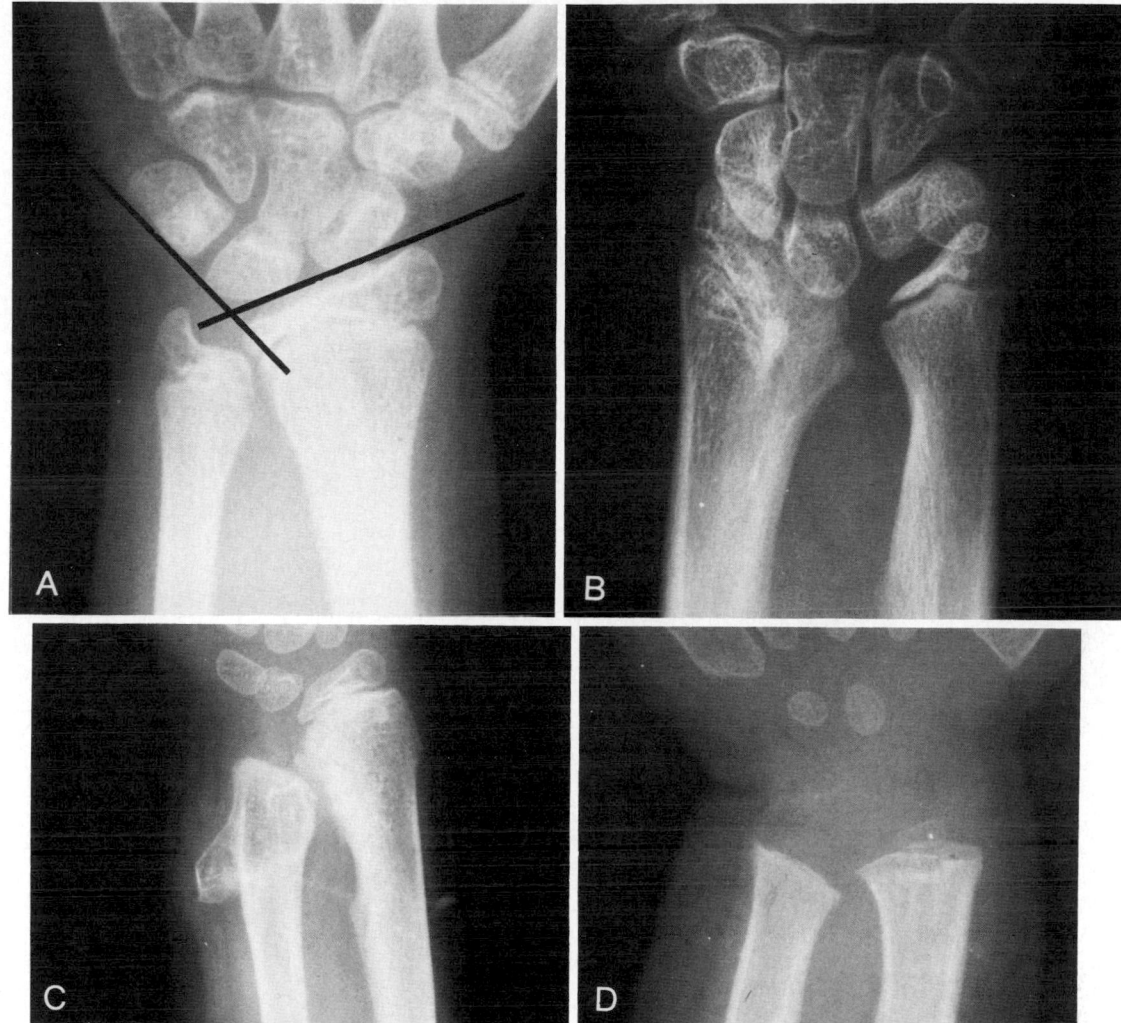

Fig. 4.86. Decreased (more acute) carpal angle. A. Decreased carpal angle in Turner's syndrome. Carpal angle (lines) measures approximately 112°. B. Decreased carpal angle and associated distal radial and ulnar deformities in dyschondrosteosis. C. Decreased carpal angle in multiple exostosis. D. Decreased carpal angle and associated slanting of distal radius and ulna in Hurler's disease.

with neurofibromatosis (Fig. 4.88B), adjacent soft tissue hemangiomas or lymphangiomas, and neurotrophic diseases such as tertiary syphilis, syringomyelia, diabetic neuropathy, etc. Most of these latter conditions tend to occur in adults, but occasionally they are encountered in children. Focal, solitary scallopings are seen with adjacent tumors (Fig. 4.88C) and after infection, trauma, or necrosis. Scalloped tarsal and carpal bones also occur in rheumatoid arthritis (synovial erosion) (Fig. 4.88D), Winchester's syndrome (a storage disease mimicking rheumatoid arthritis), pigmented villinodular synovitis, and diastrophic dwarfism.

FRAGMENTED OR IRREGULAR CARPAL-TARSAL BONES

Irregular development suggesting fragmentation of the tarsal, but not the carpal, bones is common in normal individuals. Indeed, in such cases aseptic necrosis often is erroneously suggested (Fig. 4.89). Such normal fragmentation can occur in any of the tarsals but tends to involve the cuneiforms and navicular more than the others. Fragmentation due to aseptic necrosis most commonly occurs in the tarsal navicular and is known as Kohler's disease (Fig. 4.89C). Clinically, pain is present and soft tissue swelling is demonstrable roentgenographically over the involved bone. This is a useful point in differentiating normally irregular navicular bones from those undergoing aseptic necrosis (2). This point is more than just of passing interest, for the normal navicular bone not uncommonly is irregular and sclerotic. In the hand, the carpal navicular can undergo posttraumatic aseptic necrosis, and become irregularly sclerotic, but in children this is not so common.

The tarsal and carpal bones also are irregular and

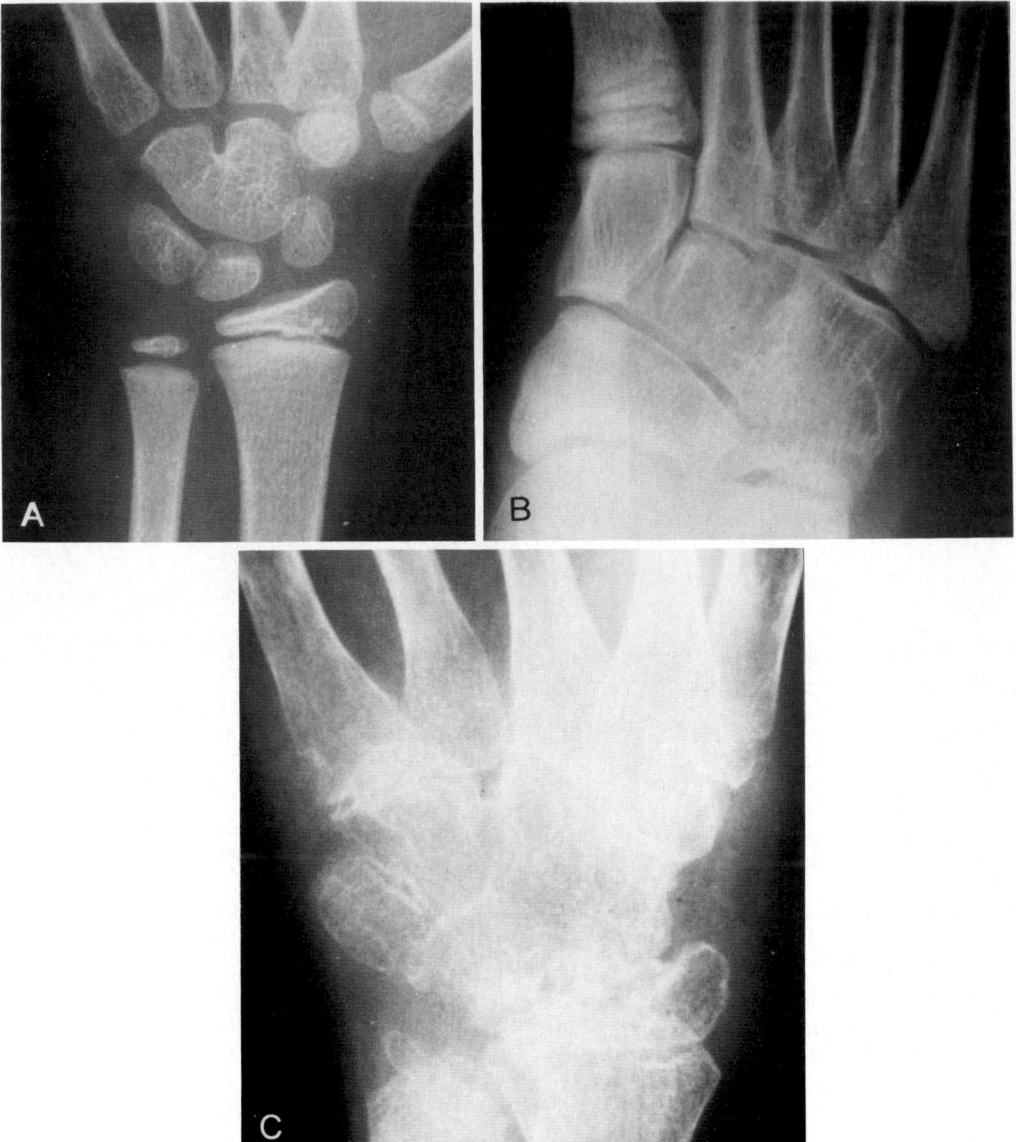

Fig. 4.87. Carpal-tarsal coalitions. A. Incidental carpal coalition. B. Multiple coalitions of the tarsal bones in a foot. C. Postinflammatory coalition in rheumatoid arthritis.

Table 4.33   Carpal-Tarsal Coalition

More Common Conditions	Less Common Conditions
Idiopathic, isolated	Diastrophic dwarfism
Ellis-van Creveld syndrome	Hand-foot-uterus syndrome
Holt-Oram syndrome	Nivergelt's mesomelic dwarf-
Acrocephalosyndactyly	ism
Arthrogryposis congenita	Otopalatodigital syndrome
Turner's syndrome	Frontometaphyseal dysplasia
Dyschondrosteosis (Made-	
lung's)	
Acquired	
Trauma	
Inflammation, infection	

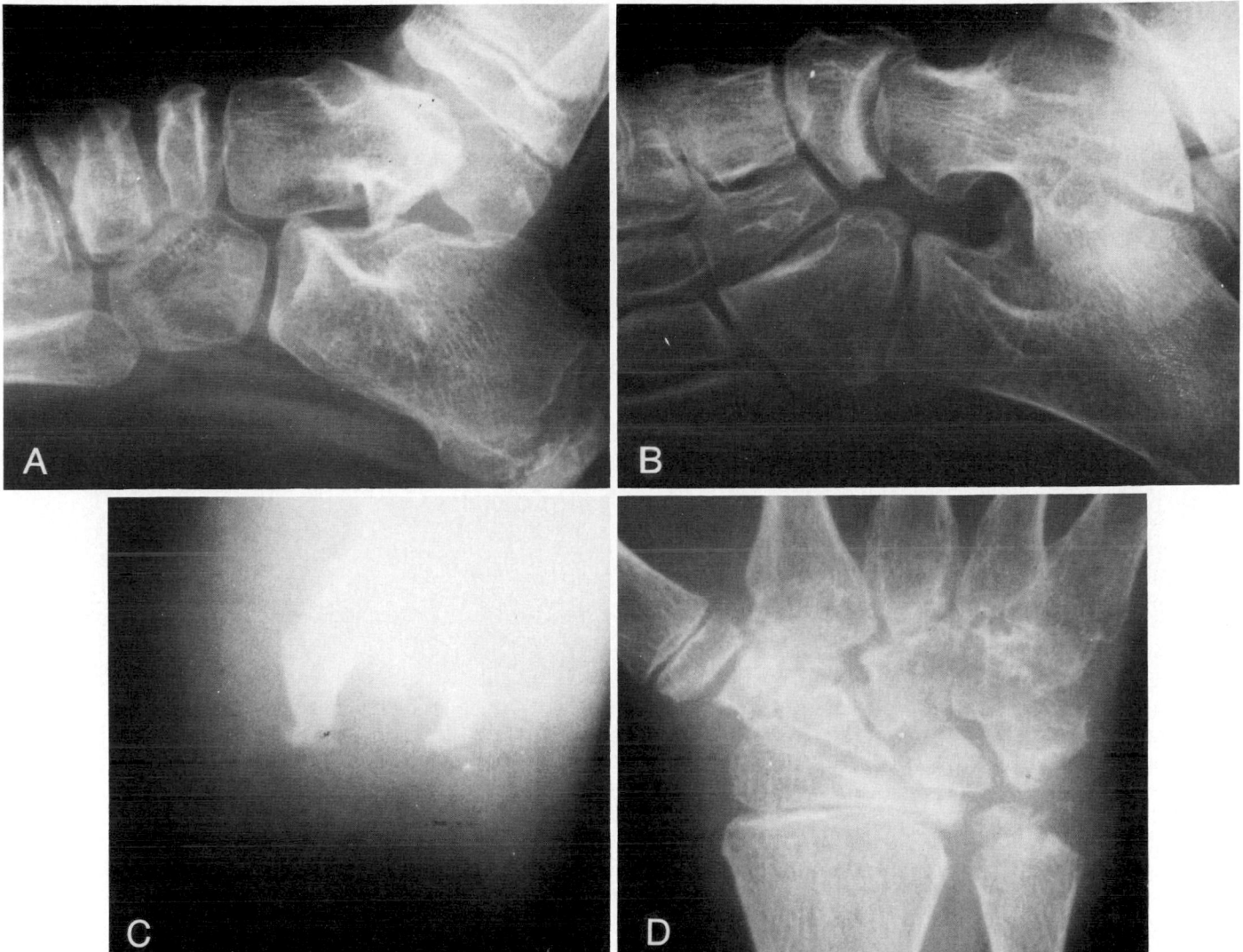

Fig. 4.88. Scalloped carpal-tarsal bones. A. Excessive scalloping of the tarsal bones in epiphyseal dysplasia. B. Similar scalloping in neurofibromatosis. C. Scalloping of calcaneus by neurofibroma. D. Scalloped, small, and irregular carpal bones in rheumatoid arthritis.

sclerotic in multiple epiphyseal dysplasia, punctate epiphyseal dysplasia (stippling and fragmentation), spondyloepiphyseal dysplasia (Fig. 4.89D), Morquio's disease (resembles spondyloepiphyseal dysplasia), after trauma or infection, in rheumatoid arthritis, and in Winchester's syndrome (storage disease mimicking rheumatoid arthritis).

References

1. Waught W: The ossification and vascularization of the tarsal-navicular and a relation to Kohler's disease. *J Bone Joint Surg* 40-B:765, 1958.
2. Weston WJ: Kohler's disease of the tarsal scaphoid. *Australas Radiol* 22:332–337, 1978.

BIPARTITE TARSAL OR CARPAL BONES

Occasionally, one of these bones will be bipartite on a congenital basis. This is especially true in early childhood, before bone formation is complete. A bipartite calcaneous is seen in Larsen's syndrome, and an acquired bipartite carpal, or tarsal, navicular can occur after aseptic necrosis.

VERTICAL TALUS

A vertical talus is seen in flat foot deformities, either idiopathic or associated with neurogenic or neuromuscular disease (Fig. 4.90). It also is seen with pes calcaneal valgus, a foot deformity commonly present in trisomy 18.

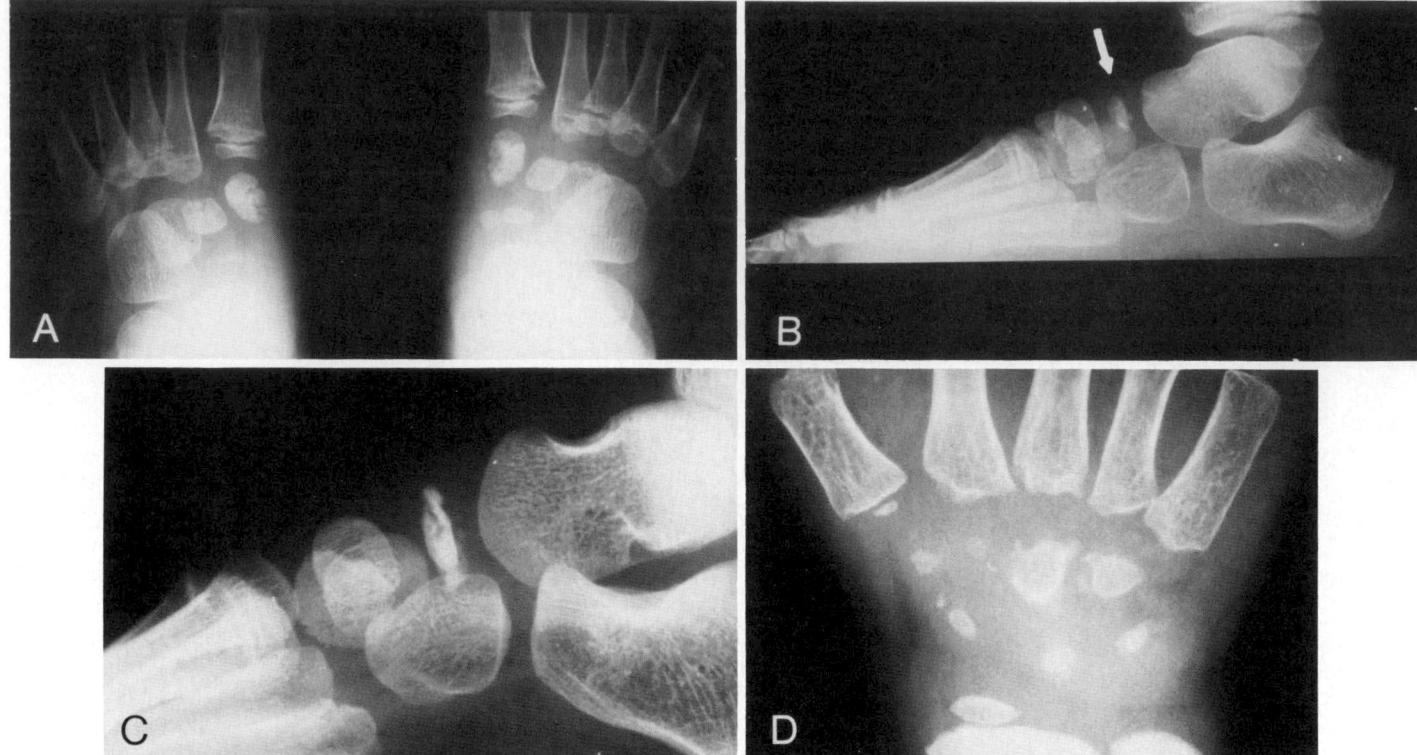

Fig. 4.89. Fragmented, irregular carpal and tarsal bones. A. Normal, irregular navicular, and cuneiform bones. B. Irregular, small navicular bone (arrow), in normal patient. C. Small, irregular and sclerotic navicular bone in Köhler's disease. Pain was present in this patient. D. Irregular, fragmented, carpal bones in spondyloephyseal dysplasia.

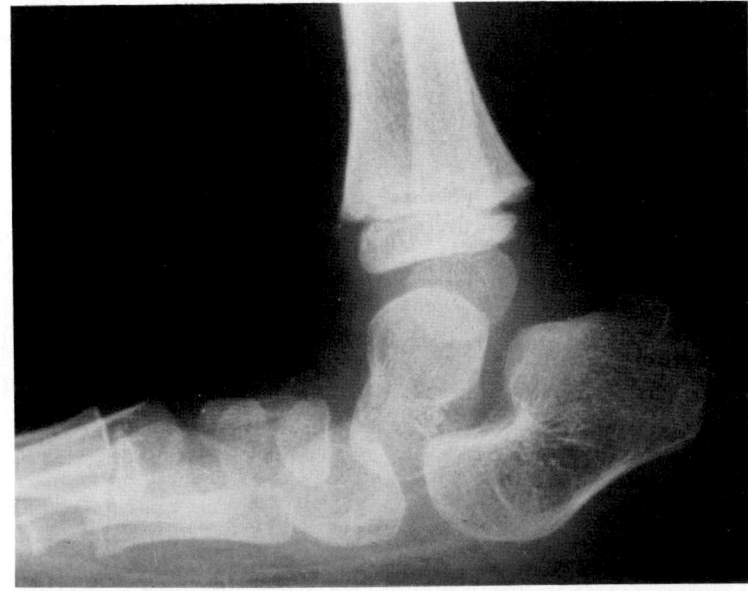

Fig. 4.90. Vertical talus. Typical vertical talus (arrow) in neurogenic flatfoot deformity.

ABNORMALITIES OF THE FLAT BONES

Patella

Perhaps the most problematic finding encountered in the patella is **normal irregularity or pseudo fragmentation during its development (Fig. 4.91A).** Indeed, when the patella begins to ossify (3–5 years), it rather routinely appears fragmented and sclerotic, and thereafter, an almost endless number of fragmentation configurations can be encountered. A bipartite patella, with two separate ossification centers also is common, and very often is bilateral. The upper outer quadrant of the patella usually is involved and the anomaly is best seen on frontal view (Fig. 4.91B). A tripartite patella is much less common.

IRREGULARITY OF THE LOWER END OF THE PATELLA

Irregularity of this kind usually denotes a chronic tendon avulsion injury or so-called Sinding-Larsen-Johansson disease (Fig. 4.91C). It is the counterpart of Osgood-Schlatter's disease of the tibial tubercle, and in addition to its occurrence in normal, active children, also commonly is seen in spastic cerebral palsy (3, 5).

DISLOCATION OF THE PATELLA

Dislocation of the patella can be acute or chronic, but chronic patellar dislocation is more common. With acute dislocation, by the time roentgenograms are obtained the patella usually reduces to normal position. However, on skyline views with 30°, 60°, and 90° knee flexion one may see an avulsed fragment of bone medially (Fig. 4.91D). With chronic dislocation, the 30°, 60°, 90° knee flexion (skyline) views are most important. With these views, patellar dislocation can be demonstrated and in many cases an associated

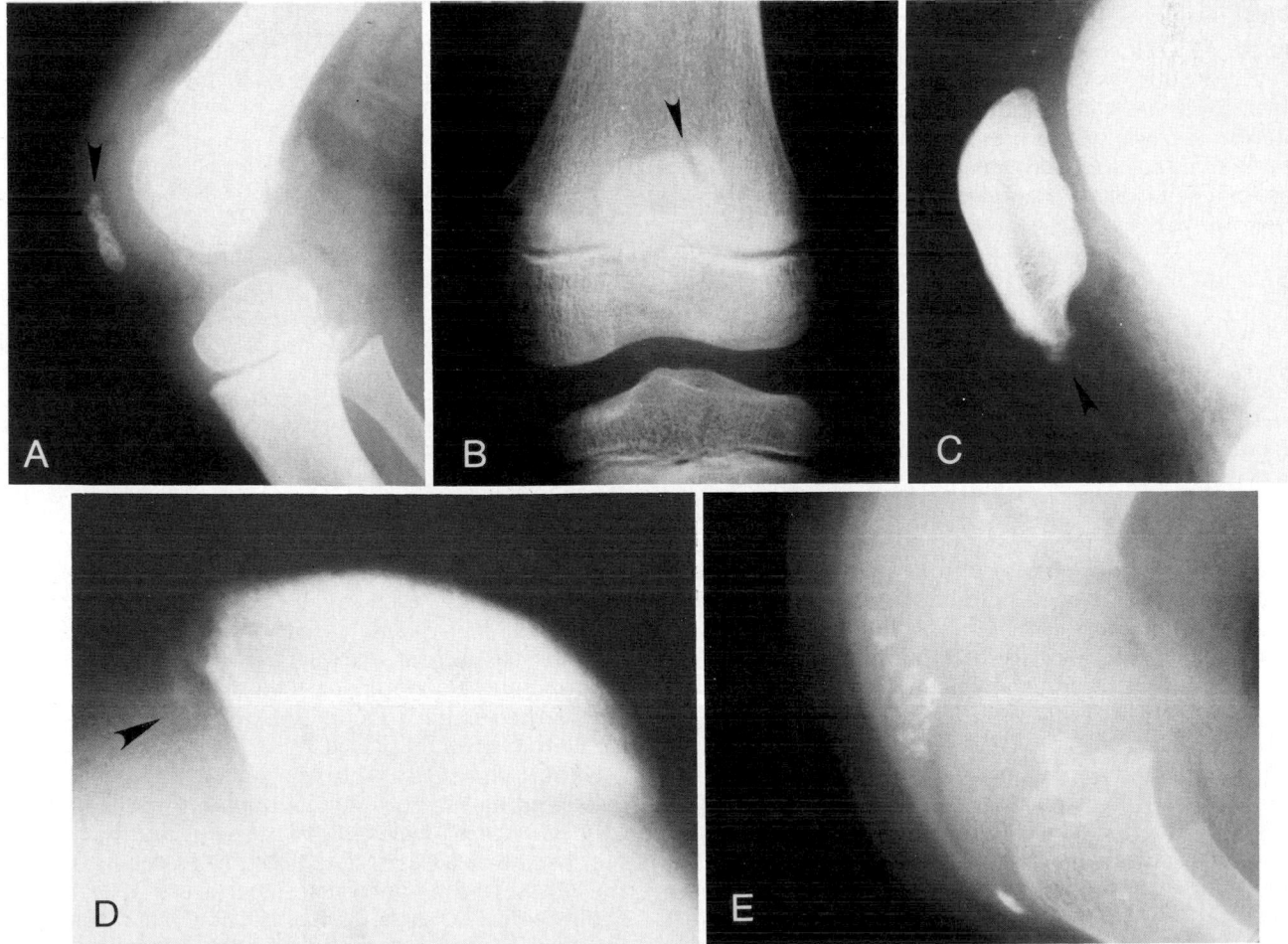

Fig. 4.91. Patellar abnormalities. A. Normal, irregular patella of young child (arrow). B. Typical fragment of bipartite patella (arrow). C. Slight fragmentation of inferior patellar pole (arrow) in Sinding-Larsen-Johansson disease. D. Small, avulsed medial fragment (arrow), with acute patellar dislocation. E. Typical stippled patella in punctate epiphyseal dysplasia.

defect on the medial undersurface of the patella is seen. The defect results from the patella riding over the condyle as it dislocates. Chronically dislocating patellae most often occur as isolated abnormalities, but also can be seen in acrocephalosyndactyly (especially Carpenter's syndrome), multiple epiphyseal dysplasia, Rubinstein-Taybi syndrome, Stickler's (hereditary arthroophthalmopathy) syndrome, and Larsen's syndrome. **Absence or hypoplasia of the patella** occurs in the nail-patella (hereditary osteoonychodysplasia) syndrome, neurofibromatosis, diastrophic dwarfism, the popliteal pterygium syndrome, birdheaded dwarfism, and on a familial basis, in otherwise normal individuals.

DEFECTS AND LYTIC LESIONS

Defects and lytic lesions of the patella are not nearly as common as they are in the long bones but they do occur. Usually they are presumed to be fibrous or cartilaginous in origin but occasionally they can be due to chronic osteomyelitis, histiocytosis X, or osteochondritis dessicans. Defects produced by other benign tumors and cysts of the patella are relatively rare. Occasionally one can encounter irregularity along the posterior surface of the patella. Although probably normal, one is never sure that the finding is not due to old osteochondritis dessicans.

FUZZY, INDISTINCT PATELLA

A fuzzy, indistinct patella can be seen with osteomyelitis and any cause of osteomalacia. **Massive destruction of the patella,** due to tumors such as Ewing's sarcoma, leukemia, metastatic disease, lymphangioma, and hemangioma, is rare.

MISCELLANEOUS ABNORMALITIES OF THE PATELLA

Punctate patellar calcifications occur in the same conditions as do stippled epiphyses (i.e., punctate epiphyseal dysplasia, the hepatorenal or Zellweger's syndrome, and Warfarin embryonopathy (see Fig. 4.91E). **Enlargement of the patella** can occur with a number of chronic arthritities, but primarily is seen with rheumatoid arthritis, hemophiliac arthropathy, and tuberculous arthritis. Much as with the epiphyses, the patellae in these conditions not only become large, but osteoporotic and glassy. In addition it has been noted that in hemophilia the patella remains rather long, but in rheumatoid arthritis it is short and squat; indeed, almost cuboid (1). **Patella alta** denotes a patellar position higher than normal, and the abnormality can be confirmed by specific measurements on lateral view (4). However, in most cases one can make a subjective judgement alone, and the problem occurs in some cases of chronic dislocation (4), spastic cerebral palsy, and on an isolated idiopathic basis.

References

1. Chlosta EM, Kuhns LR, Holt JF: The "Patellar Radio" in hemophilia and juvenile rheumatoid arthritis. *Radiology* 116:137–138, 1975.
2. Haswell DM, Berne AS, Graham CB: The dorsal defect of the patella. *Pediatr Radiol* 4:238–242, 1976.
3. Kaye JJ, Freiberger RH: Fragmentation of the lower pole of the patella and spastic lower extremities. *Radiology* 101:97, 1971.
4. Lancourt JE, Cristini JA: Patella alta and patella infera. Their etiological role in patellar dislocation, chondromalacia, and apophysitis of the tibial tubercle. *J Bone Joint Surg* 57:1112–1115, 1975.
5. Rosenthal RK, Levine DB: Fragmentation of the distal pole of the patella in spastic cerebral palsy. *J Bone Joint Surg* 59:934–939, 1977.

Clavicle

Clavicular **hypoplasia** is not uncommon and occurs with cleidocranial dysostosis, focal dermal hypoplasia (Goltz syndrome), the Holt-Oram syndrome, progeria, trisomy 13, and trisomy 18. In the latter three conditions, hypoplasia manifests primarily in **thinness of the clavicle** (Fig. 4.92A), a configuration also commonly seen on a normal basis in premature infants. In the Holt-Oram syndrome, the hypoplastic clavicles often are somewhat squat and **handlebar** in appearance (Fig. 4.92B). The configuration also can be seen in diastrophic dwarfism, the thrombocytopenia absent radius (TAR) syndrome, trisomy 18 (1), and also as a normal variation due to improper positioning of the chest (Fig. 4.92C). In cleidocranial dysostosis, the clavicle can be hypoplastic, completely absent (Fig. 4.93A), or defective in any of the thirds from which its ossification centers are derived (Fig. 4.93B). When the defect is central, it should be differentiated from

that seen with congenital pseudoarthrosis of the clavicle (Fig. 4.93C), a finding usually seen as an isolated phenomenon. In some cases of congenital pseudoarthrosis, the findings are suggestive of an ununited fracture, but in most cases, smoothness and a bulbous end of the remaining portions of the clavicle provide a clue to proper diagnosis.

Short, squat clavicles occur in any of the conditions leading to short, squat tubular bones (see Table 4.3), but the clavicles may be exceptionally short in the storage diseases (Fig. 4.92D). As far as **defects of the clavicle** are concerned, most occur after trauma and infection. Overall, however, the normal rhomboid fossa is the commonest cause of a clavicular defect. Characteristically, it is located along the lower edge of the medial aspect of the clavicle (Fig. 4.94). **Erosion of the distal end of the clavicle** occurs primarily with hyperparathyroidism (Fig. 4.95A), rheumatoid

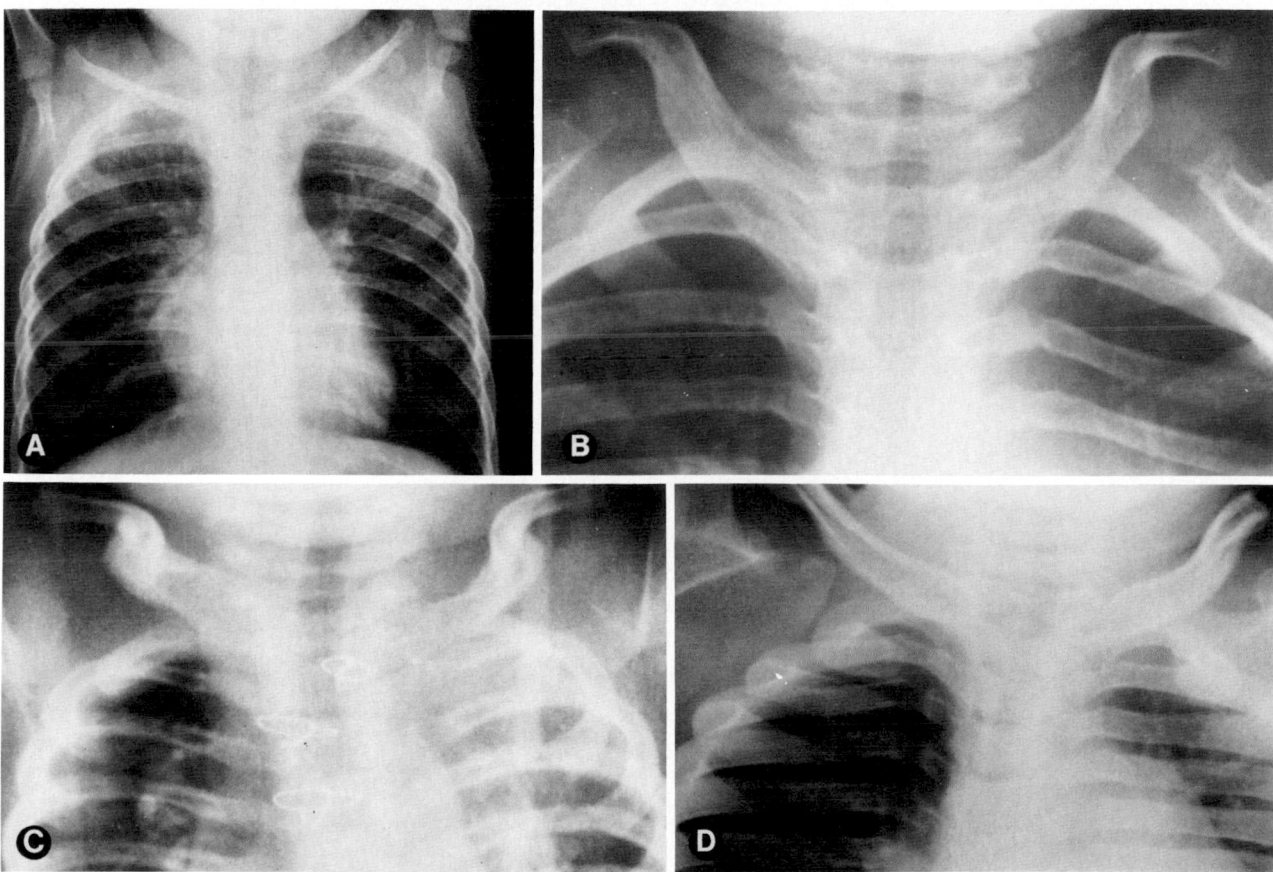

Fig. 4.92.   Hypoplasia of clavicle. A. Thin clavicles in trisomy 18. B. Hypoplastic, somewhat squat and handlebar-shaped clavicles in Holt-Oram's syndrome. C. Pseudo handlebar appearance in normal infant due to positioning with upwardly stretched arms. D. Short, squat clavicles in Hurler's syndrome.

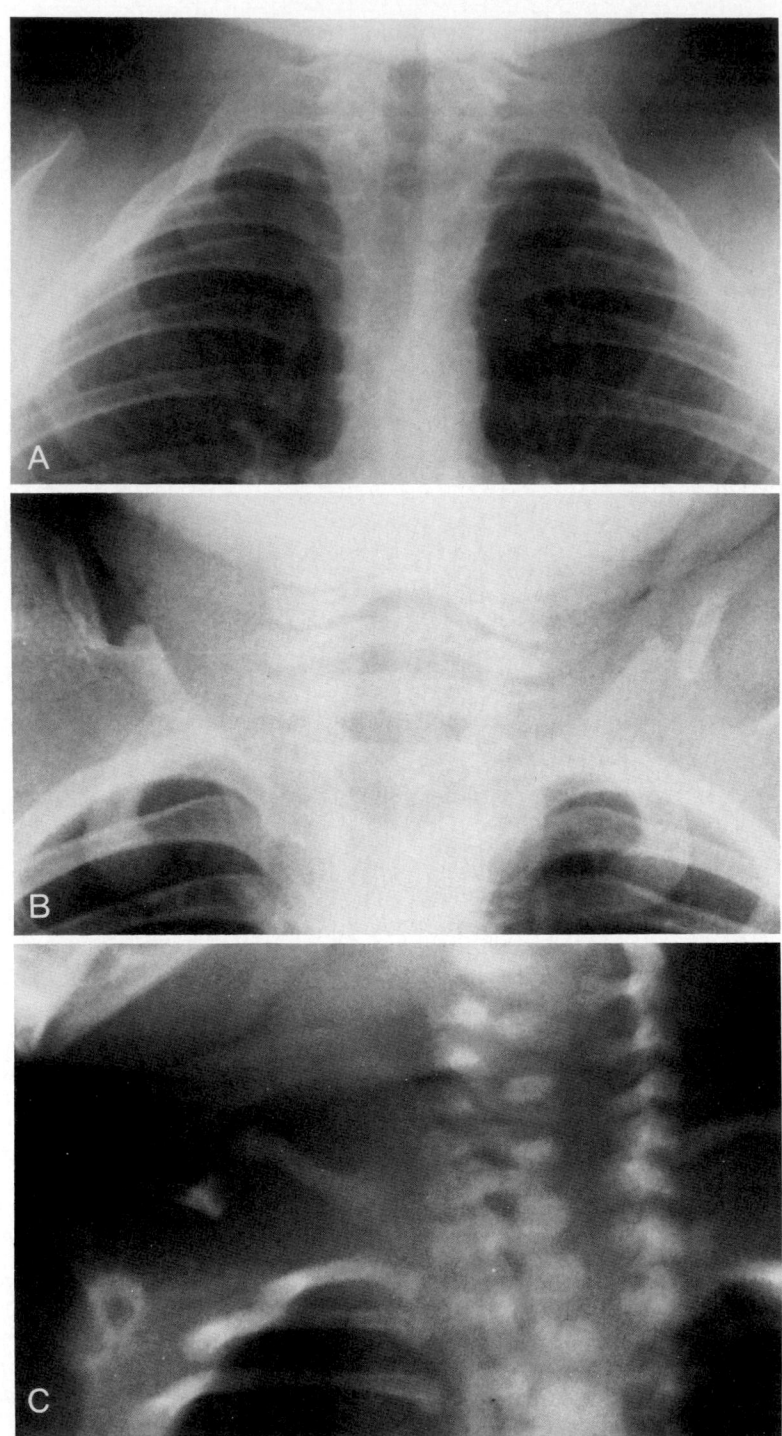

Fig. 4.93. **Absent and defective clavicles.** A. Absent clavicles; cleidocranial dysostosis. B. Hypoplastic, defective clavicles in cleidocranial dysostosis. C. Congenital pseudoarthrosis of right clavicle. Note smooth, bulbous ends of clavicular fragments.

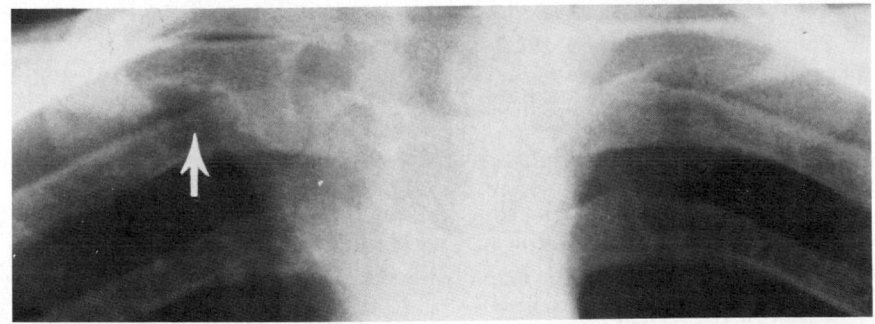

Fig. 4.94. Rhomboid fossa. Note typical, normal notch on undersurface of medial aspect of the clavicle (arrow).

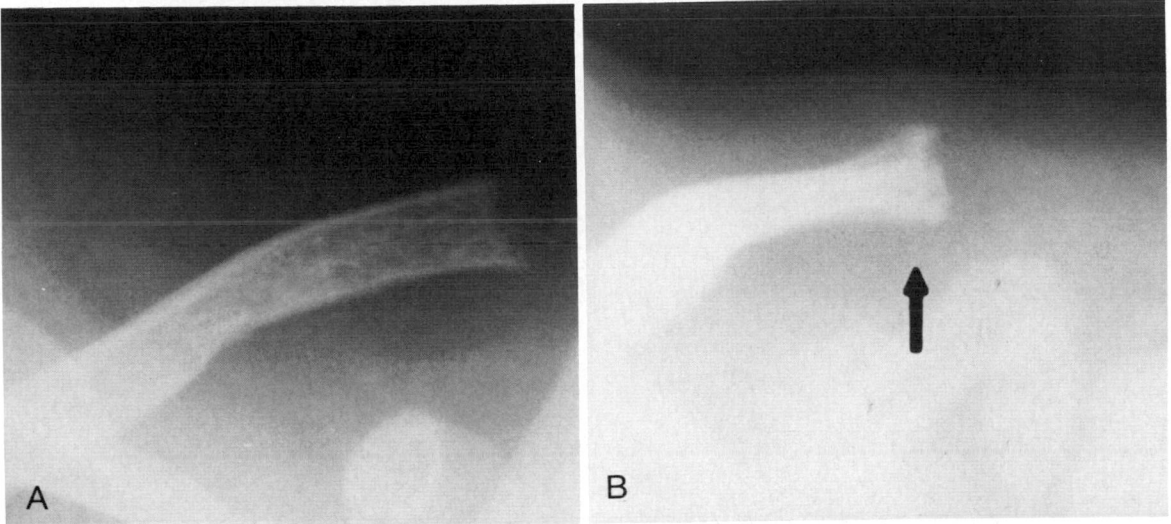

Fig. 4.95. Distal clavicular erosion and flaring. A. Note typical erosion and slight cupping of clavicle in hyperparathyroidism, secondary to renal osteodystrophy. B. Irregular, flared distal clavicle due to fracture in battered child syndrome.

arthritis, rickets, osteomyelitis, and after trauma. In the healing phase of trauma, the distal end of the clavicle can become quite bulbous and flared, and indeed the finding can be diagnostic in the battered child syndrome (Fig. 4.95B) (2). Other conditions in which distal clavicular erosion occurs include progeria, pycnodysostosis, scleroderma, gout, and the storage diseases.

Destruction, with **narrowing of the acromiclavicular joint** occurs primarily with pyogenic infections but also can be seen with rheumatoid arthritis and traumatic dislocation. **Defects and lytic lesions** of the clavicle have the same causes as do those of long bones (see p 308), and **pseudoarthrosis** of the clavicle

has been discussed earlier (p 191). In form of review, however, most commonly it is seen on a congenital, anomalous basis, and thereafter with nonunited fractures.

References

1. Igual M, Giedion A: The lateral clavicle hook: its objective measurement and its diagnostic value in Holt-Oram syndrome, diastrophic dwarfism, thrombocytopenia-absent radius syndrome and trisomy 8. *Ann Radiol* 22:136–141, 1979.
2. Kogutt MS, Swischuk LE, Fagan CJ: Patterns of injury and significance of uncommon fractures in the battered child syndrome. *Am J Roentgenol* 121:143–149, 1974.

Scapula

Enlargement of the scapula occurs with Caffey's infantile cortical hyperostosis, histiocytosis X, chronic osteomyelitis, secondary metastases and primary tumors such as Ewing's sarcoma, reticulum cell sarcoma, hemangioma, lymphangioma, and aneurysmal bone cysts (1). Caffey's disease, however, is most common

and then comes histiocytosis X. Scapular involvement in Caffey's disease may be the only lesion present in some infants and clinically is associated with swelling and redness over the area. Roentgenographically, the enlarged scapular often initially shows fuzzy margins, but thereafter, with periosteal new bone deposition, increased sclerosis around the edges is seen (Fig. 4.96A). Generally, Caffey's disease does not occur after the age of 5 months, and consequently, if one sees a similar appearance in an older infant, one should consider histiocytosis X (Fig. 4.96B).

Focal **destruction** has the same etiologies as it does in long bones, but **massive destruction of the scapula** deserves special attention. Such destruction can occur with acute osteomyelitis, metastatic disease, Ewing's sarcoma, leukemia, and lymphoma. In terms of the latter, reticulum cell sarcoma often is the offender. **Bubbly expansion of the scapula** most of-

ten occurs with healing histiocytosis X, but also can be seen with chronic osteomyelitis, lymphangiomas and hemangiomas of the scapula, fibrous dysplasia, and aneurysmal bone cyst (1). Solitary cystic lesions of the scapula have the same etiology as they do in any bone in the body, and the problem has been dealt with elsewhere (see p 308).

Smallness of the scapula occurs with many of the chondrodystrophies and dwarfing syndromes seen in infancy, but for the most part there is little specificity to the configuration. The only exception might be the small scapula with a **shallow glenoid fossa** com-

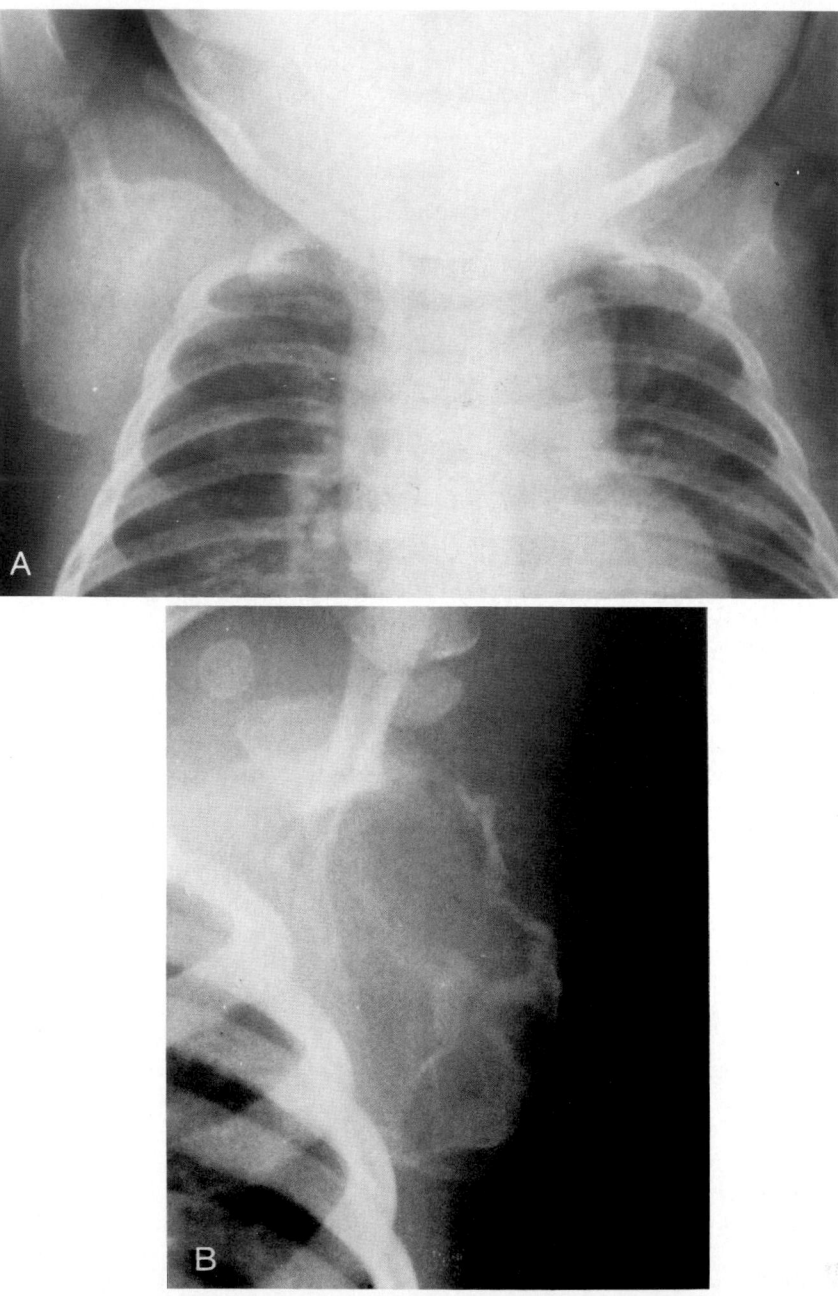

Fig. 4.96. Scapular enlargement. A. Note slightly ballooned right scapula with sclerotic edges in healing Caffey's disease. B. Markedly ballooned, destroyed scapula in histiocytosis X.

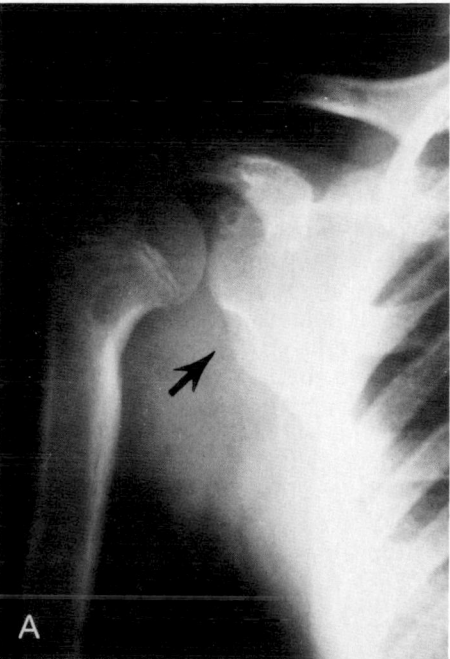

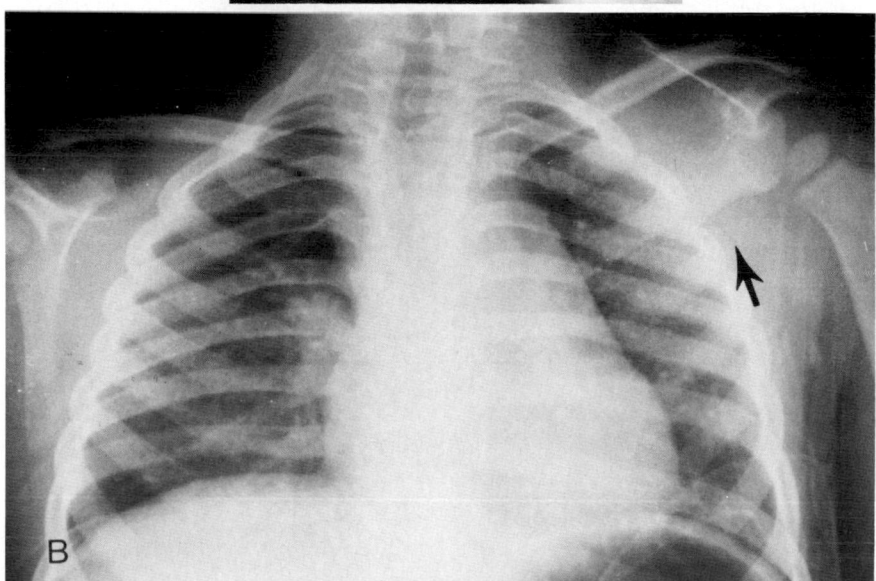

Fig. 4.97. A. **Shallow, hypoplastic glenoid fossa** (arrow) in Hurler's disease. The scapula also is hypoplastic. Note notch in upper humerus. B. **Sprengel's deformity.** Note typical upwardly rotated left scapula (arrow).

monly seen in the storage diseases (Fig. 4.97A). A **small glenoid fossa** also can be seen as the result of chronic dislocation of the shoulder (usually neurogenic disease), and of course with simple hypoplasia of the scapula. Although hypoplasia can occur on an isolated basis, it also is seen with Sprengle's deformity, a condition where the scapula is rotated and fixed in an abnormally high position (Fig. 4.97B). The findings are rather characteristic and often associated with the Klippel-Feil syndrome (fusion-segmentation anomalies of the cervical spine). In some cases an anomalous bone between the spine and scapula is seen, the so-called omo-vertebral bone.

Indistinctness of the scapular edges is seen with severe osteomalacia, and for the most part occurs with rickets and hyperparathyroidism (usually secondary in renal osteodystrophy). In some of these cases, the scapula is so soft that the bottom end becomes bent outward. Irregularity of the acromial process occurs with trauma and, in infants, is reasonably pathognomonic of the battered child syndrome (2).

References

1. Hope JW, Gould RJ: Scapular lesions in childhood. *Am J Roentgenol* 88:496–502, 1962.
2. Kogutt MS, Swischuk WE, Fagan CJ: Patterns of injury and significance of uncommon fractures in the battered child syndrome. *Am J Roentgenol* 121:143–149, 1974.

Pelvis

There are a number of findings in the pelvis which are useful in the differential diagnosis of various syndromes and dysplasias, but one of the more common is the so-called small, **squared iliac wing.** In these cases the iliac wings are smaller than normal, appear rotated outwardly, and are associated with flat acetabular roofs or angles (5). Basically, two types can be identified, and arbitrarily can be designated as A and B (Fig. 4.98). In type A, the iliac wings are more hypoplastic and outwardly rotated. They also appear very dysplastic, have deep sciatic notches, and a crinkled or irregular acetabular roof. All of these changes tend to become less pronounced as the patient grows older. In the type B wing, there is less hypoplasia and a more normal appearance of the sciatic notch and acetabular roof. However, the iliac wing still is short from top to bottom and a certain degree of outward rotation occurs. A list of conditions producing these iliac wing deformities is presented in Table 4.34, but basically, the type A iliac wing is associated with the various chondrodystrophies.

NARROWING OF THE WAIST OR LOWER PART OF THE ILIAC WING (Table 4.34)

This is a less common abnormality and usually occurs with the various storage diseases (Fig. 4.99A). However, it also occurs with trisomy 18, Larsen's syndrome, and the Melnick-Needles syndrome. In all of these cases, the roof of the acetabulum is more slanted, for the iliac wings, rather than flaring out, turn in (see Fig. 4.100C). This leads to hip dislocations, and indeed dislocation of the hips is common in the trisomy 18 and Larsen's syndromes. Increased steepness of the acetabular angle also is seen with classic congenital dislocating hip, and in the more severe cases, a pseudoacetabulum develops above the normal acetabulum. This causes the neck of the iliac wing to become even more narrowed (Fig. 4.99B). In addition to these causes, narrowing of the waist of the iliac wing can occur with bone deforming conditions such as neurofibromatosis and hemangiomas or lymphangiomas in the area (see Fig. 4.36B).

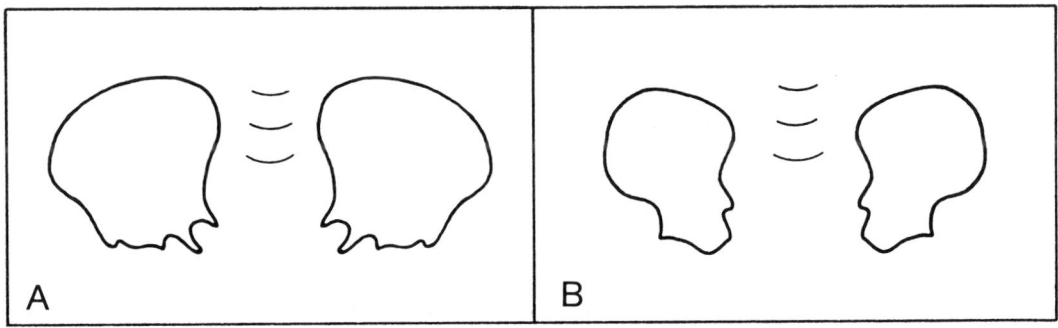

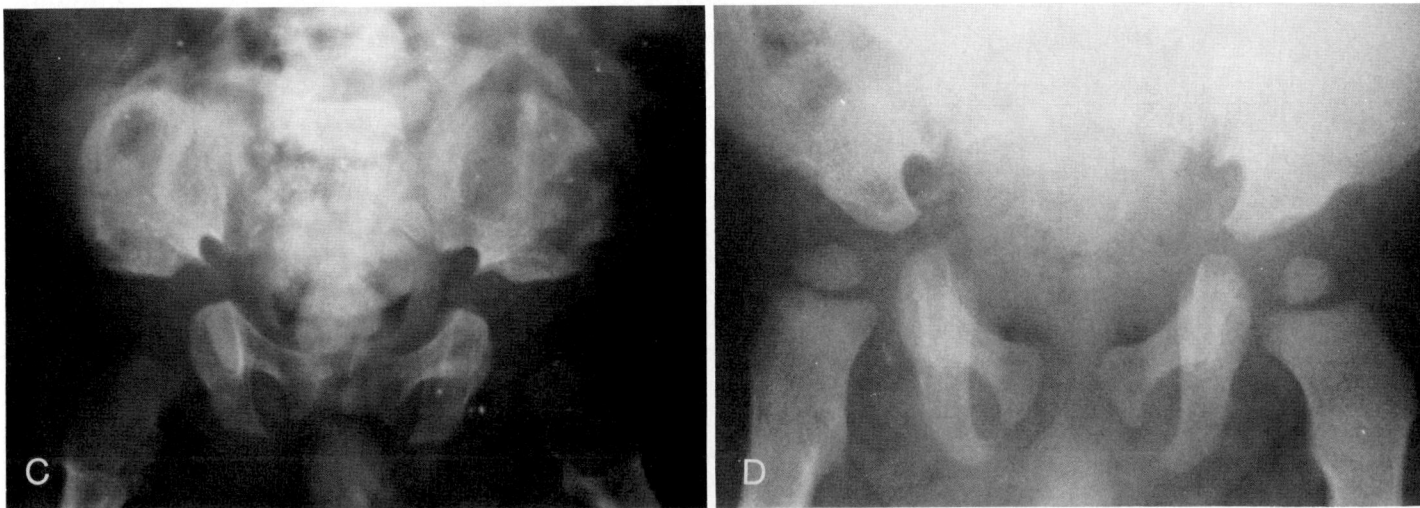

Fig. 4.98. Pelvis; squared iliac wings. A. In the **type A pelvis,** the iliac wings are markedly underdeveloped, very square, and show considerable irregularity of the acetabulum roofs. B. In the **type B pelvis,** changes are less pronounced and the iliac wings less square. C. Typical **type A pelvis** in achondroplasia. D. Typical **type B pelvis** in Hurler's disease.

Table 4.34   Small Squared and Flared Iliac Wings—Decreased Acetabular Angle

Type A
Achondroplasia
Achondrogenesis
Asphyxiating thoracic dystrophy
Ellis-van Creveld syndrome
Short rib polydactyly syndromes
Metatropic dwarfism
Kniest's syndrome
Spondyloepiphyseal dysplasia congenita
Punctate epiphyseal dysplasia (rhizomelic form)
Thanatophoric dwarfism
Morquio's disease
Severe metaphyseal dysostoses
Dyggve Melchior-Clausen syndrome
Type B
Trisomy 21 (Down's, Mongolism)
Mucopolysaccharidoses (except Morquio's)
Mucolipidoses
Other storage diseases
Cleidocranial dysostosis
Cockayne's syndrome
Acrocephalosyndactyly
Aminopterin-induced syndrome
Arthrogryposis
Cornelia de Lange syndrome
Hypophosphatasia
Popliteal pterygium syndrome
Osteo-onychodysplasia
Prune-belly syndrome
Rubinstein-Taybi syndrome
Bladder Extrophy
Sacral agenesis
Trisomy 13
Metaphyseal dysostoses (mild cases)
Osteogenesis imperfecta
Weissenbacher-Zweymuller syndrome
Narrowed iliac waist (increased acetabular angle)
Congenital dislocating hip
Trisomy 18
The storage diseases
Melnick-Needles syndrome
Hemangioma-lymphangioma of bone or soft tissue

FLAT AND STEEP ACETABULAR ANGLES

Flat acetabular angles occur in most of the chondrodystrophies demonstrating the type A pelvis and square iliac wing (see Table 4.34). Otherwise, flat acetabular angles are due to outwardly flared iliac wings and are characteristic of trisomy 21 (Fig. 4.100A). Steep acetabular angles are due to inward turning of the iliac wings and are characteristic of trisomy 18 (see Fig. 4.100C). Steep acetabular angles also occur with congenital hip dislocation (Fig. 4.100B).

DELAYED OR DEFECTIVE OSSIFICATION OF THE PUBIC BONES

This type of ossification is not uncommon in normal premature infants, but, on a pathologic basis, occurs in certain syndromes (2). For example, the pubic bones are underossified in most of the neonatal and infantile chondrodystrophies, but the finding is not utilized for specific diagnosis. On the other hand, it is a specific finding in cleidocranial dysostosis (Fig. 4.101A). It also is used as an adjunctive finding in punctate epiphyseal dysplasia, spondyloepiphyseal dysplasia congenita (Fig. 4.101B), Wolf's chromosome 4P syndrome, and the Taybi-Lindner syndrome. In all of these conditions, because the pubic bones are unossified, the **interpubic distance is increased** (see Fig. 4.101B). Other conditions where the distance is increased, but not necessarily associated with hypoplastic pubic bones include extrophy of the bladder, the cryptophalmia syndrome, the prune-belly syndrome, the Sjorgren-Larsson syndrome, Goltz syndrome, epispadias, and occasionally hypospadias. Separation of

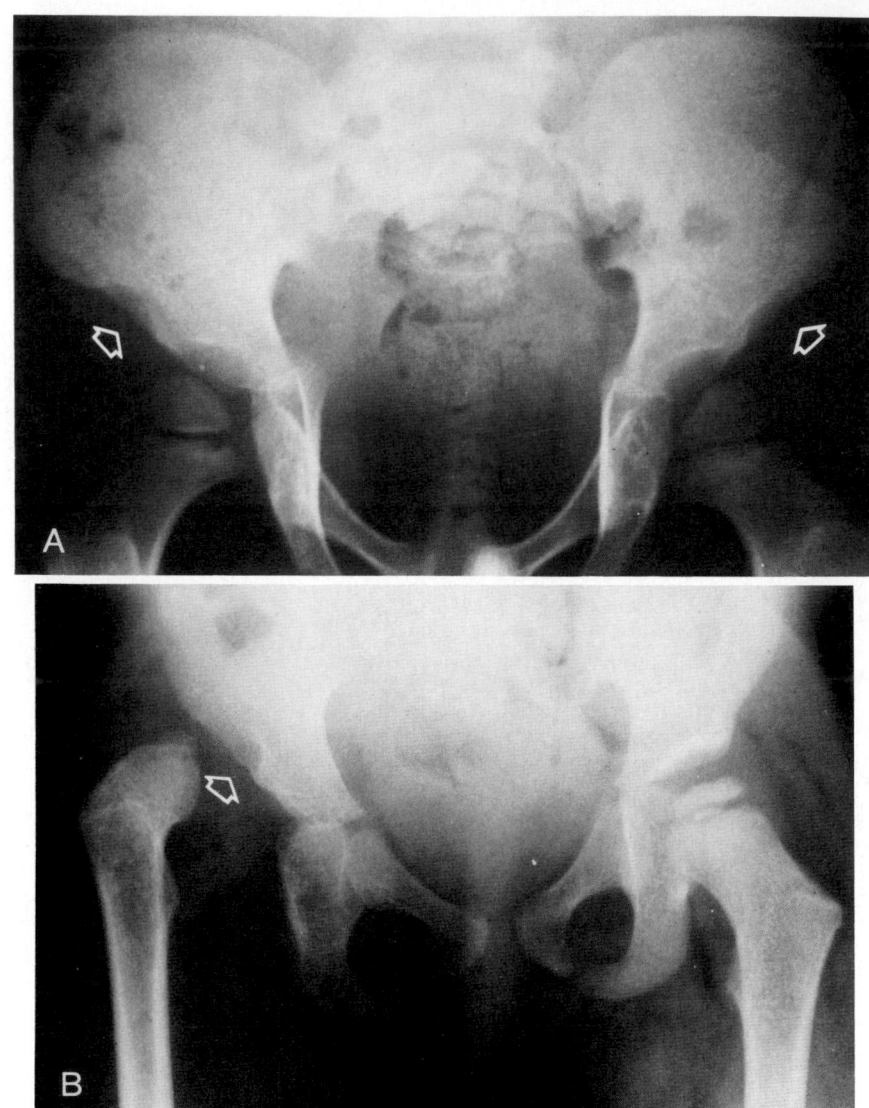

Fig. 4.99. Narrowing of waist or lower part of iliac bone. A. Narrowing (arrows) of iliac waist in Hurler's disease. B. Narrowed iliac waist (arrow) in chronic congenital hip dislocation with pseudo acetabulum formation.

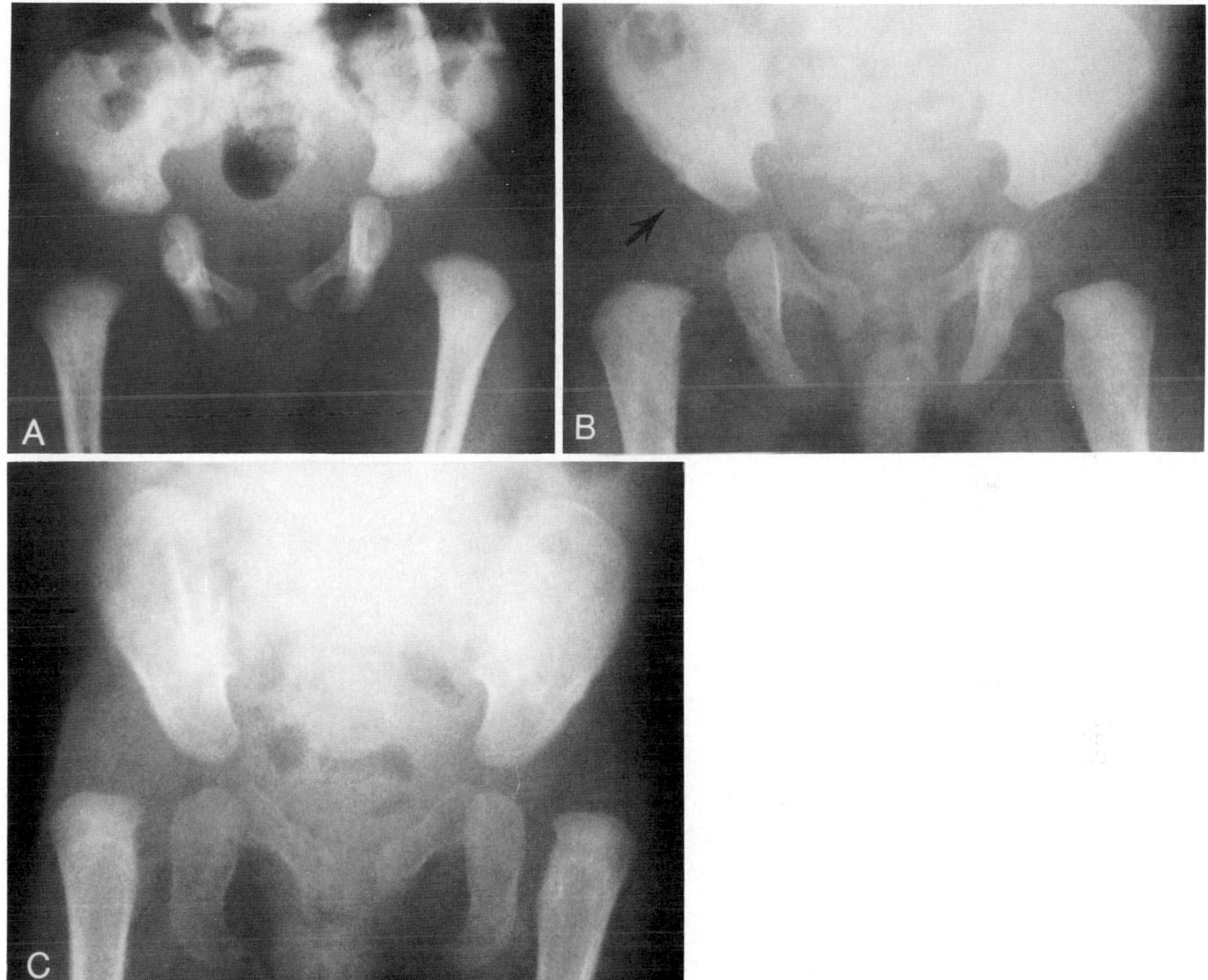

Fig. 4.100. Abnormal acetabular angles. A. Typical flat acetabular roof in trisomy 21. Also note flat acetabular roofs in achondroplasia (Fig. 4.98C). B. Increased acetabular slope in congenital hip dislocation on the right (arrow). C. Note bilateral increased acetabular slope in trisomy 18. Both hips also are dislocated.

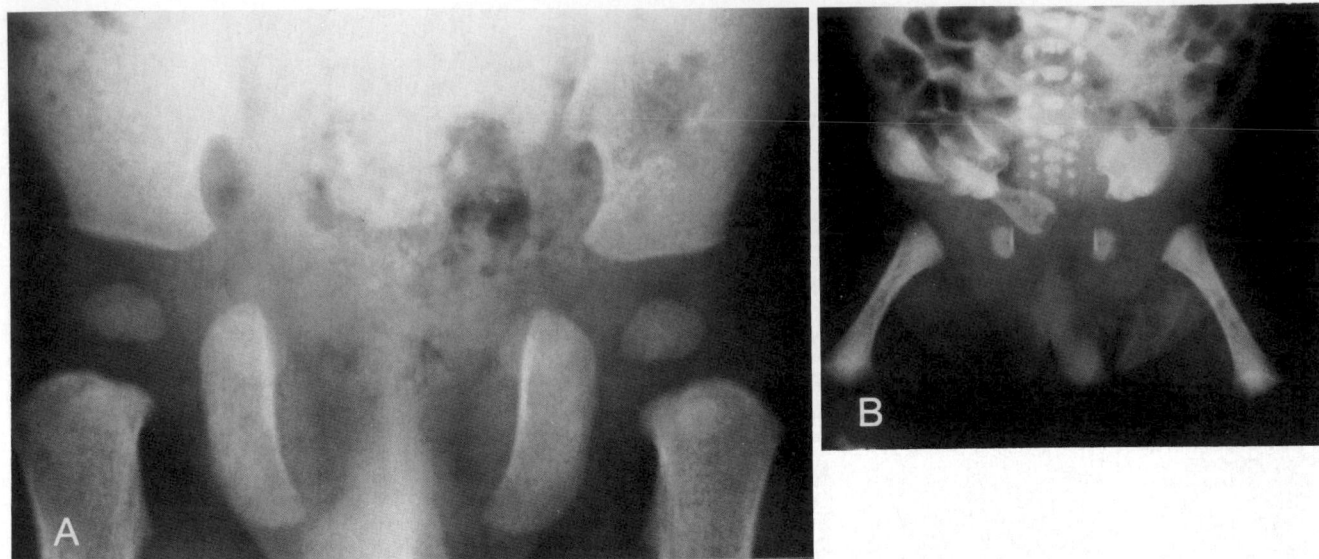

Fig. 4.101. Delayed or defective ossification of pubic bones. A. Virtual absence of pubic ramii in cleidocranial dysostosis. B. Hypoplastic pubic ramii in spondyloepiphyseal dysplasia congenita.

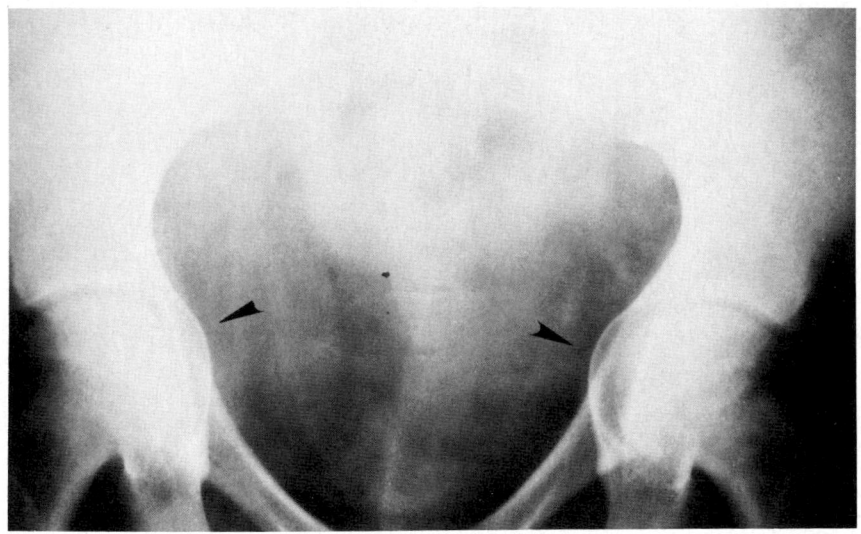

Fig. 4.102. Acetabulae protrusio. Note inward bulging of medial acetabular margins (arrows) in long standing renal osteodystrophy.

the pubic bones also can be seen with diastasis recti and has been noted in patients demonstrating anorectal, genital, and urinary tract abnormalities (3). Acquired widening of the pubic symphysis is seen after trauma, osteomyelitis, and rarely with destructive tumors.

ACETABULAE PROTRUSIO

Acetabulae protrusio is uncommon in the pediatric age group but can be seen with Turner's syndrome, osteogenesis imperfecta, Still's disease (juvenile rheumatoid arthritis), and renal osteodystrophy (Fig. 4.102).

MISCELLANEOUS ABNORMALITIES

Exostoses from the iliac wing have been dealt with elsewhere (see p 207), and so have **cortical erosions** (p 194). **Complete destruction of the pelvic bones** occurs in the same conditions as it does with any bone (i.e., acute osteomyelitis, malignant sarcomas, metastatic disease, hemangioma, lymphangioma, etc.), and

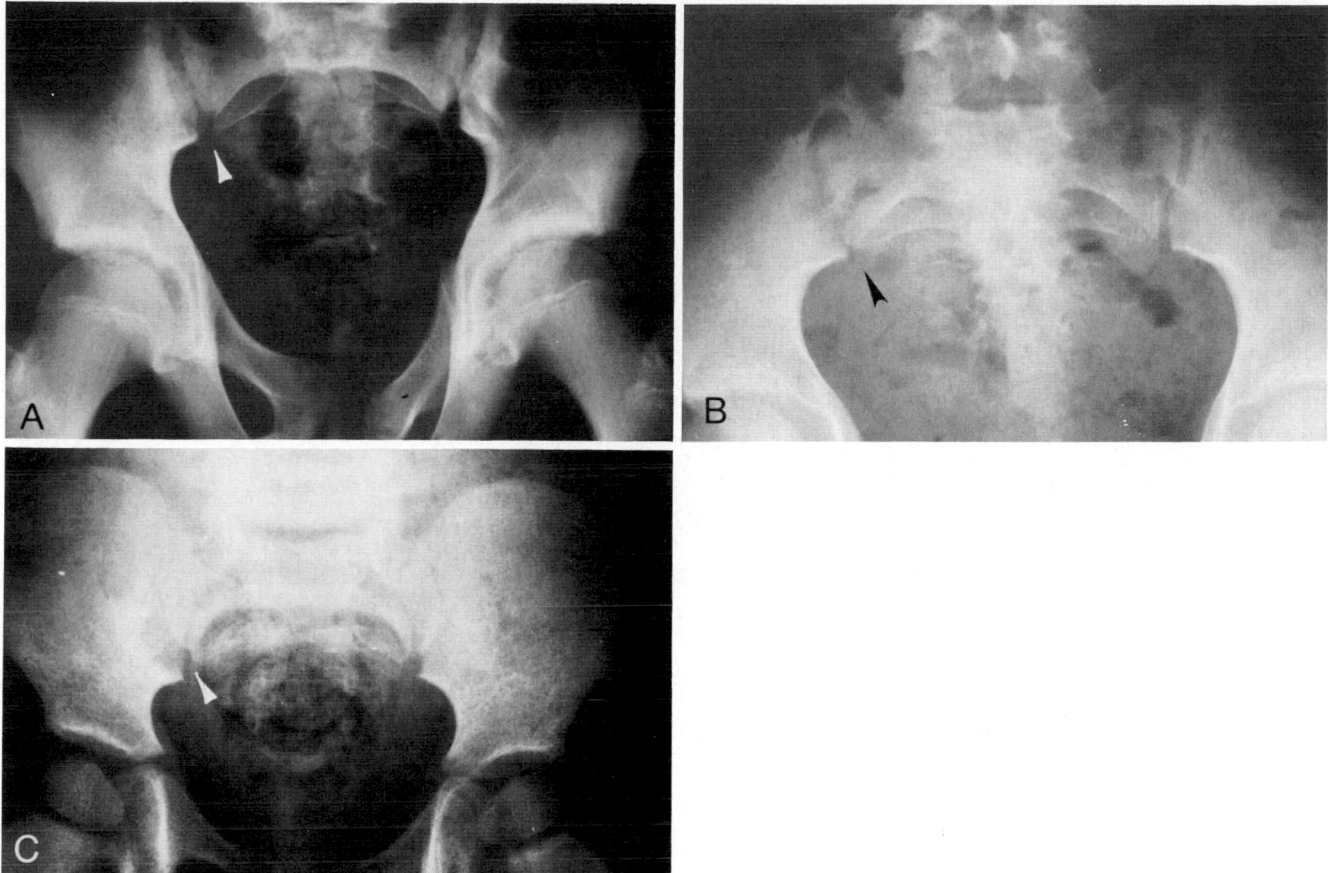

Fig. 4.103. Sacroiliac joint abnormalities. A. Widening of the sacroiliac (arrow) in pelvic trauma. B. Widened, indistinct joint in acute pyogenic infection (arrow). C. Widening of the sacroiliac joint (arrow) and adjacent bony sclerosis in healing osteomyelitis.

cysts, bony tumors, and osteomyelitis appear much the same as they do in other bones of the body.

ABNORMAL CONFIGURATIONS OF THE SACROILIAC JOINTS

These abnormal configurations are not particularly common, and apart from a variety of congenital articulation disturbances between the sacrum and iliac bone, consist primarily of **undue widening of the sacroiliac joint.** In many cases there is associated sclerosis of the joint edges and the commonest causes of this configuration are trauma (Fig. 4.103A), infection, or inflammation. Infection can be pyogenic (Fig. 4.103B) or tuberculous, while inflammation usually is due to rheumatoid arthritis. Widening secondary to acute trauma is self evident but, on a chronic basis, can be seen in the child with a longstanding limp. In these cases, the findings are the result of chronic stresses sustained by the joint as a result of the limp. In most of these conditions, the findings are difficult to distinguish one from the other (Fig. 4.103C), and when osteomyelitis is suspected, bone scanning should

be utilized (1, 3, 5). However, the bone scan will not necessarily identify that osteomyelitis is the problem, for it is a nonspecific screening modality and also is positive after trauma and conditions such as rheumatoid arthritis.

References

1. Ailsby RL, Stheli LT: Pyogenic infections of the sacroiliac joint in children: radioisotope bone scanning as a diagnostic tool. *Clin Orthop* 100:96–100, 1974.
2. Cortina H, Vallcanera A, Andres V, Gracia A, Aparici R, Mari A: The non-ossified pubis. *Pediatr Radiol* 8:87–92, 1979.
3. Muecke EC, Currarino G: Congenital widening of the pubic symphysis. *Am J Roentgenol* 103:179–185, 1968.
4. Schhad UB, McCracken GH Jr, Nelson JD: Pyogenic arthritis of the sacroiliac joint in pediatric patients. *Pediatrics* 66:375–379, 1980.
5. Taybi H, Kane P: Small acetabular and iliac angles and associated diseases. *Radiol Clin North Am* 6:215–221, 1968.
6. Trauner DA, Connor JD: Radioactive scanning in diagnosis of acute sacroiliac osteomyelitis. *J Pediatr* 87:751–753, 1975.

Sternum

Hypersegmentation of the sternum occurs in trisomy 21 (Mongolism), and **undersegmentation** in trisomy 18 (Fig. 4.104, A and B). Undersegmentation also occurs in campomelic dwarfism, Noonan's syndrome, and the Brachman De Lange syndrome and, in all of these conditions, often is associated with hypoplasia and premature fusion. A **pectus carinatum** deformity (Fig. 4.105, A and B) may result and the same problem is seen in congenital heart disease, especially the chronic cyanotic variety (2–6). Pectus carinatum also can occur as an isolated finding, but on an isolated basis **pectus excavatum** is more common (Fig. 4.105, C and D). A pectus excavatum deformity of the chest also occurs any time the bones are softened (i.e., osteomalacia, newborn with respiratory distress) and after trauma with a flail chest.

Retrosternal thickening of the soft tissues most commonly is due to some disease process in the sternum. This can be tumor, extramedulary hematopoiesis, osteomyelitis, or trauma, and often the soft tissue thickening is localized or undulating. However, it also can appear as a more uniform retrosternal arc. The latter configuration also can be seen with pleural fluid accumulations and the hypogenetic right lung syndrome (see Fig. 1.17B). A rare cause of localized thickening of the retrosternal soft tissues, just behind the manubrium, is posterior dislocation of the medial aspect of the clavicle. A congenital **bifid sternum** can occur as an incidental anomaly or with ectopia cordis (1), and lytic and destructive lesions of the sternum have the same differential diagnosis as they do with other bones of the skeleton.

References

1. Chang CH, Davis WC: Congenital bifid sternum with partial ectopia cordis. *Am J Roentgenol* 86:513–516, 1961.
2. Currarino G, Silverman FN: Premature obliteration of the sternal sutures and pigeon-breast deformity. *Radiology* 70:532–540, 1958.
3. Fischer KC, White RI, Jordan CE, Dorst JP, Neill CA: Sternal abnormalities in patients with congenital heart disease. *Am J Roentgenol* 119:530–538, 1973.
4. Gabrielsen TO, Ladyman GH: Early closure of the sternal sutures and congenital heart disease. *Am J Roentgenol* 89:975–983, 1963.
5. Kim OH, Gooding CA: Delayed sternal ossification in infants with congenital heart disease. *Pediatr Radiol* 10:219–223, 1981.
6. Lees RF, Caldicott WJH: Sternal anomalies and congenital heart disease. *Am J Roentgenol* 124:423–427, 1975.

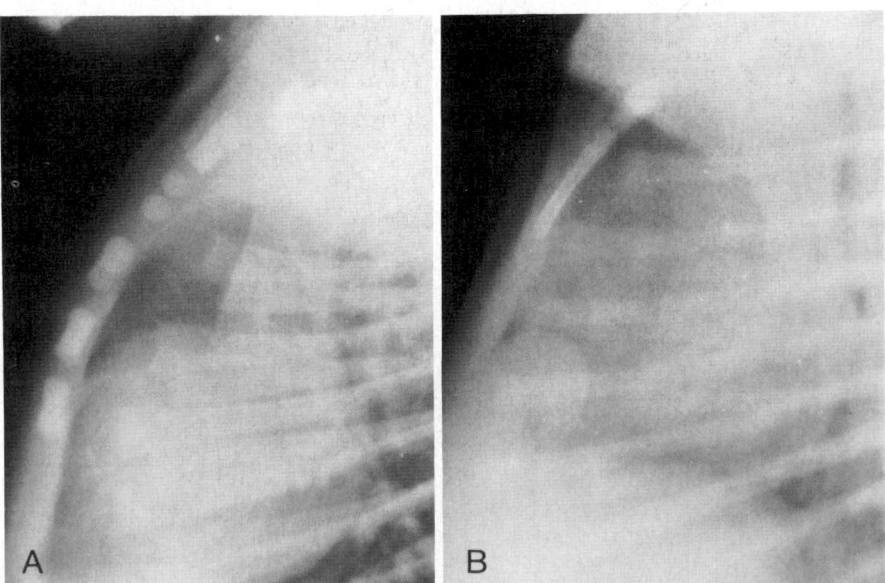

Fig. 4.104. Segmentation abnormalities of sternum. A. Note hypersegmentation of sternum in trisomy 21. B. Undersegmentation of sternum in trisomy 18.

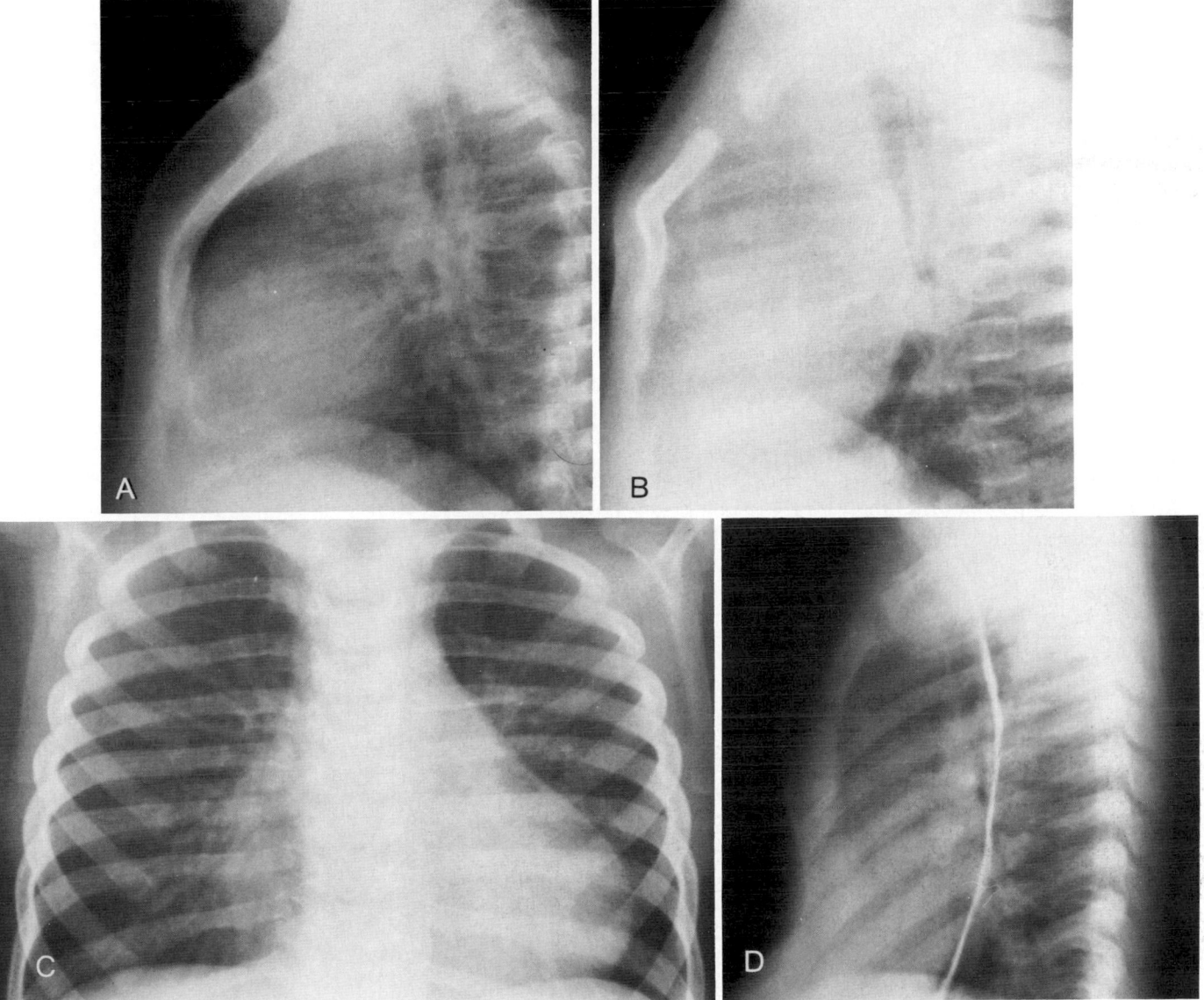

Fig. 4.105.   Pectus deformity. A. Typical bulging chest of pectus carinatum deformity in patient with congenital heart disease. B. Another patient with a pectus carinatum deformity. C. Pectus excavatum deformity leading to shift of the mediastinum to the left, downward slanting of the anterior ribs, a more horizontal position of the posterior ribs, and apparent infiltrate along the right cardiac border. D. Lateral view showing dipping sternum characteristic of the pectus excavatum deformity.

Ribs

Abnormalities of rib shape consist of under- or overtubulation, cupped or straight anterior rib ends, rib notching, twisted ribs, and rib defects (Table 4.35). Other abnormalities also occur, but basically these are no different from those which occur in other bones of the body (i.e., destructive lesions, fractures, demineralization, periosteal new bone, etc.).

Overtubulation of the ribs leads to **thin ribs,** while undertubulation causes **short squat ribs.** Basically, the same conditions producing these abnormalities in the long bones and clavicles also produce them in the

ribs, and most are documented in Tables 4.3 and 4.5. However, thin ribs are most pronounced in premature infants, trisomy 18, progeria, and osteogenesis imperfecta. **Wide, paddle-shaped ribs** constitute a specific type of rib widening where there is a short and narrow posterior, juxtaspinal segment and then broadening out of the rib to produce a paddle shape. Almost exclusively this configuration occurs in the storage diseases (Fig. 4.106), but not all of the conditions in this group of diseases produce the same degree of change and, actually, most profound changes are seen

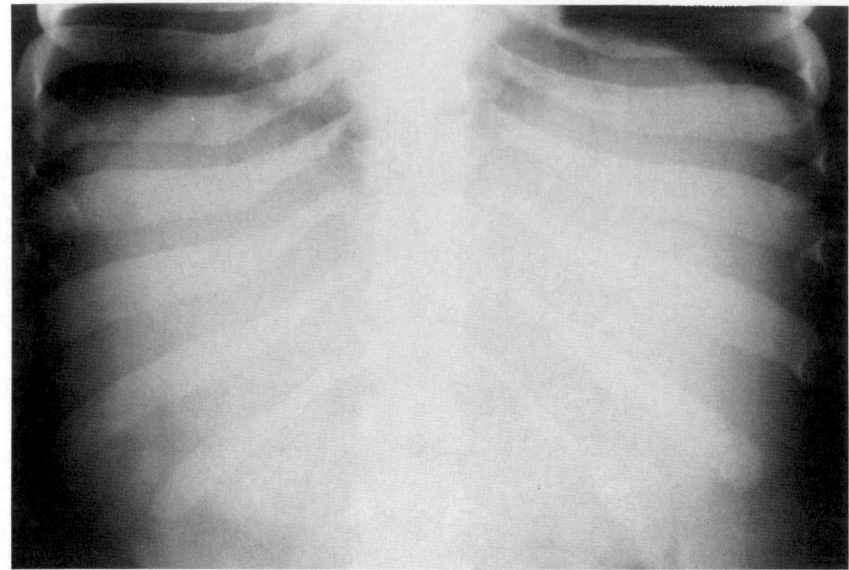

Fig. 4.106. Wide paddle-shaped ribs characteristic of Hurler's disease. Note marked narrowing proximally and considerable broadening laterally.

Table 4.35   Rib Abnormalities

A. Anterior rib cupping
   Same as metaphyseal cupping—see Table 4.24.

B. Anterior rib straightening

Hypothyroidism	}	Commonest
Osteopetrosis		
Storage Diseases		

C. Rib notching

Coarctation of aorta	}	Commonest
Postop Blalock-Taussig shunt	}	Moderately common
Normal		
Neurofibromatosis	}	Relatively rare
Melnick-Needles osteodysplasia	}	Rare
Collaterals with pulmonary valve atresia		
Superior vena cava obstruction		
AV fistula of the chest wall		
Intercostal nerve tumors		
Intercostal arteritis		
Poliomyelitis		

in Hurler's disease, Hunter's disease, mucopolysaccharidosis IV (Marateaux-Lamy), mucolipidosis II (I cell disease), and generalized gangliosidosis.

CUPPING OF THE ANTERIOR RIBS

Cupping (Fig. 4.107) is comparable to splaying of the metaphyses of the long bones and causes of both are very similar. Traumatic cupping resulting from healing costochondral injuries (Fig. 4.107C) are near pathognomonic in the battered child syndrome (3). **Undue straightening of the anterior rib ends** (Fig. 4.107D) occurs when bone growth is impaired and most often is seen with hypothyroidism, osteopetrosis, and the storage diseases (mucopolysaccharidoses, mucolipidoses, and gangliosidosis). Usually, normal anterior rib ends show slight cupping, but in these conditions they appear rather straight.

RIB NOTCHING

This is not overly common in childhood but, when seen, most often is due to coarctation of the aorta (1, 2, 9). Notches in this condition occur on the inferior surface of the ribs (most often, 4th through 8th ribs) and usually are seen in the older child (Fig. 4.108A). Even then, however, only about one half of the cases of coarctation of the aorta demonstrate the finding. The next most common cause of rib notching is normal variation, where slight undulations of the inferior rib margins may suggest notching. However, most often the finding is very subtle and overlooked. Thereafter, unilateral notching can be seen with Blalock-Taussig shunts for tetralogy of Fallot or other similar congenital heart lesions. In these cases, because the subclavian artery is anastomosed to the hypoplastic pulmonary artery, arterial flow to the involved extremity is diminished, and over the years, collateral circulation and rib notching develop. Notching or undulation of the lower rib margins also can occur with neurofibromatosis, Melnick-Needles osteodysplasia, from collateral circulation in long standing pulmonary valve atresia or pulmonary trunk agenesis

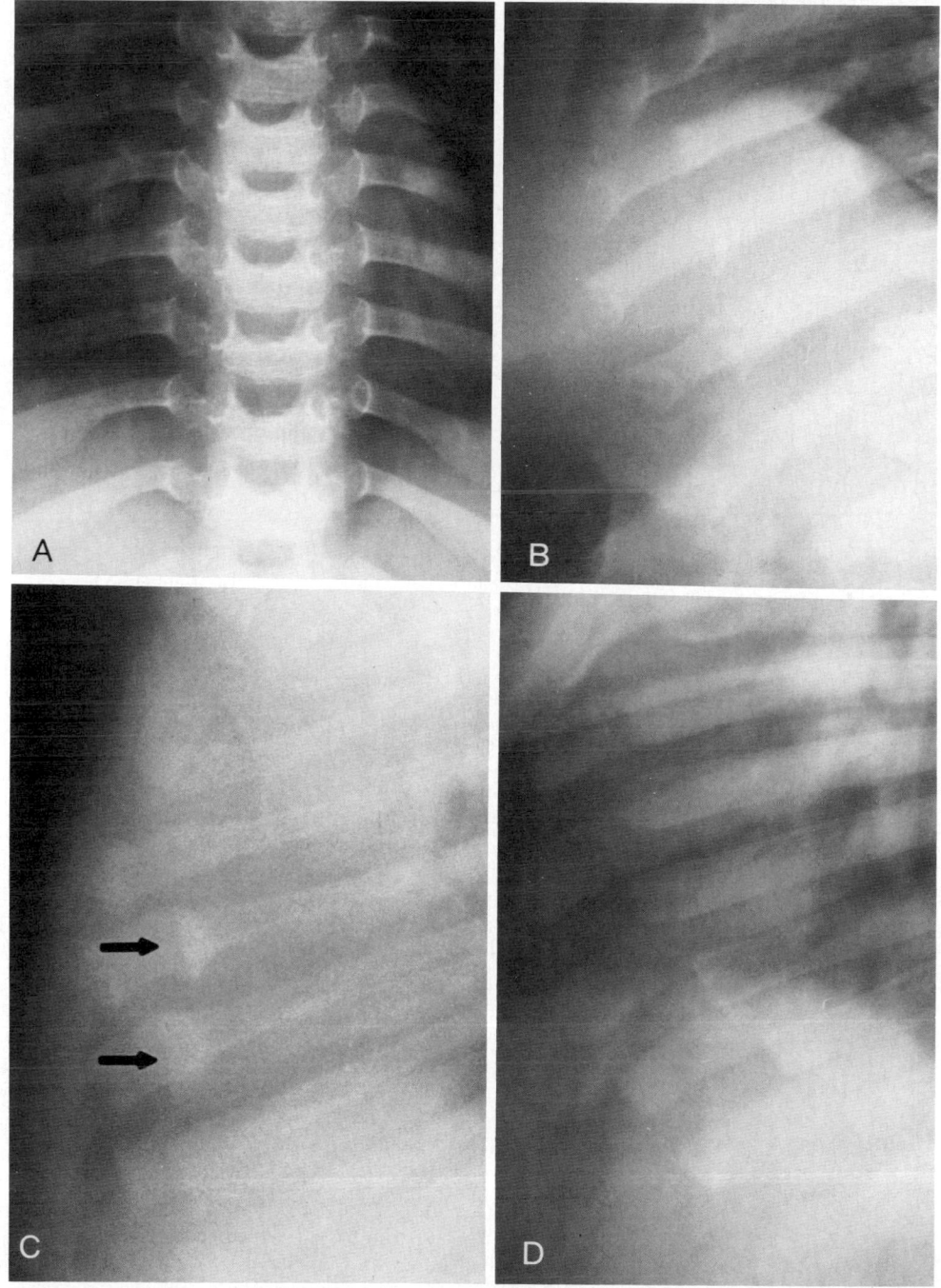

Fig. 4.107.   Cupping of the ribs. A. Cupping of the rubs in spondyloepiphyseal dysplasia. B. Same patient showing anterior cupping. C. Cupping of two ribs (arrows) in costochondral injury in battered child syndrome. D. **Undue straightening of anterior ribs.** Note flattening of the rib ends in Hurler's disease.

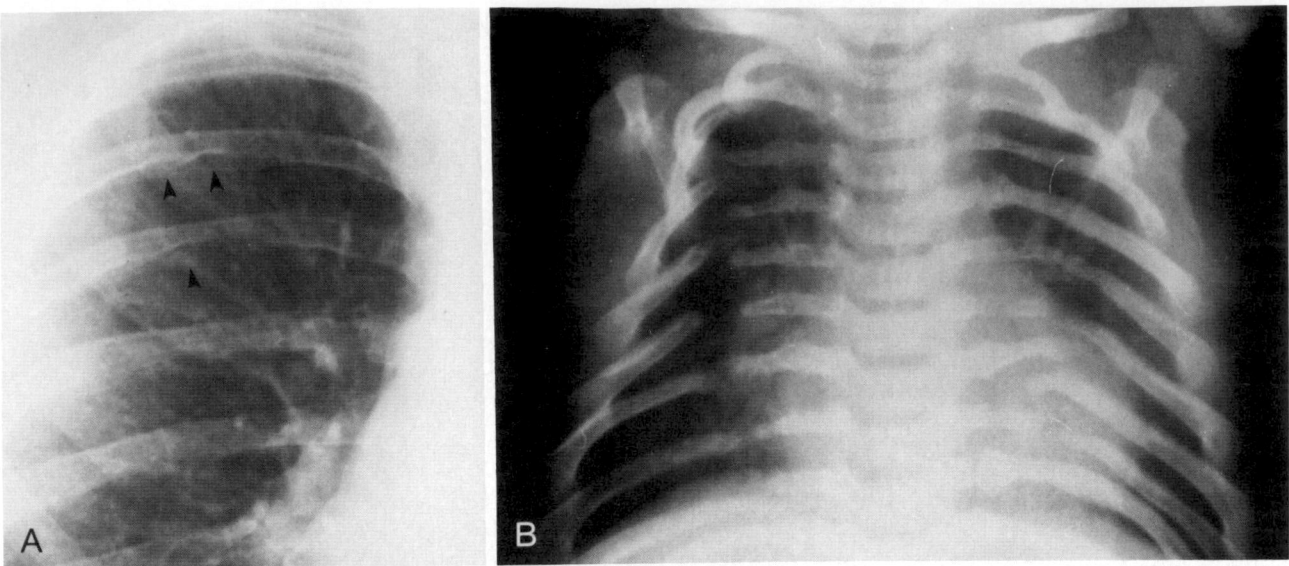

Fig. 4.108.   A. Rib notching. Typical bilateral rib notching (arrows) in coarctation of the aorta. B. **Rib defects.** Typical extensive rib defects in cerebrocostal mandibular syndrome (reproduced with permission from Williams HJ, Sane SM: *Am J Roentgenol* 126:1223–1228, 1976) (10).

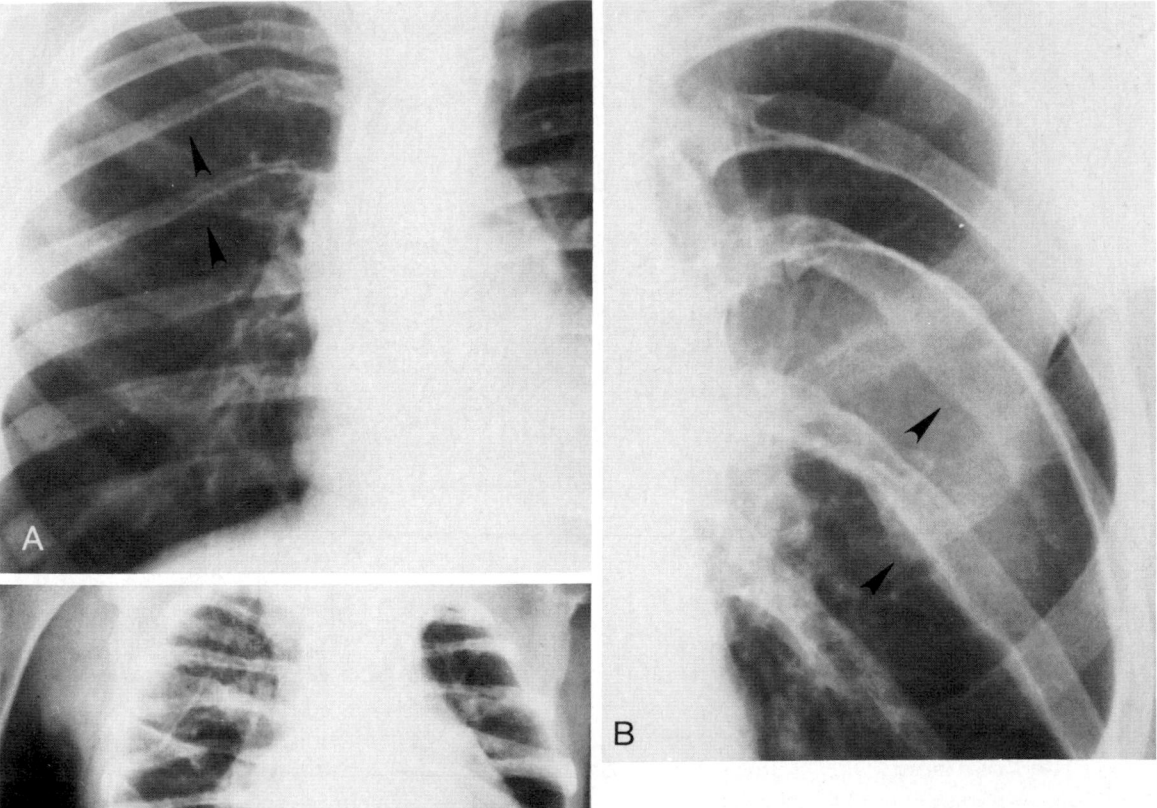

Fig. 4.109.   Twisted ribs. A. Thin, slightly twisted ribs in neurofibromatosis (arrows). B. Twisted, ribbon-like ribs in neurofibromatosis (arrows). C. Twisted, thin ribs in Melnick-Needles osteodysplasia.

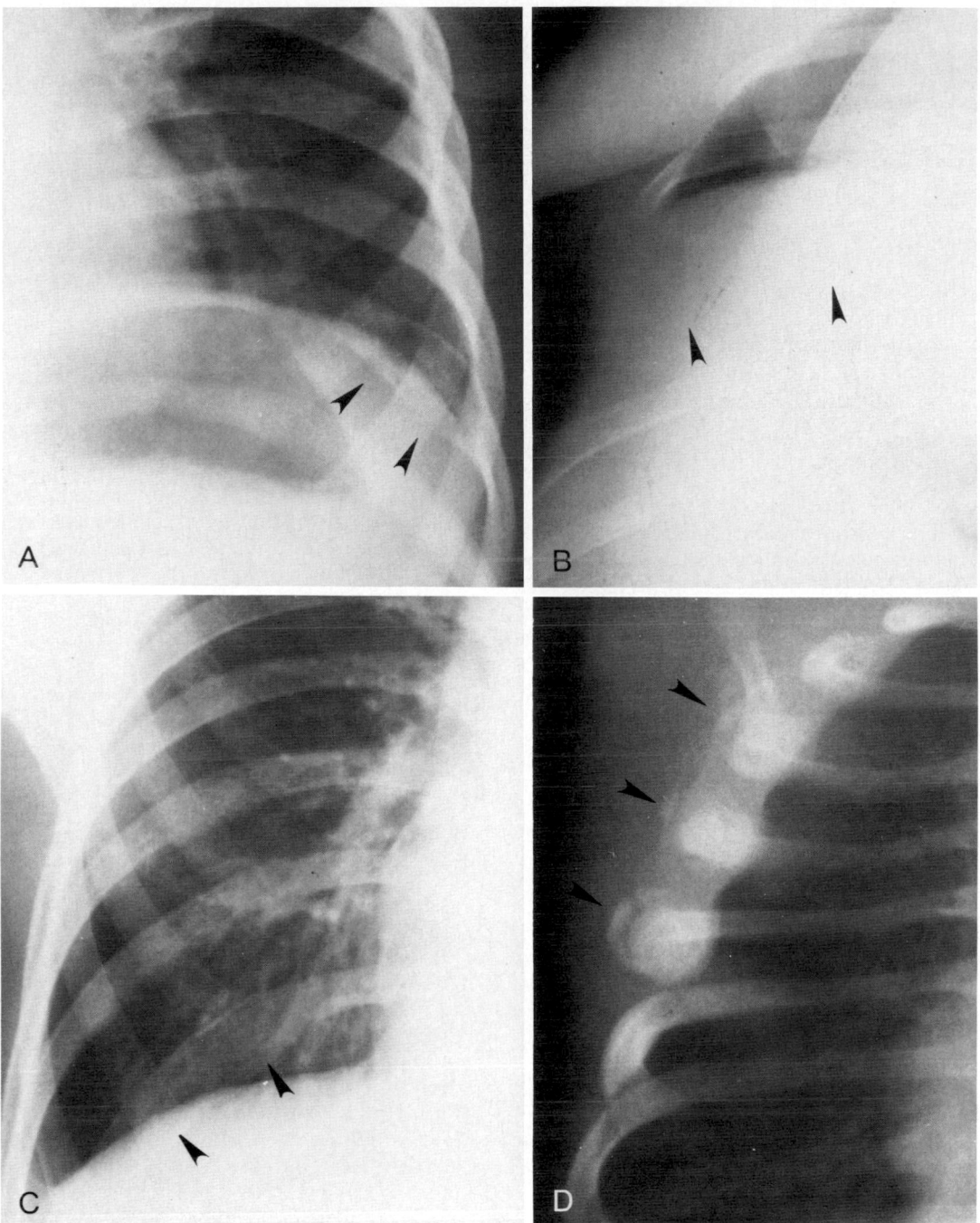

Fig. 4.110. **Massive destruction of ribs.** A. Destruction, with expansion, of rib in histiocytosis X (arrows). B. Completely destroyed rib in Ewing's sarcoma (arrows). C. Widespread destruction with moderate expansion of a rib in Ewing's sarcoma (arrows). D. **Lumpy target lesion of rib.** Multiple target lesions (arrows) of ribs due to healing rib fractures in battered child syndrome.

(i.e., the old, so-called persistent truncus arteriosis, type IV), superior vena caval obstruction, AV fistula of the chest wall, intercostal nerve tumors, intercostal arteritis, and poliomyelitis. All of these, however, are rare in childhood and, thus, on a practical basis, when rib notching is seen in a child, it either is normal,

associated with coarctation of the aorta, or secondary to a Blalock-Taussig shunt.

RIB DEFECTS

Rib defects are not particularly common in children but can be seen after infection, surgery, or fracture.

On a congenital basis, they occur in the cerebro-costo-mandibular syndrome and the finding is rather pathognomonic (Fig. 4.108B). Associated smallness of the mandible in this condition has caused most to consider it a variation of the Pierre-Robin syndrome (5, 8).

TWISTED RIBS

Twisted ribs can be seen with neurofibromatosis (Fig. 4.109, A and B), the basal cell nevus syndrome, Melnick-Needles osteodysplasia (6) (Fig. 4.109C), spondylothoracic dysplasia (4, 7), congenital hypoplasia with synostosis, and after thoracotomy. In most of these cases, the ribs also are thinned, but in neurofibromatosis, they can be wide and ribbon-like (Fig. 4.109B).

DESTRUCTIVE LESIONS

These lesions have the same differential diagnosis as they do in long, and other flat bones, but massive destruction usually occurs with osteomyelitis, histiocytosis X (Fig. 4.110A), Ewing's sarcoma (Fig. 4.110, B and C), metastatic disease, leukemia, lymphoma, and hemangioma or lymphangioma. In the latter, very often the bone is totally dissolved (i.e., vanishing bone disease—see Fig. 4.36). With Ewing's sarcoma and histiocytosis X, the destroyed rib also may be expanded (Fig. 4.110, A and C).

LUMPY, TARGET LESIONS

Lumpy, target lesions of the ribs are seen with healing rib fractures (Fig. 4.110D). The finding results from callus formation and also can be seen with rib infarction in sickle cell disease, and with healing after destruction secondary to infection or tumor. As far as fractures are concerned, most often they are sustained in the battered child syndrome.

References

1. Babbitt DP, Cassidy GE, Godard JE: Rib notching in aortic coarctation during infancy and early childhood. *Radiology* 110:169–171, 1974.
2. Gooding CA, Glickman MG, Suydam MJ: Fate of rib notching after correction of aortic coarctation. *Am J Roentgenol Radium Ther Nucl Med* 106:21–23, 1969.
3. Kogutt MS, Swischuk LE, Fagan CJ: Patterns of injury and significance of uncommon fractures in the battered child syndrome. *Am J Roentgenol* 121:143–149, 1974.
4. Kozlowski K: Spondylo-costal dysplasia—severe and moderate types (report of 8 cases). *Australas Radiol* 25:81–90, 1981.
5. Leroy JG, Devos EA, Bulcke LJV, Robbe NS: Cerebro-costo-mandibular syndrome with autosomal dominant inheritance. *J Pediatr* 99:441–443, 1981.
6. Melnick JC, Needles CF: An undiagnosed bone dysplasia: A 2 family study of 4 generations and 3 generations. *Am J Roentgenol* 97:39–48, 1966.
7. Moseley JE, Bonforte RJ: Spondylothoracic dysplasia. A syndrome of congenital anomalies. *Am J Roentgenol* 106:166–169, 1969.
8. Silverman FN, Strefling AM, Stevenson DK, Lazarus J: Cerebro-costo-mandibular syndrome. *J Pediatr* 97:406–416, 1980.
9. Sloan RD, Cooley RN: Coarctation of aorta: roentgenologic aspects of one hundred and twenty-five surgically confirmed cases. *Radiology* 61:701–721, 1953.
10. Williams HJ, Sane SM: Cerebro-costo-mandibular syndrome; long term follow-up of a patient and review of the literature. *Am J Roentgenol* 126:1223–1228, 1976.

JOINT ABNORMALITIES

Joint Space Widening

Widening of the joint space can occur because of (*a*) traumatic dislocation, (*b*) joint laxity, (*c*) synovial thickening, and (*d*) joint fluid accumulation (Table 4.36). In the pediatric age group, the latter is most common but occurs almost exclusively in the shoulder and hip (Fig. 4.111, A and B). Lateral dislocation of the humerus or femur occurs readily with fluid accumulation in these joints (1); but, in the others, the ligaments and capsules are too strong to allow much distraction of the bones. As far as the type of fluid is concerned, no specificity exists because it can be blood, serous effusion, or pus. However, traumatic effusions (hemarthroses) and pyogenic exudates are most common. Indeed, going even further, in children in the absence of trauma, pus (pyogenic exudate) should be considered the problem until proven otherwise.

Serous effusions are seen with rheumatoid arthritis, the collagenvascular diseases, tuberculous arthritis, and other chronic arthridities. In the hip one also can add toxic or transient synovitis (3) and Legg-Perthes disease. In Legg-Perthes disease, joint space widening probably is due to a combination of joint fluid accumulation and joint laxity, while in toxic synovitis, the problem is simple joint effusion. However, in the latter, only a few of the more severe cases accumulate enough fluid to develop joint space widening. Indeed, most cases demonstrate very little in the way of roentgenographic change or systemic reaction. Basically, the problem is a limp of rather rapid onset and although viral infection and/or subclinical trauma have been suspect, the condition is of unknown etiology. Transient synovitis is rare in other joints, but we believe that we have seen it in the shoulder and knee.

Hemarthroses leading to joint space widening most often occur with trauma, but occasionally can be seen with bleeding disorders, vascular synovial tumors, or with chronic inflammations of the synovium. Inflammatory synovial thickening most often occurs with tuberculous arthritis, hemophiliac arthropathy, rheumatoid arthritis, Winchester's syndrome (storage disease which looks like rheumatoid arthritis), Farber's

Table 4.36   Joint Space Widening and Narrowing

Joint space widening[a]	
Pyogenic arthritis (hip, shoulder)	
Traumatic effusion or hemarthrosis (hip, shoulder)	Commonest
Toxic (transient) synovitis (usually hip)	
Congenital dislocating hip	
Rheumatoid arthritis	
Traumatic dislocation	
Joint laxity (neurogenic-neuromuscular)	Moderately common
Tuberculous arthritis	
Fungal arthritis	
Pigmented villinodular synovitis	
Ligamentum teres rupture (hip)	
Retained cartilage fragment (hip)	
Synovial tumors	Relatively rare
Winchester's syndrome	
Congenital dislocation—other joints	
Farber's lipogranulomatosis	
Joint space narrowing	
Septic arthritis	Commonest
Rheumatoid arthritis	
Hemophiliac arthropathy	
Tuberculous arthritis	Moderately common
Degenerative arthritis (secondary)	
Slipped capital femoral epiphysis (post operative)	
Pigmented villonodular synovitis	
Fungal arthritis	
Winchester's syndrome	Relatively rare
Degenerative arthritis (primary)	
Traumatic dislocation	
Farber's lipogranulomatosis	

[a] Also use for joint dislocation.

lipogranulomatosis, and pigmented villinodular synovitis. The latter three conditions are quite rare and, in all of the conditions, it should be noted that, while synovial thickening first produces joint space widening, eventually it leads to cartilage destruction and joint space narrowing. This phenomenon occurs at different rates in the various conditions, and the slowest occurs in tuberculous arthritis. Indeed, it may take many months before any significant joint space narrowing is seen, and the reason is that there are few proteolytic enzymes produced by tuberculosis infections. With rampant pyogenic arthritis, on the other hand, proteolytic enzymes abound and joint cartilage destruction occurs rapidly. Consequently, the joint space may narrow within a few days. With rheumatoid arthritis, one may go for months or years without significant narrowing and then, with a serious exacerbation, a joint may narrow within weeks.

Traumatic dislocation with widening of the joint space is self evident and, in such cases, not only is the joint space widened, but the involved bone so out of position that the problem is relatively obvious. However, joint dislocations in childhood are less common than in adults, for most often an epiphyseal-metaphyseal fracture occurs rather than a joint dislocation. The reason for this is that, in a growing bone, the epiphyseal-metaphyseal junction is a weak area and forces are dissipated through it before they are exerted on the joint proper. Nonetheless, joint dislocations still can occur, and one of the most peculiar is that which results from rupture of the ligamentum teres in the hip. In such cases, no bony abnormality is seen, but yet there is a lateral displacement of the femur causing widening of the joint space. In other cases of traumatic dislocation of the hip, a piece of avulsed, unossified cartilage may remain in the joint. This

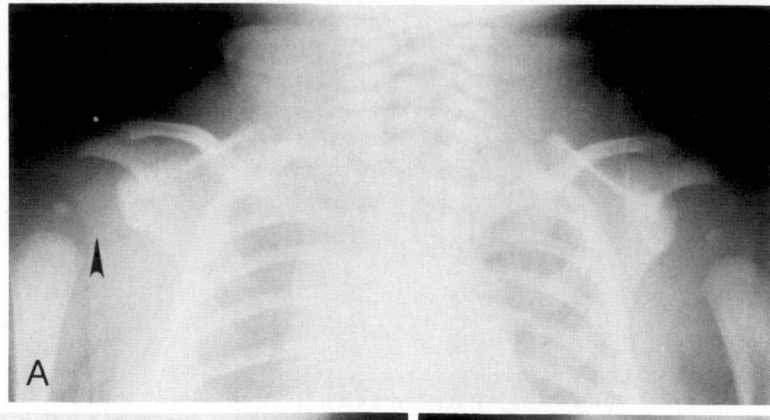

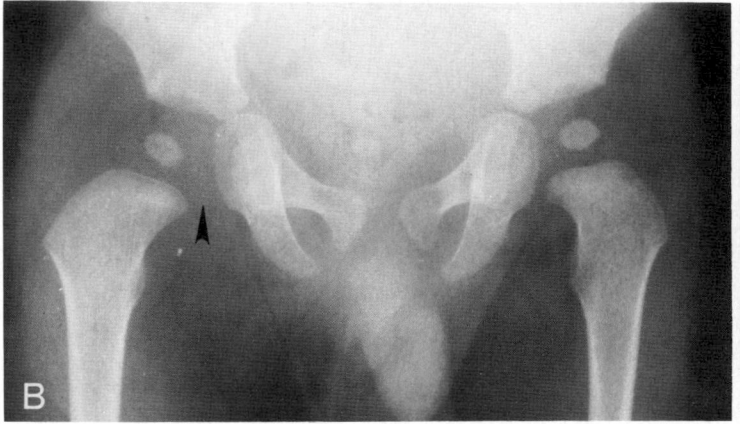

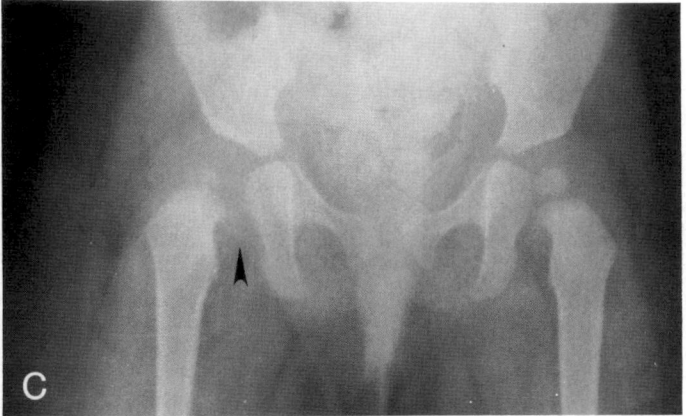

Fig. 4.111. Joint space widening. A. Typical widening of the right shoulder joint (arrow) in septic arthritis. B. Similar widening of right hip joint (arrow) in infant with septic arthritis. C. Widening of the right hip joint (arrow) with congenital dislocation. Note delayed ossification of right femoral head and increased steepness of acetabular roof.

prevents the joint from reducing and chronic joint space widening results. The finding should serve as a signal for the presence of the cartilage fragment (2), which can then be detected with CT scanning.

Congenital dislocations occur in any joint, but once again are most common in the hip (i.e., congenital dislocation of the hip). In this condition, joint space widening is associated with outward and upward displacement of the femur, dysplasia and underdevelopment of the acetabular roof, increase in its pitch, and loss of its normal cupping (Fig. 4.111C). All of these acetabular changes occur because of lack of normal femoral head articulation and are not seen with dislocation due to fluid accumulation. With fluid accumulation, the acetabular roof is normal and displacement of the femoral head is predominantly in the lateral direction. If it occurs in any other direction,

usually it is downward. Joint space widening due to laxity of the muscles and tendons around the joint almost always is due to underlying neurogenic or neuromuscular disease. However, in some cases of septic arthritis, enough destruction of the ligaments and joint capsule occurs to allow for chronic laxity and joint space widening.

References

1. Hayden CK Jr, Swischuk LE: Paraarticular soft tissue changes in infections and trauma of the lower extremity in children. *Am J Roentgenol* 134:307–311, 1980.
2. Smith GR, Loop JW: Radiologic classification of posterior dislocation of the hip: refinements and pitfalls. *Radiology* 119:569–574, 1976.
3. Neuhauser EBD, Wittenborg MH: Synovitis of the hip in infancy and childhood. *Radiol Clin North Am* 1:13–16, 1963.

Joint Space Narrowing

Joint space narrowing occurs with (*a*) traumatic joint dislocation and (*b*) joint cartilage destruction (Table 4.36). In the former, the finding is due to overlap of the dislocated bones, a finding easily demonstrable on a view taken at right angles to the one showing the narrowing. Cartilage destruction causing

joint space narrowing occurs with a number of diseases, but most often is seen with septic arthritis (Fig. 4.112A). Thereafter, one should consider rheumatoid arthritis (Fig. 4.112B), hemophiliac arthropathy, and tuberculous arthritis. However, it should be remembered that joint space narrowing with tuberculosis

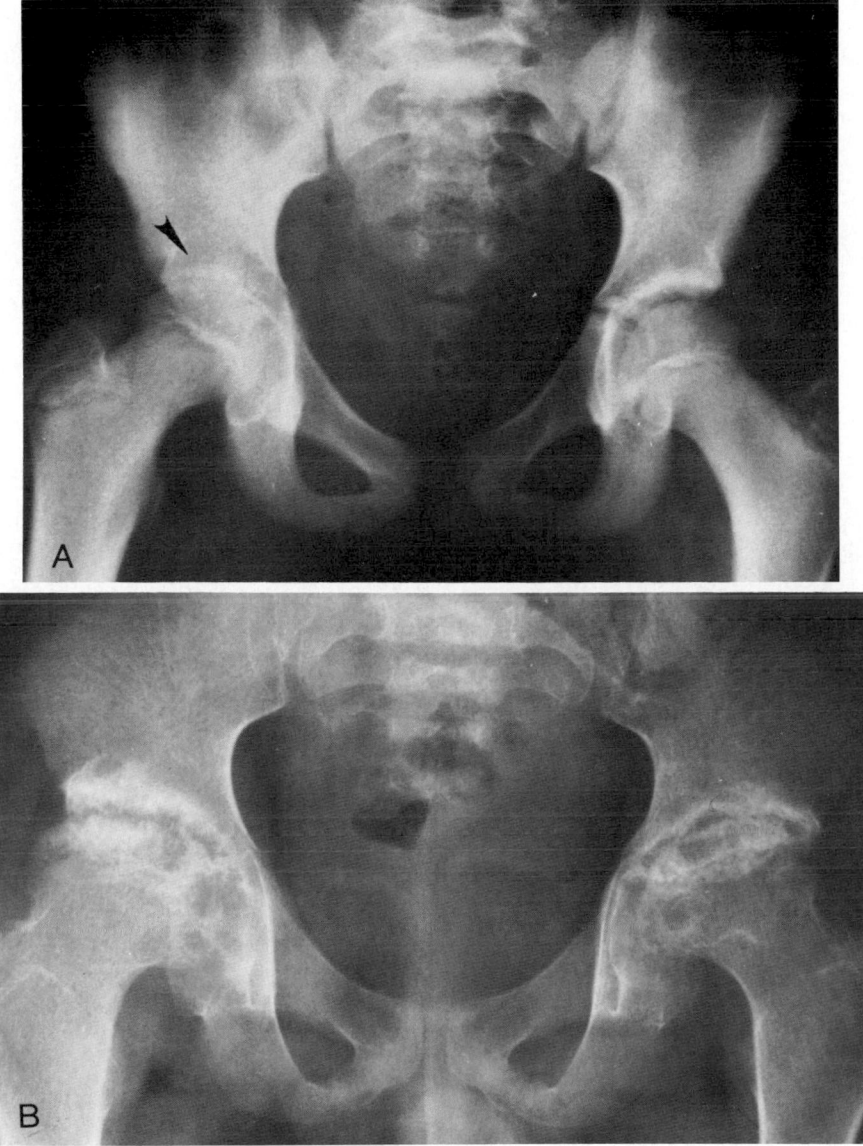

Fig. 4.112.   Joint space narrowing. A. Narrowing of the right hip joint in staphylococcal septic arthritis (arrow). B. Narrowing of both hip joints, with irregularity of the articular surfaces, in rheumatoid arthritis.

occurs only after many months. The reason is that, with tuberculosis, proteolytic enzyme activity and subsequent cartilage destruction are minimal. With septic arthritis, on the other hand, proteolytic activity is high and cartilage destruction rapid. The incidence of tuberculous arthritis varies from one geographic location to another.

Less common causes of joint space narrowing include fungal arthritis, pigmented villinodular synovitis, Winchester's syndrome, primary degenerative arthritis (very rare in children), Farber's lipogranulomatosis, Stickler's hereditary arthrophthalmopathy, and slipped capital femoral epiphysis. In the latter condition, cartilage destruction and joint space narrowing occur only after surgical intervention. It is not known just why this happens, but it is believed to result from an auto-immune phenomenon. The problem is not particularly debilitating and not overly common. Joint space narrowing with degenerative arthritis in children is rare except as it occurs secondarily, as a long term complication of Legg-Perthes disease, other causes of aseptic necrosis, septic arthritis, and trauma.

Joint Hyper and Hypomobility

These abnormalities are more readily assessed clinically than radiographically, for often there is very little in the way of roentgenographic change. As far as **hypermobility** is concerned, one should consider the following conditions: mongolism (trisomy 21), Marfan's syndrome, Morquio's disease, Ehler's-Danlos syndrome, Goltz's syndrome (focal dermal hypoplasia), hereditary arthro-ophthalmopathy or Stickler's syndrome, and the various storage diseases. In terms of joint **hypomobility**, the commonest cause, on a generalized basis, is joint contracture in arthrogryposis multiplex congenita (1) and related syndromes. Contractures also are seen in rheumatoid arthritis, punctate epiphyseal dysplasia (severe recessive form), contractural arachnodactyly, the storage diseases, hereditary arthro-ophthalmopathy (Stickler's syndrome), Winchester's syndrome, diastrophic dwarfism, metatrophic dwarfism, the more severe forms of metaphyseal dysostosis, and diabetes mellitus (2).

In terms of isolated joint **hyper or hypomobility**, the commonest causes of both are infection and trauma. However, isolated joint hypomobility also can occur with bony exostoses around the joint, congenital radial head dislocation, various congenital and acquired bony synostoses (see p 190), and Madelung's deformity of the wrist, or so-called dyschondrosteosis.

References

1. Beckerman RC, Buchino JJ: Arthrogryposis multiplex congenita as part of an inherited symptom complex: two case reports and a review of the literature. *Pediatrics* 61:417–422, 1978.
2. Grgic A, Rosenbloom AL, Weber FT, Giodano B, Malone JI, Shuster JJ: Joint contracture— common manifestation of childhood diabetes mellitus. *J Pediatr* 88:584–588, 1976.

Joint Dislocation (Table 4.37)

The same differential diagnosis as exists for joint space widening (i.e., joint fluid, trauma, lax muscles, and loose ligaments) also exists for joint dislocation. Indeed, most of the problems have been considered just a section or so back, but a few added comments regarding certain congenital dislocations might be in order. The most common congenital dislocation, of course, is congenital dislocation of the hip, and the next most common is radial head dislocation. Congenital dislocation of the hip is characterized by lateral and upward displacement of the hip, widening of the hip joint, underdevelopment of the femoral head, increased slant to the acetabular roof, and loss of cupping of the acetabular roof (see Fig. 4.111C). With radial head dislocation, proximal radioulnar synostosis commonly is associated, and the radial head is somewhat hypoplastic and bent downward (Fig. 4.113A). This type of radial head dislocation can be seen in isolated form or as part of syndromes such as the Cornelia DeLange syndrome and Noonan's syndrome. Another peculiar congenital dislocation is posterior dislocation of the proximal tibia on the distal femur or so-called genu recurvatum (Fig. 4.113B). Usually the problem results from faulty intrauterine positioning of the legs, but genu recurvatum also oc-

curs in syndromes where generalized joint dislocation is present. Posterior dislocation of the distal ulna occurs in Madelung's deformity or dyschondrosteosis (see Fig. 4.5C).

Table 4.37 Joint Dislocation

Fluid in joints[a,b]	Commonest
Traumatic[a] Congenital dislocation of the hip[a] Rheumatoid arthritis[a,b] Neurogenic-neuromuscular disease[a,b]	Moderately common
Congenital radial head dislocation[a] Madelung's deformity[a]	Relatively rare
Larsen's syndrome[b] Genu recurvatum[a] Winchester's syndrome[a,b] Farber's syndrome[b] Werner's mesomelic syndrome[b] Stickler's syndrome[b]	Rare

[a] Single joint involvement.
[b] Generalized joint involvement.

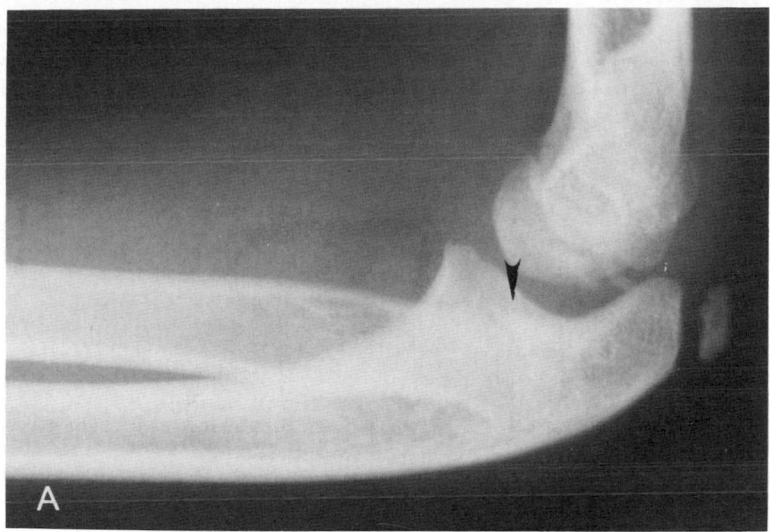

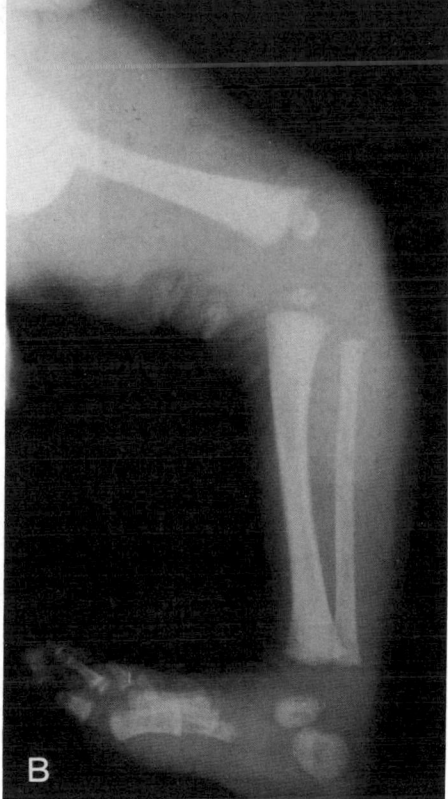

Fig. 4.113. Congenital dislocations. A. Typical appearance of congenital dislocation of the radial head (arrows). B. Genu recurvatum in neonate.

Multiple Joint Dislocations

Multiple joint dislocations are seen in conditions where neurogenic, neuromuscular, or chronic arthritic disease predisposes to joint laxity or contracture. These include conditions such as rheumatoid arthritis, Winchester's syndrome (a storage disease which resembles rheumatoid arthritis), Stickler's hereditary arthroopthalmopathy, Farber's lipogranulomatosis, and Larsen's syndrome. This latter condition is characterized by multiple joint dislocations, severe clubbed feet, and dwarfism. In addition, there is some tendency to shortening of some of the long bones, especially the distal humerus.

Joint Ankyloses

Ankyloses most commonly are acquired and secondary to infection, inflammation (i.e., rheumatoid arthritis), or trauma. Actually, most of these conditions first lead to joint space narrowing (see Table 4.36) but, with time, joint ankylosis occurs. Occasionally, ankyloses are congenital and most often this occurs around the elbow (see Fig. 4.24B). Fusion of the carpal and tarsal bones is yet another form of ankylosis and is dealt with elsewhere (see p 260).

Joint Calcification

Joint calcification can be intra or peri articular (Table 4.38). **Intra-articular calcification** is rare in children but occasionally can be seen after trauma or infection. Idiopathic calcifications of the hip joints have been demonstrated in young infants, but in follow-up are believed to have resulted from previous joint punctures (4, 5). Problems such as pseudogout, ochronosis, oxalosis, and synovial chondromatosis (1) are all uncommon in children; but, every so often, one can see a solitary calcification within a joint, usually the knee, in association with osteochondritis dissecans. This also can occur in other joints, (i.e., in the ankle from the talus), but most often, with osteochondritis dissecans, one sees only the cartilaginous defect on the articular surface of the involved bone. Acute trauma, with avulsion of pieces of an articular surface, also can lead to intra-articular calcification, and most often this occurs with cruciate ligament avulsions in the knee. Calcification of synoviomas is rare in childhood and, indeed, the tumor is, in itself, rare.

Calcification around a joint or, in other words, **periarticular calcification**, also is rare in children. However, it can be seen after burns (2), pyogenic arthritis (6), rheumatoid arthritis (3), dermatomyositis, other collagen vascular diseases, hyperparathyroidism (7), hypervitaminosis D, tumoral calcinosis, and trauma. In most of these cases, calcification is nonspecific and sheath-like in its distribution (Fig. 4.114A), but with tumoral calcinosis, the calcifications become large and flocculent (Fig. 4.114B). Some also may show calcium-fluid levels, and a similar phenomenon has been documented with para-articular calcifications in hyperparathyroidism (7).

Table 4.38 Joint Calcification

A. Intra-articular	
Traumatic avulsion Osteochondritis dissecans	Commonest
Idiopathic (in infants) Synovial chondromatosis Ochronosis Oxalosis Synovial inflammation Synovial tumors	Rare
B. Periarticular	
Collagen diseases (especially dermatomyositis)	Commonest
Trauma Infection Hypervitaminosis D Hyperparathyroidism Tumoral calcinosis (large, clumpy)	Relatively rare

References

1. Cahuzac JP, Lebarbier P, Germaneau J, Pasque M: Synovial chondromatosis in children. 4 cases. *Chir Pediatr* 20:89–93, 1979.
2. Faure C, Viatl C, Gueriot JC: Para-articular calcifications and ossifications in children with Burns. *Ann Radiol* 15:733–738, 1972. Abstract: *Radiology* 108:238, 1973.
3. Martel W, Holt JF, Cassidy JT: Roentgenologic manifestations of juvenile rheumatoid arthritis. *Am J Roentgenol* 88:400–423, 1962.
4. Nahum H, Pissarro B, Sauvegrain J: Calcification of the cartilages of the hip in infants. *Ann Radiol* 11:288–297, 1968.
5. Sauvegrain J, Millet G, Manlot G, Vacher H: Calcifications of the hip in infants and children. New cases and long-term followup. *Pediatr Radiol* 11:29–33, 1981.
6. Shawker TH, Dennis JM: Periarticular calcifications in pyogenic arthritis. *Am J Roentgenol* 113:650–654, 1971.
7. Smith FW, Junor BJR: Peri-articular calcification with fluid levels in secondary hyperparathyroidism. *Br J Radiol* 51:741–742, 1978.

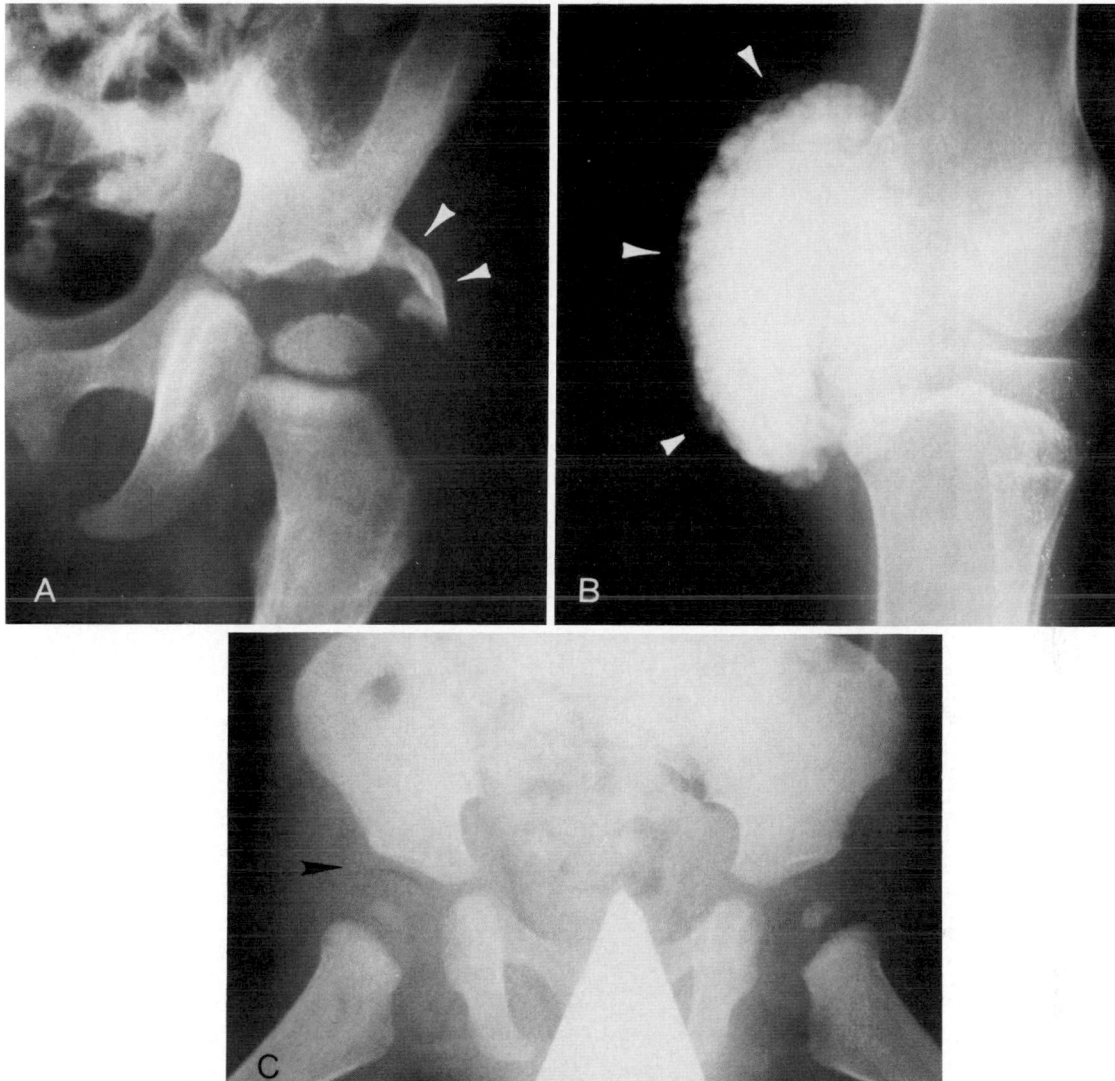

Fig. 4.114. Periarticular calcifications. A. Postseptic arthritis calcification around left hip (arrows). B. Typical large, bulky calcification (arrows) of tumoral calcinosis. C. **Gas in joint.** Typical vacuum joint (arrow). Characteristically, these air configurations are crescentic but there is debate as to whether the gas is water vapor, nitrogen, or just a vacuum.

Gas in the Joint

The commonest cause of gas in the joint (Table 4.39) is the so-called vacuum joint effect (1). When stress is applied to a normal joint, intra-articular pressures become negative and the vacuum joint results (Fig. 4.114C). There is debate as to whether the gas is nitrogen, water vapor, or an actual vacuum. The point is moot, however, for the finding is of no particular consequence, and is seen with greater frequency in patients with flaccid extremities. Intra-articular gas also can be seen after penetrating trauma postoperatively, after arthrography, and occasionally, with gas-producing organisms causing infection.

Table 4.39   Joint Gas

Normal vacuum joint	}	Commonest
Vacuum joint with hypotonia	}	Moderately common
Penetrating trauma Infection	}	Rare

Reference
1. Deffrenne P, Beraud C: Intraarticular vacuum effect. *Ann Radiol* 18:401–406, 1975.

SOFT TISSUES

Hemiatrophy and Hemihypertrophy

It is important to distinguish between these two abnormalities because, while both give rise to asymmetric limbs, in one (hemiatrophy), the affected limb is smaller than normal, and in the other (hemihypertrophy) it is larger. **Hemiatrophy** for the most part occurs with underlying, unilateral neurologic disease, and the problem is more common in the lower extremities. However, hemiatrophy also is seen in the Russell-Silver syndrome (Fig. 4.115A), a condition characterized by dwarfism, enlargement of the head, ab-

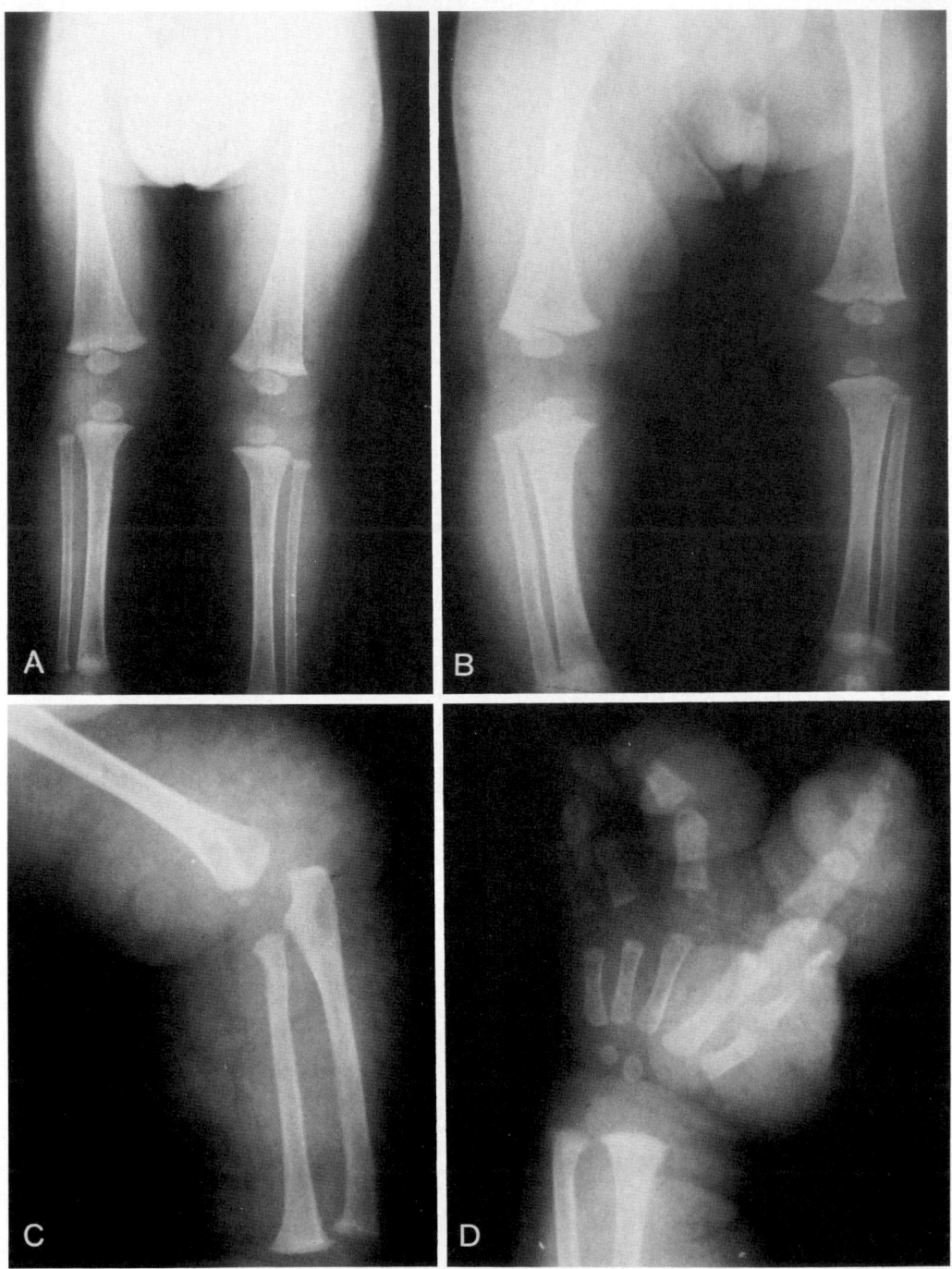

Fig. 4.115. Unequal extremity size. A. Note shorter and smaller right lower extremity in Russel-Silver dwarfism. B. Note large, slightly longer lower extremity in congenital hemihypertrophy. C. **Lymphangioma and gigantism.** Note gigantism and typical reticulation of soft tissues, and enlargement of soft tissues. D. Hand in same patient.

normal sexual development, and variable smallness of the extremities on one side of the body (1, 3). In most cases, changes are more pronounced in the lower extremity and the problem is one of congenital growth disturbance rather than neurologic deficit.

Hemihypertrophy usually also is more pronounced in the lower extremities and, although it occurs on a isolated basis (Fig. 4.115B), it also frequently is seen in association with intra-abdominal tumors. This is especially true of Wilm's tumor of the kidney, but other abdominal tumors also can be encountered. Hemihypertrophy also is seen in the Beckwith-Wiedemann (infantile gigantism) syndrome, and even with benign cystic diseases of the kidney (2, 4). In all of these cases, the involved extremity is larger than normal both in its bony and soft tissue components. The etiology of this type of hypertrophy is unknown and should not be confused with that due to localized gigantism resulting from soft tissue vascular or lymphatic tumors, or lymphatic obstruction (see Fig. 4.115, C and D, and discussion in next section).

References

1. Moseley JE, Moloshok RE, Freiberger RH: The silver syndrome; congenital asymmetry, short stature, and variations in sexual development. *Am J Roentgenol* 97:74–81, 1966.
2. Pfister RC, Weber AL, Smith EH, Wilkinson RH, May DA: Congenital asymmetry (hemihypertrophy) and abdominal disease; radiological features in 9 cases. *Radiology* 116:685–691, 1975.
3. Silver HK: Asymmetry, short stature and variations in sexual development. A syndrome of congenital malformations. *Am J Dis Child* 107:495–515, 1964.
4. Swischuk LE: *Radiology of the Newborn and Young Infant,* ed 2. Baltimore, Williams & Wilkins, 1980, p 730.

Isolated Extremity Enlargement or Gigantism

Perhaps the commonest cause of a locally enlarged extremity is a vascular or lymphangiomatous tumor, or A-V fistula of the extremity. Hyperemia in these cases causes overgrowth of all of the tissues and, in some cases, the changes are profound (Fig. 4.115, C and D). Localized gigantism also can be seen in neurofibromatosis (poorly understood mesenchymal defect is cited as the etiology), and macrodystrophialipomatosa (1). Localized gigantism also can occur with lymphatic obstruction, which can be due to congenital atresia or hypoplasia of the lymphatic channels, or compression of the lymphatics by pelvic tumors, inflammatory masses, etc. In the tropics, of course, it is also seen with filariasis or so called elephantiasis.

Hemangiomatous tumors can exist in isolated form or be seen with multiple enchondromatosis (Maffucci's syndrome) or multiple hemangioma syndromes such as the Klippel-Tetamy-Webber syndrome (2).

References

1. McCarthy DM, Dorr CA, Mackintosh CE: Unilateral localized gigantism of the extremities with lipomatosis, arthropathy and psoriasis. *J Bone Joint Surg* 51B:348–353, 1969.
2. Tetamy SA, Rogers JG: Macrodactyly, hemihypertrophy, and connective tissue nevi; report of a new syndrome and review of the literature. *J Pediatr* 89:924–928, 1976.

Muscle-Fat Ratio Abnormalities

It is relatively easy to define the muscles, subcutaneous fat, and skin of the extremities of infants and children. This being the case, one can determine whether muscle and fat are present in normal proportions, or whether one or the other is lacking or predominates (2, 4). Four basic categorizations are possible: increased muscle with normal fat, decreased muscle with excess fat, decreased fat with normal muscle, and increased fat with normal muscle (Table 4.40).

An absolute, abnormal increase in muscle bulk is not that common, but it does occur in pseudohypertrophic muscular dystrophy (Fig. 4.116A), and primary infections of the muscle such as pyomyositis (3). It also can occur on an idiopathic basis in so-called congenital muscle hypertrophy (4) and, on a focal basis, with exercise hypertrophy. Diminution of muscle bulk occurs with a number of neuromuscular diseases including Werdnig-Hoffman disease, amyotonia congenita, poliomyelitis, arthrogryposis multiplex, meningocele, brain damage, etc. In all of these cases there is muscle atrophy and, in many, an associated

Table 4.40   Muscle-Fat Ratio Abnormalities

A. Increased muscle-normal fat
Muscular dystrophy
Congenital muscular hypertrophy
Pyomyositis
Exercise hypertrophy
B. Decreased muscle-excess fat
Neurogenic disease; multiple causes
Arthrogryposis multiplex
Amyotonia congenita
Werdnig-Hoffman
Muscular dystrophy
C. Decreased fat-normal muscle
Malnutrition; cachexia[a]
Diencephalic syndrome
Total lipodystrophy
D. Increased fat-normal muscle
Exogenous obesity
Cushing's syndrome
Laurence-Moon-Biedl syndrome
Prader-Willi syndrome
Steroid therapy

[a] In late, severe stages, muscle also decreased due to protein catabolism.

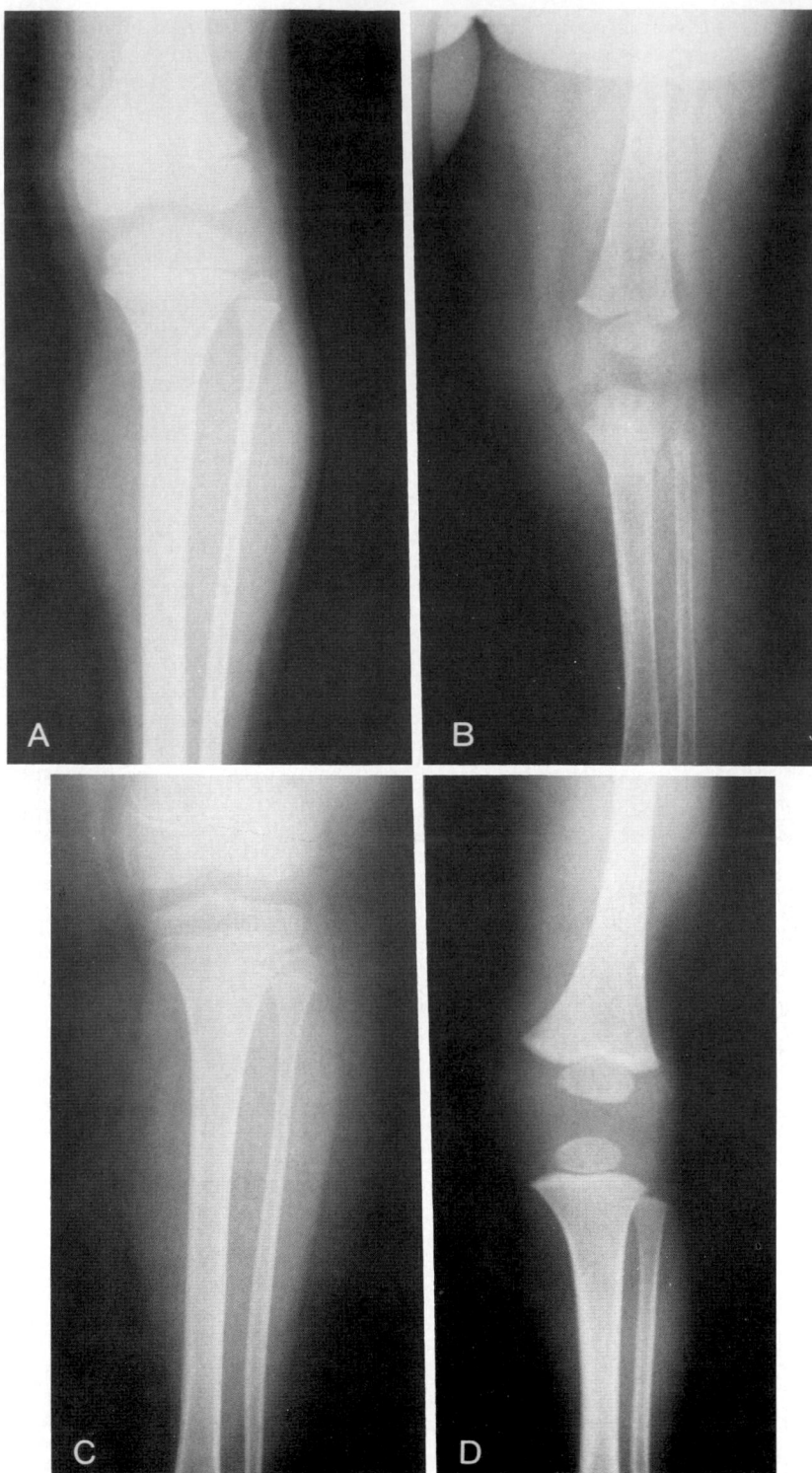

Fig. 4.116. A. **Increased muscle, normal fat.** Patient with pseudohypertrophic muscular dystrophy. Note bulbous calves. B. **Decreased muscle and increased fat.** Neurogenic disease producing thin, wasted muscles and overabundance of subcutaneous fat. C. **Excessive fat, relatively normal muscles.** Note extra fat in Prader-Willi syndrome. D. **Decreased fat, normal or increased muscle.** Note homogeneous appearance of soft tissues of legs of this patient with diencephalic syndrome. Virtually no subcutaneous fat is present. All the density is due to muscle. Clinically, the patient appeared very muscular. This is characteristic of the condition.

increase in subcutaneous fat (Fig. 4.116B). Often this increase is only relative, but in some patients it is absolute, for caloric intake is greater than their physical activity requires. Other causes of an absolute increase in subcutaneous fat include exogenous obesity, steroid therapy, Cushing's syndrome, Laurence-Moon-Biedl syndrome, and the Prader-Willi syndrome (Fig. 4.116C).

Conditions where subcutaneous fat is diminished include severe undernutrition (2), cachexia, the diencephalic syndrome (5), and total lipodystrophy (1, 6). In the diencephalic syndrome, a brain tumor is located around the anterior third ventricle, and the location of the tumor leads to hypothalamic disturbances causing abnormality of fat metabolism (Fig. 4.116D). In total lipodystrophy, a brain tumor is not present. Decreased fat is self evident in severe malnutrition, and in very severe cases with protein loss, both fat and muscle decrease.

References

1. Fairney A, Lewis G, Cotton D: Total lipodystrophy. *Arch Dis Child* 44:368–372, 1969.
2. Frank J, Klidjian MM, Karran SJ: The radiological assessment of arm muscle and fat stores in normal and malnourished patients. *Clin Radiol* 32:467–470, 1981.
3. Goldberg JS, London WL, Nagel DM: Tropical pyomyositis: a case report and review. *Pediatrics* 63:298–300, 1979.
4. Litt RE, Altman DH: Significance of the muscle cylinder ratio in infancy. *Am J Roentgenol* 100:80–87, 1967.
5. Poznanski AK, Manson G: Radiographic appearance of the soft tissues in the diencephalic syndrome of infancy. *Radiology* 81:101–106, 1963.
6. Wesenberg RL, Gwinn JL, Barnes GR Jr: The roentgenographic findings in total lipodystrophy. *Am J Roentgenol* 103:154–164, May 1968.

Reticulated Soft Tissues

Normally the interface between fat and muscle is quite sharp, but when soft tissue edema occurs reticulation of the fat is seen (Fig. 4.117). This causes obliteration of the fat muscle interface and generalized thickening of the soft tissues. Most often this is seen with infection or trauma but it also can be seen with soft tissue vascular and lymphatic tumors (see Fig. 4.115, C and D).

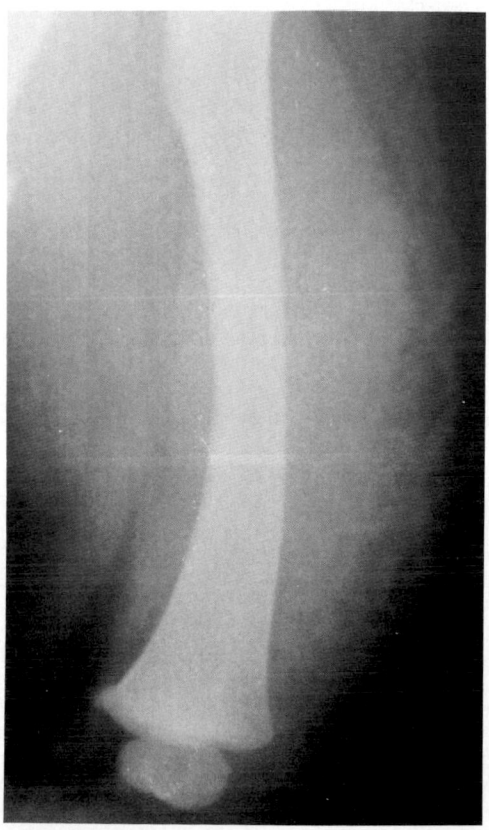

Fig. 4.117. Soft tissue reticulation. Note reticulation of soft tissues of the thigh. This is due to edema and was secondary to cellulitis.

Tendon Width Changes

The tendons of many muscles are relatively easy to visualize in infants, but most often one is dealing with the Achilles tendon in the ankle, and the infra and supra patellar tendons around the knee. As far as thickening of any of these tendons is concerned, usually it is due to trauma or inflammation (i.e., tendonitis). Almost anywhere the findings are straightforward (Fig. 4.118, A and B) but in the knee, apparent thickening of the suprapatellar tendon can be due to accumulation of fluid (pus, blood, serous effusion), in the immediately adjacent suprapatellar bursa. In such cases, the normally collapsed bursa slowly fills with fluid and distends, and in so doing it blends with the quadriceps tendon and causes it to falsely appear thickened (Fig. 4.118C). This is a very valuable finding in identifying knee joint effusions in infants and children (1).

Reference

1. Hayden CK Jr, Swischuk LE: Para-articular soft tissue changes in infections and trauma of the lower extremity in children. *Am J Roentgenol* 134:307–311, 1980.

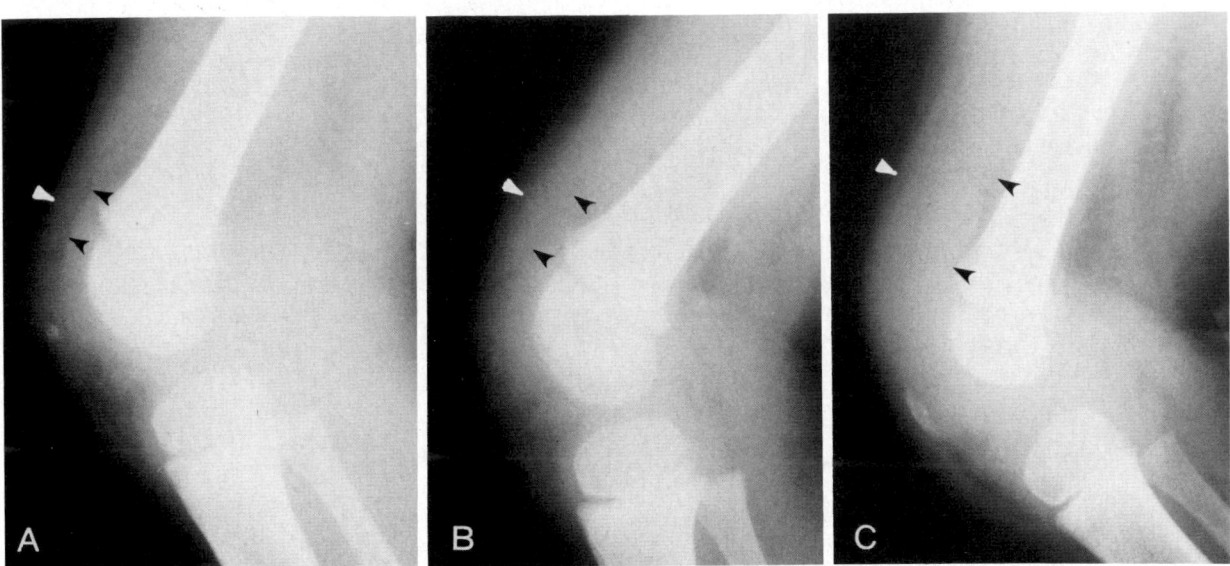

Fig. 4.118. Normal and thickened quadriceps tendon. A. Normal quadriceps tendon (arrows). B. Thickened quadriceps tendon (arrows) due to tendonitis. C. Marked pseudothickening of quadriceps tendon by massive accumulation of fluid in suprapatellar bursa (arrows) in infant with septic arthritis.

Obliterated and Displaced Fat Pads

There are numerous fat pads around the joints of the body and many are used for the detection of joint abnormality. Basically, a fat pad can be displaced or obliterated (Fig. 4.119). Obliteration is due to surrounding edema (any number of causes), and displacement (usually outward) to the presence of joint fluid. Fat pads next to bones can be displaced outward by bony masses, pus in osteomyelitis, and hematomas with trauma. All of these assessments are quite important, but their complete discussion is beyond the scope of this book. Therefore, one is referred to a number of articles and books on the subject (1–10).

References

1. Bledsoe RC, Izenstark JL: Displacement of fat pads in disease and injury to the elbow. *Radiology* 73:717–724, 1959.
2. Bohrer SP: The fat sign following elbow trauma. Its usefulness and reliability in suspecting "invisible" fractures. *Clin Radiol* 21:90–94, 1970.
3. Hayden CK Jr, Swischuk LE: Para-articular soft tissue changes in infections and trauma of the lower extremity in children. *Am J Roentgenol* 134:307–311, 1980.
4. Kohn AM: Soft tissue alteration in elbow trauma. *Am J Roentgenol* 82:867–875, 1959.
5. MacEwen DW: Changes due to trauma in the fat plane overlying the pronator quadratus muscle: A radiologic sign. *Radiology* 82:879–886, 1964.
6. Norell HG: Roentgenologic visualization of the extracapsular fat: Its importance in the diagnosis of traumatic injuries to the elbows. *Acta Radiol* 42:205–210, 1954.
7. Rogers SL, MacEwan DW: Changes due to trauma in the fat plane overlying the supinator muscle: A radiologic sign. *Radiology* 92:954–958, 1969.
8. Swischuk LE: *Emergency Radiology of the Acutely Ill or Injured Child.* Baltimore, Williams & Wilkins, 1979, pp 242–382.
9. Terry DW Jr, Ramin JE: The navicular fat stripe. A useful roentgen feature for evaluating wrist trauma. *Am J Roentgenol* 124:25–28, 1975.
10. Towbin R, Dunbar JS, Clark R: Teardrop sign: Plain film recognition of ankle effusion. *Am J Roentgenol* 134:985–990, 1980.

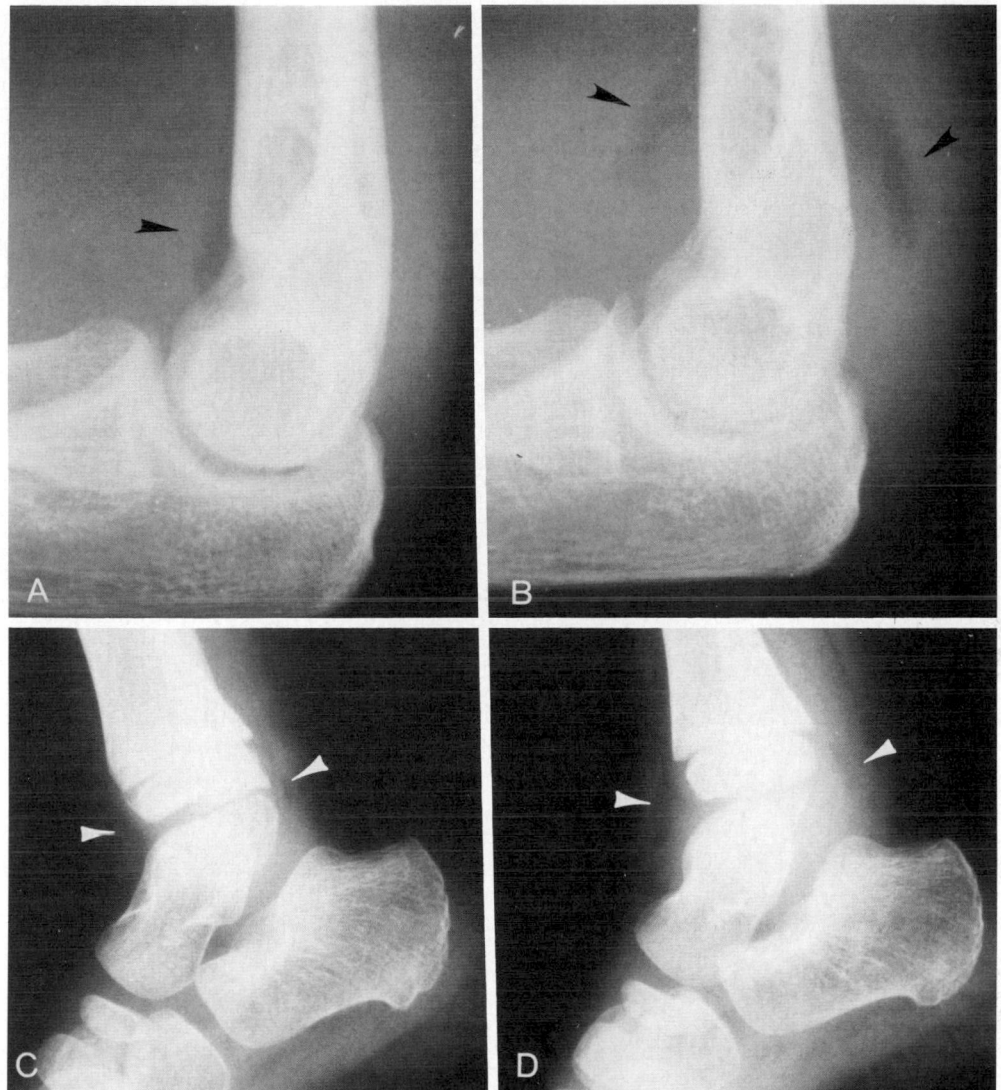

Fig. 4.119. **Fat pad abnormalities.** A. Normal anterior fat pad in elbow (arrow). B. Displacement of anterior and posterior fat pads (arrows) of the elbow by joint fluid. Normally, as in A, the posterior fat pad is not visible. C. Normal anterior and posterior ankle fat pads (arrows). D. Outwardly displaced ankle fat pads (arrows), secondary to the presence of joint fluid.

Soft Tissue Calcification and Opacities

Opacities due to **foreign bodies** can assume a variety of sizes and shapes and usually are no real problem in identification. However, some, such as glass, may or not be clearly opaque. Graphite, in a "lead" pencil usually is just faintly visible on regular roentgenograms, but most spines from spiny fishes are not visible. If they come from larger fish, and contain enough calcium, they may be visualized.

As far as **soft tissue calcification** is concerned, it can be irregular, formed, or punctate. **Irregular calcifications** occur after deep abscesses, hematomas, and with the collagen vascular diseases, namely dermatomyositis (5, 18, 20, 24). Calcification in the collagen vascular diseases usually is subcutaneous and

early on, rather delicate. Later on it can become more extensive and sheath like (see Fig. 4.120A). Irregular subcutaneous calcifications also have been noted in the basal cell nevus syndrome (17), and also can occur in the extremities after extravasation of calcium containing injections (1, 11, 14, 15, 19). This latter phenomenon commonly occurs in neonates (Fig. 4.120B). Rather extensive, irregular soft tissue calcification occurs with fat necrosis in infancy (Fig. 4.113C). This condition is of unknown etiology, but there is some feeling that it is related to both hypothermia and trauma (3, 6, 7, 21, 22). Most often these calcifications slowly disappear. Irregular calcifications in the soft tissues also can be seen with calcinosis universalis,

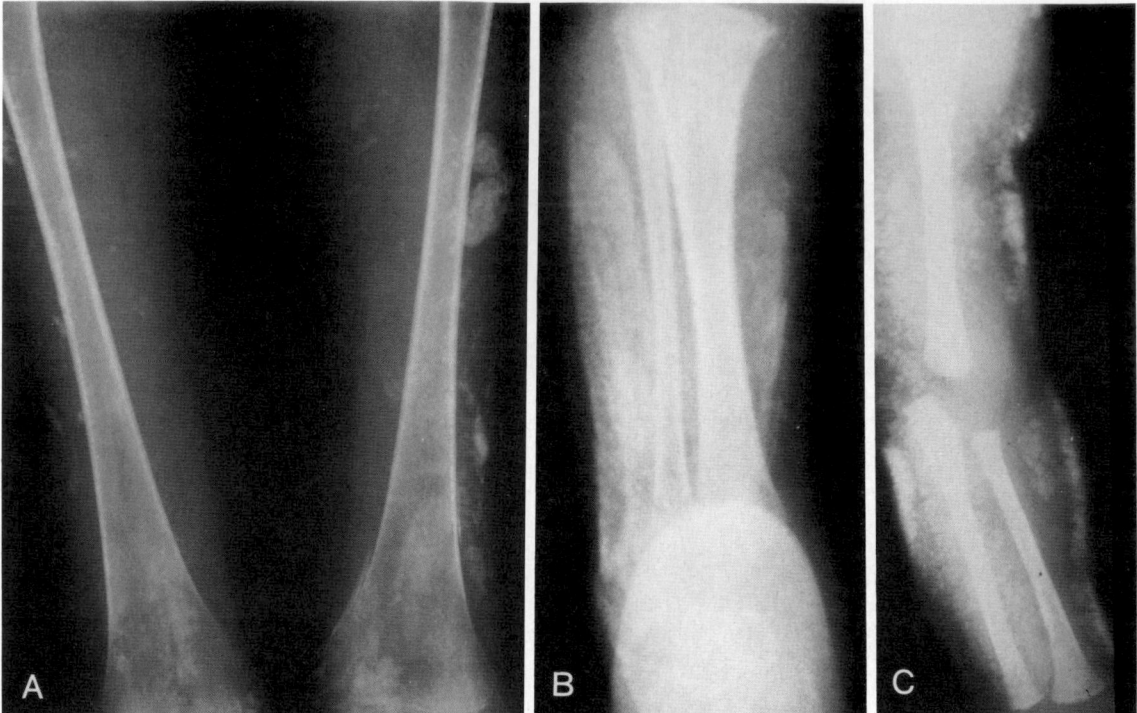

Fig. 4.120. Soft tissue calcifications. A. Typical, irregular, almost sheath-like calcifications in collagen vascular disease. B. Typical calcifications after calcium salt injections in infancy. C. Typical subcutaneous calcifications of fat necrosis in infancy.

Ehler's-Danlos syndrome, hyperparathyroidism, and hypervitaminosis D.

Formed calcifications usually occur in the muscle in the form of posttraumatic myositis ossificans (Fig. 4.121, A and B) and also may be seen after bleeding in hemophilia. In the inherited condition known as progressive myositis ossificans (23), the calcifications tend to be solid and occur around the joints or posterior spinal ligaments (Fig. 4.121, C and D). Vascular calcifications are rare in children (8, 16, 23, 25), but when seen, characteristically are tubular, linear, and parallel (Fig. 4.122A). Most often they are idiopathic and occur in infancy (2, 25), but can occur with any number of idiopathic or iatrogenic hypercalcemic states. A peculiar aortic calcification has been documented by Singleton and Merten, in a storage disease problem (20), and we have seen similar calcification in a case of supposed Gaucher's disease (see Fig. 1.48A). Punctate calcifications almost invariably are associated with hemangiomatous or lymphangiomatous tumors (Fig. 4.122B), or varices.

The large, flocculent para-articular calcifications of tumoral calcinosis (4, 9, 12, 13, 26), have been discussed elsewhere (see Fig. 4.114B). In some cases these calcifications can take the form of milk of calcium and be associated with fluid levels within the lesion (12, 13). Eventually, surgical removal of the calcified soft tissue masses is required because they interfere with joint function. Tumoral calcinosis tends to occur in families and can be associated with osteomyelitis-like

lesions of the long bones. There is no known cause for these lesions, but they are difficult to differentiate from osteomyelitis.

References

1. Berger PE, Heidelberger KP, Poznanski AK: Extravasation of calcium gluconate as a cause of soft tissue calcification in infancy. *Am J Roentgenol* 121:109–117, 1974.
2. Bird T: Idiopathic arterial calcification in infancy. *Arch Dis Child* 49:82–89, 1974.
3. Blake HA, Goyette EM, Lyter CS, Swan H: Subcutaneous fat necrosis complicating hypothermia. *J Pediatr* 46:78–80, 1955.
4. Bostrom B: Tumoral calcinosis in an infant. *Am J Dis Child* 135:246–247, 1981.
5. Budin JA, Feldman F: Soft tissue calcifications in systemic lupus erythematosus. *Am J Roentgenol* 124:358–364, 1975.
6. de Vel L, Bolin ZA: Traumatic necrosis of the subcutaneous fat of the newborn infant. *Am J Dis Child* 37:112, 1929.
7. Duhn R, Schoen EJ, Siu M: Subcutaneous fat necrosis with extensive calcification after hypothermia in two newborn infants. *Pediatrics* 41:661–664, 1968.
8. Field MH: Medial calcifications of the arteries of infants. *Arch Pathol* 42:607–618, 1946.
9. Hacihanefioglu U: Tumoral calcinosis: a clinical and pathologic study of eleven unreported cases in Turkey. *J Bone Joint Surg* 60:1131–1135, 1978.
10. Hall CM, Sutcliffe J: Fibrodysplasia ossificans progres-

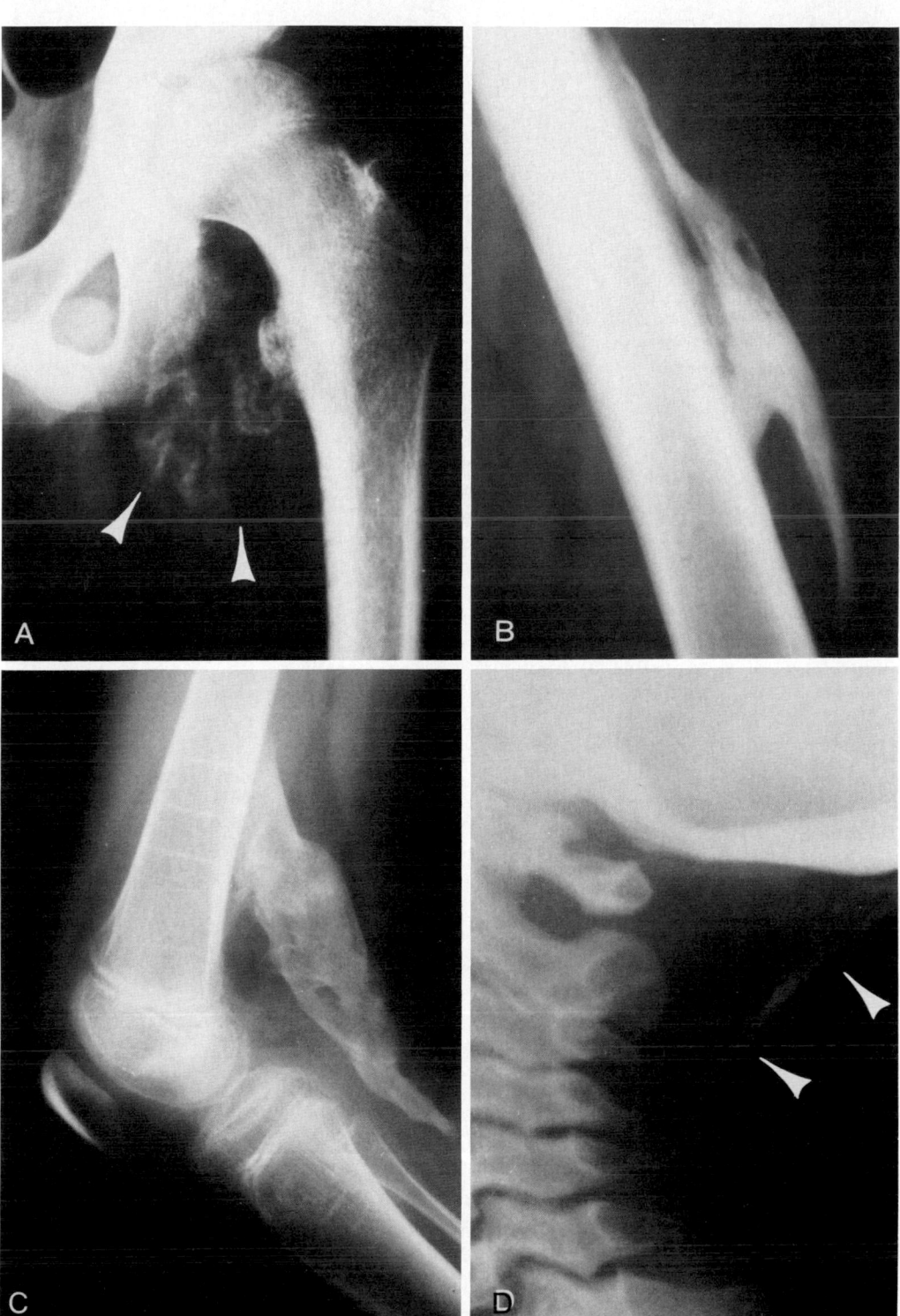

Fig. 4.121. Soft tissue calcifications. A. Irregular calcifications of myositis ossificans due to chronic tendon avulsion in neurogenic patient (arrows). B. Typical mature, traumatic myositis ossificans. C. Similar appearing solid calcifications in myositis ossificans progressiva. D. Posterior spinal ligament calcifications (arrows) in progressive myositis ossificans.

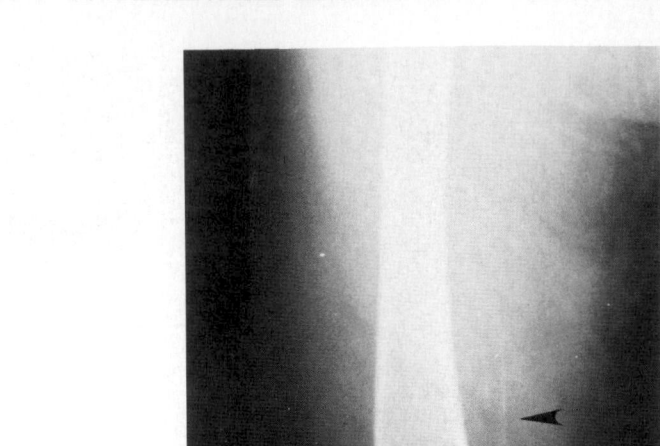
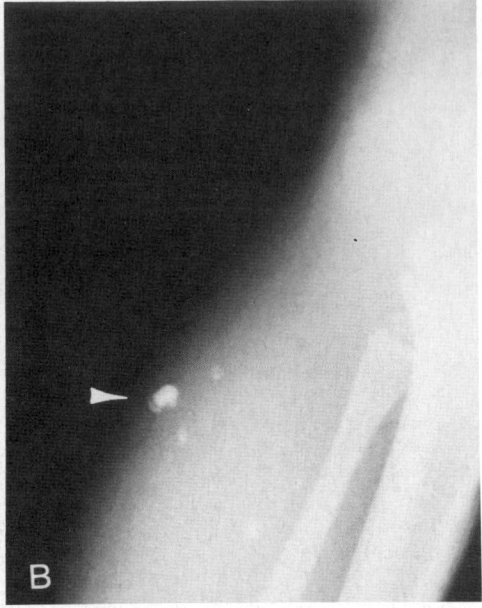

Fig. 4.122. Vascular soft tissue calcifications. A. Tubular calcifications of arteries in infancy (arrows). Courtesy A. H. Weens, M.D. B. Typical calcified phleboliths in hemangiomatous lesion of lower extremity (arrows).

siva. *Ann Radiol* 22:119–123, 1979.

11. Harris V, Ramamurthy RS, Pildes RS: Late onset of subcutaneous calcifications after intravenous injections of calcium gluconate. *Am J Roentgenol* 123:845–849, 1975.

12. Hug I, Guncaga J: Tumoral calcinosis with sedimentation sign. *Br J Radiol* 47:734–736, 1974.

13. Kolawole TM, Bohrer SP: Tumoral calcinosis with "fluid levels" in the tumoral masses. *Am J Roentgenol* 120:461–465, 1974.

14. Leape LL: Calcification of the leg after calcium infusion. *J Pediatr Surg* 5:831–833, 1975.

15. Lee FA, Gwinn JL: Roentgen patterns of extravasation of calcium gluconate in the tissues of the neonate. *J Pediatr* 86:598–601, 1975.

16. Meradjim M, de Villeneuve VH, Huber J, de Bruijn WC, Pearse RG: Idiopathic infantile arterial calcification in siblings; radiologic diagnosis and successful treatment. *J Pediatr* 92:401–405, 1978.

17. Murphy KJ: Subcutaneous calcification in nevoid basal cell carcinoma syndrome: response to parathyroid hormone and relationship to pseudohypoparathyroidism. *Clin Radiol* 20:287–293, 1969.

18. Ozonoff MB, Flynn FJ Jr: Roentgenologic features of dermatomyositis of childhood. *Am J Roentgenol* 118:206–212, 1973.

19. Ramamurthy RS, Harris V, Pildes RS: Subcutaneous calcium deposition in the neonate associated with intravenous administration of calcium gluconate. *Pediatrics* 55:802–806, 1975.

20. Sewell JR, Liyanage B, Ansell BM: Calcinosis in juvenile dermatomyositis. *Skel Radiol* 3:137–143, 1978.

21. Shackelford GD, Barton LL, McAlister WH: Calcified subcutaneous fat necrosis in infancy. *J Can Assoc Radiol* 26:203–207, 1975.

22. Sharlin DN, Koblenzer P: Necrosis of subcutaneous fat with hypercalcemia, a puzzling and multifaceted disease. *Clin Pediatr* 9:290–294, 1970.

23. Singleton EG, Holt JF: Myositis ossificans progressiva. *Radiology* 62:47–54, 1954.

24. Steiner RM, Glassman L, Schwartz MW, Vanace P: The radiological findings in dermatomyositis of childhood. *Radiology* 111:385–393, 1974.

25. Weens HS, Marin CA: Infantile arteriosclerosis. *Radiology* 67:168–174, 1956.

26. Yaghmai I, Mirbod P: Tumoral calcinosis. *Am J Roentgenol* 111:573–578, 1971.

Soft Tissue Air

Air in the soft tissues can be seen with penetrating injuries, explosions, severe contusion-abrasion injuries (Fig. 4.123A), and gas forming infections (Fig. 4.123B). Air in the soft tissues of the neck and chest usually is secondary to mediastinal emphysema resulting from some air trapping problem such as asthma (most often) or foreign body (rather rare). However, it also can be seen with blunt chest trauma and rupture or puncture of the airway (Fig.4.123C). Vascular air usually is iatrogenic and secondary to vessel catheterization but also can be seen with penetrating trauma to the heart or great vessels. In infancy, gas commonly is seen in the portal veins with necrotizing enterocolitis. It is secondary to intestinal necrosis and can be seen with other causes of bowel necrosis. Although necrotizing enterocolitis occurs predominantly in premature infants, bowel necrosis secondary to other causes of ischemia can occur in any age group.

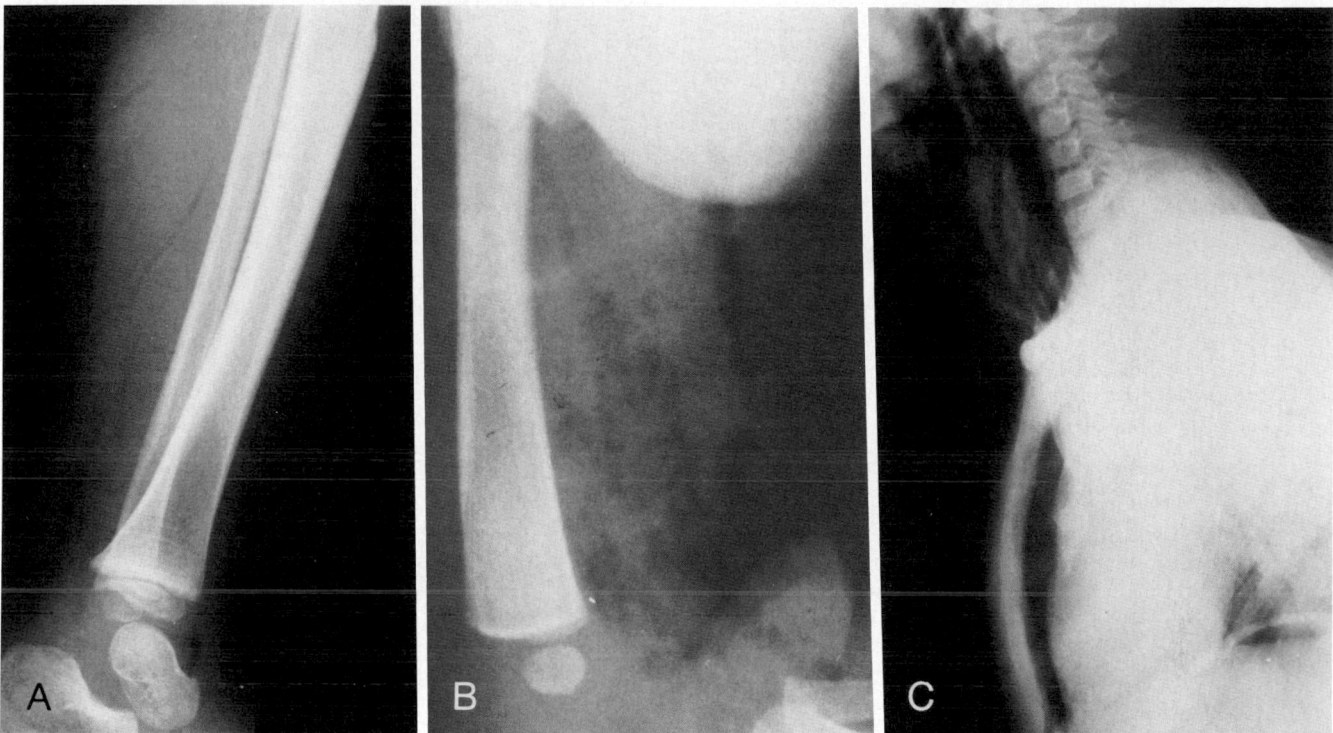

Fig. 4.123.   Soft tissue gas. A. Note gas around the ankle and in the lymphatics of the calf. This occurred after a severe contusion-abrasion of the lower leg. No open wounds of the skin were present. B. Extensive gas secondary to gas-forming infection of the soft tissues. C. Extensive subcutaneous and mediastinal air after laceration of larynx and trachea secondary to dog bite.

Soft Tissue Masses

Soft tissue masses either are well defined, or blend in with the adjacent soft tissues. When well defined, they tend to be benign tumors or cysts, but some malignant tumors can have a surprisingly well-defined margin (Fig. 4.124A). Soft tissue tumors blending with the soft tissues tend to be malignant sarcomas, vascular lesions, or inflammatory masses (Fig. 4.124B). Vascular lesions, such as hemangiomas or AV malformations, often show trailing or tortuous vessels (Fig. 4.124C). If these masses are associated with punctate calcifications, they are almost certain to be vascular or lymphangiomatous in origin. Other soft tissue tumors do not calcify very often, but occasionally one can encounter a so-called ossifying fibroma of the soft tissues. Lipomas are not particularly common in children but may produce exaggerated radiolucency on plain films and CT scans (Fig. 4.124D). This is true more of benign lipomas, for liposarcomas often do not demonstrate the typical fat density.

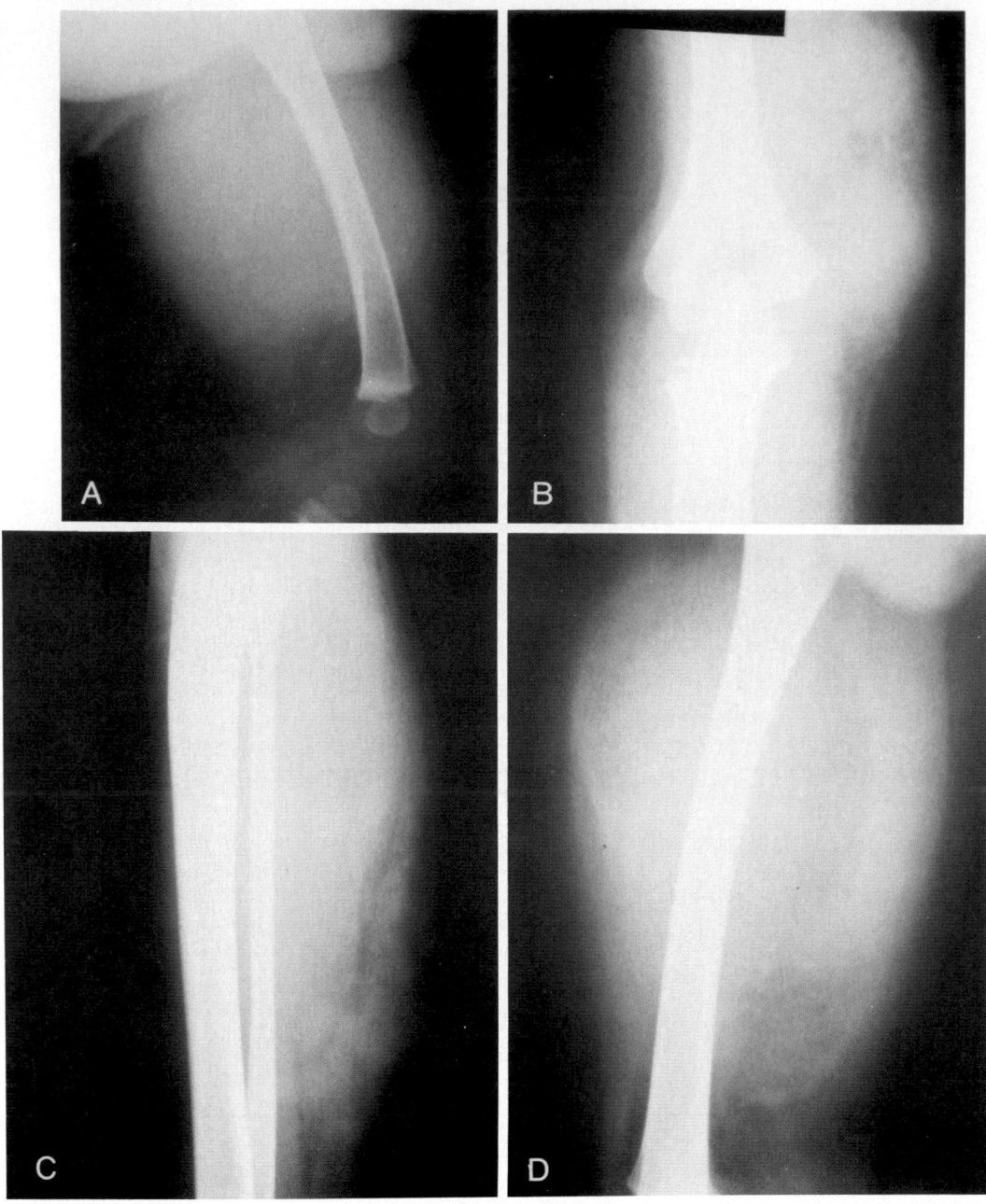

Fig. 4.124. Soft tissue masses. A. Large, relatively discrete mass due to rhadomyosarcoma in infant. B. Two inflammatory masses (inflamed nodes) around the elbow. Note indistinct margin of the masses secondary to edema. C. Large arteriovenous malformation of calf. Note tortuous and trailing blood vessels. D. Note radiolucency of this large lipoma of the thigh in a young child.

PERIOSTEAL NEW BONE DEPOSITION

Periosteal new bone is deposited in reaction to any type of periosteal irritation, and can assume one of the following configurations: (*a*) layered (single or multiple); (*b*) solid (straight, lumpy, or wavy); (*c*) spiculated (radiating outward); and (*d*) markedly elevated or ballooned (Table 4.41). Most often periosteal new bone is deposited in response to some disease arising from within the bone itself (i.e., osteomyelitis,

trauma, subperiosteal bleeding, bone infarction, bone tumor). In such cases, as the disease breaks through the cortex (i.e., pus, blood, edema, tumor), periosteal elevation occurs, and in an attempt to heal, new bone is deposited. Less commonly, the periosteum is irritated by disease, usually inflammatory, in the soft tissues or adjacent joints. As far as the joints are concerned, most often the problem is rheumatoid ar-

Table 4.41   Periosteal New Bone

Disease	Layered (Single or Multiple)	Solid (Straight, Wavy, Lumpy)	Markedly Elevated (Ballooned)	Spiculated
Infection-inflammation				
Osteomyelitis—neonatal infection (lues, rubella, etc.)	++[a]	−	−	−
Bone infarction	++	+	−	−
Cellulitis	++	+	−	−
Caffey's disease	++	++	−	−
Rheumatoid arthritis (7, 8)	+	−	−	−
Fractures-injury				
Fractures (ordinary)	++	++	−	−
Fractures (battered child)	++	++	++	−
Fractures (neurogenic)	++	++	++	−
Fractures (Pathologic)	++	+	−	−
Metabolic disease				
Rickets (healing)	++	+	−	−
Scurvy	++	−	+	−
Metabolic bone disease in premature	++	+	+	−
Hypervitaminosis D	++	−	−	−
Hypervitaminosis A	++	−	−	−
Thyroid acropachy	+	++	−	−
Gangliosidosis (infant)	++	−	++	−
Mucolipidosis II (infant)	++		++	
Hyperphosphatemia (2, 6)	++	−	++	−
Gaucher's disease (10)	++	+	−	−
Bone tumors and cysts				
Malignant—primary	++	−	−	++
Benign with fracture	++	+	−	−
Bone metastases	++	−	−	+
Leukemia-lymphoma	++	−	−	+
Hemangioma (with or without fracture)	+	+	−	+
Infantile fibromatosis (hamartomas) (11)	++	−	−	−
Miscellaneous				
Osteoarthropathy	++	++	−	−
Pachydermoperiostosis (4, 5)	++	++	−	−
Neurofibromatosis	−	−	+	−
Macrodystrophia lipomatosa	+	+	−	−
Normal infants (prematures)	++	−	−	−
Vascular soft tissue tumors	+	+	−	−
Mastocytosis (early stages)	+	−	+	−
Prostaglandin E treatment	++	−	−	−
Venous stasis	+−	++	−	−

[a] ++, quite common; +, occasional; −, rare or never.

thritis. In the soft tissues the problem can be cellulitis, deep abscess, pyomyositis, venous stasis, or vascular tumor. Periosteal new bone deposition also can be seen in rickets, but only in its healing stages. Before healing, although osteoid is formed, in the absence of adequate amounts of calcium, it does not become radio-opaque. With healing, however, calcium is deposited along the now elevated appearing periosteum, and pathologic periosteal bone deposition is suggested.

Another time when periosteal new bone deposition

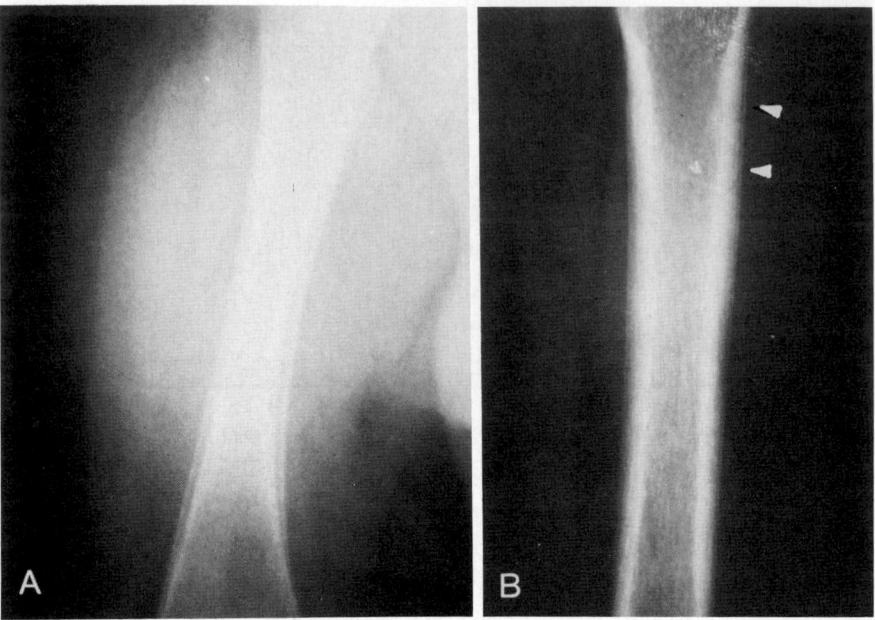

Fig. 4.125. True versus pseudoperiosteal new bone deposition. A. Note typical, true periosteal new bone deposition in premature infant. B. Pseudoperiosteal new bone deposition (arrows) secondary to demineralization revealing last layer of normally deposited cortical bone.

occurs under somewhat unusual circumstances is when it is deposited as a reaction to some distant, non-bony disease process. It then is termed idiopathic hypertrophic osteoarthropathy (3) and, as in the adult, the initiating problem can be an intrathoracic tumor (3), some other distant tumor (9), pulmonary infection (1, 3, 12), chronic intestinal or liver disease (3), or cyanotic heart disease (19). With the latter, chronic hypoxia is considered the underlying factor, but in the other conditions no specific etiology has been determined. However, circulating toxins or nonspecific neurogenic disturbances often are suggested as possible etiologies. Finally it should be mentioned that when a bone becomes demineralized, the last layer of normal periosteal new bone, previously deposited, becomes visible as a thin, white line (Fig. 4.125). In such cases it should be noted that the apparent layer of periosteal new bone does not bulge or deviate away from the cortex; rather it remains in complete alignment with the cortex and attests to its normal heritage. With pathologic deposition, the reverse is true.

In general, when one or another of the foregoing periosteal new bone configurations is seen, some underlying disease should be present, but while this is almost irrevocably true in older children, in the very young infant periosteal new bone deposition can be normal (14). Indeed, this is the only time when it can be normal, and actually, the phenomenon is quite common. Basically it occurs between the ages of 2 and 6 months (peaks at 3 months), more often in premature infants, and is believed to represent nothing more than exuberant normal diaphyseal new bone apposition (18). It must be differentiated from pathologic periosteal new bone formation, and for the most part one can do this on the basis of its configuration and favorite locations. In this regard, it is a phenomenon of the long bones and most often is seen in the femora (Fig. 4.125A), tibiae, and humeri. In the tibiae, it tends to occur medially more than laterally, and in all the bones it is primarily diaphyseal. In other words, the layer of periosteal new bone is deposited along the diaphysis and disappears before it gets to the metaphysis. Similar diaphyseal new bone deposition preponderance occurs in Caffey's disease (infantile cortical hyperosteosis) but, generally, concomitant clinical symptoms establish the latter diagnosis. With normal periosteal new bone, no symptoms are present and roentgenographic identification often is incidental.

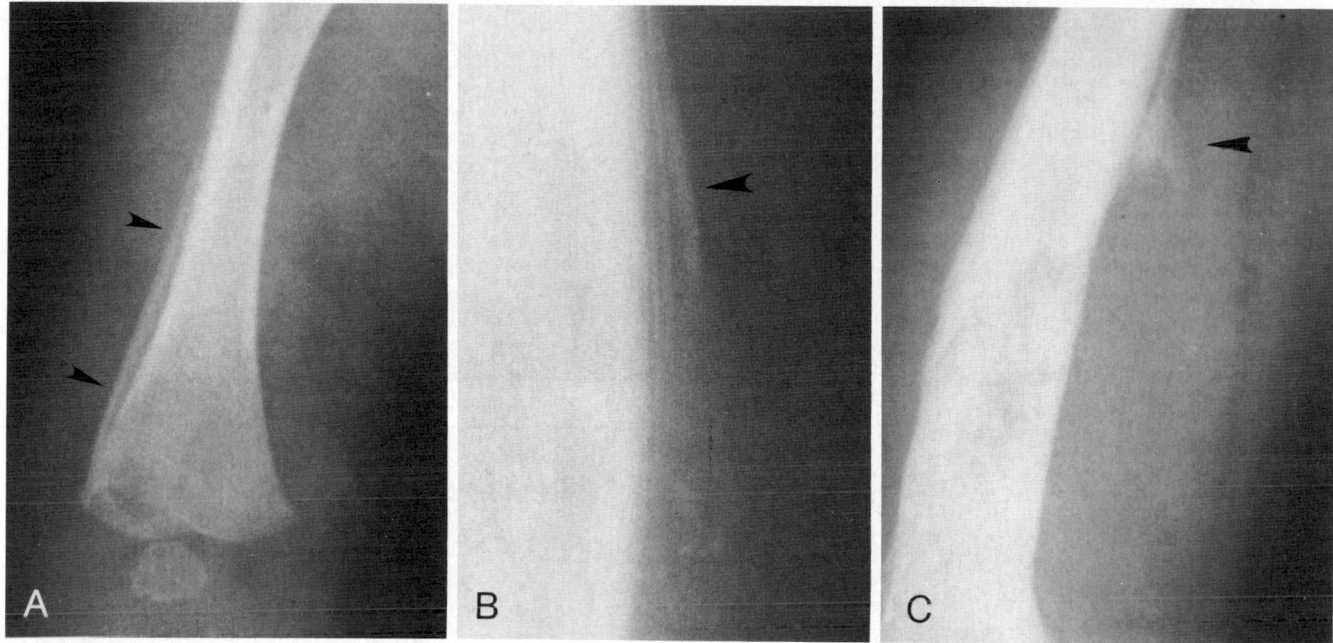

Fig. 4.126. Layered periosteal new bone. A. Single layer of periosteal new bone (arrows) in infant with osteomyelitis. Note destructive lesion in distal metaphysis. B. Multiple layers of periosteal new bone in patient with Ewing's sarcoma. Also note Codman's triangle (arrow). C. Codman's triangle in patient with healed, chronic osteomyelitis (arrow).

Layered Periosteal New Bone

Thin, layered periosteal new bone can occur in single or multiple layers (Fig. 4.126). Its appearance belies a rather active and/or acute disease process; i.e., acute osteomyelitis, bone infarction (usually sickle cell disease), malignant bone tumors (both primary and secondary), leukemia and lymphoma, healing fractures (ordinary and pathologic), more aggressive histiocytosis X, and indolent soft tissue inflammations and infections (15). In those cases where the disease process involves the metaphyses, periosteal new bone deposition extends down to the epiphyseal-metaphyseal junction, and when it is extremely aggressive, cortical breakthrough causes such rapid periosteal elevation that an acute triangle is formed at the point of maximal elevation. This has been termed Codman's Triangle (Fig. 4.126), and although it can be seen with any aggressive lesion, it is most characteristic of malignant bone tumors. Other causes of layered periosteal new bone deposition are listed in Table 4.41.

Solid, Straight, Wavy, or Lumpy Periosteal New Bone

This form of periosteal new bone deposition indicates a slow disease process (Fig. 4.127) and, consequently, is not seen with malignant bone tumors or the usual case of osteomyelitis or bone infarction. However, if bone infection is low grade, or a benign tumor is associated with pathologic fracturing, solid new bone deposition can be seen. Such new bone deposition can be straight or undulating (i.e., lumpy or wavy) and, when the latter, chronic venous stasis, long standing infection (either bony or soft tissue), or chronic stress fractures also should be considered. Solid, rather straight, periosteal new bone deposition in the fingers occurs with thyroid acropachy, but the problem is rare in children (16), and solid periosteal bone deposition can be seen in histiocytosis X (see Fig. 4.127A).

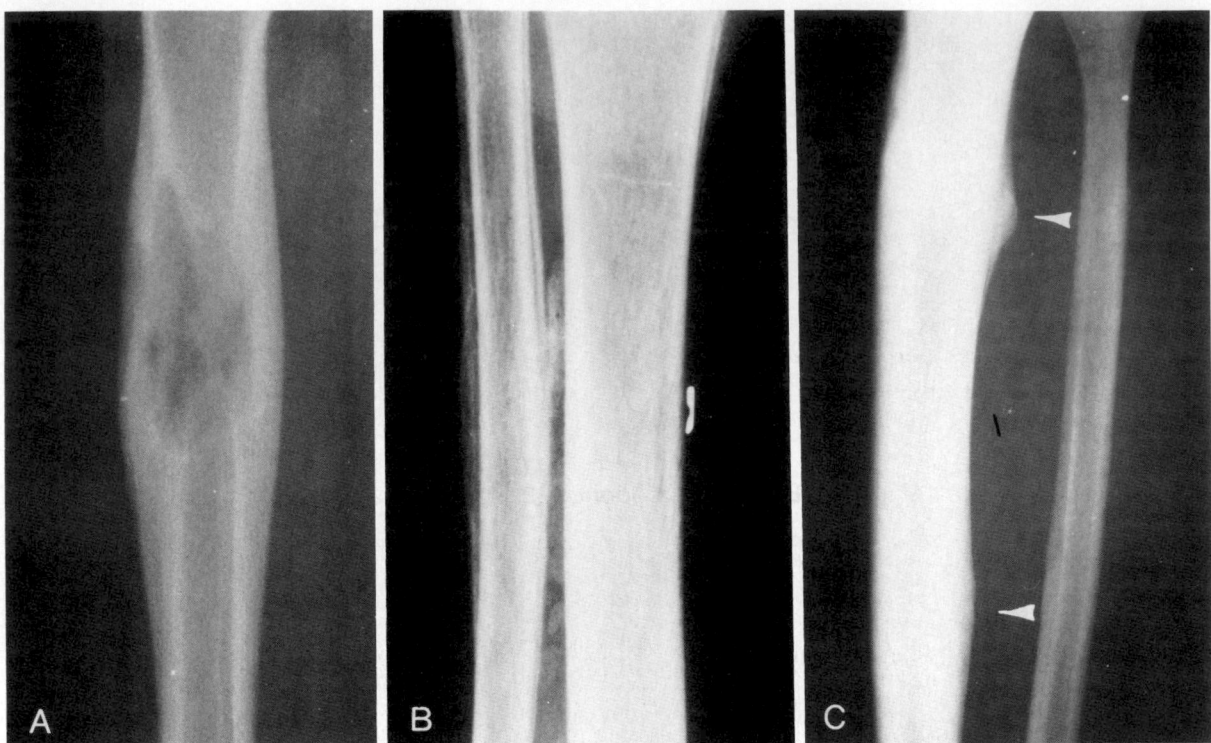

Fig. 4.127. Solid, straight, wavy, or lumpy periosteal new bone. A. Solid, dense periosteal new bone in histiocytosis X. B. Solid, thick single layer of periosteal new bone deposition with chronic soft tissue infection. C. Lumpy periosteal new bone deposition in healing stress fractures (arrow).

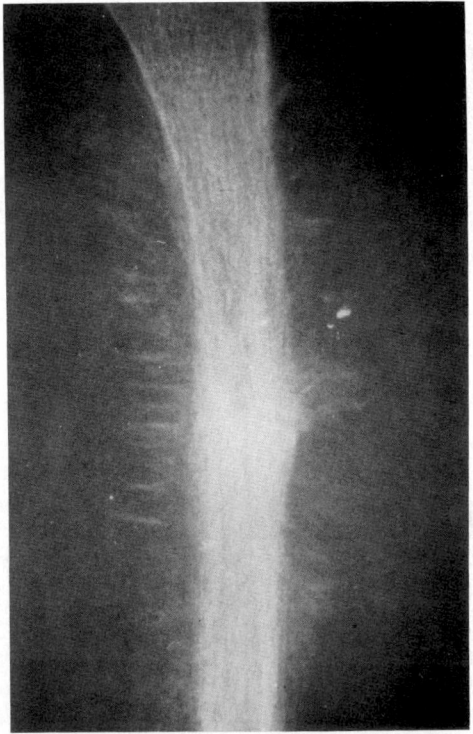

Fig. 4.128. Spiculated periosteal new bone. Typical spiculations in malignant bone tumor (arrow). Ewing's sarcoma.

Spiculated Periosteal New Bone

In the long bones, spiculated periosteal new bone deposition reflects a very abrupt and rapid elevation of the periosteum. For this reason, it is virtually synonymous with malignant bone tumor, either primary (more common), or secondary (Fig. 4.128). In such cases, periosteal elevation occurs at a rate just slow enough to allow new bone deposition on perpendicularly oriented fibers located between the elevated periosteum and underlying cortex. These fibers, called Sharpey's fibers, provide a lattice for calcium deposition which, because of its perpendiular orientation, leads to spiculation. Such spiculation is not seen with osteomyelitis, bone infarction, or trauma, probably because periosteal elevation is too rapid or abrupt. In addition, in osteomyelitis, it also has been suggested that proteolytic activity of the exudate leads to destruction of the fibers, but this would not explain why spiculated bone is not seen with periosteal elevations secondary to bone infarction or hemorrhage. All of this notwithstanding, however, when spiculated periosteal new bone is seen one should think of malignant bone tumors such as Ewing's sarcoma, osteosarcoma, fibrosarcoma, chondrosarcoma, metastatic disease, leukemia, and occasionally even lymphoma. The only benign tumor which produces some degree of spiculation with any consistency is hemangioma of the bone.

Markedly Elevated (Ballooned) Periosteal New Bone

In these cases, periosteal new bone takes the form of a single, often undulating, layer, widely removed from the shaft (Fig. 4.129). In some cases, the periosteum is pulled so far away that ballooning occurs. Almost always, the finding is due to extensive periosteal bleeding and most often is seen with neurogenic fractures and fractures in the battered child syndrome. In both instances, excessive motion around the fracture site predisposes to marked subperiosteal bleeding and periosteal elevation. Similar bleeding, usually spontaneous or due to minor trauma, also occurs in bleeding disorders, neurofibromatosis (20), and of course, is classic in scurvy. Scurvy, however, is quite rare these days. Ballooned periosteal new bone deposition also occasionally is seen in mastocytosis in its early stages.

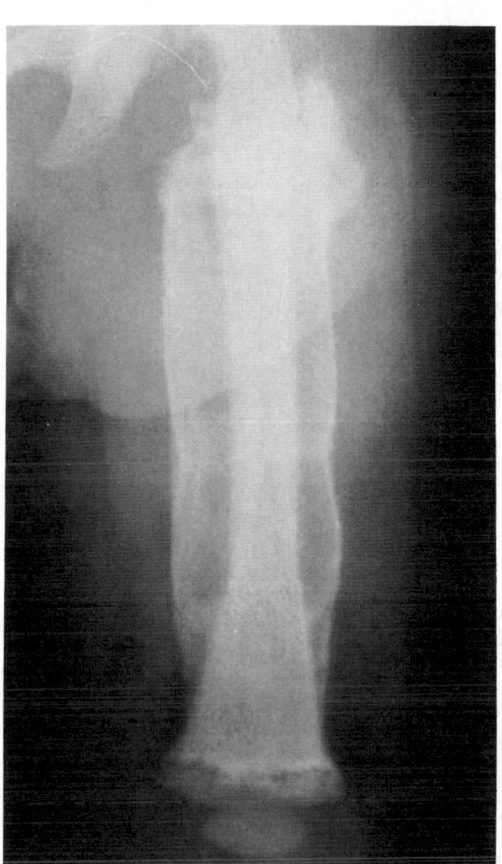

Fig. 4.129.   Ballooned, periosteal new bone. Typical ballooning in massive subperiosteal bleeding in battered child syndrome (arrows).

References

1. Athreya BH, Borns P, Rosenlund ML: Cystic fibrosis and hypertrophic osteoarthropathy in children. *Am J Dis Child* 129:634–637, 1975.
2. Caffey J: Familial hyperphosphatasemia with ateniosis and hypermetabolism of growing bone. *Progr Pediatr Radiol* 4:438–468, 1973.
3. Cavanaugh JJA, Holman GH: Hypertrophic osteoarthropathy in childhood. *J Pediatr* 66:27–40, 1965.
4. Chamberlain DS, Whitaker J, Silverman F: Idiopathic osteoarthropathy and cranial defects in children (familial idiopathic osteoarthropathy). *Am J Roentgenol* 93:408–415, 1965.
5. Currarino G, Tierney RC, Giesel RG, Weihl C: Familial idiopathic osteoarthropathy. *Am J Roentgenol* 85:633–644, 1961.
6. Dunn V, Condon VR, Rallison ML: Familial hyperphosphatasemia; diagnosis in early infancy and response to human thyrocalcitonin therapy. *Am J Roentgenol* 132:541–545, 1979.
7. Goel KM, Rawson SP, Shanks RA: Radiological assessment of fifty patients with juvenile rheumatoid arthritis: correlation with clinical and laboratory abnormalities. *Pediatr Radiol* 2:51–60, 1974.
8. Kapusta MA, Sedlezky I: Periostitis: an early diagnostic sign of juvenile rheumatoid arthritis. *J Can Assoc Radiol* 18:268, 1967.
9. Kay CJ, Rosenberg MA, Burd R: Hypertrophic osteoarthropathy and childhood Hodgkin's disease. *Radiology* 112:177–178, 1974.
10. Miller JH, Ortega JA, Heisel MA: Juvenile Gaucher disease simulating osteomyelitis. *Am J Roentgenol* 137:880–882, 1981.
11. Morettin LB, Mueller E, Schreiber M: Generalized ha-

martosis (congenital generalized fibromatosis). *Am J Roentgenol* 114:722–734, 1972.

12. Nathanson I, Riddlesberger MM Jr: Pulmonary hypertrophic osteoarthropathy in cystic fibrosis. *Radiology* 135:649–651, 1980.
13. Seibert JJ, Byrne WJ, Golladay ES: Development of hypervitaminosis A in a patient on long-term parenteral hyperalimentation. *Pediatr Radiol* 10:173–174, 1981.
14. Shopfner CE: Periosteal bone growth in normal infants. *Am J Roentgenol* 97:154–163, 1966.
15. Swischuk LE, Jorgenson F, Jorgenson A, Capen D: Wooden splinter induced "pseudotumors" and "osteomyelitis-like lesions" of bone and soft tissues. *Am J Roentgenol* 122:176–179, 1974.
16. Thomas J, Collipp PJ, Sharma RK: Thyroid acropathy.

Am J Dis Child 125:745–746, 1973.
17. Ueda K, Saito A, Nakano H, Aoshima M, Yokota M, Muraoka R, Iwaya T: Brief clinical and laboratory observations: cortical hyperostosis following long-term administration of prostaglandin E in infants with cyanotic congenital heart disease. *J Pediatr* 97:834–836, 1980.
18. Volberg FM Jr, Whalen JP, Krook L, Winchester P: Lamellated periosteal reactions: A radiologic and histiologic investigation. *Am J Roentgenol* 128:85–87, 1977.
19. Wastie ML, Wong HO, Ang AH: Hypertrophic osteoarthropathy in cyanotic congenital heart disease. *Australas Radiol* 17:276–279, 1973.
20. Yaghmai I, Tafazoli M: Massive subperiosteal hemorrhage in neurofibromatosis. *Radiology* 122:439–441, 1977.

BONE TUMORS, CYSTS, AND TUMOR-LIKE LESIONS

In analyzing bone tumors, cysts and tumor-like lesions, the following roentgenographic features should be considered: (*a*) whether the lesion is single or multiple; (*b*) whether it is metaphyseal, diaphyseal, or epiphyseal; (*c*) whether it occurs in a flat bone, long bone, or both; (*d*) the type and rate of bone destruction it produces; (*e*) whether calcification or ossification are associated; (*f*) whether it is central (medullary) or eccentric (cortical); and (*g*) whether or not there is an associated soft tissue mass.

Single or Multiple Lesions

For the most part, multiple lesions occur with fibrous dysplasia, multiple enchondromatosis or Ollier's disease (unilateral predominance of the enchondromas in this condition is common), multiple osteochondromatosis (no unilateral predominance), histiocytosis X, osteomyelitis, metastatic disease, leukemia, lymphoma, and benign cortical defects. The latter lesions are very common in children and are completely innocuous. Most often they are seen in the knees and ankles, and their characteristics are discussed in greater detail in the next section.

Location of the Lesion

It is helpful to note whether a lesion occurs in a **long or flat bone** and, if in a long bone, whether it is **diaphyseal, metaphyseal, or epiphyseal.** Thereafter, one should determine whether the lesion is **central (medullary) or eccentric (cortical).** Primarily **diaphyseal** lesions are not that common, but of those malignant, Ewing's sarcoma should be considered first. On the benign side of the ledger, one should consider histiocytosis X and possibly fibrous dysplasia. With osteomyelitis, bone infarction, most other bone tumors, metastatic disease, and bone cysts, the **metaphyses** are favored.

As far as **eccentricity of a lesion** is concerned, most lesions are central, and located in the medullary cavity of the bone. However, benign cortical defects and their related lesion, the nonossifying fibroma, characteristically are eccentric (Fig. 4.130A). These tumors, probably one and the same, are separated primarily by size. When they are large and cystic, they are termed nonossifying fibromas, and when small and less prominent, they go by the name of benign cortical defects. Both can exist in the same individual, and many times, especially with benign cortical defects, the lesions are multiple. They occur primarily around the knees and ankles, and although benign cortical defects may appear cyst-like en face, on tangent their cortical location is clearly apparent (see Fig. 4.66D). Once these roentgenographic criteria are met for a solitary lesion, the diagnosis virtually is assured. When low grade osteomyelitis produces such a defect, differention may be more difficult, but clinical symptoms should separate the two conditions. In addition, in osteomyelitis the defect almost always extends to the epiphyseal line. Indeed, very often the adjacent epiphysis is involved, and so is the joint. When nonossifying fibromas are large, they are susceptible to pathologic fracture, but this does not occur with the smaller ones or with benign cortical defects. With time, both lesions tend to disappear spontaneously, and thus, neither lesion requires any specific therapy. The natural course is for the lesions to become obliterated by healing and bony sclerosis (Fig. 4.130B).

In contradistinction to benign cortical defects and nonossifying fibromas, benign, unicameral, bone cysts characteristically are central. They expand the cortex and are quite radiolucent (Fig. 4.130C), and because they are expansile their cortex becomes quite thin and susceptible to pathologic fracture. Histologically, they

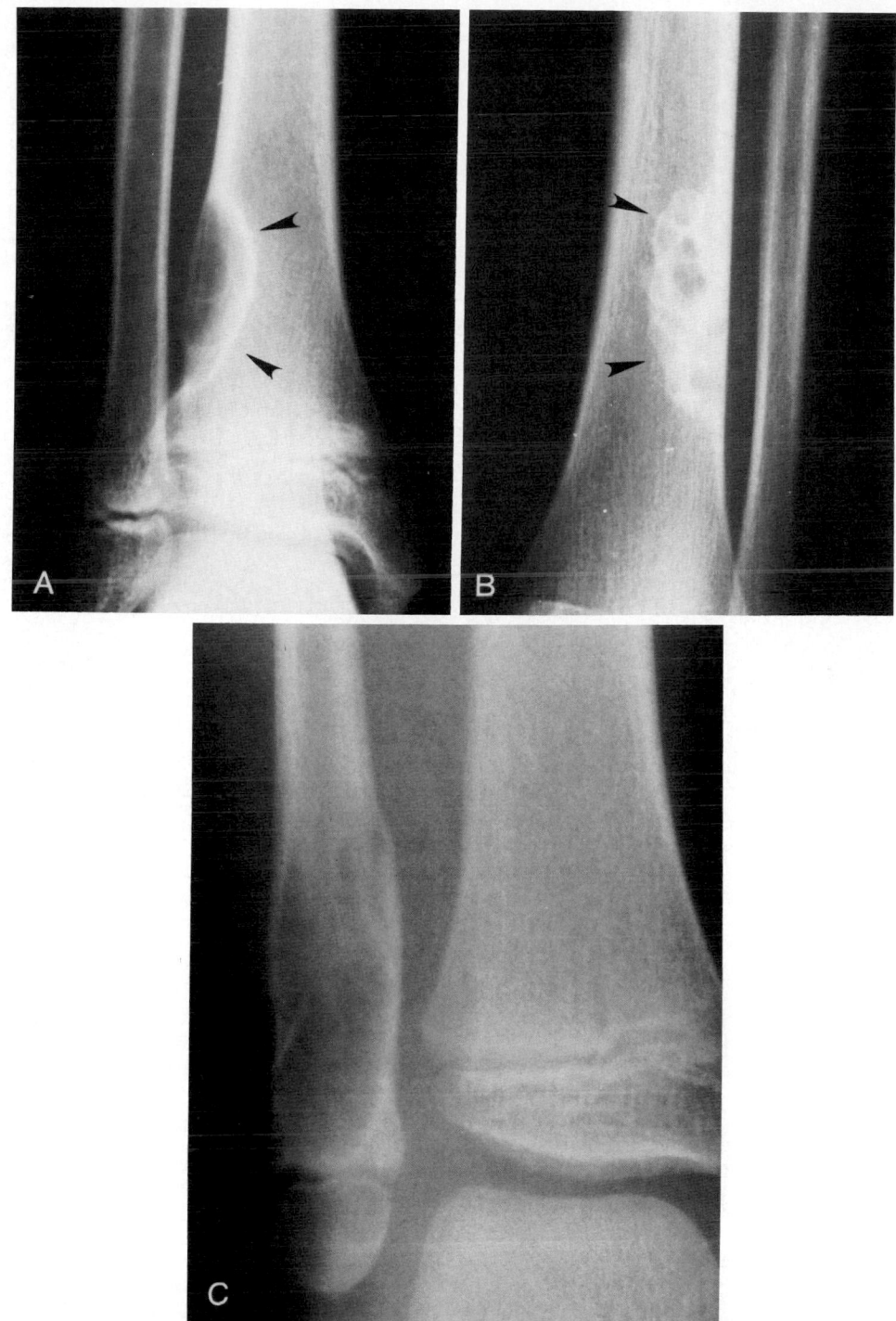

Fig. 4.130. Solitary bone lesion; value of location. A. Typical eccentric location of nonossifying fibroma (arrows). B. Another typical eccentric nonossifying fibroma in its healing stage (arrows). C. Typical central, metaphyseal location of benign bone cyst. A pathologic fracture is present and there is a pushed-in fragment of bone, seen on end.

are full of serous fluid, and consequently, when such fractures occur, a piece of the cyst wall can fall into the cyst cavity. Roentgenographically, the phenomenon results in the so-called "fallen fragment" (27), or "tumbling bullet" (33) signs (Fig. 4.130C). Bone cysts, much as nonossifying fibromas and benign cortical defects, heal by slow, spontaneous obliteration, but often the process is hastened by repeated fracturing or surgical filling with bone chips. More recently, however, steroid injections seem to accomplish the same objective (9). Overall, bone cysts have a tendency to recur, at least until the patient passes out of adolescence. Eighty percent occur in the proximal humerus and femur (23), but they can occur in other long bones (30) and even in flat bones.

Lesions located within the **epiphysis** are far less common than those seen in the metaphysis. When they do occur, they usually are accounted for by one of the following conditions: osteomyelitis (12) (Fig. 4.131A), osteochondritis dissecans, histiocytosis X (rather rare in epiphysis), benign bone cysts (also rare in epiphysis), normal epiphyseal defects (common in knees), monoarticular rheumatoid arthritis (Fig. 4.131B), tuberculous arthritis (10), fungal arthritis, traumatic avulsions, and rarely, intraosseous ganglions (see Table 4.21). Tumors causing epiphyseal

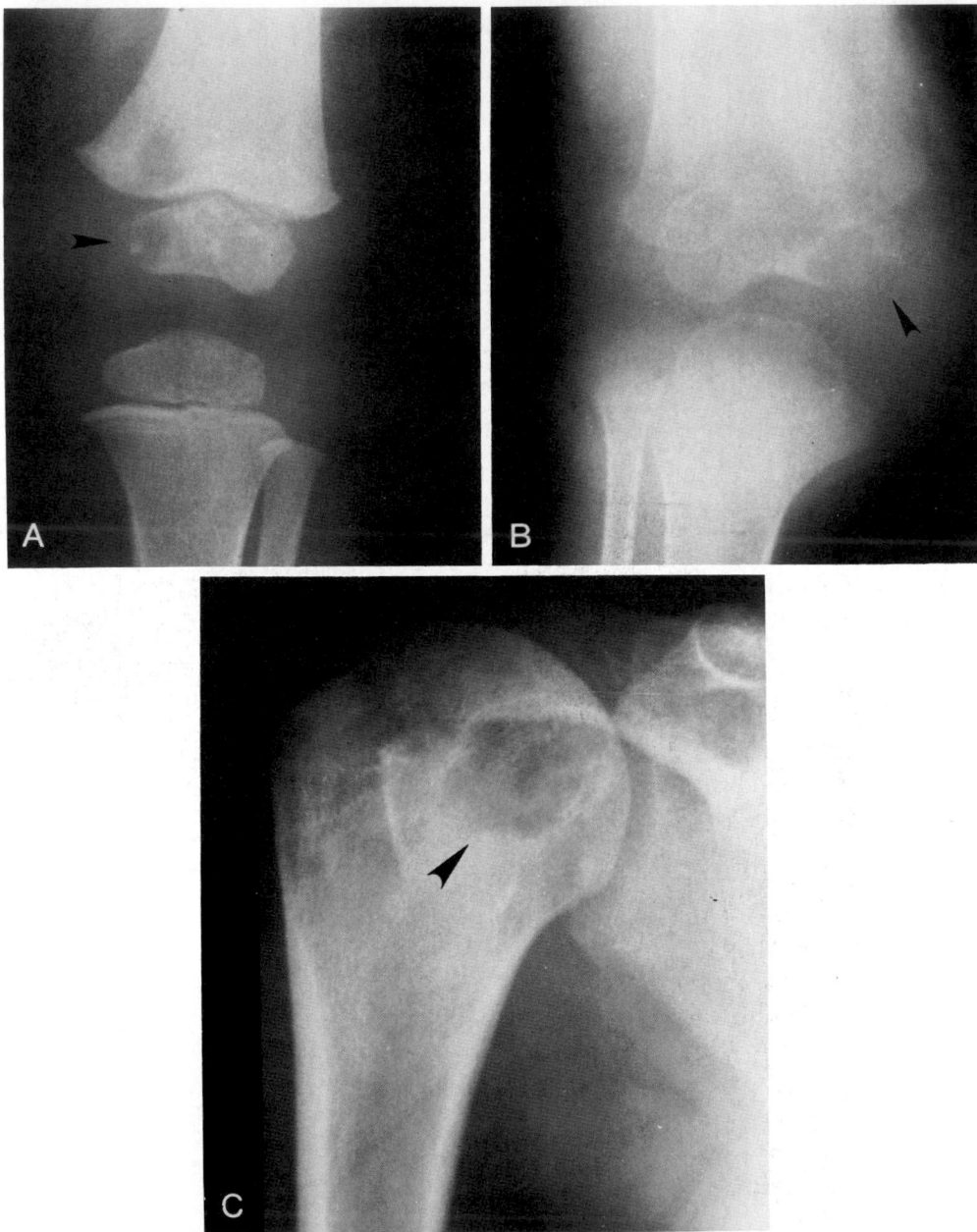

Fig. 4.131. Solitary bone lesions; epiphyseal location. A. Note radiolucent defect in the distal femoral epiphysis (arrow). Above it is another radiolucent defect in the metaphysis. Both were caused by osteomyelitis. B. Large defect in distal femur secondary to erosion in monarticular rheumatoid arthritis (arrow). C. Classic appearance of chondroblastoma in young adult (arrow). Note its epiphyseal-metaphyseal location. For other lesions producing epiphyseal defects, see Figure 4.54.

defects are rare, except for chondroblastomas. This tumor, more a problem of older children, characteristically involves the epiphysis and extends across the epiphyseal line into the metaphysis (Fig. 4.131C). The other tumor, notoriously involving the epiphysis, is the giant cell tumor. However, this is not a common tumor in children, and furthermore, does not produce an isolated epiphyseal defect.

Type and Rate of Bone Destruction

Bone destruction can be rapid or slow, and can occur from diseases arising from within the bone, or from those arising in adjacent tissues. The latter, for the most part, occurs with soft tissue bone tumors, chronic tendon avulsions, and periosteal lesions such as the rare periosteal sarcoma and the posttraumatic giant cell tumor (subperiosteal hematoma). Soft tissue radiography, zero radiography, CT and NMR scanning are quite useful for delineating many of these lesions. Arteriography also can be employed, but is utilized primarily for defining the degree of vascularity in, or around a tumor.

As far as destruction from within is concerned, it can be (a) aggressive and moth-eaten, (b) aggressive and homogeneous, or (c) slow, and variably expanding (Figs. 4.132–135). The more active the destructive process, the less distinct and sclerotic is the margin of the lesion, and conversely, the slower the rate of destruction, the more discrete and sclerotic is the margin. When rapid destruction results in a moth-eaten appearance of the bone, and the cortex is penetrated, the term permeative is applied. Cortical penetration also commonly occurs with aggressive homogenous destruction, and in either case, when this happens periosteal elevation and new bone deposition is seen. For the most part, diseases producing moth eaten destruction include acute osteomyelitis, metastatic disease, leukemia, lymphoma, malignant bone tumors, and bone infarction (Fig. 4.132).

Aggressive destruction leading to a more homogeneous pattern of destruction (Fig. 4.133) is seen with osteomyelitis, acute or treated with antibiotics (5, 29), bone infarction, some cases of leukemia, lymphoma, or metastatic disease, and the histiocytosis X-eosinophilic granuloma group of lesions (Fig. 4.133). When these lesions are sharp-edged or "punched out", and their margins, nonsclerotic, one should first consider histiocytosis X and then osteomyelitis, especially fungal (Fig. 4.134). Other conditions to be considered include all of the neonatal infections (i.e., rubella, CID, lues), multiple fibromatosis or hamartosis of bone, fibrous dysplasia, malignant fibrous histiocytoma, osteitis fibrosa cystica, bone infarcts associated with pancreatitis, and intraosseous bleeding with blood dyscrasias such as hemophilia. When **homogeneous bone destruction is focal, and associated with considerable sclerosis of its margins**, a slower disease process should be inferred, and then one should consider lesions such as bone cysts, low grade osteomyelitis (Brodie's abscess), fibrous dyspla-

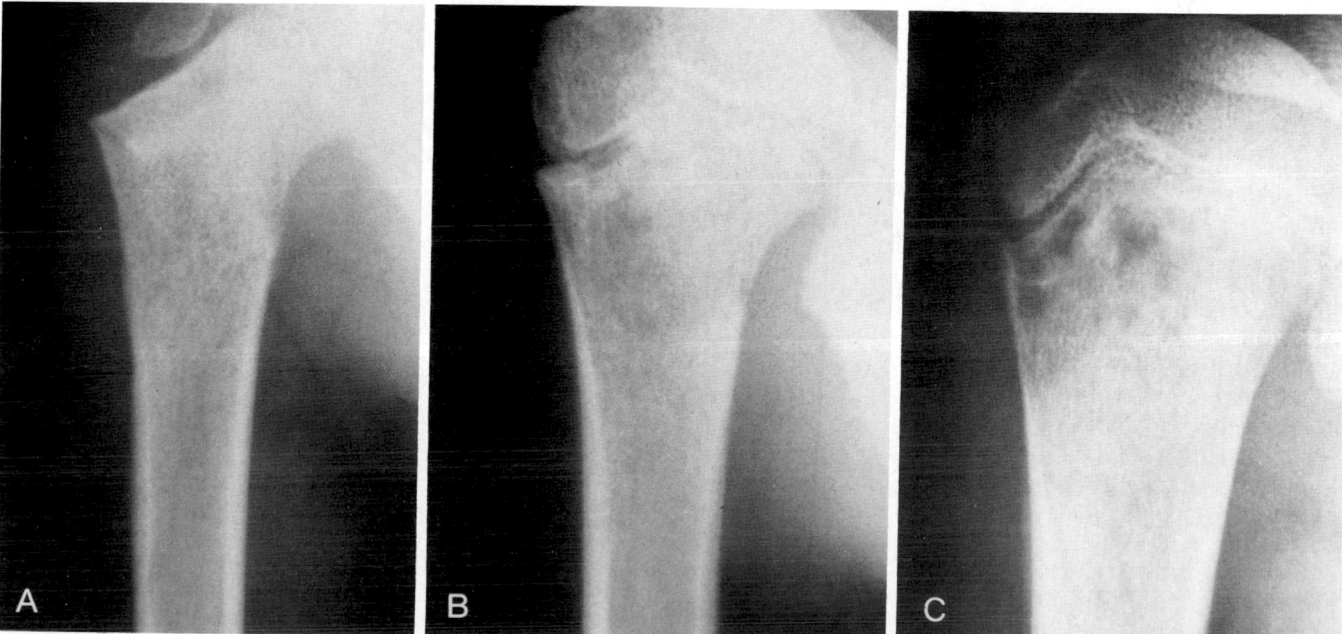

Fig. 4.132. Bone destruction; aggressive-motheaten appearance. A. Typical motheaten, coarsely trabeculated, destruction due to tumor (metastatic neuroblastoma). B. Similar appearance due to acute osteomyelitis (arrow). C. More extensive and coarse appearing destruction in osteomyelitis.

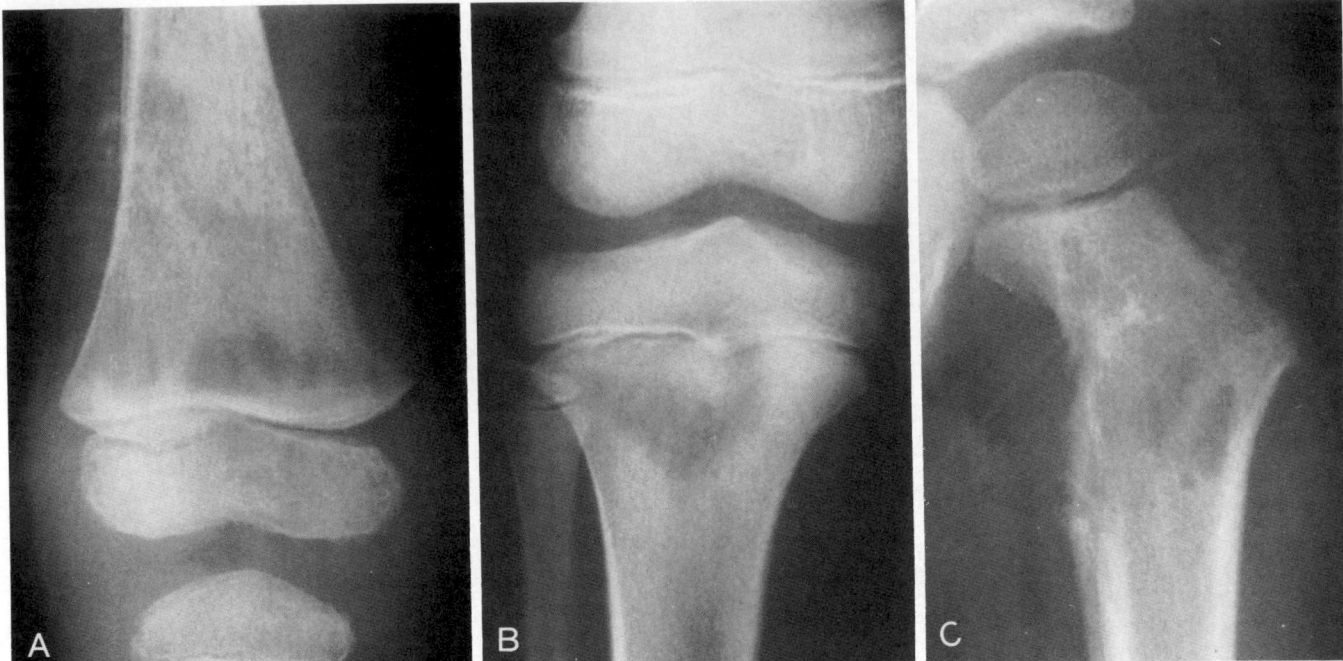

Fig. 4.133. Bone destruction; aggressive homogeneous appearance. A. Rather homogeneous bone destruction in metastatic neuroblastoma. Also note permeative pattern in some areas. B. Aggressive, rather homogeneous destruction in osteomyelitis. C. Homogeneous destruction in histiocytosis X. In all cases, note lack of any significant peripheral sclerosis.

sia, chondromyxoid fibroma, hemangioma, lymphangioma, and intraosseous ganglion (Fig. 4.135). The densest, thickest, margins are seen with Brodie's abscess, some cases of chondromyxoid fibroma, fibrous dysplasia, and intraosseous ganglions. The thinnest sclerotic margins are seen with unicameral bone cysts, aneurysmal bone cysts, giant cell tumors, some cases of fibrous dysplasia, hemangiomas, lymphangiomas, and a few enchondromas.

When any of the foregoing, slow growing lesions are multiloculated, the two best possibilities are unicameral bone cyst (all compartments communicate and thus the cyst is still unicameral), or fibrous dysplasia (Fig. 4.136). Somewhat similar configurations can be seen with multiple enchondromatosis, malignant fibrous histiocytoma, the brown tumor of hyperparathyroidism, giant cell tumors, aneurysmal bone cysts, and hemangiomas or lymphangiomas of bone (Fig. 4.136C). Less commonly, one might encounter chondromas or chondromyxoid chondromas producing multiloculated lesions. However, the latter tend not to be so multiloculated and their sclerotic margins are broader. Occasionally, histiocytosis X lesions also can appear somewhat multiloculated (Fig. 4.136D).

Finally, a note may be made regarding certain bone tumors which produce rather elongated lesions. For the most part, these are benign tumors and include fibrous dysplasia and multiple enchondromas (Ollier's disease). In fibrous dysplasia, the lesions are quite variable and may be associated with areas of radiolucency, bone expansion, cystic change, sclerosis, or smudgy, expanded bone (Fig. 4.137). With multiple enchondromatosis, the lesions often consist of broad, radiolucent stripes extending for some distance into the diaphysis of the long bones (Fig. 4.138). Some of these lesions become somewhat bulbous, and occasionally may be difficult to distinguish from osteochondroma or exostoses. Multiple enchondromatosis, or Ollier's disease, tends to be predominantly, if not entirely, unilateral in its distribution, and eventually some of the cartilaginous lesions may calcify in characteristic cartilaginous, popcorn fashion (Fig. 4.139).

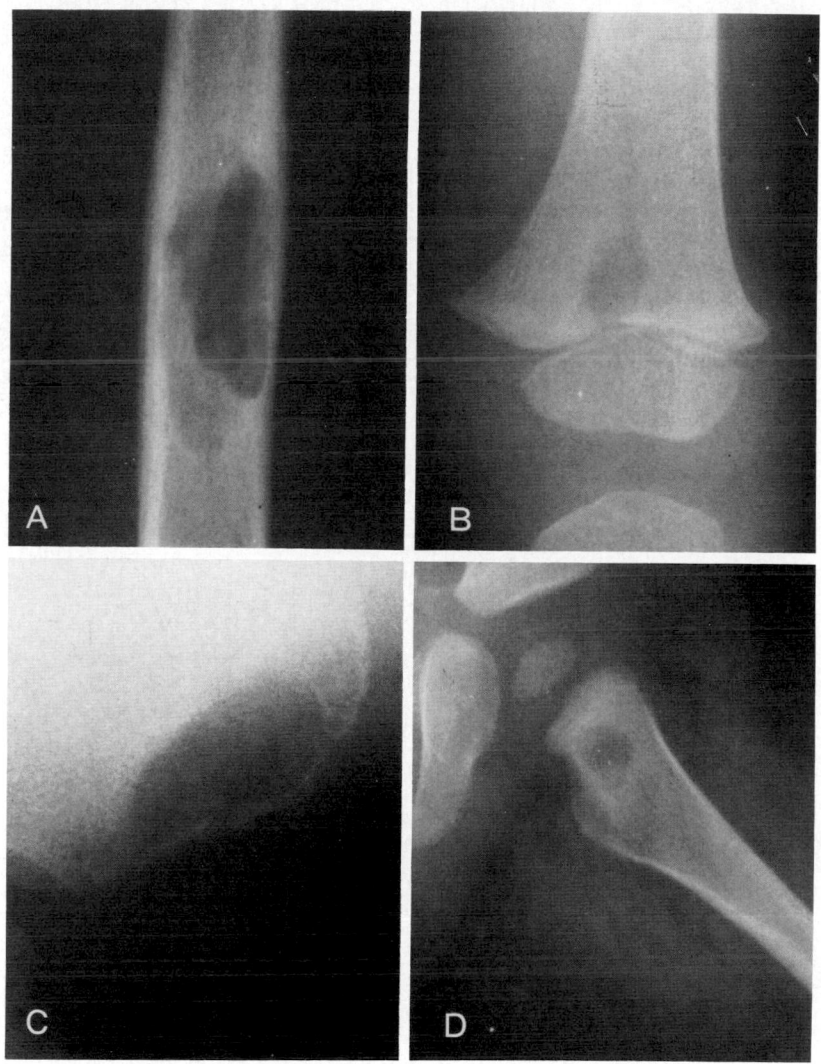

Fig. 4.134. Punched out lytic lesions. A. Typical punched out lesion of histiocytosis X (arrows). Often these lesions are more dramatically displayed in the calvarium. B. Smaller lesion of histiocytosis X. C. Somewhat similar lesion in the iliac wing of a patient with disseminated coccidiomycosis. D. Small focus of osteomyelitis.

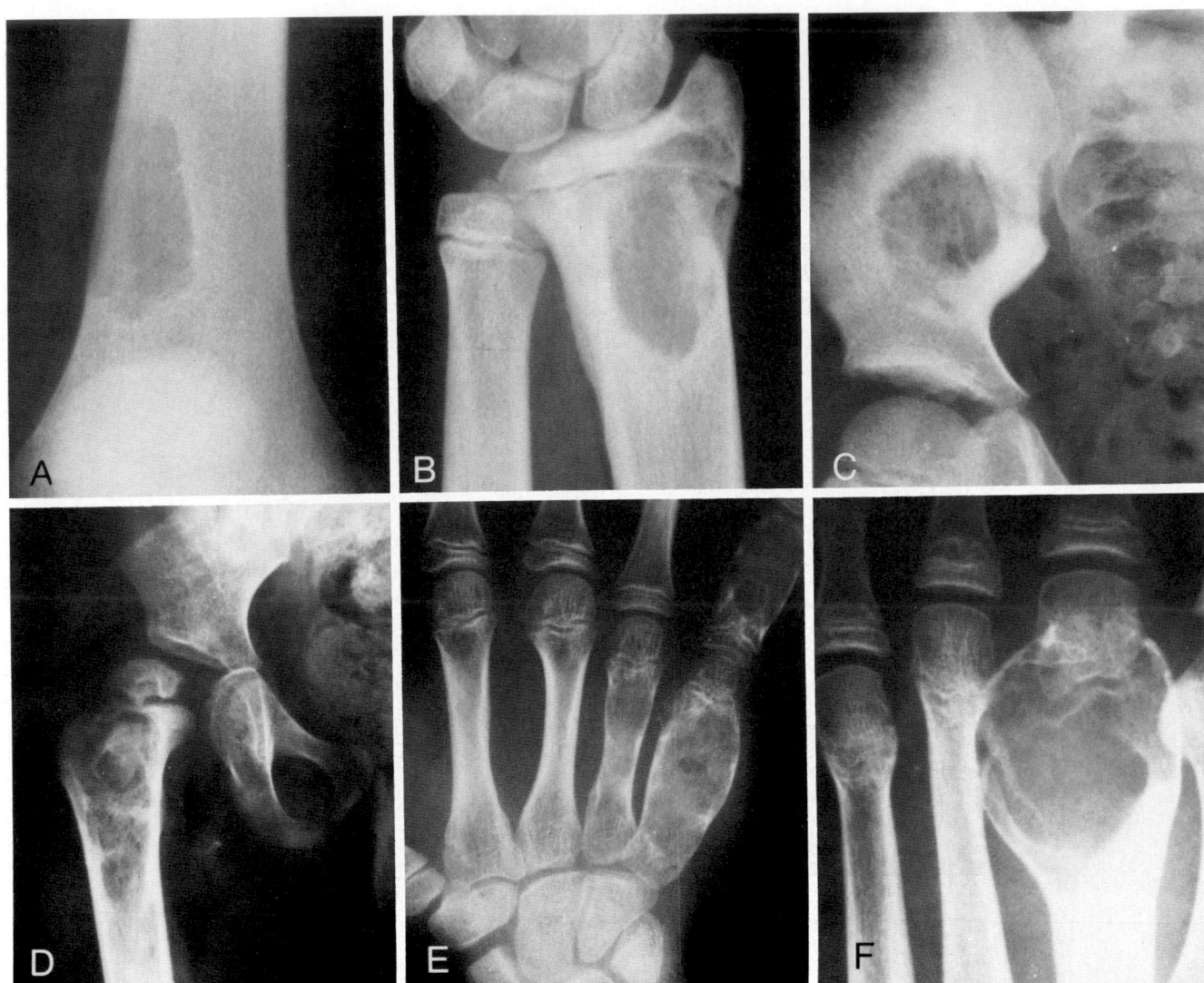

Fig. 4.135. Bone destruction; nonaggressive. A. Slow bone destruction with minimal destruction in nonossifying fibroma. B. Slow destruction with more sclerosis in low grade osteomyelitis (i.e., Brodie's abscess). Note extension into epiphysis. C. Slow destruction with sclerosis in benign bone cyst of iliac wing. D. Slow destruction with considerable sclerosis in chronic, cystic tuberculosis of the bone. Also note epiphyseal involvement. E. Slow destruction with expansion of bones in multiple enchondromatosis. F. Slow destruction with marked expansion in solitary enchondroma.

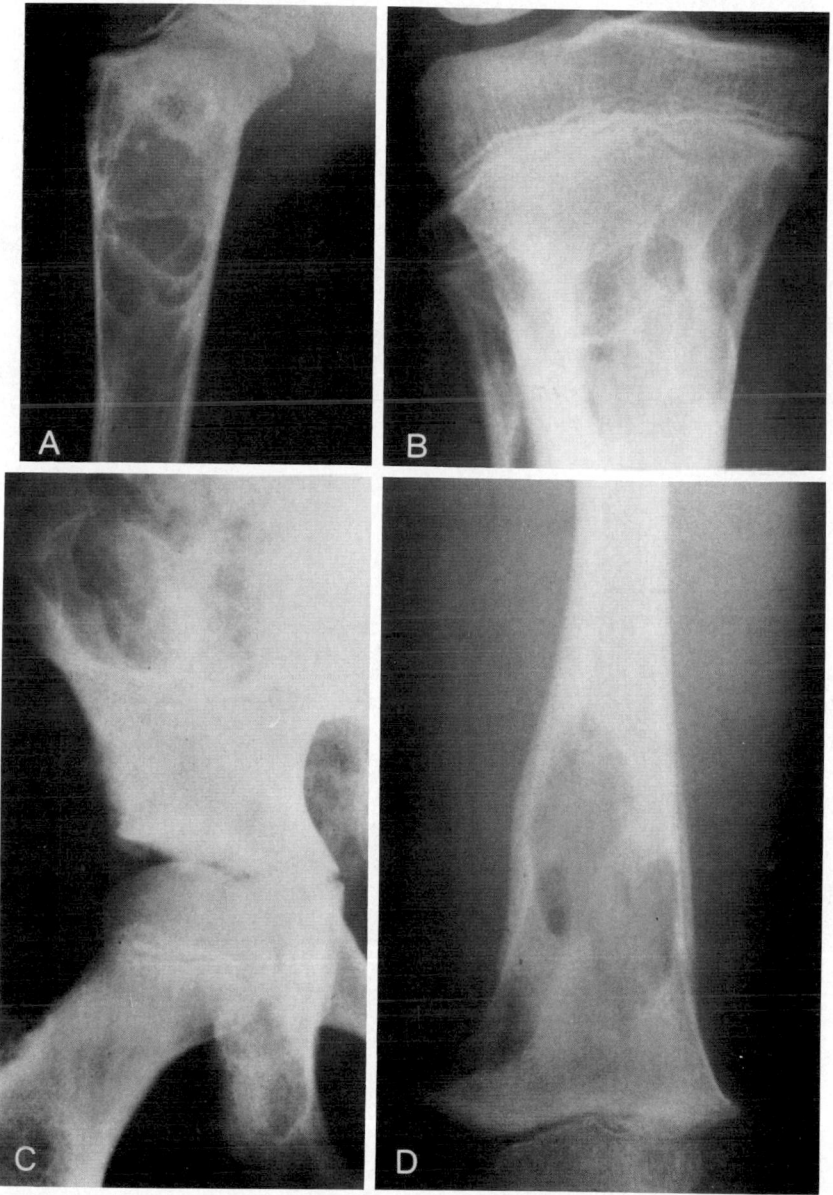

Fig. 4.136. Multiloculated cystic lesions. A. Multiloculated unicameral bone cyst. B. Multiloculated fibrous dysplasia, with pathologic fracture. C. Multiloculated lymphangioma of bone. D. Somewhat multiloculated cystic destruction in histiocytosis X.

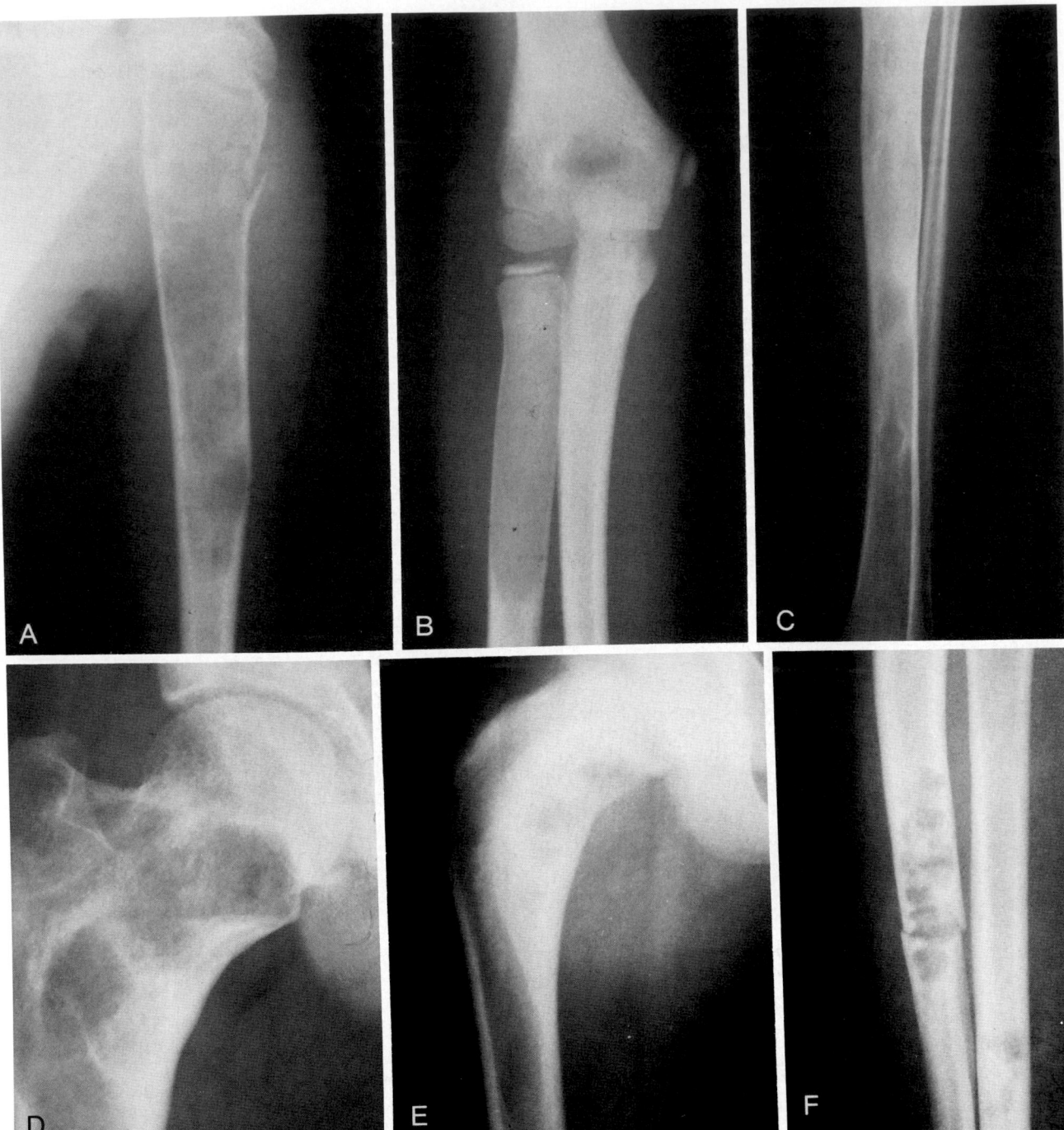

Fig. 4.137. Fibrous dysplasia; various lesion types. A. Long multiloculated, expanding lesion of fibrous dysplasia of humerus. Note pathologic fracture. B. Long expanding lesion of radius with smudgy, ground glass appearance. C. Long, mixed lytic and blastic lesion of tibia in fibrous dysplasia. D. Multiloculated, expanding lytic lesion of upper femur. E. Sclerosing, slightly loculated lesion in another patient. F. Small locules in multiloculated lesion of fibrous dysplasia with pathologic fracture.

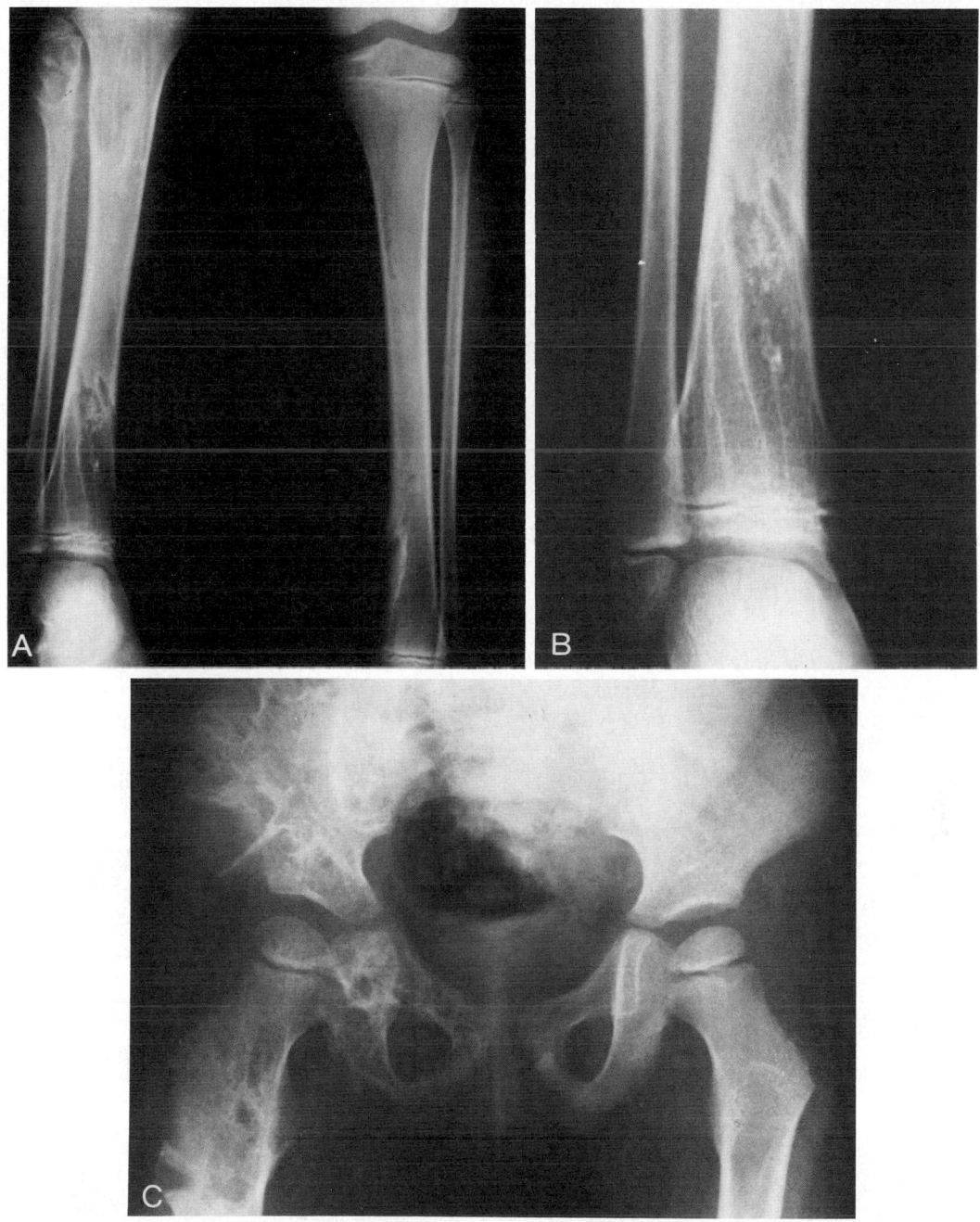

Fig. 4.138.   Lesions of multiple enchondromatosis. A. Note unilateral predominance of long radiolucent lesions in the tibial metaphyses on the right. B. Closeup of lower tibial lesion to show elongated pattern of tumor. C. Another patient with less linear enchondromas. Note unilateral distribution.

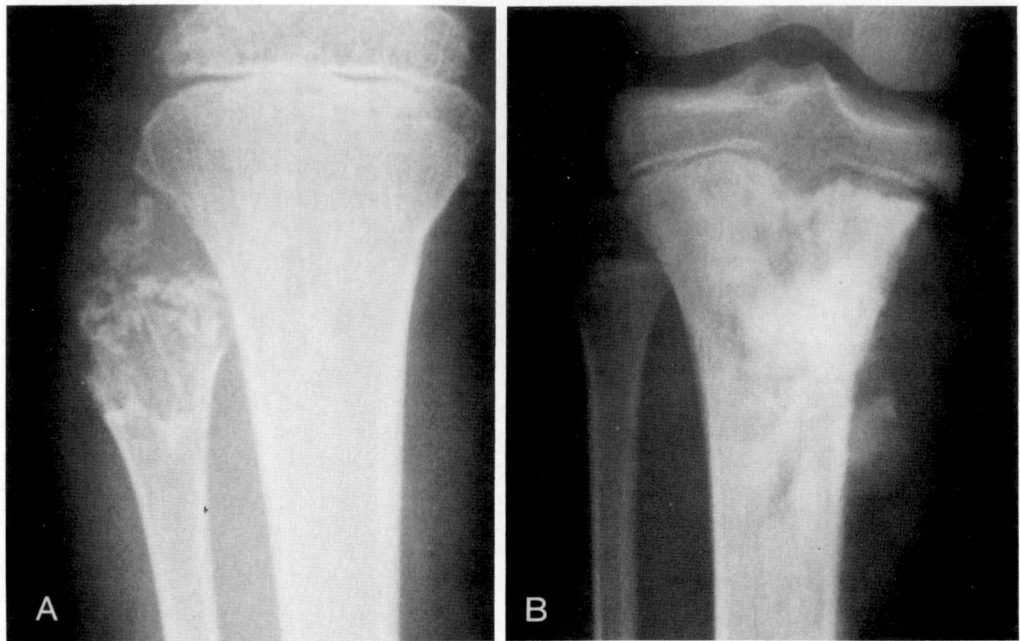

Fig. 4.139. Calcification—ossification in bone tumors. A. Typical, irregular calcification of cartilage in enchondroma. Patient with Ollier's disease. B. Sclerosis due to new bone formation in osteogenic sarcoma of tibia.

Calcification or Ossification

Very few bone lesions calcify or ossify and almost always, when calcifications are seen they are irregular, and in some type of cartilage tumor (i.e., enchondroma, chondroblastoma; Fig.4.139A). Ossification, often profound, is characteristic of osteogenic sarcoma and usually is rather formless (Fig. 4.139B). Metastatic lesions from osteogenic sarcoma also can ossify and these are best known in the lung. Punctate calcifications are pathognomonic of hemangiomatous or lymphangiomatous tumors, but these tumors most often are soft tissue tumors and involve the bones only secondarily. The calcifications, of course, are calcified phleboliths (see Fig. 4.122B).

Soft Tissue Components

Soft tissue components of a bony lesion result only when the disease process within the bone breaks through the cortex and extends into the soft tissues. This occurs, for the most part, with infection and malignant bone tumors. Occasionally, expansile bone cysts or benign bone tumors become so large that they produce associated bulging of the soft tissues, but there is no actual extension of the lesion into the soft tissues if no fracture occurs.

References

1. Brant EE, Jordan HH: Radiologic aspects of hemophilic pseudotumors in bone. *Am J Roentgenol* 115:525–539, 1972.
2. Brower AC, Culver JE Jr, Keats TE: Diffuse cystic angiomatosis of bone: report of two cases. *Am J Roentgenol* 118:456–463, 1973.
3. Carlson DH, Wilkinson RH, Bhakkavisiam A: Aneurysmal bone cysts in children. *Am J Roentgenol* 116:644–650, 1972.
4. Cohen H, Haller JO, Friedman AP: Pancreatitis, child abuse, and skeletal lesions. *Pediatr Radiol* 10:175–177, 1981.
5. Davis LA: Antibiotic modified osteomyelitis. *Am J Roentgenol* 103:608–610, 1968.
6. Echeverria J, Kaude JV: Multifocal tuberculous osteomyelitis. *Pediatr Radiol* 7:238–240, 1978.
7. Feldman F, Johnston A: Intraosseous ganglion. *Am J Roentgenol* 118:328–343, 1973.
8. Feldman, F, Lattes R: Primary malignant fibrous histiocytoma (fibrous xanthoma) of bone. *Skeletal Radiol* 1:145–160, 1977.
9. Fernbach SK, Blumenthal DH, Poznznski AK, Dias LS, Tachdjian MO: Radiographic changes in unicameral bone cysts following direct injection of steroids: a report of 14 cases. *Radiology* 140:689–695, 1981.
10. Goldblatt M, Cremin BJ: Osteoarticular tuberculosis: its presentation in colored races. *Clin Radiol* 29:669–677, 1978.
11. Goluboff N, Cram R, Ramgotra B, Singh A, Wilkinson GW: Polarthritis and bone lesions complicating traumatic pancreatitis in two children. *Can Med Assoc J* 118:924–928, 1978.
12. Green NE, Beauchamp RD, Griffin PO: Primary subacute epiphyseal osteomyelitis. *J Bone Joint Surg* 63A:107–114, 1981.
13. Hollingworth P, Isaacs D, Dydder G: Recurrent osteo-

lytic lesions and subcutaneous fat necrosis in association with a developmental pancreatic cyst. *Arch Dis Child* 54:790–792, 1979.

14. Keating JP, Shackelford GD, Shackelford PG, Ternberg JL: Pancreatitis and osteolytic lesions. *J Pediatr* 81:350–353, 1972.
15. Kozlowski K: Brodie's abscess in the first decade of life. *Pediatr Radiol* 10:33–37, 1980.
16. Kozlowski K, Middleton RWD: Aneurysmal bone cysts—review of 10 cases. *Australas Radiol* 24:170–175, 1970.
17. Krill CE Jr, Mauer AM: Pseudotumor of calcaneus in christmas disease. *Pediatrics* 77:848–855, 1970.
18. Kubicz S: Radiological aspects of aneurysmal bone cysts in children. *Ann Radiol* 13:211–218, 1970.
19. Kushner DC, Weinstein HJ, Kirkpatrick JA: The radiologic diagnosis of leukemia and lymphoma in children. *Semin Roentgenol* 15:316–334, 1980.
20. Mainzer F, Hanagi H, Steinbach HL: The variable manifestations of multiple enchondromatosis. *Radiology* 99:377–388, 1971.
21. Locher GW, Kaiser G: Giant-cell tumors and aneurysmal bone cysts of ribs in childhood. *J Pediatr Surg* 10:103–108, 1975.
22. McLeod RA, Beabout JW: The roentgenographic features of chondroblastoma. *Am J Roentgenol* 118:464–471, 1973.
23. Norman A, Schiffman M: Simple bone cysts: factors of age dependency. *Radiology* 124:779–782, 1977.
24. Prentice AID: Variations on fibrous cortical defect. *Clin Radiol* 25:531–533, 1974.
25. Pullan CR, Alexander JW, Halse PC: Aneurysmal bone cyst—a report of three cases. *Arch Dis Child* 53:899–901, 1979.
26. Reilly BJ, Davidson JW, Bain H: Lymphangiectasis of the skeleton: a case report. *Radiology* 103:385–386, 1972.
27. Reynolds J: The "fallen fragment sign" in the diagnosis of unicameral bone cysts. *Radiology* 92:949–953, 1969.
28. Schajowicz F, Alello C, Francone M, Giannini R: Cystic angiomatosis. *J Bone Joint Surg* 60:100–106, 1978.
29. Season EH, Miller PR: Primary subacute pyogenic osteomyelitis in long bones in children. *J Pediatr Surg* 11:347–353, 1976.
30. Shulman HS, Wilson SR, Harvie JN, Cruickshand B: Unicameral bone cyst in a rib of a child. *Am J Roentgenol* 128:1058–1050, 1977.
31. Simmons CR, Harle TS, Singleton EB: The osseous manifestations of leukemia in children. *Radiol Clin North Am* 6:115–130, 1968.
32. Steiner GC: Fibrous cortical defect and nonossifying fibroma of bone: a study of the ultrastructure. *Arch Pathol* 97:205–210, 1974.
33. Taxin RN, Feldman F: The tumbling bullet sign in a post-traumatic bone cyst. *Am J Roentgenol* 123:140–143, 1975.

SYNDROMOLOGY

The identification of syndromes, dwarfs, etc., is an important part of pediatric radiology but there are so many syndromes to remember, and so many findings to consider, that the problem becomes overwhelming. Of course, if one deals with the problem on a regular basis, identification is a little easier, but never is it without difficulty at all. For this reason, one needs to devise some system of analysis and, in this regard, one might begin by noting that the most useful information is derived from examination of the long bones, hands, pelvis, and spine. Additional information is available from examination of the skull, feet, and other flat bones, but almost always, if one cannot make a diagnosis from the bones noted in the first group, difficulty persists. Differential diagnoses, and more details, for the various skeletal findings to be noted in the ensuing discussion are available throughout this chapter and in a number of currently available syndrome books (1–4). The following is a brief resume only, and only one possible approach to the evaluation of syndromes.

Long Bone Findings

One of the first long bone observations to be made concerns bone length, and while occasionally the bones are too long, most often the problem is shortening. In this regard, once shortening is noted, one should try to determine whether it is the proximal (humerus, femur), middle (tibia, fibula, radius-ulna), or distal (hands, feet), segment of the extremity which bears the brunt of the shortening. Proximal segment predominance is referred to as rhizomelic, and middle segment as mesomelic shortening. Distal segment shortening, as a predominant or isolated phenomenon, is rather uncommon and then generally is referred to as peripheral dysostosis. For a list of conditions presenting with overly long or short bones, see Tables 4.3 and 4.5.

After major segment predominance has been assessed, one should try to decide whether the problem in the individual bone is diaphyseal, metaphyseal, or epiphyseal. Diaphyseal predominance is easiest to assess because in such cases the metaphyses and epiphyses appear normal or near normal. Abnormal **diaphyseal changes** can be grouped as follows: (a) thin or overtubulated bones (see Table 4.5); (b) short, squat or undertubulated bones (see Table 4.3); and (c) diaphyseal sclerosis caused by periosteal deposition (see p 161). **Metaphyseal abnormalities** consist of (a) splaying, (b) cupping, (c) widening, and (d) irregularity (see Tables 4.23–4.26). **Abnormalities of the epiphysis** usually consist of (a) smallness, (b) fragmentation or irregularity, and (c) calcification (see Tables 4.15–4.21). In most instances, it is relatively easy to determine whether the epiphysis or metaphysis is bearing the brunt of the abnormality; but, in some cases, epiphyseal maldevelopment is so profound that secondary metaphyseal changes are induced (i.e., it is surmised that, because the epiphysis is underdeveloped, injury to the growth plate results and causes subsequent metaphyseal growth disturbance). In such cases, it is important to appreciate that the epiphyseal changes are the primary problem because, otherwise, an erroneous diagnosis will result. For the most part, this phenomenon occurs with the pseudoachondroplasia syndromes, and almost always one is dealing with multiple epiphyseal dysplasia or spondyloepiphyseal dysplasia (see Fig. 4.4B).

Hand and Foot Abnormalities

With these abnormalities, it is the hand which pays off more than the foot, for hand changes are easier to assess and usually more striking. Changes in the hands include the following: a spade-shaped hand, shortening of the metacarpals (either selective or generalized), shortening of various phalanges, shortening of the thumb, triphalangeal thumb, incurving of the fifth digit, cone-shaped epiphyses, polydactyly, and syndactyly (see Tables 4.28–4.31). In addition to assessing the small bones of the hands and feet, the carpal and tarsal bones should be assessed for irregularity, smallness, scalloping, and fusion (see Table 4.33).

Pelvic Changes

For the most part, pelvic changes are most useful for the diagnosis of the various chondrodystrophies, storage diseases, and certain chromosomal abnormalities. Although in the past, much was made regarding these pelvic configurations, currently they are used less than other abnormalities of the skeletal system. Nonetheless, one still should be familiar with the differential diagnosis for (a) short, squared off iliac wings; (b) iliac wings with a narrow waist; (c) increased and decreased acetabular angles; and (d) absence of portions of the pubic bones (see Table 4.34).

Spine Abnormalities

Assessment of the spine can be very helpful in establishing diagnoses in confusing syndromes and dwarfing conditions. However, as with the rest of the skeleton, one should have some idea as to which findings are most helpful. In this regard, it is worthwhile looking at the following: (a) the C_1-C_2 area for abnormalities of the dens (see Table 6.25); (b) the presence or absence of clefting abnormalities of the vertebral bodies (see Table 6.7); and (c) the shape of the vertebral bodies. Abnormal shapes consist of (a) platyspondylia (for various types; see Table 6.10), (b) cuboid vertebrae (see Table 6.11), (c) round or bullet-shaped vertebrae (see Table 6.14), and (d) notched or beaked vertebrae (see Table 6.16). In addition, one should determine whether the vertebral column is narrowed or normal in diameter. This is important in identifying achondroplasia and some of the other chondrodystrophic dwarfs where the vertebral canal is narrowed (see Table 6.18).

Miscellaneous Findings

In the long bones, miscellaneous findings include congenital dislocations, synostoses, and abnormalities of mineralization (i.e., demineralization and increased sclerosis). All of these features have been covered in earlier sections. Other abnormalities include exostoses, calcification of cartilage, and twisted bones. The latter, almost exclusively occur in the Melnick-Needles syndrome, but also can be seen with neurofibromatosis. Exostoses are seen in a variety of conditions (see p 207), but on a diagnostic basis they are used most often in the multiple exostosis syndrome and in the nail patella syndrome where they take the form of iliac wing exostoses (horns) or Fong's lesion. Calcification of cartilage occurs in punctate epiphyseal dysplasia, Zellweger's hepatorenal syndrome, and Warfarin embryonopathy (see Fig. 4.43). In these cases, as well as calcification of the epiphyseal cartilages, calcification of the cartilages in the pelvis and spine also occurs.

References

1. Poznanski AK: *The Hand in Radiologic Diagnosis*. Philadelphia, W. B. Saunders, 1974.
2. Smith DW: *Recognizable Patterns of Human Malformations: Genetic, Embryologic and Clinical Aspects*. Philadelphia, W. B. Saunders, 1970.
3. Spranger JW, Langer LO Jr, Weidemann HR: *Bone Dysplasias: An Atlas of Constitutional Disorders of Skeletal Development*. Philadelphia, W. B. Saunders, 1974.
4. Taybi H: *Radiology of Syndromes*. Chicago, Year Book Medical Publishers, 1975.

BONE AGE DETERMINATION

Bone age determination is an important part of pediatric radiology and almost everyone uses the Greulich-Pyle tables (3) for its determination. For the most part, these suffice; but other methods of bone age determination are available and, of these, probably the most sensitive is the Elgenmark method (2). In this method, all the ossification centers of the epiphyses and carpal and tarsal bones are counted on one side of the body, and then the total is compared to what should be normal. However, only occasionally does one require this much refinement in bone age determination, and actually, if one is doing a lot of bone age work, one can memorize certain key ossification centers to facilitate rapid assessment. With this method, one still can obtain a reasonably accurate

estimate of bone age and, for the most part, the centers include: (a) the capitate and hamate of the wrist; (b) the distal radial and ulnar epiphyses; (c) the epiphysis of the proximal phalanx of the thumb; (d) the pisiform bone; (e) the sesamoid of the thumb; (f) the epiphyses of the terminal phalanges; and, in the elbow: (a) the capitellum; and (b) the radial head epiphysis (Fig. 4.140).

In addition to the foregoing considerations, one or two other practical points about bone age determination might be made. For example, one should appreciate that girls mature more quickly than do boys and, as age progresses, the difference becomes greater. Furthermore, rate of bone maturation differs somewhat from one race to another (Blacks mature faster than

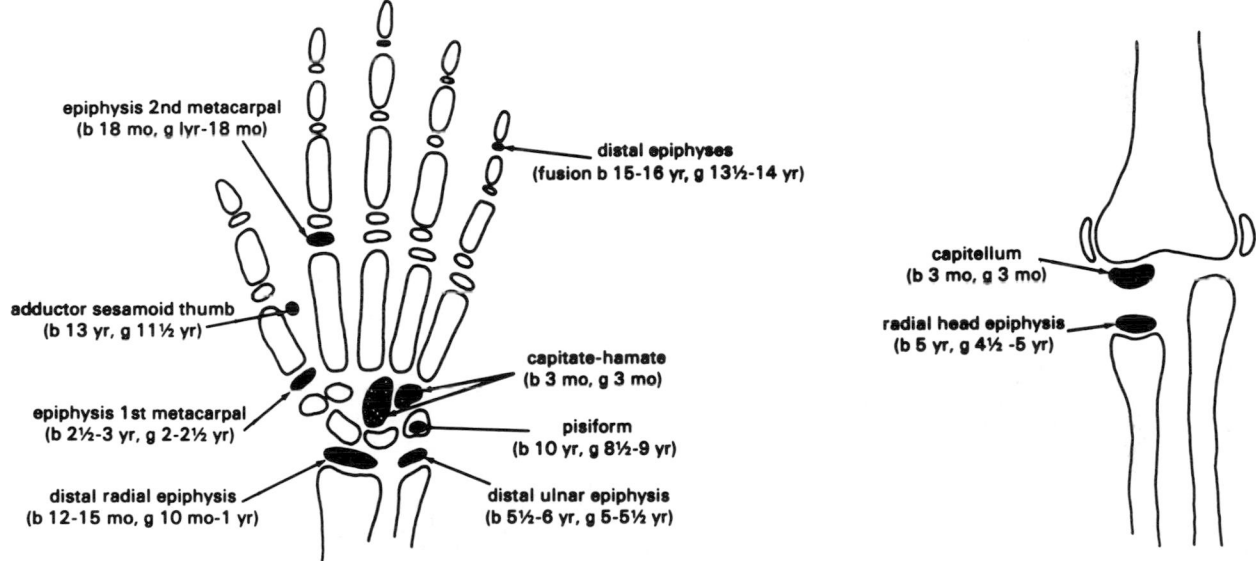

Fig. 4.140. Bone age determination. Utilizing the above data, one can arrive at a reasonably accurate bone age estimate.

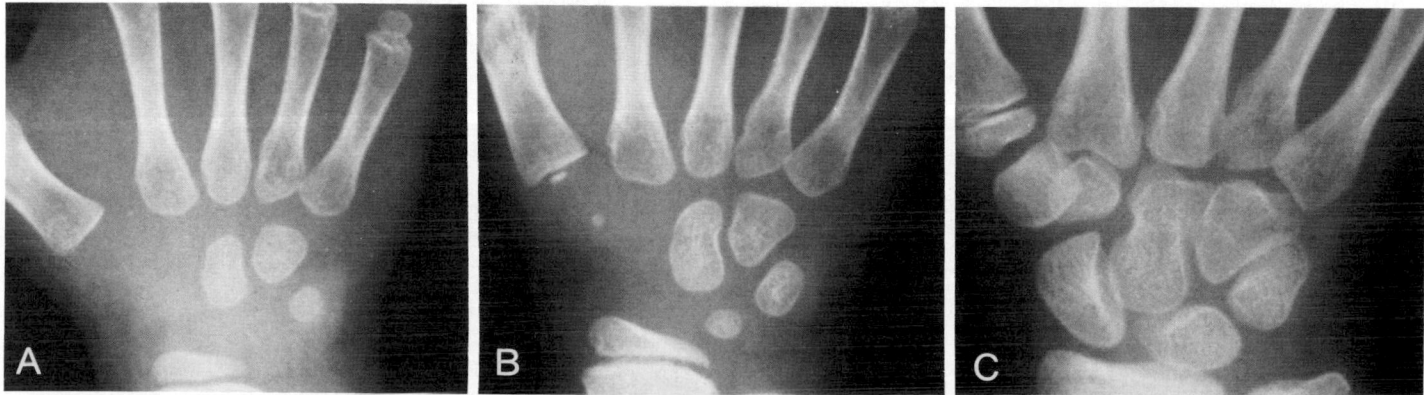

Fig. 4.141. Maturation of carpal bones. A. Young infant with rather round carpal bones. B. Maturation leads to more angular configuration of these bones. C. More maturity leads to larger and much more angular, adult appearing, bones.

Whites), and to some extent from one socioeconomic group to another (lower groups mature slower). More important, however, is the fact that, in certain endocrinological abnormalities, the ossification centers come in less regularly and, in some cases, seemingly haphazardly. In other words, one center might come in unexpectedly, and yet another, which should have come in, is delayed. In these cases, it is important to assess as many centers as possible (this is the time to use the Elgenmark method) and, in addition, to appreciate how mature the individual bones appear. This is best accomplished with the carpal bones which appear more and more angular as they become more mature (Fig. 4.141). In infants they are round and smooth while in teenagers they are quite angular. Nonetheless, in some cases, it is still difficult to estab-

lish an absolutely accurate bone age, and then it probably is more important to note degree of change from one examination to another.

References

1. Caffey J: *Pediatric X-Ray Diagnosis*, ed 6. Chicago, Year Book Medical Publishers, 1972, vol 2, pp 815–895.
2. Elgenmark O: Normal development of the ossific centers during infancy and childhood: Clinical, roentgenologic and statistical study. *Acta Paediatr* 33 (Suppl 1): 1946.
3. Greulich WW, Pyle JS: *Radiographic Atlas of Skeletal Development of Hand and Wrist*, ed 2. Stanford, Stanford University Press, 1959.
4. Sontag LW, Snell D, Anderson M: Rate of appearance of ossification centers from birth to the age of five years. *Am J Dis Child* 58:949–1956, 1939.

Advanced and Delayed Bone Age

Bone age deviations from normal are numerous and can be seen with endocrinologic, metabolic, and dysplastic bone disease. Most of the conditions producing such changes are listed in Table 4.42, and the information has been derived from experience and a number of extensive publications on the subject (1–3).

Table 4.42 Altered Bone Age

A. Retarded bone age
- Achondrogenesis
- Achondroplasia
- Aminopterin-induced syndrome
- Camptomelic syndrome
- Carpenter syndrome (acrocephalopolysyndactyly)
- Cephaloskeletal dysplasia (Taybi-Linder syndrome)
- Cerebrohepatorenal syndrome (Zellweger's syndrome)
- Chondrodysplasia punctata
- Chondroectodermal dysplasia (Ellis-van Crevald syndrome)
- Cleidocranial dysostosis
- Cloverleaf skull syndrome
- Cornelia de Lange syndrome
- Cushing's syndrome
- Diastrophic dwarfism
- Epiphyseal dysplasia (multiple and spondylo)
- Failure to thrive-malnutrition (nonspecific)
- Fanconi's anemia
- Generalized gangliosidosis
- Hypothyroidism
- Infants of toxemic mothers
- Leprechaunism
- Lesch-Nyhan syndrome
- Lightwood's syndrome
- Lorain-Levi syndrome
- Mesomelic dwarfism (Nievergelt type)
- Metatropic dwarfism
- Morquio's disease
- Mucolipidoses
- Mucopolysaccharidoses
- Noonan's syndrome
- Pierre Robin syndrome
- Prader-Willi syndrome
- Riley-Day syndrome
- Rubella, congenital
- Rubinstein-Taybi syndrome
- Russell-Silver syndrome
- Saldino-Noonan syndrome
- Small for gestational age neonate
- Spondyloepiphyseal dysplasia
- Thanatophoric dwarfism
- Trisomy 18
- Trisomy 21
- Turner's syndrome
- Von Gierke's syndrome
- Weill-Marchesani syndrome
- Wilson's syndrome
- XXXXY syndrome

B. Accelerated bone age
- Acrodysostosis
- Adrenogenital syndrome
- Asphyxiating thoracic dystrophy
- Beckwith-Wiedemann syndrome
- Chondroectodermal dysplasia
- Cockayne's syndrome
- Cushing's syndrome
- Diastrophic dwarfism
- Homocystinuria
- Hyperthyroidism
- Lawrence-Seip syndrome
- Marshall's syndrome
- McCune-Albright syndrome
- Majewski syndrome
- Peripheral dysostosis
- Saldino-Noonan syndrome
- Sotos' syndrome
- Typus edinburgenesis

C. Dysharmonic maturation
- Asphyxiating thoracic dystrophy
- Chondroectodermal dysplasia
- Diastrophic dwarfism
- Saldino-Noonan syndrome

References

1. Kuhns LR, Finnstrom O: New standards of ossification of the newborn. *Radiology* 119:655–660, 1976.
2. Smith DW: *Recognizable Patterns of Human Malfor-*mations: *Genetic, Embryologic and Clinical Aspects.* Philadelphia, W. B. Saunders, 1970.
3. Taybi H: *Radiology of Syndromes.* Chicago, Year Book Medical Publishers, 1975.

RICKETS: ROENTGENOGRAPHIC DIFFERENTIAL DIAGNOSIS

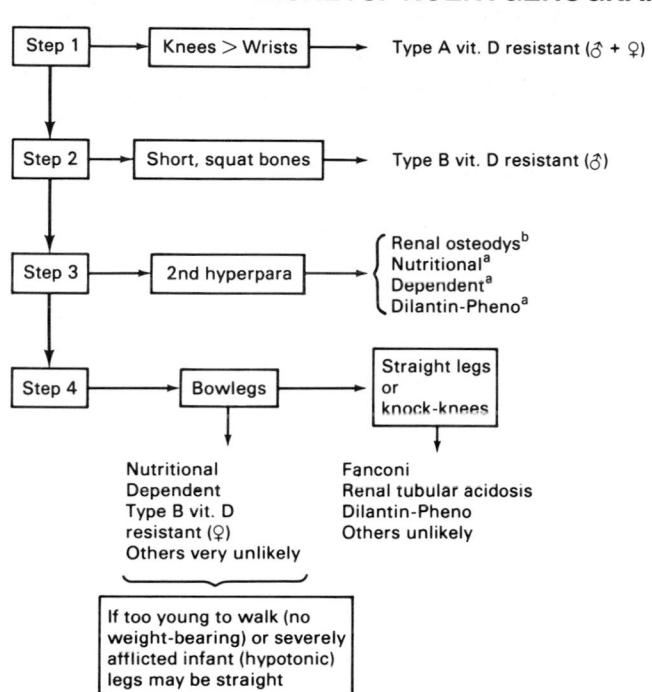

Rickets has a number of causes and roentgenographically can be mimicked by conditions such as metaphyseal dysostosis and hypophosphatasia. However, once one decides that rickets is the problem, very often the type can be determined from roentgenographic examination of the knees and wrists alone (2). This can be accomplished by the application of the following four steps (Fig. 4.142).

Fig. 4.142. Roentgenographic scheme for diagnosis of rickets. Step 1 identifies patients with type A hypophosphatemic vitamin D-resistant rickets. **Step 2** identifies type B hypophosphatemic vitamin D-resistant rickets in males. Females with this form of rickets are not identified in this step, and with all other patients pass on to the next step. **Step 3** identifies patients with renal osteodystrophy and the occasional case of severe nutritional, dependent, or dilantin-phenobarb rickets. **Step 4** deals with the remaining patients and allows one to offer a practical, short differential diagnosis in each instance. [a]A few severe cases only; [b]accounts for most cases.

Step 1. Distribution of Epiphyseal-Metaphyseal Change

In this step, one must decide whether the rachitic changes are uniformly distributed throughout the skeleton or most prominent in the lower extremities. This is a very important determination for it serves to specifically identify a certain group of patients with hypophosphatemic vitamin D resistant rickets (2). The preponderance of lower extremity changes in these patients has been known for some time, and their characteristically bowed legs, with medial widening of the epiphyseal plates of the distal femur and proximal tibia also are well known (Fig. 4.143A). In the more severely afflicted individuals, similar changes are seen in the proximal femur and distal tibia, but in the upper extremity, changes usually are entirely absent. If they occur, they consist of nothing more than slight broadening or cupping of the ulna (Fig. 4.143B).

Widening of the epiphyseal plates medially is a stress-related phenomenon and occurs medially because, with bowed legs, stresses are more pronounced medially (1). Such an increase in stress probably im-pairs already abnormal bone growth even further. Support for this concept exists in the fact that, if these patients present with straight legs, epiphyseal plate widening is uniform from side to side and, if knee-knees occur, widening of the epiphyseal plates occurs laterally. This would be expected because, with knee-knees, increased stresses are more pronounced through the lateral aspect of the epiphyseal-metaphyseal junction. However, most cases of this type of hypophosphatemic rickets, designated type A (2), show bowing and medial epiphyseal plate widening.

Unfortunately, not all patients with hypophosphatemic vitamin D-resistant rickets show the foregoing discrepancy of knee and wrist findings. Indeed, there are some patients who demonstrate equal changes in the upper and lower extremities and a rather severe modeling error of the long bones. This undertubulation error results in very short, squat bones, and this type of rickets is identified by step 2.

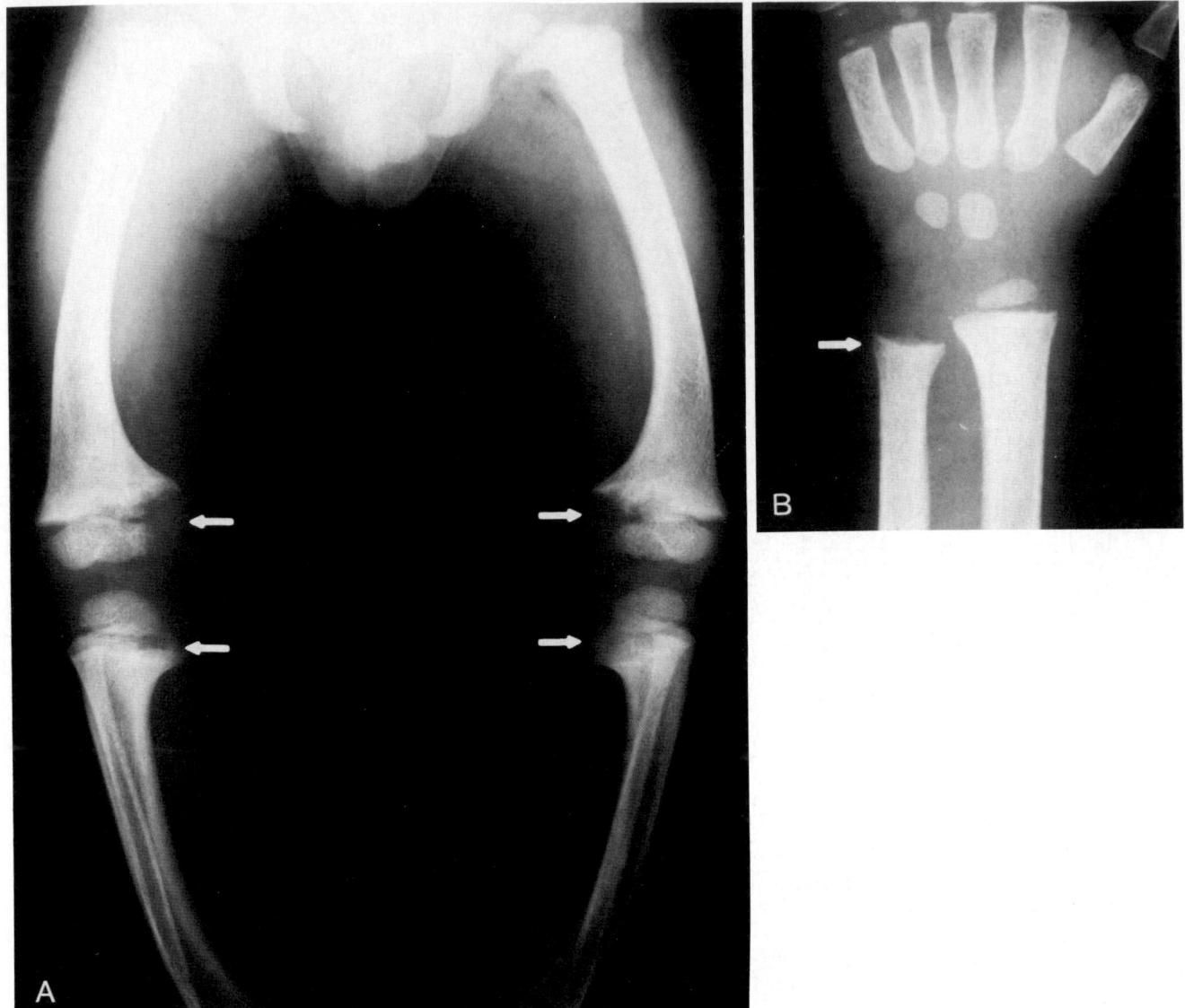

Fig. 4.143. Rickets: step 1. Identifies type A hypophosphatemic rickets. Note characteristic bowing of lower extremities and widening of the medial aspects of the epiphyseal plates (arrows). B. Wrist is almost normal; only slight cupping of the ulna (arrow) is seen. In most cases, not even this finding is present.

Step 2. Presence or Absence of a Generalized Modeling Error Leading to Short, Squat Bones

Very severe cases of any type of rickets can result in some bone growth impairment, but when severe shortening of the long bones is seen, one should begin to suspect the second type of hypophosphatemic vitamin D resistance, that is type B rickets (2). Overall, the bones in these patients have a rather distinctive appearance (Fig. 4.144) because all of the bones appear quite short and squat. Very often the humerus seems to take the brunt of the abnormality and appears club-like, indeed, rather similar to that seen in Hurler's disease (Fig. 4.144).

The changes just described for this type of hypophosphatemic rickets are seen in males. In females, the findings are not nearly as striking and this discrepancy reflects the sex-linked inheritance pattern in hypophosphatemic vitamin D-resistant rickets (i.e., males generally show greater change than do females). However, because the females do not show the same findings they usually are not identified in step 2; rather they are identified in step 4.

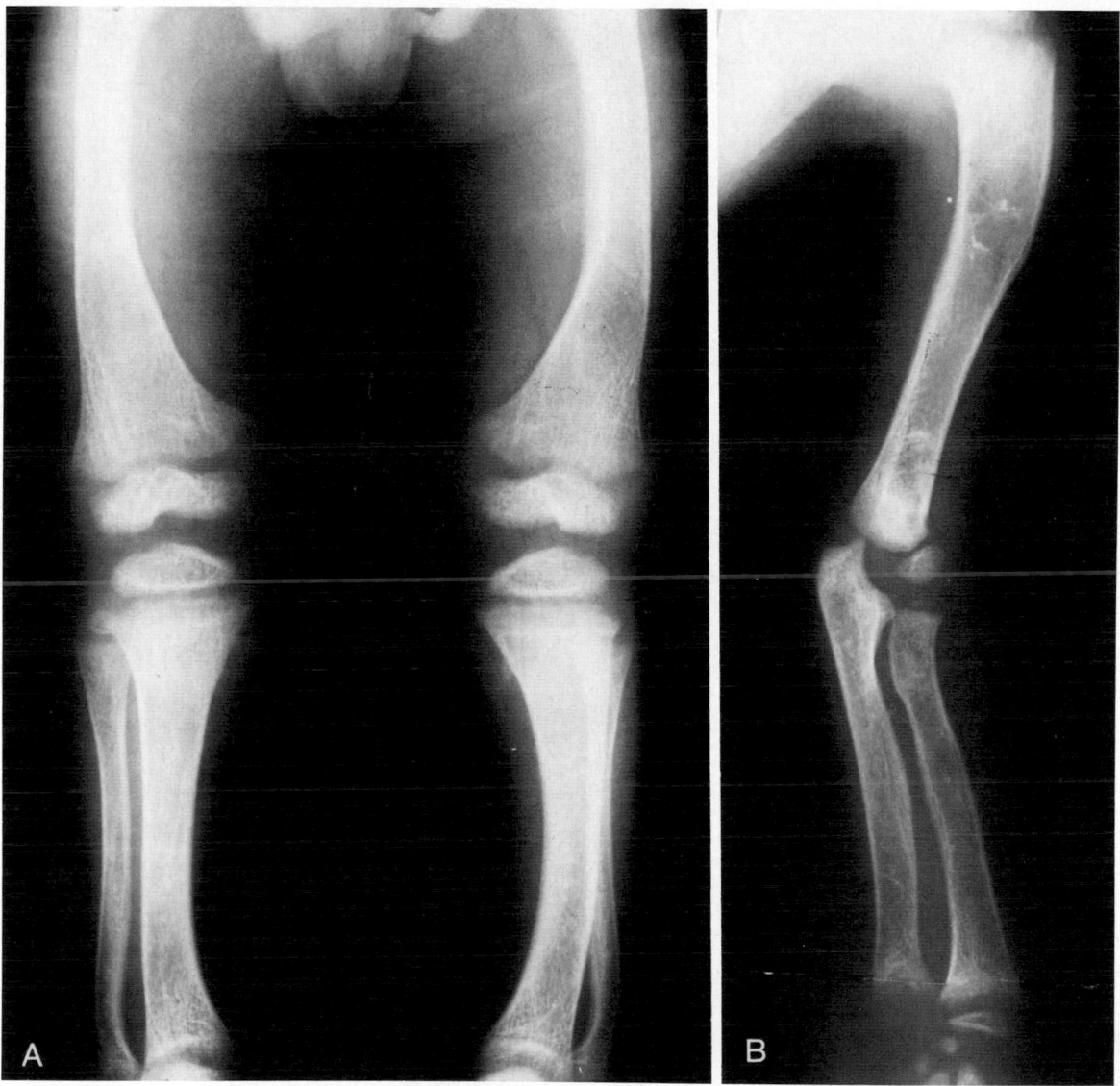

Fig. 4.144. Step 2. Identifies type B hypophosphatemic rickets—male. A. Note short, squat undertubulated bones. Also note bowing and uniformity of epiphyseal-metaphyseal change. B. Upper extremity showing similar findings. Note that changes in the wrist are equal to those in the knees and the Hurler-like appearance of the humerus.

Step 3. Presence of Secondary Hyperparathyroidism

Roentgenographic evidence of secondary hyperparathyroidism in a patient with rickets usually denotes the presence of renal osteodystrophy. Hyperparathyroidism in these patients occurs because their renal diseases are such that there is impairment of both tubular and glomerular function. Impairment of glomerular function leads to phosphorous retention and this causes the parathyroid glands to overreact and secondary hyperparathyroidism to develop. Invariably, secondary hyperparathyroidism becomes the predominant feature in the bones of these patients (Fig. 4.145).

Secondary hyperparathyroidism manifests in subperiosteal bone resorption, endosteal bone resorption, and generalized bony demineralization. Subperiosteal and endosteal resorption of bone most often is seen in the (a) middle phalanges of the hands; (b) upper, inner proximal tibial metaphyses; (c) femoral neck; (d) distal clavicles; (e) distal radius and ulna; and (f) lamina dura of the teeth. These findings are well known and generally not present in any other type of rickets. However, we have noted that they can occur in infants with nutritional or dependent rickets, and older children with dilantin-phenobarb rickets. All of these

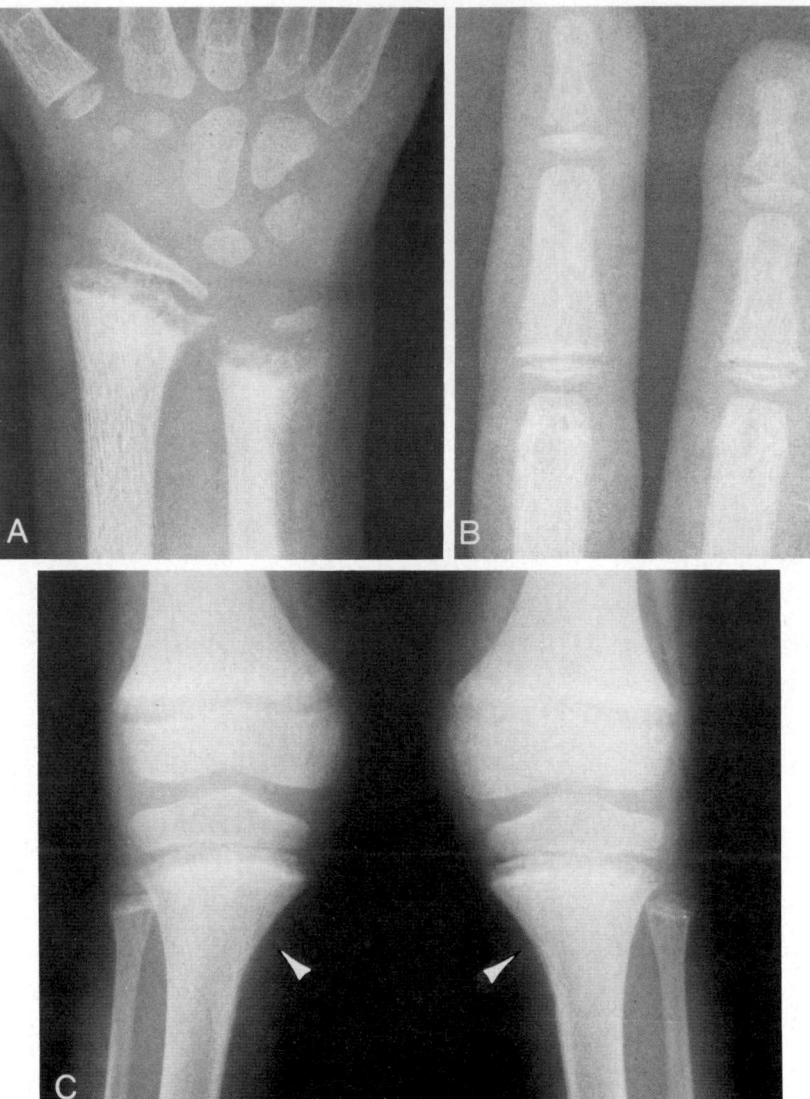

Fig. 4.145.   Rickets: step 3. Identifies secondary hyperparathyroidism. A. Note typical coarse trabecular pattern, loss of cortical distinction, and subperiosteal resorption in the distal ends of the long bones. B. Note subperiosteal bone resorption over the phalanges. C. Subperiosteal bone resorption present along the upper medial tibial aspects (arrows).

patients, however, have very severe rickets and we believe that secondary hyperparathyroidism in them is induced by the prolonged and profound hypocalcemia present when rickets is this severe. This point notwithstanding, however, secondary hyperparathy-roidism generally is a feature of patients with renal disease causing glomerular dysfunction. This leads to renal osteodystrophy and the identification of this condition is the main function of step 3. All patients remaining at this point pass on to step 4.

Step 4. Presence or Absence of Bowlegs, Knock-Knees, or Straight Legs

Whether bowlegs, knock-knees, or straight legs are determined to be present in rickets is surprisingly valuable in their further differentiation. Bowlegs generally occur in patients who have normal muscle tone and are ambulant. If they are not ambulant, mild, or no bowing at all is seen, and if a patient is nonambu-lant and has poor muscle tone, straight legs result. If hypotonia and ambulation exist together, knock-knees develop. One can use these observations to further differentiate one form of rickets from another (Fig. 4.146).

Generally speaking, bowlegs occur in patients with both types A and B hypophosphatemic vitamin D-resistant rickets, and the majority of patients with

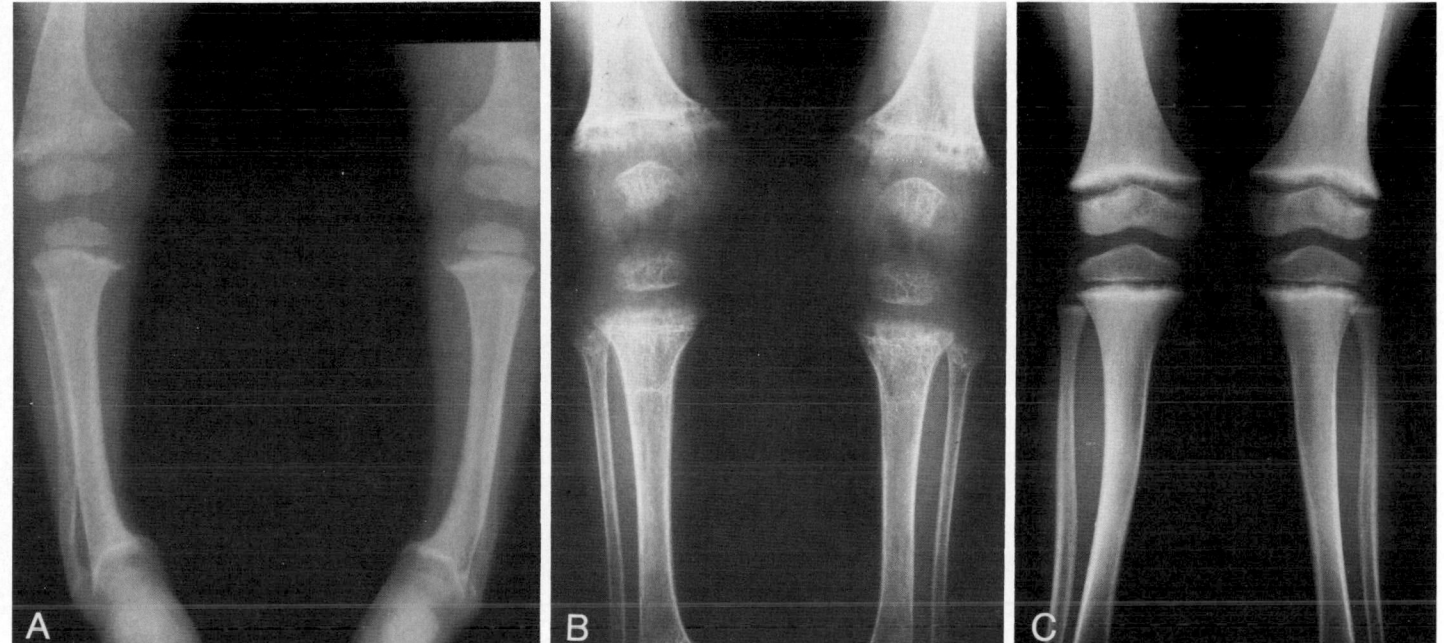

Fig. 4.146. Rickets: step 4. Further differentiation based on presence or absence of bowlegs, knock-knees, or straight legs. A. Bowlegs in patient with dependent rickets. This patient was ambulant. B. Straight legs in patient with very severe dependent rickets. Patient was virtually nonambulant. C. Knock-knees in patient with Fanconi (cystinosis) rickets. This patient was ambulant and hypotonic.

nutritional or dependent rickets. If, however, patients with the latter two forms are too young to walk, or so severely afflicted that they are not ambulant, they show straight legs, or mild bowing only. Other patients showing straight legs, and almost all those showing knock-knees, include patients with Fanconi's syndrome (with or without cystinosis), renal tubular acidosis, Dilantin-phenobarb rickets, and renal osteodystrophy. For the most part, these patients are chronically ill and have decreased muscle tone.

The scheme just outlined deals with untreated rickets presenting after the age of 6 months. Under 6 months of age, only certain forms of rickets are manifest and these include congenital (maternal vitamin D deficiency) rickets, rickets secondary to prematurity (metabolic disease of the premature), and rickets secondary to proximal renal tubular acidosis. In terms of

our classification, all of these patients would demonstrate a uniform distribution of epiphyseal-metaphyseal change, straight legs or mild bowing only (they are nonambulant), no signs of secondary hyperparathyroidism, and no evidence of a modeling error of the long bones. All would be identified in step 4 as would patients with rickets secondary to hormonally active bone tumors or other bone lesions producing distant rachitic changes.

References

1. Bateson EM: Non-rachitis bow leg and knock-knee deformities in young Jamaican children. *Br J Radiol* 39:92–101, 1966.
2. Swischuk LE, Hayden CK Jr: Rickets: a roentgenographic scheme for diagnosis. *Pediatr Radiol* 8:203–208, 1979.

Chapter 5

HEAD

SIZE ABNORMALITIES

When making head size assessments, and the skull is enlarged, it is important to determine whether it is enlarged out of proportion to the face or whether both are enlarged proportionately. The latter is less common and most often is seen in normal, but large children and on a pathologic basis in gigantism. In terms of calvarial enlargement, out of proportion to face size, the problem can be (a) absolute calvarial enlargement or (b) relative enlargement because of hypoplasia of the jaw and face. The latter problem is discussed in Chapter 2 and this section deals only with absolute calvarial enlargement.

Large Head (Table 5.1)

The commonest cause of an enlarged head in the pediatric age group is hydrocephalus (Fig. 5.1). For the most part this occurs in infancy because, when hydrocephalus develops in older children and adolescents, calvarial enlargement is only minimal or absent (i.e., for enlargement of the head to occur the sutures must still be open). The etiology of hydrocephalus may be congenital or acquired and, although calvarial configurations differ in some of the conditions, final diagnosis generally is relegated to CT scanning, NMR or, in early infancy, ultrasonography. Congenital causes include aqueductal stenosis, stenosis of the foramen of Monroe (unilateral ventricular enlargement), the Arnold Chiari malformation (downward displacement of the medulla and fourth ventricle), and Dandy-Walker cyst (obstruction of the foramina of the fourth ventricle). The most common cause of hydrocephalus, however, is acquired, and due to meningeal adhesions secondary to meningitis. Adhesions also can result from trauma-induced subarachnoid bleeding (common in the battered child syndrome) and occasionally with bleeding secondary to blood dyscrasias. In premature neonates, bleeding usually is secondary to prematurity and hypoxia. In all of these cases, adhesions lead to decreased CSF fluid absorption and subsequent hydrocephalus, and a similar phenomenon can occur when the meninges are infiltrated in the storage diseases.

Hydrocephalus also can result from tumors and cysts compressing and obstructing the normal CSF pathways, and these same tumors and cysts, if large enough, can produce calvarial enlargement because of size alone. Finally, hydrocephalus should be differentiated from hydranencephaly, another cause of calvarial enlargement. In this rare condition, there is virtual complete destruction of the brain in utero (except for the mid-brain), and all that remains is a membranous sac. As the sac becomes filled with fluid, the calvarium enlarges.

Subdural hematoma is another relatively common cause of calvarial enlargement and, when bilateral, produces characteristic biparietal widening of the skull (see Fig. 5.7D). Enlargement of the head also is seen in a number of syndromes, and in most of these conditions it is the brain that is large. Conditions to be considered include cerebral gigantism or Soto's syndrome, the Russell Silver dwarf (hemiatrophy) syndrome, the Beckwith-Wiedemann syndrome, the various craniometaphyseal dysostoses, and most of the chondrodystrophies (i.e., achondroplasia, achondrogenesis, thanatrophoric dwarfism, Kniest's syndrome, and metatrophic dwarfism). Enlargement of

Table 5.1 Large and Small Head

Large head	
Hydrocephalus	Commonest
Subdural hematoma	
The chondrodystrophies	Moderately common
Calvarial thickening (see Table 5.2)	
Cleidocranial dysostosis	Relatively rare
Craniometaphyseal dysostosis	
Pyle's disease	
Beckwith-Wiedemann syndrome	
Russell-Silver dwarf	
Storage diseases	
Neurofibromatosis	
Familial megalencephaly	Rare
Lipomatosis-hemangiomatosis syndrome	
Large brain tumor or cyst	
Hydranencephaly	
Small head	
Brain atrophy	Commonest
Poor brain growth (multiple causes)	
Universal craniosynostosis	Relatively rare

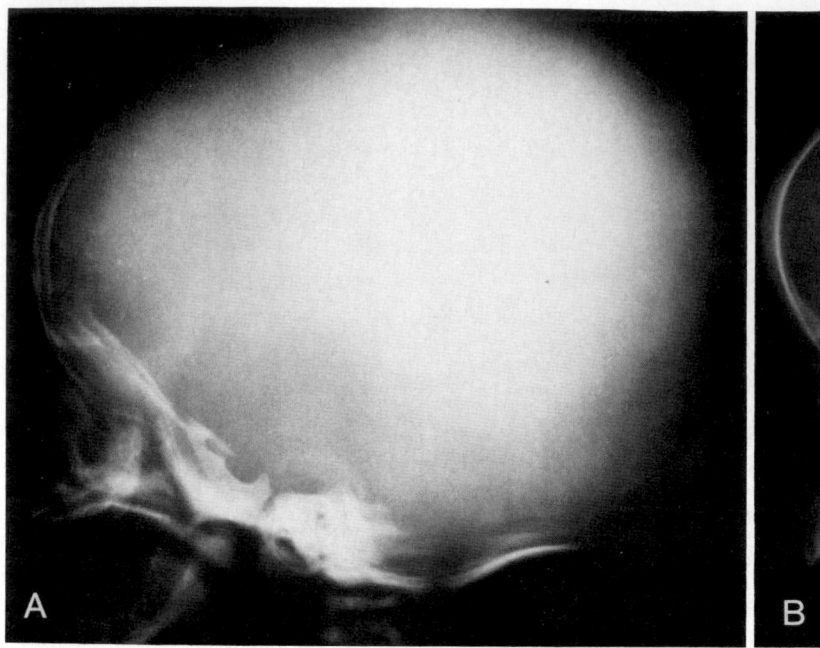
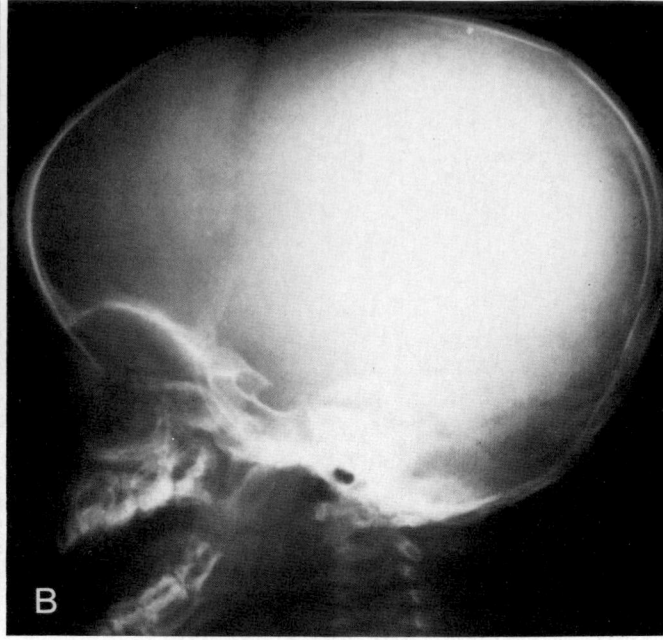

Fig. 5.1. Large head. A. Large head in hydrocephalus. In this patient the face appears small because the head is so large. B. Large head in patient with achondroplasia. There is a certain degree of maxillary hypoplasia in this condition but still the head is larger than normal. Also note the elongated sella, a common finding in achondroplasia.

the head also is seen in neurofibromatosis (5, 6, 8) but the etiology is unknown. A similar phenomenon has been documented with multiple cutaneous hemangiomas (7) and lipomas (9).

Familial macroencephaly due to megalencephaly is a relatively rare cause of calvarial enlargement. The condition is characterized by a large brain and mental retardation (3), but a benign form, without retardation recently also has been documented (2). Calvarial enlargement due to enlargement of the brain also occurs with the storage diseases (i.e., the mucopolysaccharidoses, mucolipidoses, and generalized gangliosidosis). Finally it should be noted that the head also can enlarge anytime the calvarial bones become excessively thickened (see later section on this subject).

References

1. Asch AJ, Myers GJ: Benign familial macrocephaly; report of a family and review of the literature. *Pediatrics* 57:535–539, 1976.
2. Day RE, Schutt WH: Normal children with large heads—benign familial megalencephaly. *Arch Dis Child* 54:512–517, 1979.
3. DeMeyer W: Megalencephaly in children. *Neurology* 22:634–643, 1972.
4. Fitz CR, Harwood-Nash DC, Boldt DW: The radiographic features of unilateral megalencephaly. *Neuroradiology* 15:145–148, 1978.
5. Holt JF, Kuhns LR: Macroencephaly in neurofibromatosis. *Ann Radiol* 18:458, 1975.
6. Holt JF, Kuhns LR: Macrocranium and macrocephaly in neurofibromatosis. *Skeletal Radiol* 1:25–28, 1976.
7. Stephan MJ, Hall BD, Smith DW, Cohen MM Jr: Macrocephaly in association with unusual cutaneous angiomatosis. *J Pediatr* 87:353–359, 1975.
8. Weichert KA, Dine MS, Benton C, Silverman FN: Macrocranium and neurofibromtosis. *Radiology* 107:163–166, 1973.
9. Zonana J, Rimoin DL: Macrocephaly with multiple lipomas and hemangiomas. *Pediatrics* 89:600–603, 1976.

Small Head (Table 5.1)

Roentgenographic assessment of the small head initially is made from the lateral skull film. However, when doing so, one should exercise some caution because, in some cases while the head appears small on lateral view (short from front to back), on frontal view it is compensatorily wide. In some cases this is due simply to postural change (i.e., prolonged lying on one's back) and actual head circumference may be normal. On the other hand, when a head is small in both parameters the most common cause is brain atrophy (Fig. 5.2A). In such cases, calvarial smallness is associated with progressive narrowing of the sutures, thickening of the calvarium and, in more advanced cases, overgrowth of the air-filled paranasal sinuses and mastoid air cells (see Fig. 5.5D). In addition, one usually sees loss of normal inner table convolutions and, in advanced cases, a small sella. All of these changes are due to decreased intracranial pressure and are distinctly different from those seen when the head is small because of primary, universal craniosynostosis. In these cases, since all the sutures fuse prematurely, the head becomes round and small,

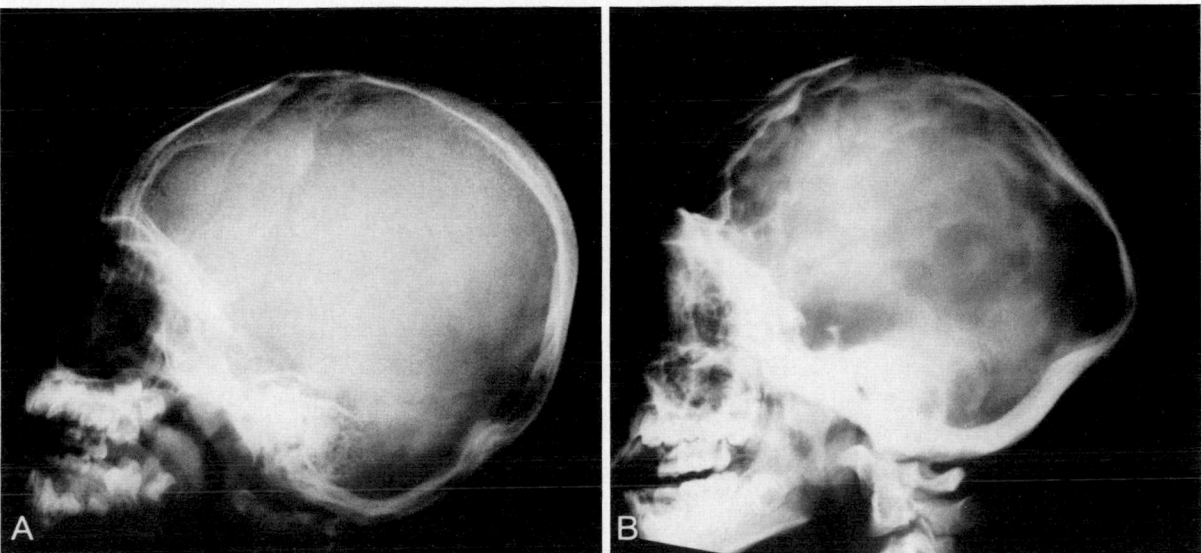

Fig. 5.2. Small head. A. Note that the head is small in proportion to the face. Also note absence of convolutional markings and rather poorly defined cranial sutures. In addition the calvarium is slightly thickened. These findings are consistent with decreased intracranial pressure and this patient had brain atrophy. B. Small head in universal craniosynostosis. Note how pronounced the inner table convolutions appear (increased intracranial pressure), and also note enlargement of the sella. All of the sutures are obliterated because they closed prematurely.

but at the same time intracranial pressure increases. Indeed, virtually every finding (except for spreading of the sutures) of chronically increased intracranial pressure is present; i.e., markedly increased innner

table convolutions, demineralization of the dorsum of the sella and posterior clinoids, and even enlargement of the sella (Fig. 5.2B).

ABNORMAL CALVARIAL CONFIGURATIONS

Generally, abnormal calvarial configurations consist of the following: (*a*) deformity associated with primary craniosynostosis; (*b*) postural flattening; (*c*) unilateral smallness; (*d*) frontal bossing; (*e*) biparietal bossing; and (*f*) localized bulging.

Deformity with Craniosynostosis

To undertake a lengthy discussion on primary craniosynostosis would be beyond the scope of this book, but it might at least be noted that, for each suture synostosed, a specific calvarial deformity results (2, 5, 6). These are summarized in Table 5.2, but in addition it might be noted more than one suture can be involved in some patients. In such cases, calvarial configurations can be most bizarre and, in this regard, one of the most bizarre is the so-called clover leaf or Kleeblattschädell skull (1, 3, 4, 7). In this condition the skull bulges, in clover leaf fashion, over the bregma and both parietal regions (see Fig. 5.7). The deformity can occur in isolated form or in association with other anomalies, and has been recorded with thanatophoric dwarfism (4).

Roentgenographically, when a suture closes prematurely, one usually sees one or more of the following: (*a*) the specific calvarial deformity for the suture; (*b*) narrower than normal sutures with unusually sharp edges; (*c*) sclerosis along the suture edges; (*d*) actual bony fusion (usually incomplete bridging) of

Table 5.2 Calvarial Configurations in Primary Craniosynostosis

Suture	Calvarial Configuration	Descriptive Terms
Sagittal	Long, narrow head	Scaphycephaly or dolichocephaly
Bilateral coronal	Short, wide head, hypertelorism, proptosis, small anterior fossa	Brachycephaly or bradycephaly
Metopic	Frontal wedging or keel-shaped head	Trigonocephaly
Bilateral lambdoid	Shallow posterior fossa; prominent bregma	Turricephaly
Unilateral coronal	Unilateral, frontal flattening, uptilting of orbit and tilting of nasal septum	Plagiocephaly
Unilateral lambdoid	Unilateral posterior flattening	Plagiocephaly
All sutures	Small, round head	Microcephaly

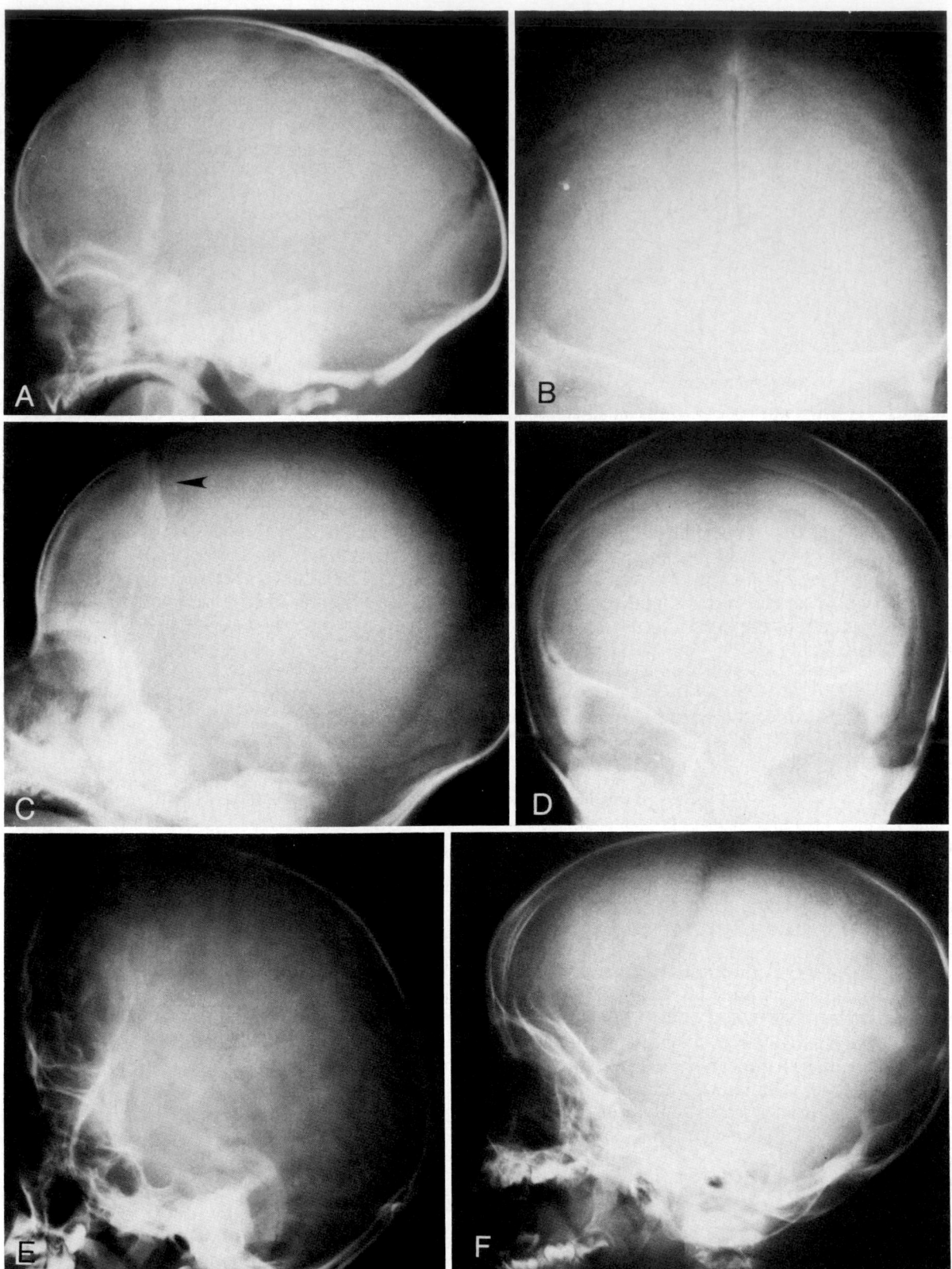

Figure. 5.3.   Calvarial deformity; craniosynostosis. A. Typical elongated head in saggital synostosis. Also note thickening of the upper aspect of the parietal bone. B. Frontal view showing very sharp, straight saggital suture, partially bridged. C. Unusually sharp-edged, partially obliterated coronal sutures in bilateral coronal synostosis (arrows). D. Frontal view showing biparietal widening and upward slanting of the sphlenoid bones and orbits to give the characteristic harlequin appearance of bilateral coronal synostosis. In unilateral synostosis, similar changes are seen on one side only. E. Longstanding coronal synostosis in Crouzon's syndrome. Note marked brachycephaly, pronounced flattening of the front of the head and increased convolutional markings over the frontal region. F. Note flattening of the inferior, occipital region, characteristic of lambdoid synostosis.

the suture; (*e*) bony ridging along the suture; and (*f*) locally increased convolutional markings (Fig. 5.3). The latter finding is variable and due to pressure from the locally crowded brain. In isolated, sagittal synostosis, because such confinement of the brain is minimal, convolutional markings usually are normal. They are more prominent with coronal and lambdoid synostosis (especially if unilateral) and with multiple suture involvement (Fig. 5.3E). When all sutures are involved, microcephaly also is present, and this leads to severe confinement of the brain. Indeed, inner table convolutions usually are markedly increased and intracranial pressures elevated.

References

1. Angle CR, McIntire MS, Moore RC: Cloverleaf skull; kleeblattschädell-deformity syndrome. *Am J Dis Child* 114:198–202, 1967.
2. Ebel KD: Craniostenosis-roentgenological and craniometric features. *Pediatr Radiol* 2:1–14, 1974.
3. Feingold M, O'Connor JF, Berkman M, Darling DB: Kleebattschädell syndrome. *Am J Dis Child* 118:589–594, 1969.
4. Iannaccone G, and Gerlini G: The so-called "Cloverleaf skull syndrome." A report of 3 cases with a discussion of its relationships with thanatophoric dwarfism and the craniostenoses. *Pediatr Radiol* 2:175–184, 1974.
5. Nathan MH, Collins VP, Collins LC: Premature unilateral synostosis of the coronal suture. *Am J Roentgenol* 85:433–446, 1961.
6. Swischuk LE: *Radiology of the Newborn and Young Infant*, ed 2. Baltimore, Williams & Wilkins, 1980, pp 736–755.
7. Wollin DG, Binnington VI, Partington MW: Cloverleaf skull. *J Can Assoc Radiol* 19:148–154, 1968.

Postural Flattening

Basically, there are two types of postural flattening and both occur over the occiput; i.e., (*a*) asymmetric flattening and (*b*) symmetric flattening. The first is more common and results from the infant lying on its back and keeping its head rotated to one side. This occurs in neurologically compromised infants but also in some perfectly normal infants who just seem to prefer lying that way. Flattening of the entire occiput usually is seen in retarded children who constantly lie on their backs (Fig. 5.4). Although the finding occasionally can be seen in some normal infants (inherited calvarial shape) and some who are not retarded (i.e., perhaps just chronically immobilized), most often it is seen in the retarded child.

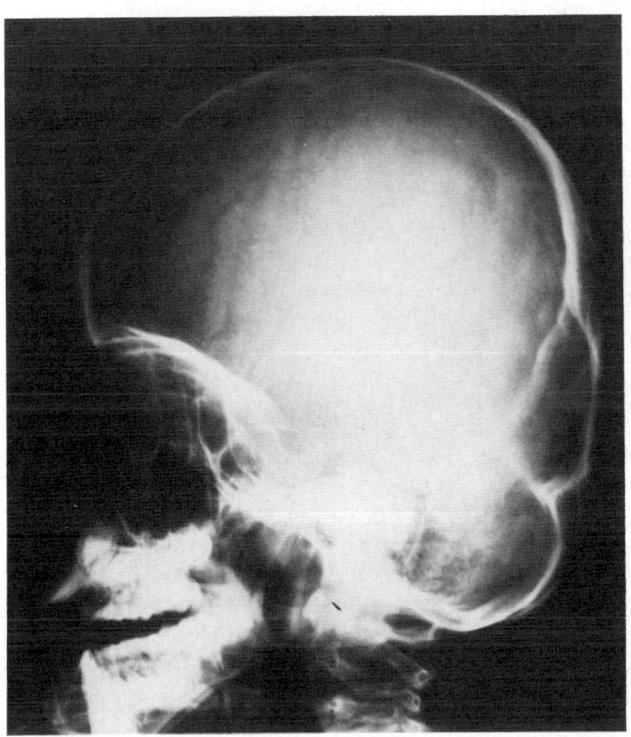

Fig. 5.4. Postural flattening. Characteristic flattening of the occiput in retarded child, chronically lying on its back.

Unilateral Small Head

To a minor degree, unilateral calvarial smallness is present in many, if not most, normal individuals. This type of asymmetry continues into the face, but to the casual observer usually goes unnoticed. When more severe, it becomes more apparent clinically and roentgenographically, and then must be differentiated from unilateral smallness due to underlying brain atrophy. In these cases, the brain is atrophic on one side, and

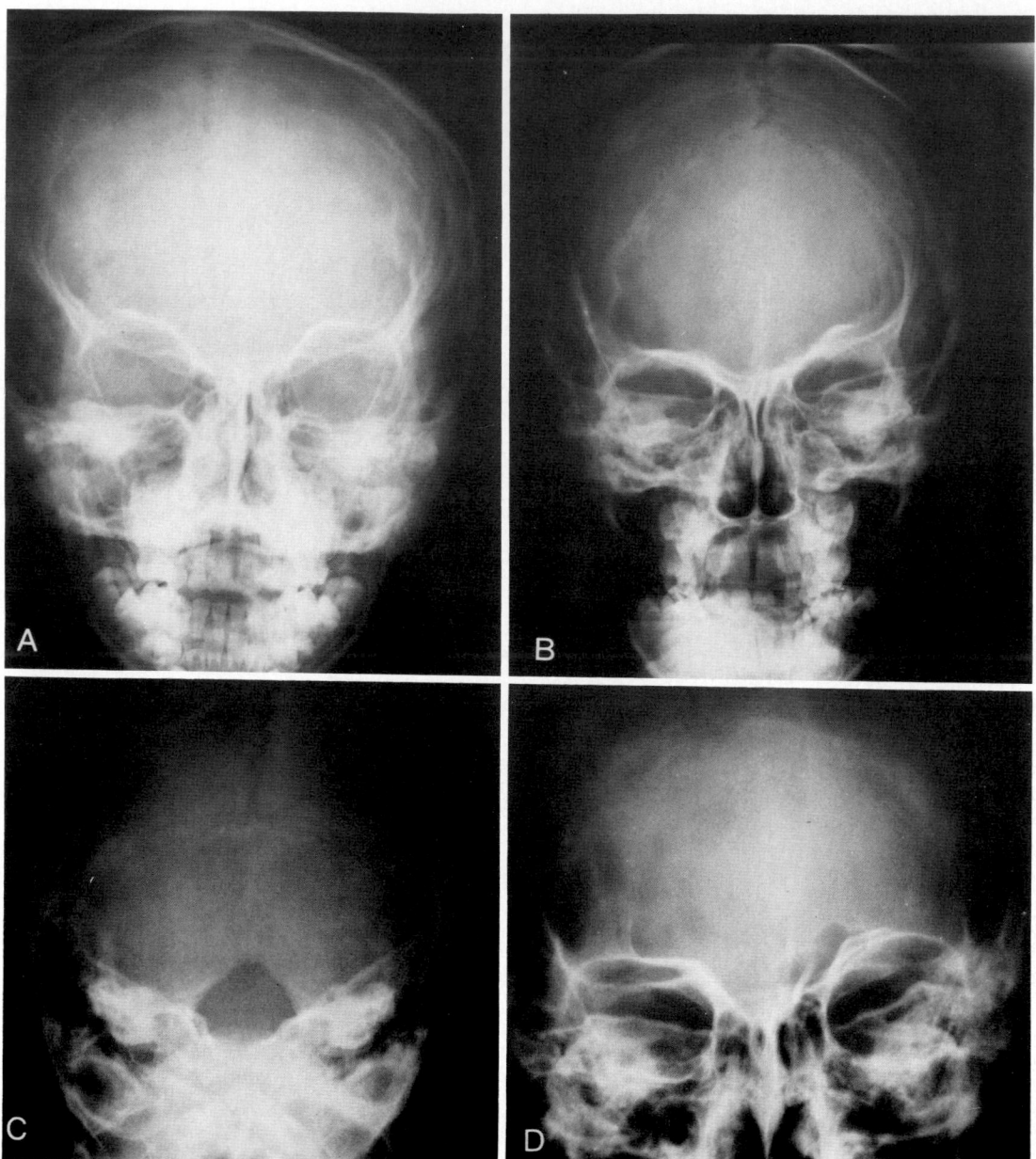

Fig. 5.5. Unilateral calvarial smallness; atrophy. A. Note flattening the left. B. Another patient demonstrating elevation of the sphenoid wing on the left. C. Same patient demonstrating slight elevation of the left petrous bone due to unilateral atrophy. D. Unequal orbits and early sinus development on the left, due to atrophy. Note high position and roundness of orbital roof on left.

in addition to the calvarium being smaller on that side, the ipsilateral bones often are thickened, and the petrous pyramid and sphenoid wing elevated (Fig. 5.5). There also may be associated upward slanting of the orbit and secondary enlargement of the paranasal sinuses and mastoid air cells on the involved side. The entire complex of findings is known as the Dyke, Davidoff-Masson syndrome (1), and underlying brain atrophy is clearly demonstrable with CT scanning.

Unilateral smallness of the calvarium also occurs with unilateral lambdoid or coronal synostosis (see previous section), and in the Silver dwarfing syndrome. In this latter condition, also known as congenital hemiatrophy, the more profound changes occur in the lower extremities. However, the upper extremities also may be small and, in some cases, the ipsilateral side of the skull also is small. Other features of the syndrome include gonadal abnormalities and inguinal hernias (2–4). When the head is enlarged in these patients, but one side still smaller than the other, the condition is referred to as the Russell-Silver syndrome. Both conditions are interrelated and probably one and the same.

References

1. Dyke CG, Davidoff LM, Masson CG: Cerebral hemiatrophy with homolateral hypertrophy of the skull and sinuses. *Surg Gynecol Obstet* 57:588–600, 1933.
2. Marks LJ, Bergeson PS: The Silver-Russell syndrome. *Am J Dis Child* 131:447–451, 1977.
3. Moseley JE, Moloshok RE, Freiberger RH: The Silver syndrome; congenital asymmetry, short stature, and variations in sexual development. *Am J Roentgenol* 97:74–81, 1966.
4. Silver HK: Asymmetry, short stature and variations in sexual development. A syndrome of congenital malformations. *Am J Dis Child* 107:495–515, 1964.

Frontal Bossing

Frontal bossing is a common finding in children and seldom is normal. Most often it occurs with the chondrodystrophic dwarfs (achondroplasia, achondrogenesis, thanatophoric dwarfism, metatrophic dwarfism, diastrophic dwarfism, etc.) and hydrocephalus (Fig. 5.6). However, it also is seen with cleidocranial dysostosis, pyknodysostosis, megalencephaly, the storage diseases, chronic subdural hematoma (biparietal widening is more common), and with thickening of the frontal bone as seen with the chronic anemias, healing rickets, hypophosphatasia, etc. (see section on thickening of the calvarium).

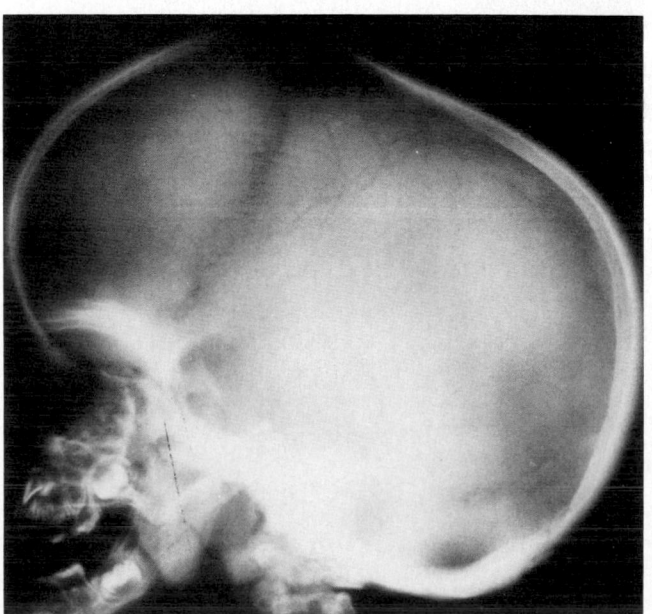

Fig. 5.6. Frontal bossing. Characteristic frontal bossing in achondroplasia. This patient also had large ventricles.

Biparietal Bossing

Biparietal bossing is not as common as frontal bossing and, as far as syndromes are concerned, the one best known to produce such bossing is bilateral coronal synostosis, isolated, or associated with Crouzon's disease (see Fig. 5.3D). Gross, biparietal (actually bitemporal) bossing is seen in the rare cranio-synostosis syndrome known as cloverleaf skull or Kleeblattschädel (Fig. 5.7, A and B). Rather prominent biparietal bossing also is seen in cleidocranial dysostosis (Fig. 5.7C), pyknodysostosis, and chronic bilateral subdural hematoma (Fig. 5.7D).

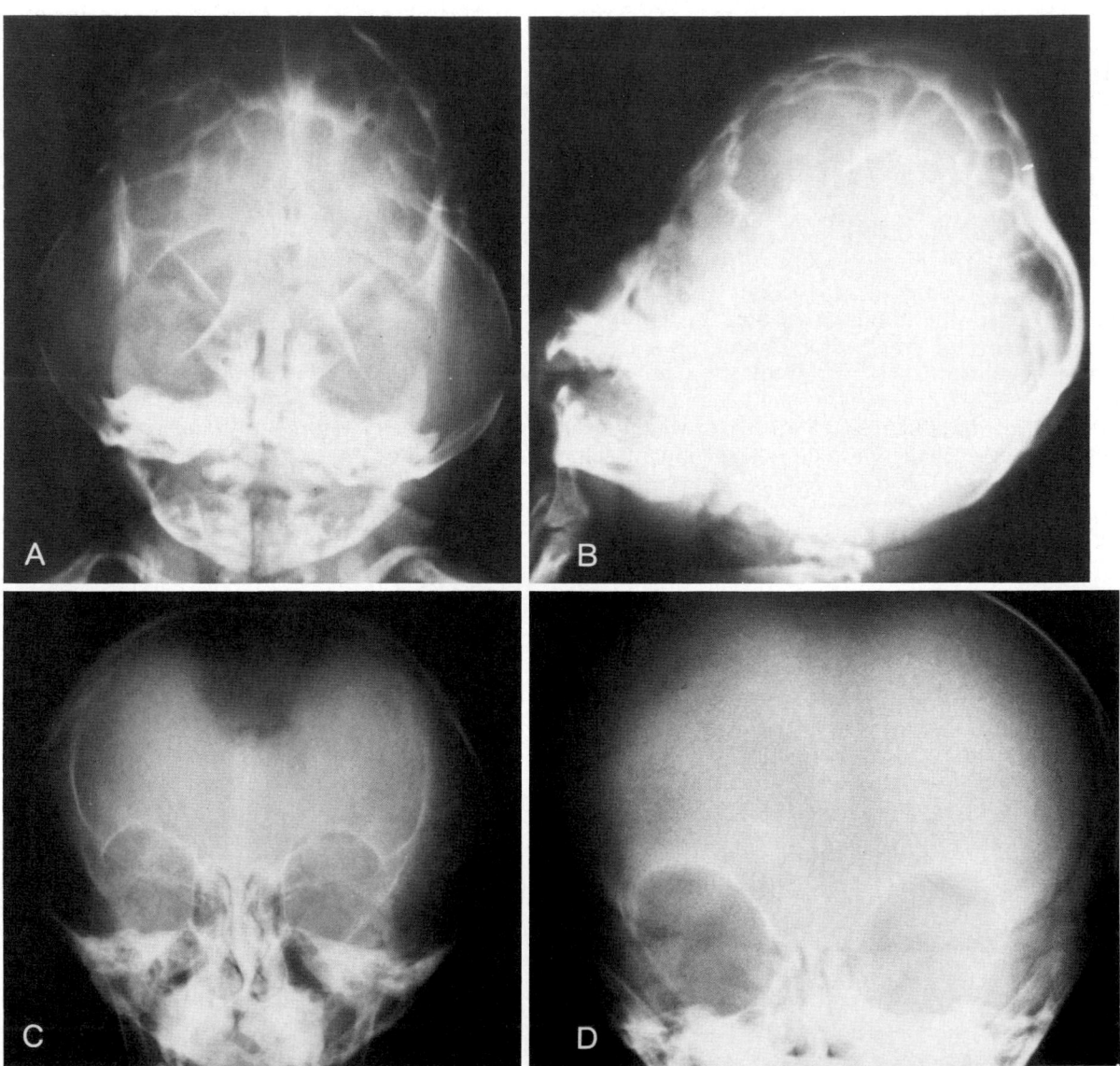

Fig. 5.7. Biparietal bossing. A. Pronounced biparietal (actually bitemporal) bulging in cloverleaf skull. B. Lateral view to show bulging of the upper portion of the calvarium, the third component of the cloverleaf. Also, note prominent convolutions characteristic of this craniosynostosis syndrome. C. Biparietal prominence in cleidocranial dysostosis. D. Biparietal prominence in chronic bilateral subdural hematoma.

Localized Bulges

These can result from lesions causing pressure erosion of the calvarium from within, lesions of the calvarium itself, or scalp abnormalities. Those conditions involving the scalp include a variety of tumors and cysts, and localized subgaleal bleeds. Most often the findings are self-evident, and underlying calvarial abnormality may or may not be present. This depends on whether the overlying lesion is causing any destruction or erosion of the bone. As far as calvarial lesions are concerned, the most common problem is a cephalohematoma. When healed, the degree of bulging is minimal and, roentgenographically, one sees localized thickening and sclerosis of the calvarium only (see Fig. 5.10A). In early infancy, before the cephalohematoma has fully healed, the bulge may be more profound and clinically misinterpreted for a depressed skull fracture. The reason for this is that the edge of the calcifying cephalohematoma feels much like the edge of a depressed fracture (Fig. 5.8A).

Other causes of localized calvarial bulging include intradiploic dermoid cysts, histiocytosis X, fibrous dysplasia, chronic anemias, metastatic lesions (Fig. 5.8C), and rarely, primary calvarial bone tumors. In chronic anemia, the entire calvarium is thickened in many cases, but in others only a small part is affected, and then a localized calvarial bulge results. This is most likely to occur with iron deficiency and sickle cell anemia.

Intracranial lesions producing localized bulging of the skull also usually produce inner table thinning. The problem must be long standing and conditions leading to the finding include porencephalic cysts (Fig. 5.8B), arachnoid cysts, large intracranial tumors and, occasionally, unilateral subdural hematomas. With the latter condition, bulging usually is subtle and, as far as tumors are concerned, they usually are large and occur in infancy.

A leptomeningeal cyst, although not causing actual bulging of the calvarium, does cause a scalp bulge. In such cases, a skull fracture leads to tearing of the dura, and through this tear, the arachnoid membrane herniates. Slowly, as the herniation pulsates, there is erosion of the calvarium along the fracture site. Eventually, an elongated or rounded area of bone destruction results. It has a discreet but not overly sclerotic edge (see Fig. 5.29D) and a fluctuant overlying mass. Often there is some degree of adjacent focal brain atrophy in these patients, a finding readily demonstrable with CT scanning.

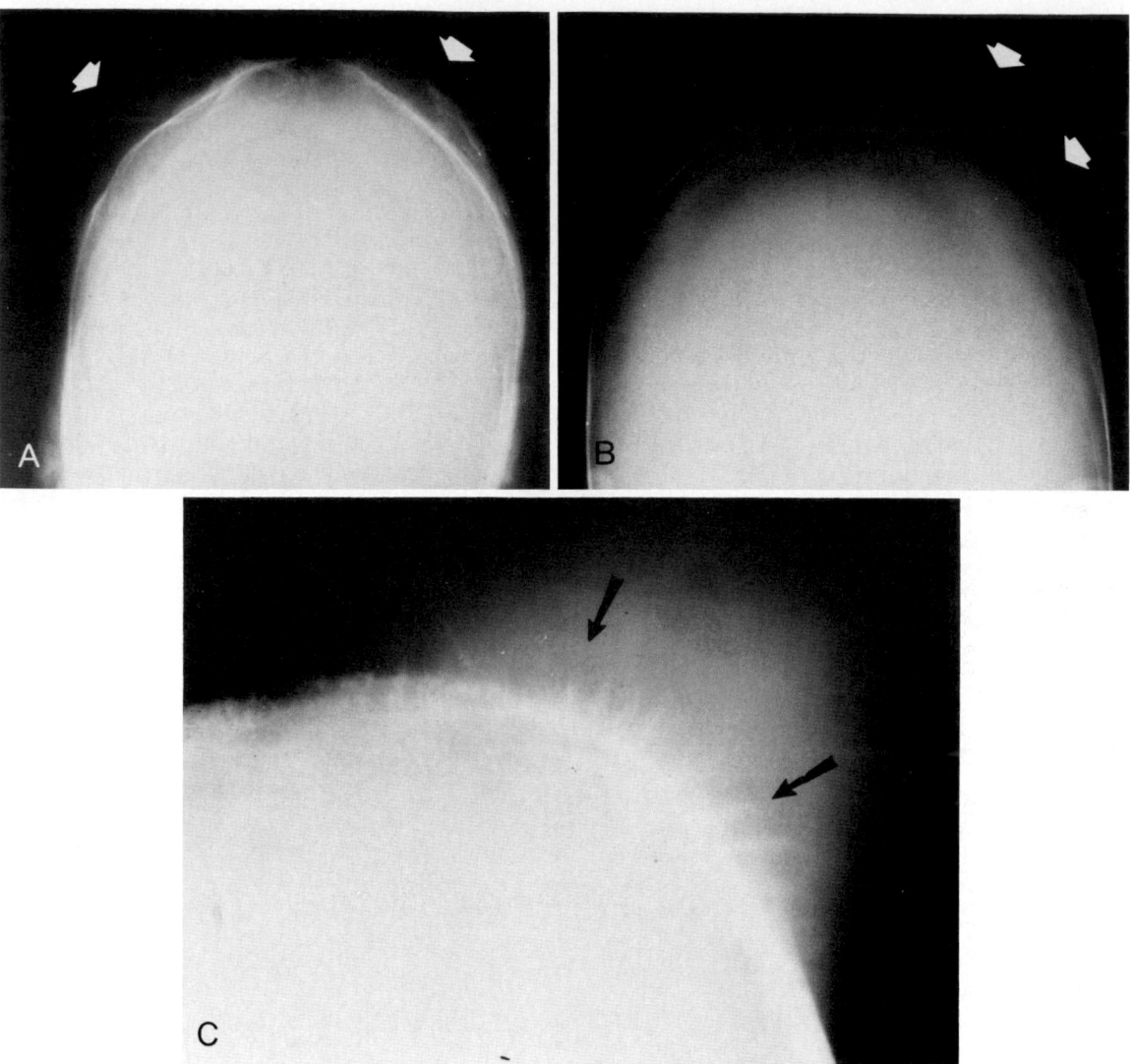

Fig. 5.8. Localized bulges. A. Note bilateral, calcifying cephalohematomas (arrows). The rim of the one on the right is incompletely calcified and clinically can be misinterpreted for a depressed skull fracture. B. Localized bulging of the calvarium (arrows), due to large congenital porencephalic cyst. C. Localized bulging with spiculation of bone due to metastatic neuroblastoma (arrows).

THICKENING OF THE CALVARIUM

Thickening of the calvarium can be generalized, confined to the base, or focal in the vault. Furthermore, in some cases it can be associated with homogeneous sclerosis, while in others, sclerosis is spotty. In still others vertical striations of the diploë exist. Conditions producing these combinations of changes are listed in Tables 5.3 and 5.4.

Table 5.3 Generalized Calvarial Thickening (with or without Sclerosis)

A. Homogeneous sclerosis

Normal
Decreased intracranial pressure
    Brain atrophy
    Posthydrocephalus shunting
	Commonest

Dilantin therapy Hypervitaminosis D Hypoparathyroidism Pseudohypoparathyroidism Idiopathic hypercalcemia Storage diseases Osteopetrosis Healing rickets (with bossing)	Relatively uncommon
Acrodysostosis Cockayne's syndrome Craniometaphyseal dysplasia (Pyle's disease) Jansen's metaphyseal dysostosis Lawrence-Seip syndrome Osteopathia striata Otopalatodigital syndrome Pyknodysostosis Van Buchem's osteosclerosis Fluorosis Melorheostosis Kenny-Caffey syndrome (tubular synosis) Myelosclerosis Myotonic dystrophy	Rare

B. Nonhomogeneous sclerosis, or no sclerosis

Chronic anemia[a] Thalassemia, sickle cell, iron deficiency anemia, hereditary spherocytosis	Commonest
Hyperparathyroidism Active and healing rickets	Moderately common
Dilantin therapy Polycythemia Metastatic disease[b]	Relatively uncommon
Hyperphosphatasia Hypophosphatasia Leukemia—lymphoma[b]	Rare

[a] Often show vertical striations.
[b] May show vertical striations.

Table 5.4 Localized Thickening of the Calvarium

Localized thickening of the calvarium
    Cephalohematoma; healed[a]
    Trauma[a]
	Commonest

Fibrous dysplasia[b] Anemia[c] Chronic infection[a] Cerebral hemiatrophy[a]	Moderately common
Meningioma[b,c] Hemangioma[a,b,c] Other primary bone tumors[b]	Rare
Base of the skull thickening Bony dysplasias	Commonest
Fibrous dysplasia[b]	Moderately common
Meningioma[b] Chordoma of clivus Chronic infection of nasopharynx[a]	Rare
Other tumors of clivus	Very rare

[a] Sclerotic.
[b] Sclerotic or lytic.
[c] Vertical striations.

Generalized Thickening

The commonest cause of generalized calvarial thickening, **associated with homogeneous, increased density** of bone, is normal variation. Thereafter, one should consider one of a number of sclerosing bony dysplasias (Fig. 5.9A), or long-standing decreased intracranial pressure (1, 6, 13). The latter occurs with cerebral atrophy and after successful shunting for hydrocephalus. In either case, it is the prolonged decrease in intracranial pressure which leads to inward growth of the calvarium and thickening of the bones (Fig. 5.9B). In atrophy, the phenomenon also is referred to as hyperostosis cranii ex vacuo. Generalized thickening, with increased density of the calvarium also is seen in healing renal osteodystrophy, especially in patients on dialysis.

Generalized calvarial thickening, with **nonhomogeneous sclerosis or no sclerosis** at all, is seen in a number of metabolic and hematologic conditions (Table 5.3). In the hematologic conditions, in addition to thickening, the diploë of the calvarial bones also shows vertical striation (Fig. 5.9C). As far as this phenomenon is concerned, most commonly it is seen with chronic anemias such as sickle cell disease, iron deficiency anemia, thalassemia, congenital spherocytosis, and polycythemia (2, 5, 11, 12, 17). The changes often are more focal with iron deficiency and sickle cell anemia than with the other anemias. Occasionally

similar, focal findings are seen with leukemia, lymphoma, or metastatic disease, and almost always, the latter is metastatic neuroblastoma. In some cases of metastatic neuroblastoma, in addition to the vertical striations in the calvarium, spiculated periosteal new bone is seen, and the sutures usually are spread. The latter results from the fact that, in addition to the bony metastases, meningeal implants are present and cause increased intracranial pressure. In all of these hypertrophied marrow, or infiltrative problems, the vertical, diploic striations result from pressure atrophy of smaller trabeculi. A similar phenomenon, but with concentric lamellations, recently has been described with sickle cell disease (19), and we have seen it with neuroblastoma metastases (see Fig. 5.10D).

When metabolic disease produces thickening of the calvarium, no striations are seen, but the bones may show patchy sclerosis. For the most part, the following conditions should be considered: hyperparathyroidism (18), hyperphosphatemia, hypophosphatasia, and healing rickets. In hyperparathyroidism the skull may appear very mottled, the so-called salt and pepper skull (Fig. 5.9D), and with hyperphosphatemia, the thick skull may be lamellated. Generalized irregular thickening of the calvarium can be seen in fibrous dysplasia (Fig. 5.9E), and the findings also can be focal (see Fig. 5.11D).

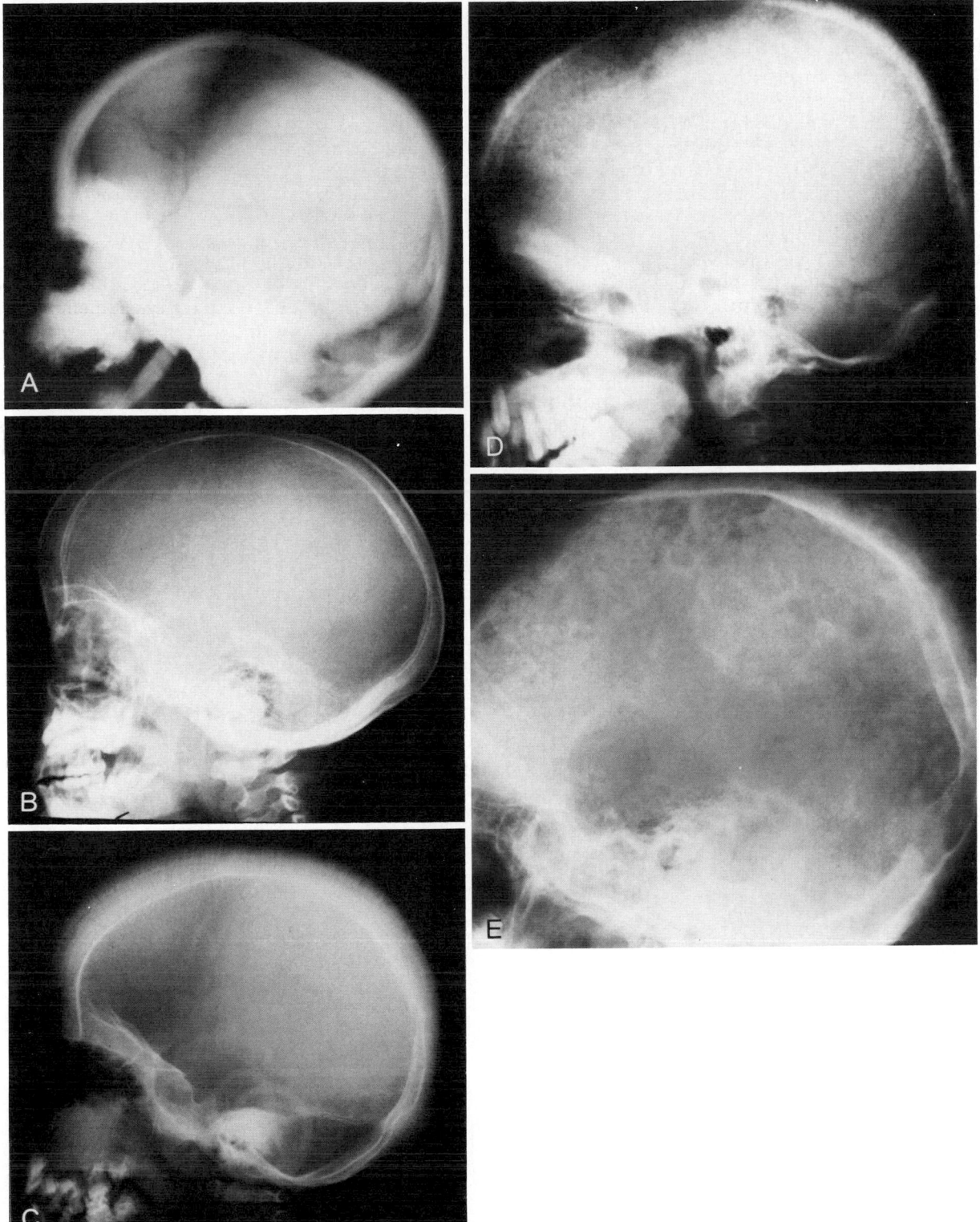

Fig. 5.9. Generalized calvarial thickening. A. Typical thickening of the calvarium with increased sclerosis in osteopetrosis. B. Thickening of the calvarium secondary to decreased intracranial pressure in brain atrophy. C. Thickening due to Cooley's anemia. Note vertical striations. D. Thickened, salt and pepper skull in hyperparathyroidism (secondary hyperparathyroidism in renal osteodystrophy). E. Fibrous dysplasia with generalized, irregular thickening of the calvarium. Note predominant lucency, but some alternating areas of sclerosis.

Localized Thickening of the Skull

Thickening of the skull on a localized basis, much as with generalized thickening, may or may not be associated with sclerosis. When **sclerosis is present,** however, the most common problem is a healing cephalohematoma (Fig. 5.10A). Most often this is a problem in the postnatal period but it also can be seen in older infants. A peculiar such circumstance occurs in the frontal bone in chronic head-bangers (20) and we have seen a similar problem in a young child who was battered in the form of repeated insults to the temples. Localized sclerosis with thickening also can occur with chronic osteomyelitis, adjacent cellulitis, healing histiocytosis X, tuberous sclerosis (Fig. 5.10B), the chronic anemias (especially sickle cell disease and iron deficiency anemia), leukemia, and metastatic neuroblastoma. The latter three also usually show vertical striations (Fig. 5.10C), but also can show concentric lamellations (Fig. 5.10D).

Very large areas of increased sclerosis and thickening of the calvarium almost always are due to the hyperostotic form of fibrous dysplasia. Very often the base and frontal regions of the skull are involved (see Fig. 5.11, D and E). Focal thickening, with sclerosis of the skull due to other bone tumors, is rather uncommon but can be seen with some hemangiomas (Fig. 5.10E), osteomas and, rarely, with osteogenic sarcoma.

Localized thickening **without sclerosis** is not particularly common and most often is seen with fibrous dysplasia. It also can be seen with the rare meningioma occurring in childhood (Fig. 5.10F). Thickening and sclerosis of most or all of one side of the calvarium in association with ipsilateral smallness of the calvarium, reflects underlying cerebral atrophy or the so-called Dyke, Davidoff Masson syndrome.

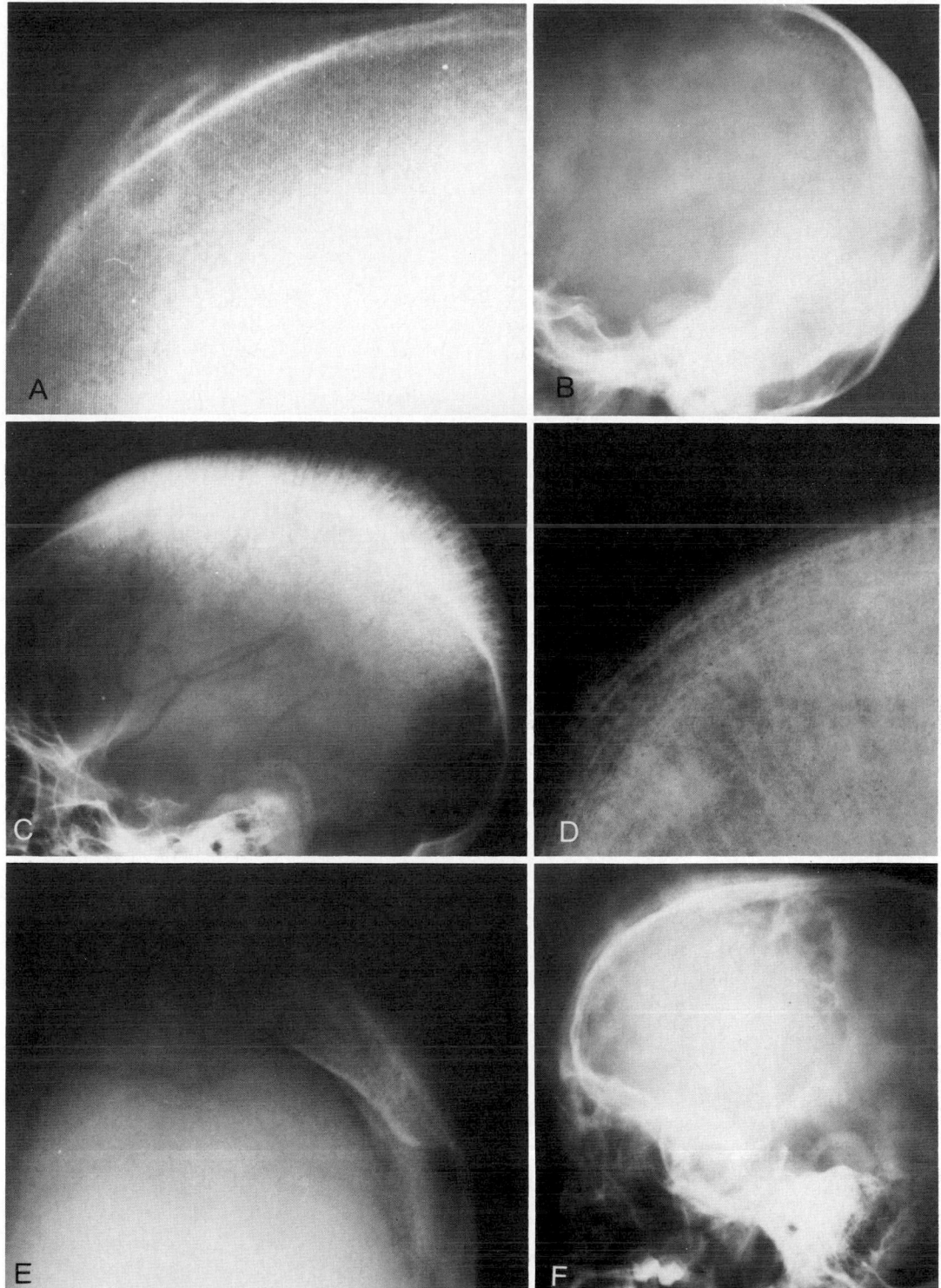

Fig. 5.10. Localized thickening of the calvarium. A. thickening of the calvarium due to partially healed cephalohematoma. B. Occipital thickening in tuberous sclerosis. C. Localized thickening, with vertical striations in sickle cell disease. D. Localized thickening with concentric lamellations in metastatic neuroblastoma. E. Localized thickening with some honeycombing and striations in osseous hemangioma. F. Frontal thickening, with lysis, in menigioma.

Thickening of the Base of the Skull

Predominant thickening of the skull base occurs with bony dysplasias such as osteopetrosis (Fig. 5.11A), craniometaphyseal dysplasia (including Pyle's disease), Englemann-Camurati's diaphyseal dysplasia, Melnick-Needles osteodysplasia, Jansen's metaphyseal dysostosis (7), cleidocranial dysostosis, the otopalatodigital syndrome (Fig. 5.11B), and melorheostosis. Tumors or tumor-like conditions leading to thickening of the base of the skull include fibrous dysplasia (most common), meningioma, chordoma of the clivus (8, 10), chondrosarcoma (4), and tumors of the nasopharynx. Thickening of the base of the skull also can occur with chronic nasopharyngeal infections (14), but all of these conditions are rare in children. Chondromas can be identified by the calcification with which they are associated (Fig. 5.11C), and fibrous dysplasia can be lytic or sclerotic (Fig. 5.11, D and E). Meningioma usually is lytic.

References

1. Anderson R, Kieffer SA, Wolfson JJ, Peterson HO: Thickening of the skull in surgically treated hydrocephalus. *Am J Roentgenol* 110:96–101, 1970.
2. Burko H, Mellins HZ, Watson J: Skull Changes in iron-deficiency anemia simulating congenital hemolytic anemia. *Am J Roentgenol* 86:447–452, 1961.
3. Caffey J: Cooley's erythroblastic anemia: some skeletal findings in adolescents and young adults. *Am J Roentgenol* 65:547, 1951.
4. Cook PL, Evans PG: Chondrosarcoma of the skull in Maffucci's syndrome. *Br J Radiol* 50:833–836, 1977.
5. Dykstra OH, Halbertsma T: Polycythemia vera in childhood. *Am J Dis Child* 60:907–916, 1940.
6. Griscom NT, Kook Sang, O: The contracting skull; inward growth of the inner table as a physiologic response to diminution of intracranial content in children. *Am J Roentgenol* 110:106–110, 1970.
7. Holthusen W, Holdt JF, Stoeckenius M: The skull in metaphyseal chondrodysplasia type jansen. *Pediatr Radiol* 3:137–144, 1975.
8. Kendall BE, Lee BCP: Cranial chordomas. *Br J Radiol* 50(598):687–698, 1977.
9. Lee KF, Lin SR, Hodes PH: New roentgenologic findings in myotonic dystrophy; an analysis of 18 patients. *Am J Roentgenol* 115:179–185, 1972.
10. Lim GHK: Clivus chordoma with unusual bone sclerosis and brainstem invasion. *Australas Radiol* 19:242–250, 1975.
11. Marlow A, Fairbanks VF: Polycythemia vera in an 11 year old girl. *N Engl J Med* 263:950–952, 1960.
12. Moseley JE: Skull changes in chronic iron deficiency anemia. *Am J Roentgenol* 85:649–652, 1961.
13. Moseley JE, Rabinowitz JG, Dziadiw R: Hyperostosis cranii ex vacuo. *Radiology* 87:1105–1107, 1966.
14. Nemir RL, Branom-Genieser N, Balasubramanyam P:Extensive sclerosis of the base of the skull due to primary nasal tuberculosis. *Pediatr Radiol* 8:42–44, 1979.
15. Paling MR, Hyde I, Dennis NR: Osteopathia striata with sclerosis and thickening of the skull. *Br J Radiol* 54:344–348, 1981.
16. Powell JW, Weens HS, Wenger NK: The skull roentgenogram in iron deficiency anemia and in secondary polycythemia. *Am J Roentgenol* 95:143–147, 1965.
17. Shahidi NT, Diamond LK: Skull changes in infants with chronic iron deficiency anemia. *N Engl J Med* 262:137–139, 1960.
18. Steinback HL, Young DA: The roentgen appearance of pseudohypoparathyroidism (PH) and pseudo-pseudo-hypoparathyroidism (PPH), differentiation from other syndromes associated with short metacarpals, metatarsals, and phalanges. *Am J Roentgenol* 97:49–66, 1966.
19. Williams AO, Lagundoye SB, Johnson CL: Lamellation of the diploe in the skulls of patients with sickle cell anemia. *Arch Dis Child* 50:948–952, 1975.
20. Williams JP, Fowler GW, Pribram HF, Delaney CA, Fish CH: Roentgenographic changes in headbangers. *Acta Radiol Diagn* 13:37–42, 1972.

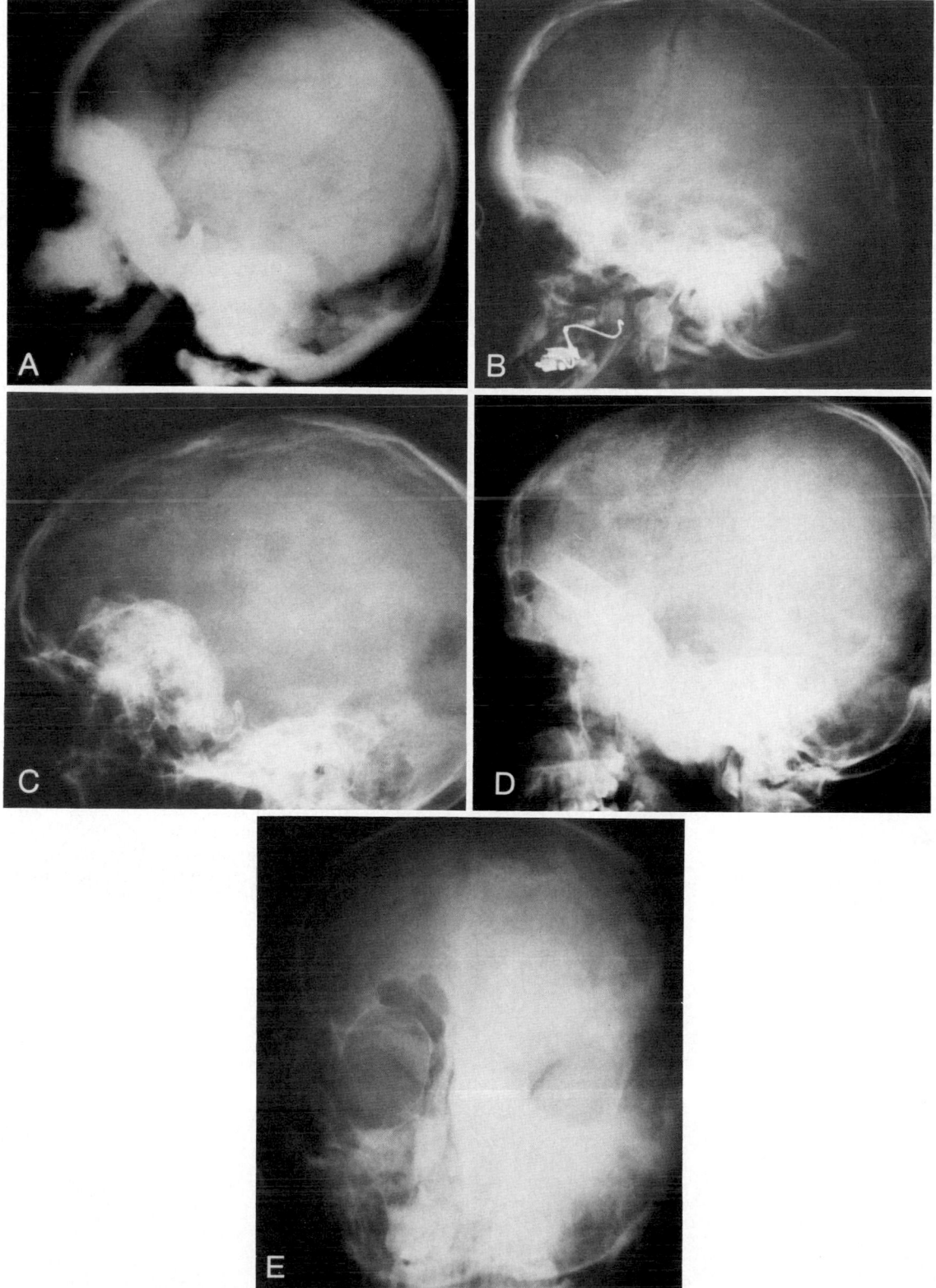

Fig. 5.11.   Thickening of the base of the skull. A. Thickening and sclerosis of the skull base in osteopetrosis. All of the other bones, including the facial bones, also are sclerotic and slightly thickened. B. Basal sclerosis and thickening in otopalatodigital syndrome. C. Thickening due to enchondroma (arrows). D. Marked sclerosis of the base of the skull in fibrous dysplasia. E. Frontal view in same patient showing marked frontal and periorbital sclerosis and thickening.

THINNING OF THE CALVARIUM

Thinning of the calvarium, just as thickening, can be generalized or localized (Table 5.5). **Localized thinning** usually is due to some slowly growing and eroding intracranial lesion; i.e., a porencephalic cyst (Fig. 5.12A), an arachnoid or leptomeningeal cyst, or a tumor. However, similar thinning can be seen with chronic subdural hematomas and unilateral hydrocephalus due to unilateral foramen of Monroe obstruction. The plain film findings in all of these conditions, of course, are nonspecific.

Aneurysmal bone cysts also can produce localized thinning of the calvarium (Fig. 5.12B), and isolated thinning of a sphenoid wing, or other parts of the calvarium, occurs with neurofibromatosis (Fig. 5.12, C and D). The latter is believed to be secondary to a nonspecific, mesenchymal defect of bone development. This type of bone abnormality is common in neurofibromatosis, and when the defect in the sphenoid bone is extensive, only a membrane remains, and pulsating exophthalmus results.

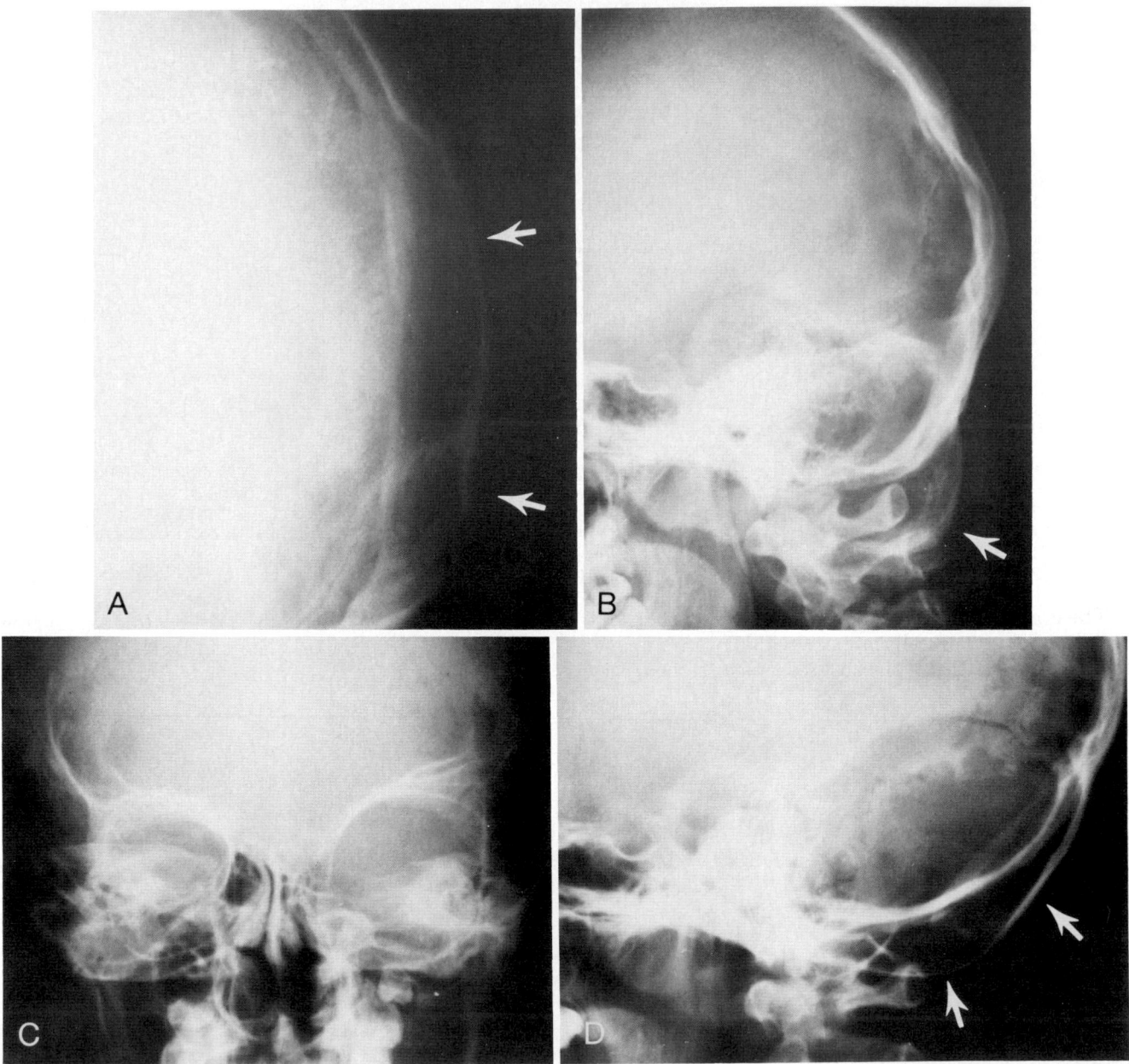

Fig. 5.12. Thinning of the calvarium; localized. A. Note localized thinning of the calvarium, due to acquired proencephalic cyst (arrows). Also note calcification, just above the area of thinning. B. Thinning due to expanding aneurysmal bone cyst (arrows). C. Absence of sphenoid wing on the left, due to thinning. Also note that the left orbit is large in this patient with neurofibromatosis. D. Occipital thinning in neurofibromatosis (arrows).

As far as **generalized thinning** of the calvarium is concerned, it almost always is part of some bone dysplasia or syndrome (Table 5.5). However, the problem also normally occurs in infancy, in the premature infant. The most common dysplasia to produce calvarial thinning is osteogenesis imperfecta, but other conditions to be considered include the aminopterin-induced syndrome, cleidocranial dysostosis in infancy, hypophosphatasia, Melnick-Needles osteodysplasia, progeria, some of the trisomies, and long standing hydrocephalus.

Table 5.5 Thinning of the Calvarium

A. Generalized	

Long standing hydrocephalus (untreated)
    Osteogenesis imperfecta
    Normal, in prematures
	Commonest

Advanced rickets
    Craniolacunia or lacunar skull
    Trisomies
	Moderately common

Cleidocranial dysostosis Hypophosphatasia	Relatively rare

Aminopterin-induced syndrome
    Melnick-Needles syndrome
    Progeria
	Rare

B. Localized	
Intracranial cysts	Commonest
Neurofibromatosis Chronic subdural hematoma	Moderately common
Localized or unilateral hydrocephalus Intracranial tumor	Relatively rare

ABNORMALITIES OF THE SUTURES

The cranial sutures are visible and open throughout childhood, but normally appear wider in infants. As far as abnormalities of the sutures are concerned, they can appear either (a) too wide or (b) too narrow. Furthermore, either problem can be seen on a generalized basis, or to involve one or two sutures only.

Sutures Too Wide (Table 5.6)

Generalized widening of the sutures may be real and due to increased intracranial pressure, or only apparent and due to underossification of the calvarial bone edges (Fig. 5.13). As far as the latter is concerned, most often one is dealing with some form of demineralizing metabolic bone disease, or a bony dysplasia where membranous bone ossification is impaired. These conditions are listed in Table 5.6. On a normal basis, delayed ossification causing unduly wide appearing sutures is common in premature infants.

On a pathologic basis, spreading of the sutures occurs from any number of causes of increased intracranial pressure; meningitis, cerebritis, abscess, intracranial hemorrhage, cerebral edema, brain tumor, hydrocephalus, hydraencephaly, megalencephaly, expanding cysts, subdural hematoma or hygroma, pseudotumor cerebri (10), lead encephalopathy, hypervitaminosis A encephalopathy (3), and other encephalopathies. In addition, we have seen actual suture spread (not just bone underossification) in active rickets, but do not know its cause. At any rate, in any of these cases, suture spread appears about the same and, when marked, is easy to assess (Fig. 5.13).

Lesser degrees of spread are more of a problem, especially in children under 2 to 3 yr where a certain degree of prominence of the coronal suture is normal (8, 9). Most likely this type of spread is physiologic and attests to the relatively rapid growth of the brain at this age. As an aid to differentiating this type of suture spread from pathologic spread, one should look at the sagittal suture. If the sagittal suture also is wide, pathologic spread usually is present, but if the sagittal suture is normal, physiologic spread is more likely. Physiologic spreading of the sagittal suture does not

Table 5.6 Wide Sutures

Normal (neonate-all)	
Normal (infant-coronal)	
Intracranial bleeding, contusion[a]	
Intracranial infection[a]	Commonest
Intracranial edema	
Hydrocephalus[a]	
Intracranial tumor[a]	
Rickets[b]	
Prematurity[b]	
Intrauterine growth failure[b]	Moderately common
Intrauterine infections[b]	
Encephalopathy[a]	
Deprivational dwarfism[a]	
Large intracranial cysts[a]	
Hypothyroidism[b]	
Cleidocranial dysostosis[b]	Relatively rare
Hyperparathyroidism[b]	
Osteogenesis imperfecta[b]	
Megalencephaly[a]	
Hydraencephaly[a]	
Aminopterin-induced syndrome[b]	
Hypophosphatemia[b]	
Pachydermoperiostosis[b]	
Progeria[b]	Rare
Pycnodysostosis[b]	
Jansen's type Metaphyseal dysostosis[b]	
Treated hypothyroidism[a]	
Pseudotumor cerebri[a]	

[a] Increased pressure.
[b] Pseudospread due to defective ossification.

occur as readily as it does with the coronal suture. Indeed, it is questionable as to whether physiologic spread of the sagittal suture ever occurs. In addition to these considerations, it should be noted that, after the age of 3 months, if the width of the coronal suture in its uppermost portion is over 3 mm, increased pressure is said to be likely (5). Evaluation of the sutures in the neonate is even more difficult, because the normal sutures can be quite wide: up to 1 cm or more. They can have this appearance for up to 1 month after birth, but usually somewhere during the first month of life the sutures become more "normal" in appearance.

Another time when generalized calvarial suture spread is seen is after head trauma. Of course, if there is significant intracranial injury (i.e., intracranial hemorrhage, subdural hematoma, etc.), a rise in intracranial pressure is not unexpected and neither is suture spread. However, spreading of the sutures also can occur in the absence of such injury and, indeed, in the absence of calvarial fracture. Furthermore, many of these children have few, if any, significant clinical symptoms. It is difficult to explain why the sutures should spread under these circumstances, especially when CT scans are normal. The phenomenon,

however, does occur and probably is related to the increase in brain mass noted after closed head injuries in children (11). This phenomenon does not occur in adults, but in infants and children has been ascribed to posttraumatic, increased blood flow, which then causes increased brain mass, and increased intracranial pressure. Consequently, one can see spreading of the sutures and yet no obvious intracranial abnormality, and in patients in whom we have observed this phenomenon, sutures return to normal after a few weeks or sooner.

Finally, it should be noted that generalized suture spread, at times rather marked, occurs in deprivational dwarfism (1, 2, 4, 6). In these children, while they are emotionally deprived, growth of the body is retarded and so is that of the brain. Actually, there is some indication that there exists a temporary impairment of growth hormone production, but whatever the cause, when these children are removed from their deprived environment, rebound growth of the body and brain occur. So exhuberant is this phenomenon that intracranial pressures rise and the sutures spread. It is important not to misinterpret this exaggerated normal phenomenon for a pathologic state. Similar rebound growth can be seen under other circumstances where body and brain growth are impaired for some time; for example, treated hypothyroidism.

Localized spread of one or more sutures almost invariably is related to calvarial trauma. In such cases, a fracture may extend directly into the suture, or the suture only, can "fracture" or "widen." The term "diastatic sutural fracture" is applied to this type of injury, and then it is important to compare the involved suture with that on the other side (Fig. 5.13D). Of course, if the suture is unpaired, interpretation is a little more difficult.

References

1. Afshani E, Osman M, Girdany BR: Widening of cranial sutures in children with deprivational dwarfism. *Radiology* 109:141–144, 1973. Year Book of Radiology, 1975, p 390.
2. Capitanio MA, Kirkpatrick JA: Widening of the cranial sutures, a roentgen observation during periods of accelerated growth in patients treated for deprivation dwarfism. *Radiology* 92:53–59, 1969.
3. Lippe B, Hensen L, Mendoza G, Finerman M, Welch M: Chronic vitamin A intoxication. *Am J Dis Child* 135:634–636, 1981.
4. Marks HG, Borns P, Steg NL, Stine SB, Stroud HH, Vates TS: Catch-up brain growth demonstration by CAT scan. *J Pediatr* 93:254–257, 1978.
5. Segall HD, Mikity VG, Rumbaugh CL, Bergeron RT, Scanlan RL, Teal JS: Cranial sutures in the first two years of life-normal measurements and the "sprung suture." *Am Soc Neuroradiol Abstr* (10th Annu Meeting Neuroradiol) 4:124–132, 1972.
6. Sondheimer FK, Grossman H, Winchester P: Suture diastasis following rapid weight gain; pseudo-pseudotumor cerebri. *Arch Neurol* 23:314–318, 1970.
7. Swischuk LE: *Emergency Radiology of the Acutely Ill or*

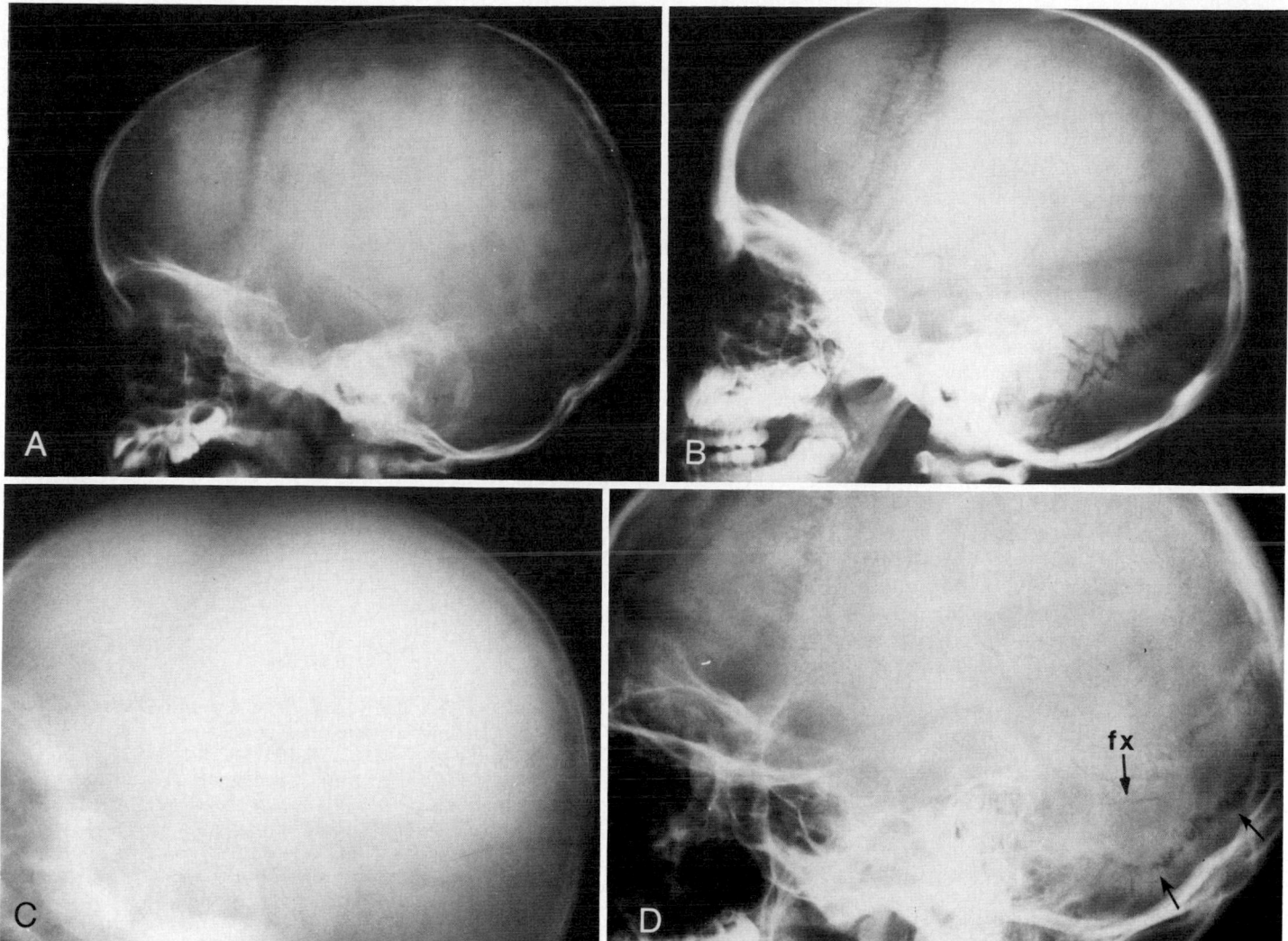

Fig. 5.13.   Sutures too wide. Note typical widening of the coronal suture due to increased intracranial pressure. Patient with neuroblastoma. B. Prominent (more radiolucent than normal) sutures in patient with hypothyroidism. C. Indistinct, apparently wide coronal suture in patient with severe vitamin D-dependent rickets. D. **Spread sutures—focal.** Note unilateral prominence of lambdoid suture (arrows). The patient had head trauma. Also note fracture (upper arrow).

Injured Child. Baltimore, Williams & Wilkins, 1979, p 391.

8. Swischuk LE: The growing skull. *Semin Roentgenol* 9:115–124, 1974.

9. Swischuk LE: The normal pediatric skull: variations and artifacts. *Radiol Clin North Am* 10:277–290, 1972.

10. Weisberg LA, Chutorian AM: Pseudotumor cerebri of childhood. *Am J Dis Child* 131:1243–1248, 1977.

11. Zimmerman RA, Bilaniuk LT, Bruce D, Dolinskas C, Orbrist W, Kuhl D: Computed tomography of pediatric head trauma: acute general cerebral swelling. *Radiology* 126:403–408, 1978.

Narrowed or Obliterated Sutures

Sutures can become narrowed, or frankly obliterated, on a primary or secondary basis, but the latter probably is more common (Table 5.7). Primary obliteration or synostosis has been dealt with earlier (see Table 5.2), and is common. Its etiology is unknown, but the general feeling is that it is related to an abnormality of dural development in the fetus. Any of the sutures in almost any combination can be involved and, radiographically, in addition to calvarial deformity, one can see (a) narrower and sharper than normal sutures, (b) variable sclerosis along the suture edges and, in some cases (c) actual bony bridging (see Fig. 5.3). Primary craniosynostosis usually is seen in isolated form (10) but it also can be seen with certain syndromes. For example, the coronal and sagittal sutures frequently are involved in Crouzon's craniosynostosis and in the acrocephalosyndactyly syndromes (Apert's, Pfieffer's Carpenter's, etc.). Presumed primary, but perhaps secondary, synostosis also is seen in Jansen's metaphyseal dysostosis, the Rubinstein-Taybi syndrome, punctate epiphyseal dysplasia, the aminopterin-induced syndrome, and the idiopathic hypercalcemia or Williams' syndrome.

When suture synostosis occurs on a secondary basis, the problem is (a) decreased intracranial pressure or (b) some bony hypermebabolic state (2). Decreased intracranial pressure can occur with brain atrophy or after shunting for successfully treated hydrocephalus (1, 3, 4, 6, 8). In either case, because intracranial pressure is decreased on a prolonged basis, the calvarial bones, rather than being kept apart, are allowed to approach each other and narrow the sutures. Even-

tually, they fuse and become obliterated. In addition, in these cases, the calvarium becomes thickened, the sella becomes small, and the paranasal sinuses and mastoid air cells may show compensatory overgrowth. The findings are quite different from primary synostosis (compare Fig. 5.14, A and B).

Hypermetabolic conditions leading to premature synostosis of the calvarium include hyperthyroidism (5, 7, 9), healing rickets, hypophosphatasia (in active or healing stage), and hypervitaminosis D. Premature closure of the sutures also occurs in the various storage diseases and chronic anemias (Fig. 5.14C). It is not known why the phenomenon occurs in storage diseases, but it may be that there also is some degree of hypermetabolism present. Decreased intracranial pressure seems unlikely because most of these patients demonstrate megalencephaly rather than small atrophic brains. In the chronic anemias, local hypermetabolism, secondary to bone marrow overgrowth, probably is the cause of premature suture closure (see Fig. 5.14C).

Table 5.7 Narrowed or Obliterated Sutures

Primary synostosis (Table 5.2) Decreased intracranial pressure[a] Atrophy Shunted hydrocephalus	Common
Healing rickets[a]	Moderately common
Storage diseases[a] Chronic anemias[a] Hyperthyroidism[a] Crouzon's disease Acrocephalosyndactyly syndromes	Relatively rare
Hypervitaminosis D[a] Hyperparathyroidism[a] Hypophosphatasia[a] Idiopathic hypercalcemia[a] Jansen's metaphyseal dysostosis Rubenstein-Taybi syndrome Punctate epiphyseal dysplasia Aminopterin-induced syndrome	Rare

[a] Secondary synostosis.

References

1. Anderson R, Kieffer SA, Wolfson JJ, Long D, Peterson HO: Thickening of the skull in surgically treated hydrocephalus. *Am J Roentgenol* 110:96–101, 1970.
2. Duggan C, Keener E, Brit G: Secondary craniosynostosis. *Am J Roentgenol* 109:277–293, 1970.
3. Griscom NT, Kook Sang O: The contracting skull; inward growth of the inner table as a physiologic response to diminution of intracranial content in children. *Am J Roentgenol* 110:106–110, 1970.
4. Hattner RS, Putman C, Shames DM: Decompression hyperostosis: cranial hyperostosis mimicking bilateral subdural hematoma on brain scintography. *Radiology* 115:673–674, 1975.
5. Johnsonbaugh RE, Bryan RN, Hierlwimmer Ulf R, Georges LP: Premature craiosynostosis: A common complication of juvenile thyrotoxicosis. *J Pediatr* 93:188–191, 1978.
6. Kaufman B, Weiss MH, Young HF, Nulsen FE: Effects of prolonged cerebrospinal fluid shunting on the skull and brain. *J Neurosurg* 38:288–297, 1973.
7. Menking FWM, Schmid WU, Ebel KD, Holthusen WH, Schmidt WWT: Premature craniosynostosis associated with hyperthyroidism. *Ann Radiol* 15:279–284, 1972.
8. Moseley JE, Rabinowitz JG, and Dziadiw R: Hyperostosis cranii ex vacuo. *Radiology* 87:1105–1107, 1966.
9. Riggs W Jr, Wilroy RS Jr, Etteldorf JN: Neonatal hyperthyroidism with accelerated skeletel maturation, craniosynostosis, and brachydactyly. *Radiology* 105:621–625, 1972.
10. Tait MV, Gilday DL, Ash JM, Boldt DJ, Harwood-Nash DCF, Fitz CR, Barry J: Craniosynostosis; correlation of bone scans, radiographs and surgical findings. *Radiology* 133:615–621, 1979.

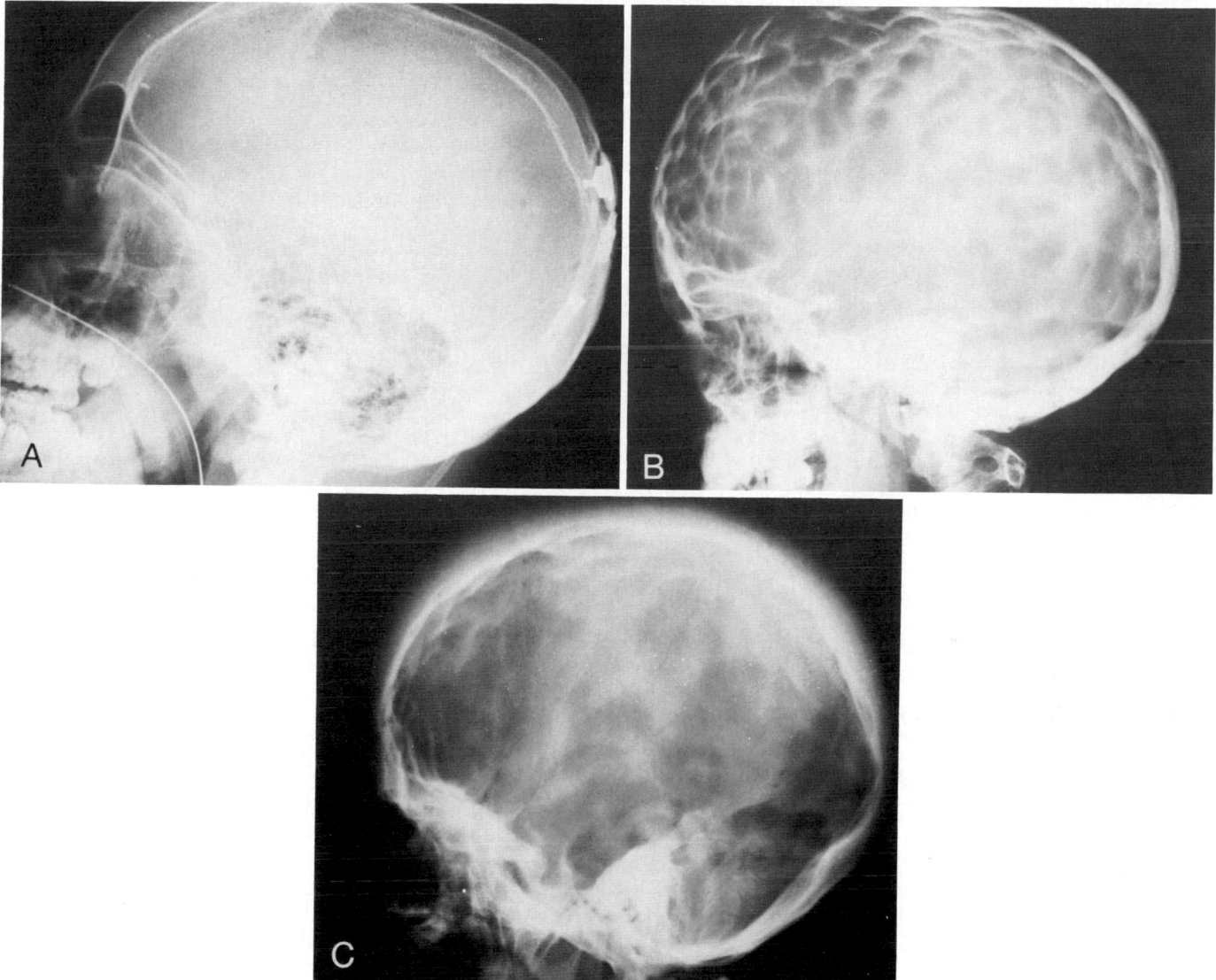

Fig. 5.14. Obliterated or prematurely fused sutures. A. Note absence of sutures in this retarded patient with a small head, thickened calvarium, and overgrowth of the sinuses and mastoid air cells. B. Obliterated sutures in primary craniosynostosis. Note increased convolutional markings due to brain crowding and increased pressure. C. Obliterated sutures, increased intracranial pressure, and exaggerated convolutional markings in secondary synostosis in patient with chronic anemia due to stematocytosis.

CONVOLUTIONAL MARKING ABNORMALITIES

Inner table convolutions are a normal feature of the childhood skull and result from the gyri of the normally pulsating brain pounding against the inner table. Usually they are not present at birth but become variably prominent after the first year of life. In terms of pathologic change, convolutional markings can be-come too prominent or not be prominent enough. Generally, when they are too prominent, there is some problem with increased intracranial pressure and when they are not prominent enough, decreased intracranial pressure is the culprit (Table 5.8).

Table 5.8   Convolutional Marking Abnormalities

A. Increased	
Normal	} Commonest
Chronic increased intracranial pressure	
Lacunar skull	} Moderately common
Primary synostosis (local)	
Primary synostosis—universal	
Secondary synostosis—universal	
Rickets	
Hypophosphatasia	} Relatively rare
Hyperthyroidism	
Chronic anemia	
Cloverleaf skull (primary synostosis)	
Metaphyseal dysostosis	
B. Decreased	
Atrophy	} Commonest
Shunted hydrocephalus	
Severe failure to thrive	} Moderately common
Deprivational dwarfism	
Hypothyroidism	} Relatively rare

Increased Convolutional Markings

The commonest cause of increased inner table convolutional markings is chronically increased intracranial pressure, but the finding is a late manifestation of the problem. Consequently, it should be seen in association with other signs of chronically increased intracranial pressure; for example, spread sutures, demineralization of the sella, truncation of the posterior clinoids and, in some cases, actual sellar enlargement (Fig. 5.15A). It is most important to note these additional features as they serve to distinguish children with chronically increased intracranial pressure from some who are perfectly normal, but yet demonstrate alarmingly prominent convolutional markings (3). In the latter case, the findings are entirely normal and not associated with any signs of chronically increased intracranial pressure (Fig. 5.15B).

In most cases of chronically increased intracranial pressure, the problem is some slowly expanding intracranial lesion (i.e., tumor, cyst, hydrocephalus). In such cases there is time for increased convolutions to develop, and this is important because, if spread is acute (i.e., intracranial bleed, meningitis, brain abscess, cerebritis), no increase in convolutional markings occurs. Another time when increased convolutional markings are seen is with universal craniosynostosis (Fig. 5.15C). In these cases, premature union of the calvarium causes it to be small and unable to accommodate the normally growing brain. As a result intracranial pressures rise and inner table convolutions become more prominent. Such a phenomenon can occur with primary or secondary synostosis, and the latter occurs in conditions such as healing rickets, hypophosphatasia, hypercalcemia, and in chronic anemias such as Cooley's anemia. In all of these cases, it is believed that local bone hypermetabolism predisposes to closure of the sutures.

Locally increased convolutional markings are less common, and not so dire a finding. Most commonly the problem is premature closure of one, or perhaps, two cranial sutures causing localized crowding of the brain (Fig. 5.15D).

Lacunar skull, craniolacunia, or Lückenschadel

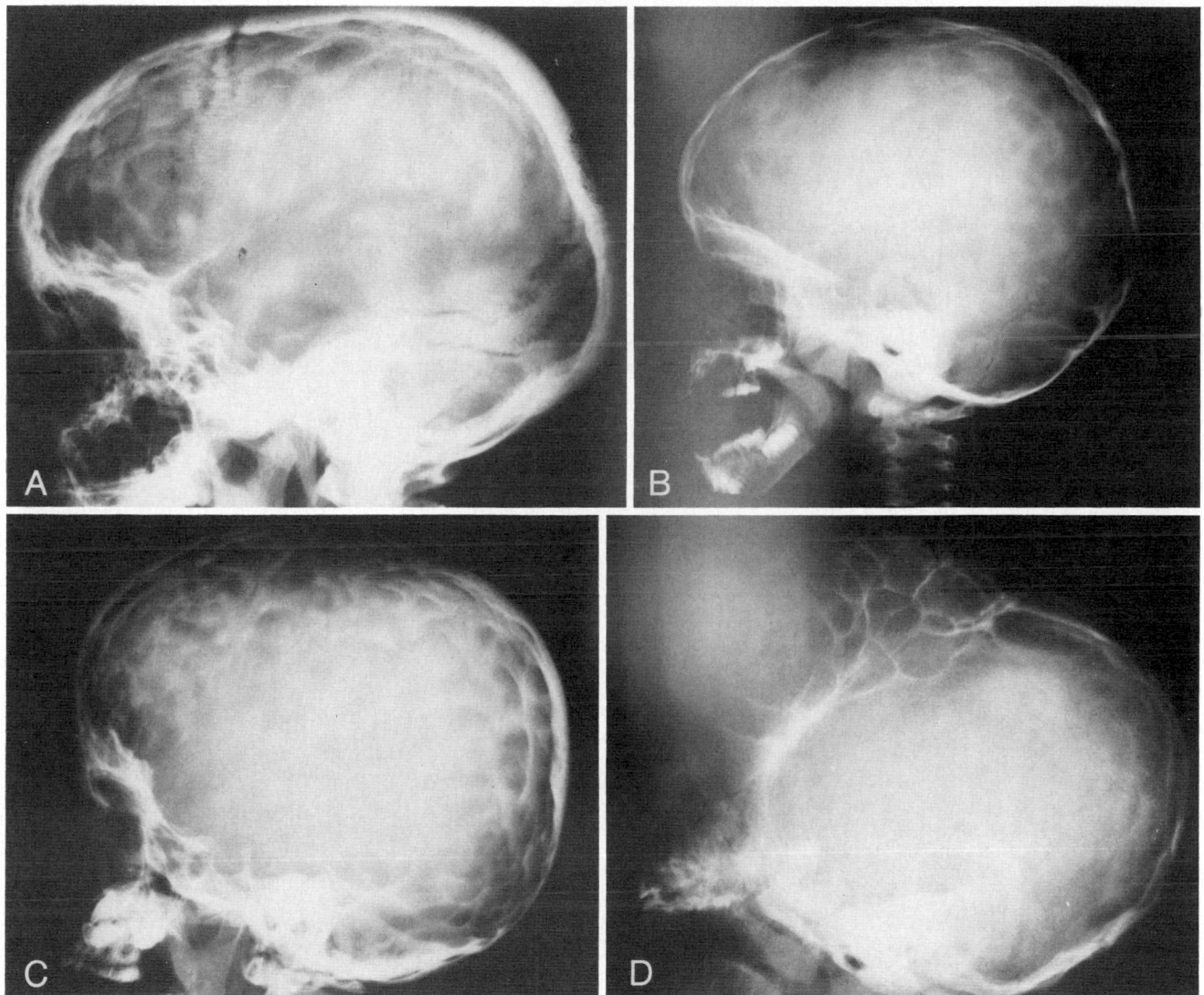

Fig. 5.15. **Increased convolutional markings.** Increased convolutional markings due to chronically increased intracranial pressure. Patient with longstanding brain tumor. Note spread sutures, and enlarged sella. B. Normal patient with prominent convolutional markings. Note normal sutures and normal sella. C. Increased convolutional markings in premature synostosis of the sutures. Note absence of suture visualization, and slight enlargement of the sella. D. Localized increased convolutional markings due to brain crowding in focal synostosis of the sutures.

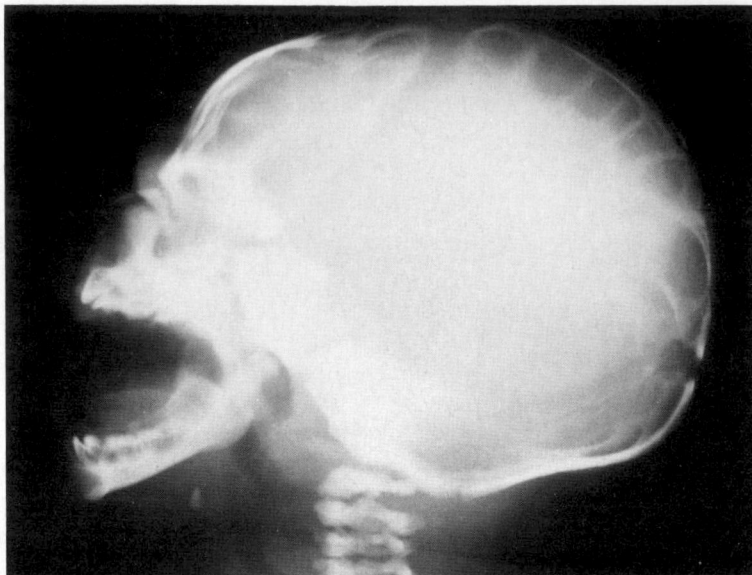

Fig. 5.16. Increased convolutions; lacunar skull. Typical inner table calvarial defects of lacunar skull. These are not due to increased pressure and are not the same as the increased convolutions seen in Figure 5.15.

skull represents another condition where inner table markings are increased. However, the problem is not increased intracranial pressure but rather faulty inner table bone formation (Fig. 5.16). Lacunar skull is seen almost exclusively in patients with meningoceles, meningomyeloceles, or encephaloceles, and then, only in neonates. Only rarely does it occur otherwise. By the age of 6 to 8 months, virtually no remaining lacunar skull is present in any infant, regardless of whether the head becomes larger or smaller. It is important to note this, for many patients with lacunar skull have associated hydrocephalus (Arnold-Chiari malformation, aqueduct stenosis), and it is tempting to assign the increased convolutional pattern to chronically increased intracranial pressure. However, this is not so; the problem is defective bone formation associated with focal dural defects.

Decreased Convolutional Markings

As noted earlier, it is normal for convolutional markings to be sparse or absent in neonates and young infants in their first year of life. Indeed, even up to the age of 3 or 4 yr, some children show very little in the way of inner table convolutional markings, but thereafter, at least some should be present. However, when the brain fails to grow normally (i.e., brain atrophy, severe failure to thrive, deprivational dwarfism, hypothyroidism), inner table convolutional markings become less prominent (see Fig. 5.14A). In any of these conditions, if the problem is reversible, once appropriate treatment is instituted, convolutional markings usually return (Fig. 5.17) and, indeed, in some cases become quite prominent. This does not occur with brain atrophy.

Another relatively common cause of decreased inner table convolutional markings is shunted hydrocephalus. In these cases, with successful shunting, intracranial pressures are decreased and, because of this, the calvarium becomes inwardly thickened, the sutures prematurely closed, and convolutional markings less prominent or absent.

References

1. McRae DL: Observations on craniolacunia. *Acta Radiol Diagn* 5:55–64, 1966.
2. Shopfner CE, Jabbour JT, Vallion RM: Craniolacunia. *Am J Roentgenol* 93:343–349, 1965.
3. Macaulay D: Digital markings in the radiographs of the skull in children. *Br J Radiol* 24:647–652, 1951.

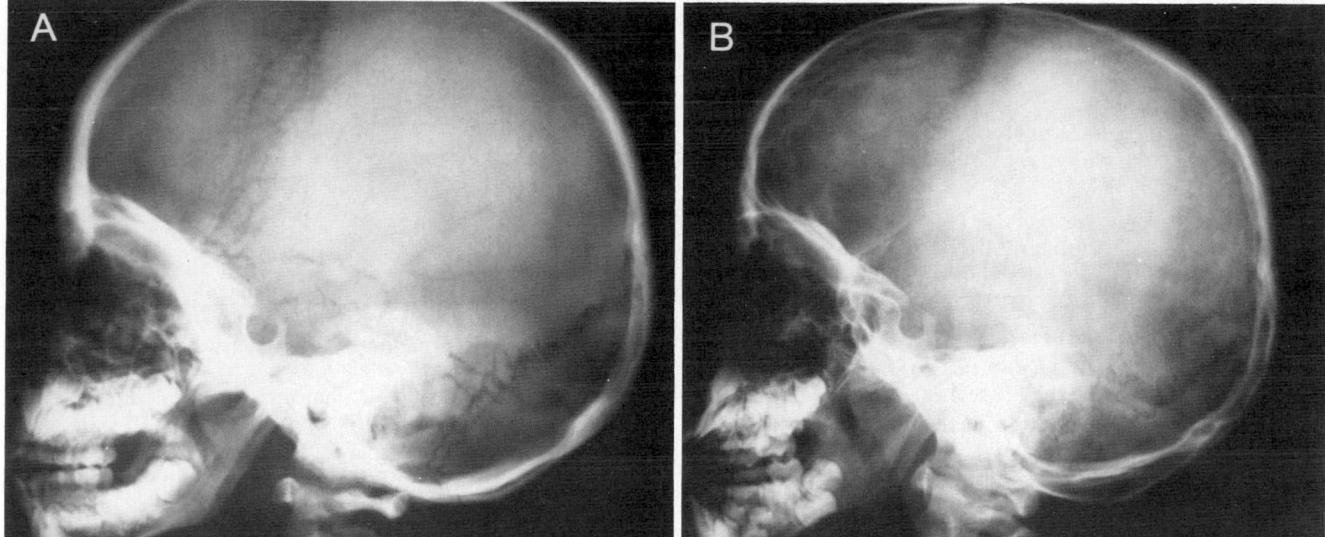

Fig. 5.17. Decreased convolutional markings. A. Patient with hypothyroidism and paucity of convolutional markings. Also note prominence of the sutures and slight roundness of the sella. B. After treatment note increase in convolutional markings, slight spread of the sutures and change in sellar configuration. All of these changes are due to maturation and accelerated brain growth.

ABNORMALITIES OF CALVARIAL DENSITY

For the most part the same conditions causing increased or decreased density of the skeleton cause the findings in the calvarium (see Table 4.1 and 4.2). In those cases where abnormalities of calvarial density are accompanied with thickening of the skull, one is referred to Table 5.3. Multiple or patchy calvarial densities can be seen on a normal basis and are due to variable thickness of the calvarium. However, scattered areas of increased density also are seen in tuberous sclerosis (1), acromegalic gigantism and, occasionally, with metastatic disease, leukemia, or lymphoma. In addition, patchy calvarial densities, alternating with areas of radiolucency, are seen in more florrid cases of hyperparathyroidism.

Reference

1. Medley BE, McLeod RA, Houser OW: Tuberous sclerosis. *Semin Roentgenol* 11:35–54, 1976.

RADIOLUCENT LINES IN THE CALVARIUM

The commonest radiolucent lines in the calvarium are those caused by vascular grooves, sutures, synchondroses, and fractures (4). A detailed discussion of all possible appearances of these structures is beyond the scope of this book, and is covered in detail, elsewhere (7). The following comments are merely a resume.

Normal sutures are the structures which most commonly cause radiolucent lines in the calvarium of children, but usually pose a problem only when rotation of the skull places them in a peculiar projection. As a safeguard, then, it behooves one to know the positions into which these sutures are projected with rotation of the head. In addition, it is important to note that most of the troublesome sutures (squamosal, lambdoid, other posterior fossa sutures), are paired, and such pairing should be sought for constantly. Utilizing this rule, even if a suture appears as a fracture, if it is located in the expected position, and if it is one of a pair, then most likely it is a suture. If, on the other hand, one already has identified both sutures of any given pair, and another similar line is seen, even though it is located where one might expect a suture, it should be a fracture.

Knowledge of normal, accessory sutures is next most important and, for the most part, these include the posterior parietal fissure, intraparietal accessory suture (near horizontal in the parietal bone) (2, 6, 7), the basal synchondroses (3), the metopic suture (8), and the midline occipital fissure (1). With intraparietal and posterior parietal fissures, the fact that these structures often are paired and, indeed, quite symmetric is helpful. In addition, the posterior parietal fissure occurs in the lower third of the parietal bone and, consequently, if a similar finding is seen in the upper part of the parietal bone, a fracture should be suspected. Intraparietal sutures are quite common and most tend to be relatively horizontal in position. However, occasionally vertical intraparietal sutures are encountered and in some cases so many of these sutures are present that an eggshell fracture of the calvarium is mimicked. In any of these cases, if one cannot make a decision as to whether a radiolucent line(s) is a fracture, other findings, such as type of injury, location of injury, overlying soft tissue swelling, can be utilized. Ultimately, if none of these potentially helpful considerations produce results, one may resort to a bone scan; fractures should be positive and sutures negative.

Vascular grooves producing radiolucent lines in the calvarium are not a problem if they are tortuous or branching, but if they are straight, they also can be misinterpreted for fractures. In this regard, one of the most commonly misinterpreted vascular grooves is that which occurs in the frontal bone. It is produced by the supraorbital artery, and when it is straight, or gently curving, it can mimic a fracture. Diploic veins over the parietal bone are no particular problem because they have a stellate configuration, but the superficial branch of the temporal artery, as it crosses the temporal bone can be mistaken for a fracture. The middle meningeal artery usually is recognized for what it is, and only its posterior branch as it travels horizontally, commonly is misinterpreted for a fracture.

As far as fractures are concerned, usually they occur at, or near, the site of injury. However, if the injury is a broad surface injury, the fracture may occur in curvilinear fashion, at some distance away from the point of impact. Nonetheless, fractures usually are not great problems in identification. If depressed, a V-shaped configuration of the fracture line, sclerosis along one of the fracture line edges, and increased density of some of the depressed fragments can aid in diagnosis. Increased density in these cases results from overlapping of the fracture fragments or visualization of the fragments on tangent.

References

1. Franken EA: The midline occipital fissure: diagnosis of a fracture versus anatomic variants. *Radiology* 93:1043–1046, 1969.
2. Shapiro R: Anomalous parietal sutures and the pipartite parietal bone. *Am J Roentgenol* 115:569–577, 1972.
3. Shopfner CE, Wolfe TW, O'Kell RT: The intersphenoid synchondrosis. *Am J Roentgenol* 104:184–193, 1968.
4. Swischuk, L.E.: The growing skull. *Semin Roentgenol* 9:115–124, 1974.
5. Swischuk, L.E.: The normal newborn skull. *Semin Roentgenol* 9:101–113, 1974.
6. Swischuk, L.E.: The normal pediatric skull variations artifacts. *Radiol Clin N Am* 10:227–290, 1972.
7. Swischuk, L.E.: *Emergency Radiology of the Acutely Ill or Injured Child.* Baltimore, Williams & Wilkins, 1979, pp 383–421.
8. Torgerson, J.: A roentgenologic study of the metopic suture. *Acta Radiol* 33:1–11, 1950.

ABNORMALITIES OF THE SELLA

The sella can be larger than normal, smaller than normal, or of abnormal shape. If it is larger, pathology is present, but if it is smaller, pathology may or may not be present. Indeed, most often it is not. Abnormal shapes of the sella many times are just normal variations, but there are a few specific configurations which should strongly suggest a pathologic condition. All of these features of the sella are discussed in ensuing paragraphs and summarized in Table 5.9.

Table 5.9 Sellar Size Abnormalities and Configurations

Sellar size abnormalities		Sellar configurations	
A. Large sella		Types	Causes
Intrasellar tumor Chronically increased pressure with tumor or hydrocephalus	} Commonest	A. Stretched sella	1. Normal (common) 2. Enlarging head (common)
Nelson's syndrome Hypothyroidism	} Relatively rare	B. Scooped or Omega sella	1. Optic chiasm tumor (most common) 2. Pituitary fossa tumor (relatively rare) 3. Unilateral normal (relatively rare)

Empty sella syndrome
    Intrasellar cyst (congenital, acquired)
    Chronic pressure with universal craniosynostosis
	} Rare	C. Boat-shaped or J-shaped sella	1. Normal (most common)
			2. Chiasmatic or intrasellar tumor (relatively rare)
			3. Intrasellar cyst (rare)

B. Small sella Normal	} Commonest	D. Dysplastic sella	1. Neurofibromatosis (most common)

Atrophy
    Shunted hydrocephalus
    Hypopituitarism
	} Moderately common		

Large Sella

The commonest cause of a large sella in the pediatric age group is an intrasellar tumor. Such a tumor may arise within the sella itself (adenoma—Fig. 5.18A) (11), or from the para-sellar regions. The best example of the latter is the craniopharyngioma. The common occurrence of calcification (irregular or curvilinear) in this tumor aids in its diagnosis (Fig. 5.18B). The sella also can enlarge in the late stages of chroincally increased intracranial pressure, but the finding usually takes months to develop (see Fig. 5.15, A and C). In such cases, enlargement probably results from bone erosion secondary to intrasellar subarachnoid space distension and dilation.

The sella also enlarges in response to rebound hypertrophy of the pituitary gland secondary to end organ failure. For example, after bilateral adrenal ablation, rebound hypertrophy of the pituitary gland is known as Nelson's syndrome (3, 6, 14, 15). A similar phenomenon occurs with hypothyroidism (1, 12, 13). In either condition, if rebound hypertrophy is long standing, an actual adenoma may develop in the pituitary gland. In most cases of rebound hypertrophy, the enlarged sella is quite round, and in hypothyroidism has been termed the "cherry" sella (see Fig. 5.13B) (12).

The sella also can enlarge when a subarachnoid cyst enters the pituitary fossa. However, the problem is quite rare. Nonetheless, such cysts can be congenital or acquired and the latter occurs after intracranial bleeds, infections, or infiltration with the storage diseases (10). Dilation of the arachnoid space in the pituitary fossa, as occurs in the empty sella syndrome, is relatively rare in children (8, 9).

Finally, the sella can enlarge on a nontumor basis, in neurofibromatosis. In such cases the finding represents yet another manifestation of the mesenchymal, developmental defect present in this condition. Although the sella may appear as though it contains a tumor, enlargement is merely a manifestation of bizarre bone formation (see Fig. 5.21).

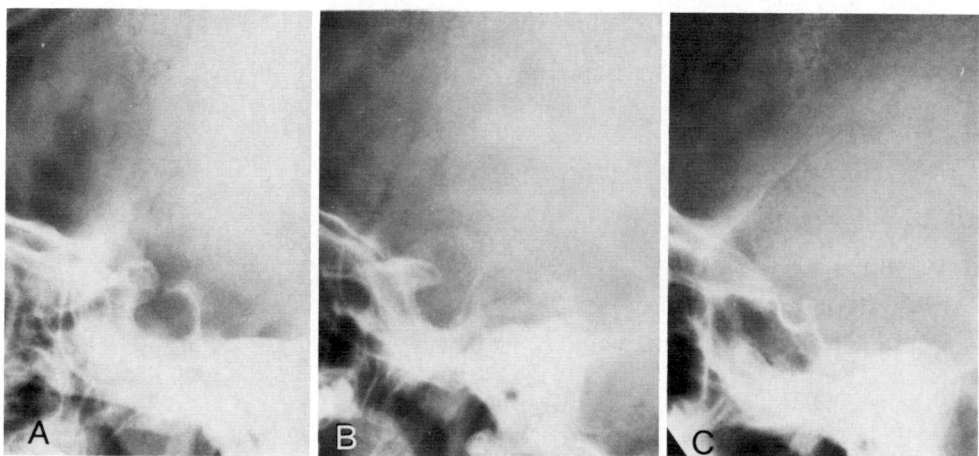

Fig. 5.18. Small and large sellas. A. Large sella due to adenoma of pituitary gland. B. Large sella due to craniopharyngioma. Note curvilinear intra and suprasellar calcification. C. Small sella in normal child. A small sella also can be seen in hypopituitarism.

Small Sella

The commonest cause, by far, of a smaller than normal sella is normal variation (Fig. 5.18C). However, in children, a small sella also commonly is seen in hypopituitarism and with decreased intracranial pressure (4, 13). The latter can occur with brain atrophy or after successful shunting for hydrocephalus. In either case, the sella becomes small in response to chronically decreased intracranial pressure. The phenomenon is exactly opposite to that which occurs when the sella enlarges in response to chronically increased intracranial pressure. With decreased intracranial pressure, other findings accompany the small sella, and these include (a) inward thickening of the calvarium, (b) absence of convolutional markings, and (c) prominence of the paranasal sinuses and mastoid air cells.

Shape Abnormalities

Shape abnormalities of the sella inlcude (a) the strctched sella, (b) the scooped or omega sella, (c) the boat-shaped or J sella, and (d) the dysplastic sella (Fig. 5.19). In addition to this, one may encounter a number of nonspecific and, usually, not important changes in configuration of the anterior clinoids, the middle clinoids, and the bridged sella (Fig. 5.20). The stretched sella often is misinterpreted for the J-shaped

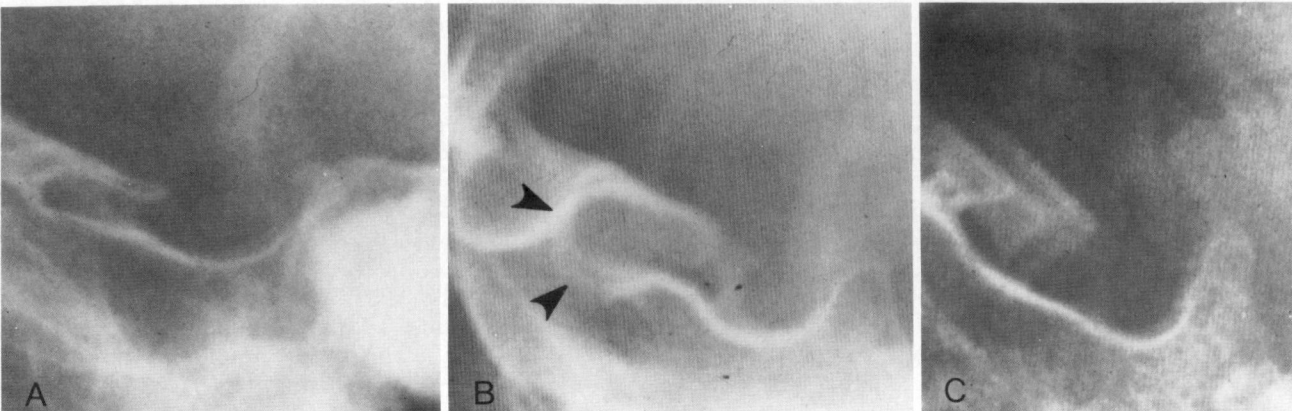

Fig. 5.19. Sellar shape abnormalities. A. Typical stretched sella. B. Typical scooped or omega sella. C. Boat-shaped or J sella. See text for conditions associated with these sellar configurations.

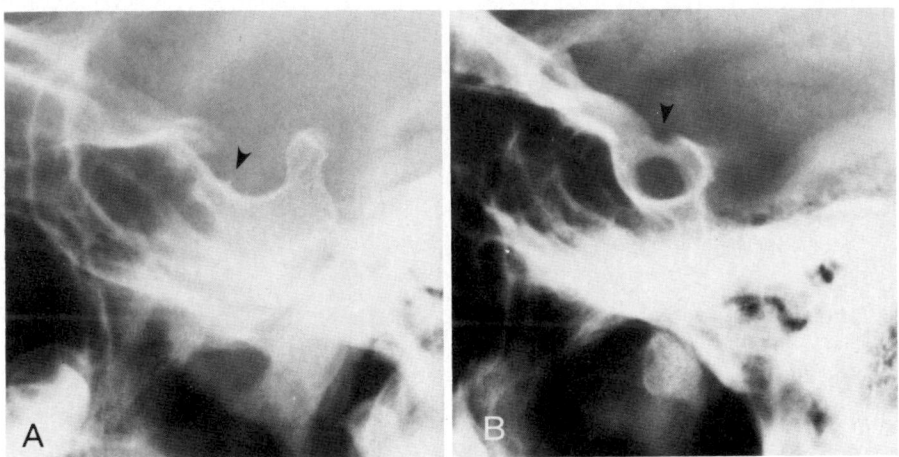

Fig. 5.20. Miscellaneous sellar abnormalities. A. Note small, middle clinoids (arrow). Many times these are larger. B. Typical bridged sella due to ossification of diaphragma sella (arrows). Often the sella also is small in these patients. Neither of these findings is of any clinical significance.

sella, but the two should be separated for they represent changes due to different problems. **The stretched sella** most often occurs in normal children, but it also is seen with any cause of calvarial enlargement. In these latter cases it seems that, as the calvarium enlarges, there is undue stretching to the base of the skull and, subsequently, elongation of the chiasmatic sulcus, flattening of the tuberculum sellae, and shallowness of the pituitary fossa. The stretched sella is seen in the various storage diseases, chondodystrophic dwarfs, hydrocephalus, and megalencephaly.

As far as the **scooped or omega sella** is concerned, almost always it denotes the presence of a tumor in the optic chiasm. Most often the tumor is an optic glioma but it can be a neurofibroma or any other tumor that might occur in the area. Only occasionally is it seen in the normal individual, and then it is usually unilateral.

The J or boat-shaped sella differs from the stretched sella in that the tuberculum sellae is com-

pletely flattened or eroded and the entire sella more boat shaped. This type of sellar configuration occasionally is seen in normal children; more often it occurs when an optic glioma extends into the pituitary fossa or an intrasellar tumor extends into the optic chiasm. Occasionally, it can be seen with a subarachnoid cyst doing the same thing.

As far as a **dysplastic sella** is concerned, the most common problem is neurofibromatosis. Indeed, except for a few minor congenital variations in configuration of the sella, neurofibromatosis virtually is the sole culprit. In this regard, sellar configurations are almost endless (Fig. 5.21).

References

1. Bellini MA, Neves I: The skull in childhood myxedema: its roentgen appearance. *Am J Roentgenol* 76:495–498, 1956.
2. Burrows EH: The so-called J-sella. *Br J Radiol* 37:661–669, 1964.

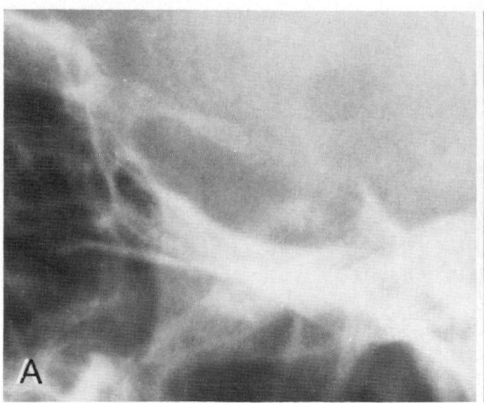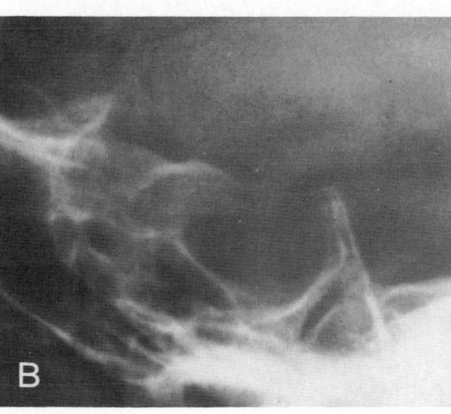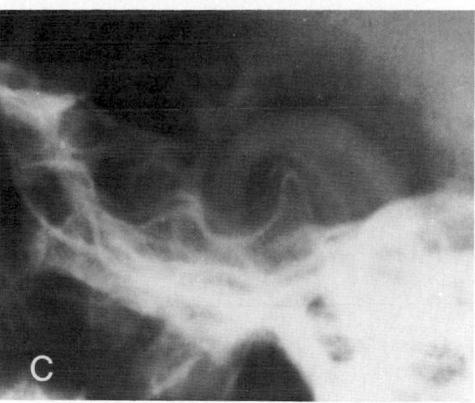

Fig. 5.21. Dysplastic sella. A–C. Three cases of sellar and, in some cases, adjacent sphenoid wing dysplasia in neurofibromatosis. None of these patients had intra or parasellar tumors.

3. Danziger J, Wallace S, Handel S, Samaan NB: The sella turcica in primary end organ failure. *Radiology* 131:111–115, 1979.
4. Fisher RL, DiChiro G: The small sella turcica. *Neuroradiology* 91:996–1008, 1964.
5. Fournier AM, Denizet D: La selle turcique en omega. *Marseille Med* 102:503–509, 1965.
6. Hopwood NJ, Kenny FM: Incidence of Nelson's syndrome after adrenalectomy for Cushing's disease in children. *Am J Dis Child* 131:1353–1356, 1977.
7. Kier EL: "J" and "Omega" shape of sella turcica. *Acta Radiol* 9:91–94, 1969.
8. Kaufman B: The "empty" sella turcica—a manifestation of the intrasellar subarachnoid space. *Radiology* 90:931–941, 1968.
9. Merle P, Georget, AM, Goumy P, Jarlot, D: Primary empty sella turcica in children. Report of two familial cases. *Pediatr Radiol* 8:209–212, 1979.
10. Neuhauser EBD, Griscom NT, Gilles FH, Crocker AC: Arachnoid cysts in the hurler-hunter syndrome. *Ann Radiol* 11:453–469, 1968.
11. Richmond IL, Wilson CB: Pituitary adenomas in childhood and adolescence. *J Neurosurg* 49:163–168, 1978.
12. Swischuk LE, Sarwar M: The sella in childhood and hypothyroidism. *Pediatr Radiol* 6:1–3, 1977.
13. Swischuk LE, Sarwar M: The sella turcica (some lesser known dynamic features). *CRC Crit Rev Diagn Imaging* 11:37–55, 1978.
14. Weinstein, M, Tyrrell, B., Newton, T.: The sella turcica in Nelson's syndrome. *Radiology* 118:363–365, 1976.
15. Young LW, Lim GHK, Forbes GB, Bryson MF: Postadrenalectomy pituitary adenoma (Nelson's syndrome) in childhood: clinical and roentgenologic detection. *Am J Roentgenol* 126:550–559, 1976.

FORAMEN MAGNUM ABNORMALITIES

Foramen magnum abnormalities consist primarily of size and configuration disturbances (Table 5.10). These abnormalities usually are visible on plain films but are more clearly demonstrated with regular tomography and, currently, computerized tomography. As far as size is concerned, the foramen magnum can be too large or too small, and as far as configuration is concerned, the main problem is asymmetric smallness. For the most part, the latter occurs with fusion (occipitalization) of C_1 to the base of the skull (Fig. 5.22A). In such cases, union of C_1 to the base of the skull is bony, and in some cases the narrowed foramen magnum can produce pressure on the brain stem and upper cervical cord. This is aggravated by the frequently associated finding of upward displacement of the dens, or so-called basilar invagination (see Fig. 5.23).

Enlargement of the foramen magnum is seen with cervical-occipital meningoceles, the Arnold-Chiari malformation, syringobulbia, and posterior fossa cysts extending into the spinal canal. The most common of these cysts is the Dandy Walker cyst (Fig. 5.22B), but

Table 5.10   Foramen Magnum Abnormalities

A. Enlargement	
Arnold-Chiari malformation Cervical occipital encephaloceles	Commonest
Dandy-Walker cyst	Moderately common

Other posterior fossa cysts
    Cervical cord tumor
    Syringobulbia
    Posterior fossa tumor
	Rare

B. Small foramen magnum	
Chondrodystrophies	Commonest
Bilateral or unilateral occipitalization	Relatively rare
C. Irregular foramen magnum	
Normal neonatal ossicles	Commonest
Unilateral or bilateral occipitalization	Moderately common

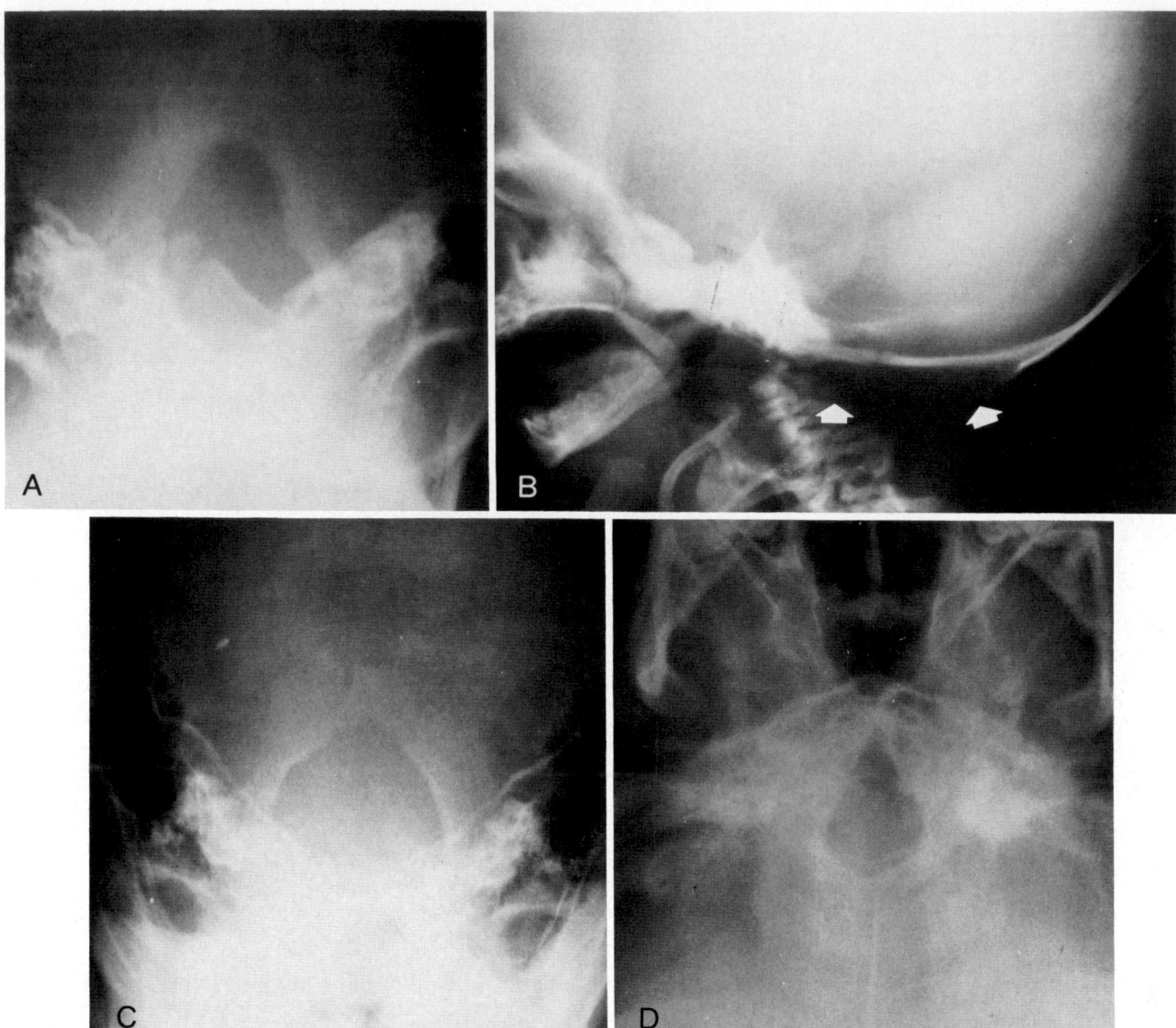

Fig. 5.22. Abnormalities of the foramen magnum. A. Asymmetrically deformed, small foramen magnum secondary to unilateral occipitalization of C1. B. Large foramen magnum in Dandy-Walker cyst, with extension into the cervical spine (arrows). C. Large foramen magnum in older patient with Arnold-Chiari malformation. D. Small foramen magnum in achondroplasia.

overall the Arnold-Chiari malformation is the most common cause of a large foramen magnum (Fig. 5.22C). In this condition it is the downward displacement of the fourth ventricle and medella which cause enlargement of the foramen magnum. In the Dandy-Walker cyst, congenital obstruction of the foramina of the fourth ventricle cause its dilation and, when it becomes large enough, it can extend into the cervical canal and cause enlargement of the foramen magnum. Other cysts of the posterior fossa, herniating through the foramen magnum, are rather uncommon and so are tumors and cysts of the cervical spine rising upward and enlarging the foramen magnum. A final cause of enlargement of the foramen magnum is un-

derdevelopment of the upper cervical spine, especially the posterior elements, and concomitant underdevelopment of the foramen magnum.

A smaller than normal foramen magnum usually is seen in the chondrodystrophies and, of these, achondroplasia is the most common (Fig. 5.22D). Others include achondrogenesis, thanatophoric dwarfism, metatrophic dwarfism, and diastrophic dwarfism. In any of these conditions, it is failure of adequate growth of the cartilaginous base of the skull which leads to constriction of the foramen magnum. In milder cases the abnormality is of no serious consequence, but when severe, hydrocephalus can result (2). The foramen magnum also may be smaller than normal with occipitalization of C_1 (Fig. 5.22A) and, finally, it should be noted that the foramen magnum often is normally irregular in the neonate. Ossification of the base of the skull is incomplete and, thus, many extra ossification centers and irregularities of ossifications result (1). These are of no particular consequence and should be recognized as such.

References

1. Caffey J: The accessory ossicles of the supra-occipital. *Am J Roentgenol* 70:401–412, 1953.
2. Cohen ME, Rosenthal AD, Matson DD: Neurologic abnormalities in achondroplastic children. *J Pediatr* 71:367–376, 1967.

BASILAR INVAGINATION

In the condition known as basilar invagination, the odontoid process protrudes into the foramen magnum and, consequently, there is compression of the upper cervical cord and medulla. The commonest cause is congenital occipitalization of C_1, a condition where the atlas is fused to the occiput of the skull. Union can be fibrous, cartilaginous, or bony, and it is the close apposition of the atlas to the base of the skull which causes the dens to ride high (Fig. 5.23). Basilar invagination, due to hypoplasia of C_1, is seen in syndromes such as achondroplasia, Morquio's disease, trisomy 21, etc. In these cases, occipitalization usually is not present, but severe hypoplasia of C_1 causes the remainder of the cervical spine, including the dens, to ride high.

A less common cause of basilar invagination in the pediatric age group is softening of the base of the skull. The most common cause of such softening is osteogenesis imperfecta, but the problem also can occur in hyperparathyroidism (primary or secondary with renal osteodystrophy), severe rickets, and in some cases of hypophosphatasia.

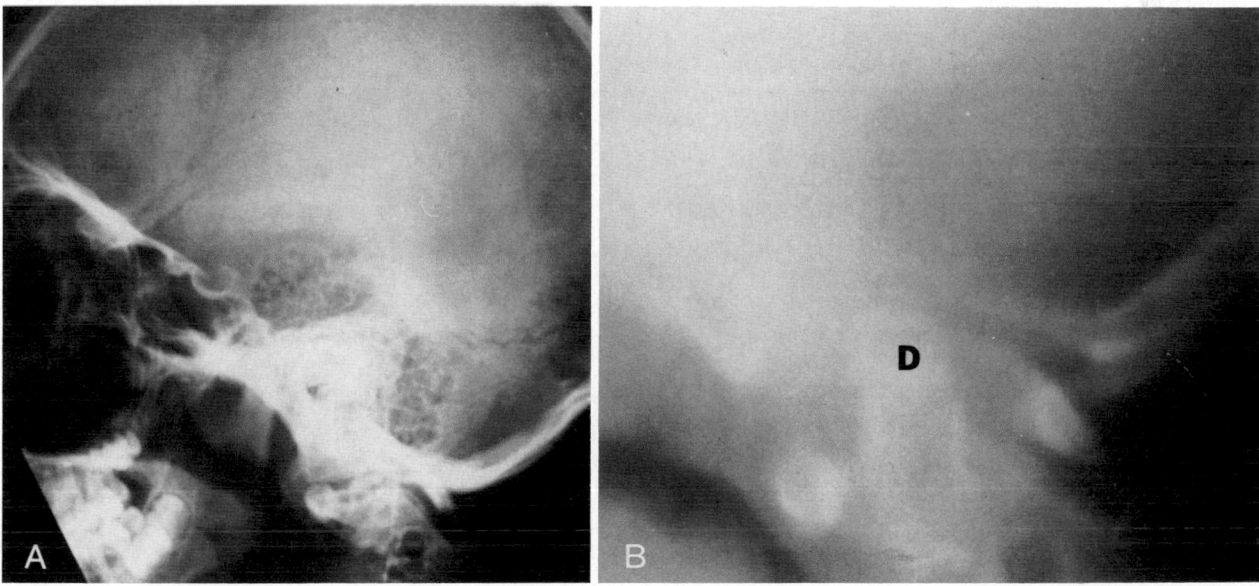

Fig. 5.23. Basilar invagination. A. Note difficulty in defining normal anatomy of the base of the skull, C1, and the dens. **B.** Laminagram showing invagination of dens (D) into foramen magnum. This patient had occipitalization of C1.

BASAL ANGLE ABNORMALITIES

The basal angle of the skull, measured as the angle between the lines drawn from (*a*) the clivus to the tuberculum sella and (*b*) the tuberculum to the nasion (base of nose), usually measures from 131° to 135°. In some conditions it is increased while in others it is decreased. Basically, it is increased (more acute) in Mongolism or trisomy 21, Turner's syndrome, acromegaly, craniosynostosis (coronal usually), and occasionally in hypothyroidism (1). It is decreased (flatter) in Klinefelter's syndrome, the XXX syndrome, and eunuchoidism (1). It also is decreased in platybasia, as seen in cleidocranial dysostosis, and bone softening conditions such as osteogenesis imperfecta, hyperparathyroidism, severe rickets, and hypophosphatasia. An example of an inceased basal angle is present in Figure 5.3C, a case of coronal craniosynostosis.

References

1. Rzymski K, Kosowicz J: Abnormal basal angle of the skull in sex chromosome aberrations. *ACTA Radiol* 17:669–675, 1976.

ABNORMALITIES OF THE ANTERIOR FONTANELLE

The anterior fontanelle, of course, should be open at birth and remain open for a few months after birth. Eventually, as the infant grows older, it becomes smaller and finally is obliterated. In infancy, two common deviations from this sequence of events can occur; i.e., the anterior fontanelle can be too big or too small. When **too large,** almost always there is associated delayed ossification of the membranous bones of the calvarium. This is a common phenomenon in the normal premature infant and, occasionally, is seen in normal, full term infants. Pathologically, it occurs with neonatal rubella and, indeed, almost any cause of intrauterine growth failure (2), hypothyroidism, and bony dysplasias where defective ossification of the bone is present (Table 5.11). An example of the latter is seen in Figure 5.24A, a case of cleidocranial dysostosis. The anterior fontanelle also is large when the calvarium enlarges, but the fact that it is large in such cases is no problem. Another relatively common cause of an overly large anterior fontanelle is lacunar skull. In these patients, a temporary cranium bifidum (ossification defect in the mid-frontal bone) exists and this defect continues into the anterior fontanelle.

An **overly small** anterior fontanelle occasionally is seen in perfectly normal infants, but more often occurs with primary or secondary premature closure of the cranial sutures, atrophy of the brain (Fig. 5.24B), and decreased intracranial pressure secondary to shunting of hydrocephalus. The latter two examples, of course, are merely examples of secondary premature synostosis.

Finally, it might be noted that occasionally one can encounter one or more extra bones in the anterior fontanelle (Fig. 5.24C). Usually this finding is of no particular cosequence, and these bones can be seen in completely normal patients (1) or in patients with hydrocephalus. Large and small anterior fontanelles, and an anterior fontanelle bone are demonstrated in Figure 5.24.

References

1. Girdany BR, Blank E: Anterior fontanelle bones. *Am J Roentgenol* 95:148–153, 1965.
2. Philip AGS: Fontanel size and epiphyseal ossification in neonates with intrauterine growth retardation; preliminary communication. *J Pediatr* 84:204–207, 1974.

Table 5.11 Anterior Fontanelle Abnormalities

A. Large fontanelle	

Premature—normal
   Intrauterine infections
   Trisomy 21 mongolism
	Commonest

Hypothyroidism (Cretinism)
   Severe rickets
   Trisomy 18
   Osteogenesis imperfecta
   Cranium bifidum with lacunar skull
	Moderately common

Epiphyseal dysplasia punctata (Conradi's disease) Cliedocranial dysostosis	Relatively rare

Aminopterin-induced syndrome
   Cerebrohepatorenal syndrome (Zellweger)
   Congenital scalp defect syndrome
   Cutis laxa
   Hypophosphatasia
   Hallerman-Streiff syndrome
   Melnick-Needles (osteodysplasia syndrome)
   Otopalatodigital syndrome
   Pachydermoperiostitis
   Progeria
   Rubinstein-Taybi syndrome
	Rare

B. Small fontanelle	

Craniosynostosis (primary)
   Brain atrophy (secondary synostosis)
   Shunted hydrocephalus (secondary synostosis)
	Commonest

Craniosynostosis (secondary)
   Chronic anemias
   Rickets
   Hypophosphatasia
	Moderately common

Normal variation	Rare
C. Anterior fontanelle bone	
Normal	Commonest
Large head (hydrocephalus)	Moderately common

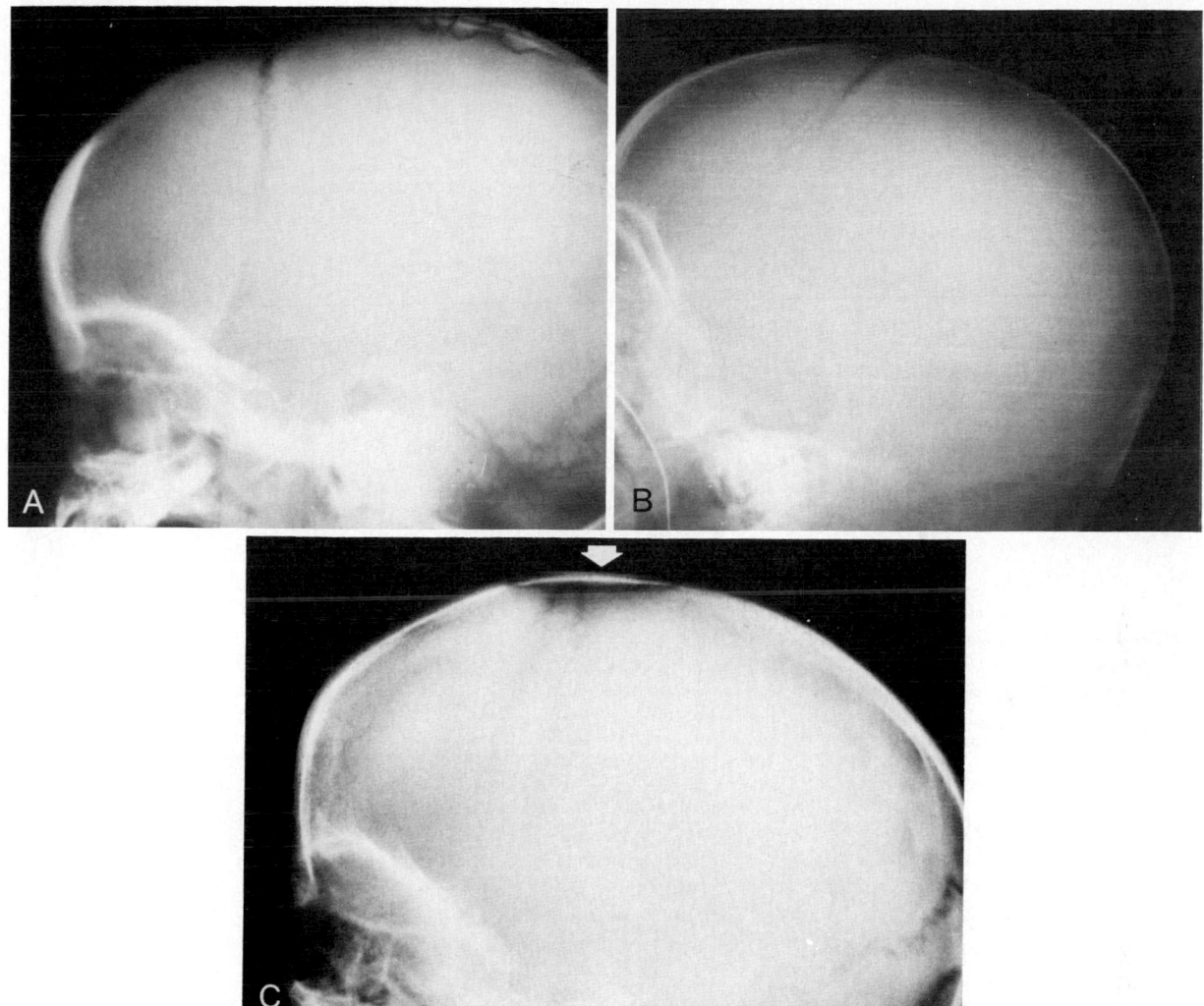

Fig. 5.24. Anterior fontanelle abnormalities. A. Large anterior fontanelle due to underossification in cleidocranial dysostosis. B. Small anterior fontanelle secondary to premature closure of sutures in brain atrophy. C. Anterior fontannelle bone (arrows).

WORMIAN BONES

Wormian bones are intrasutural bones and, although they commonly occur in normal infants, also are seen in pathologic states (Fig. 5.25) (Table 5.12). Most often they are seen along the lambdoid suture and, as far as pathologic conditions are concerned, the ones most commonly encountered are osteogenesis imperfecta and cleidocranial dysostosis. Others include: pycnodysostosis, hypophosphatasia, pachydermoperiostosis, some trisomies, idiopathic acro-osteolysis, progeria, cretinism, hypothyroidism, and the Hallermann-Streiff, aminopterin-induced, kinky hair (Menke's), otopalitaldigital, and Prader-Willi syndromes. As a side point, it also has been noted that excess wormian bone formation occurs in some patients with gross central nervous system abnormalities (1). However, it may be that many of these infants have lesser known chromosomal abnormalities.

Reference

1. Pryles CV, Khan AJ: Wormian bones. *Am J Dis Child* 133:380–382, 1979.

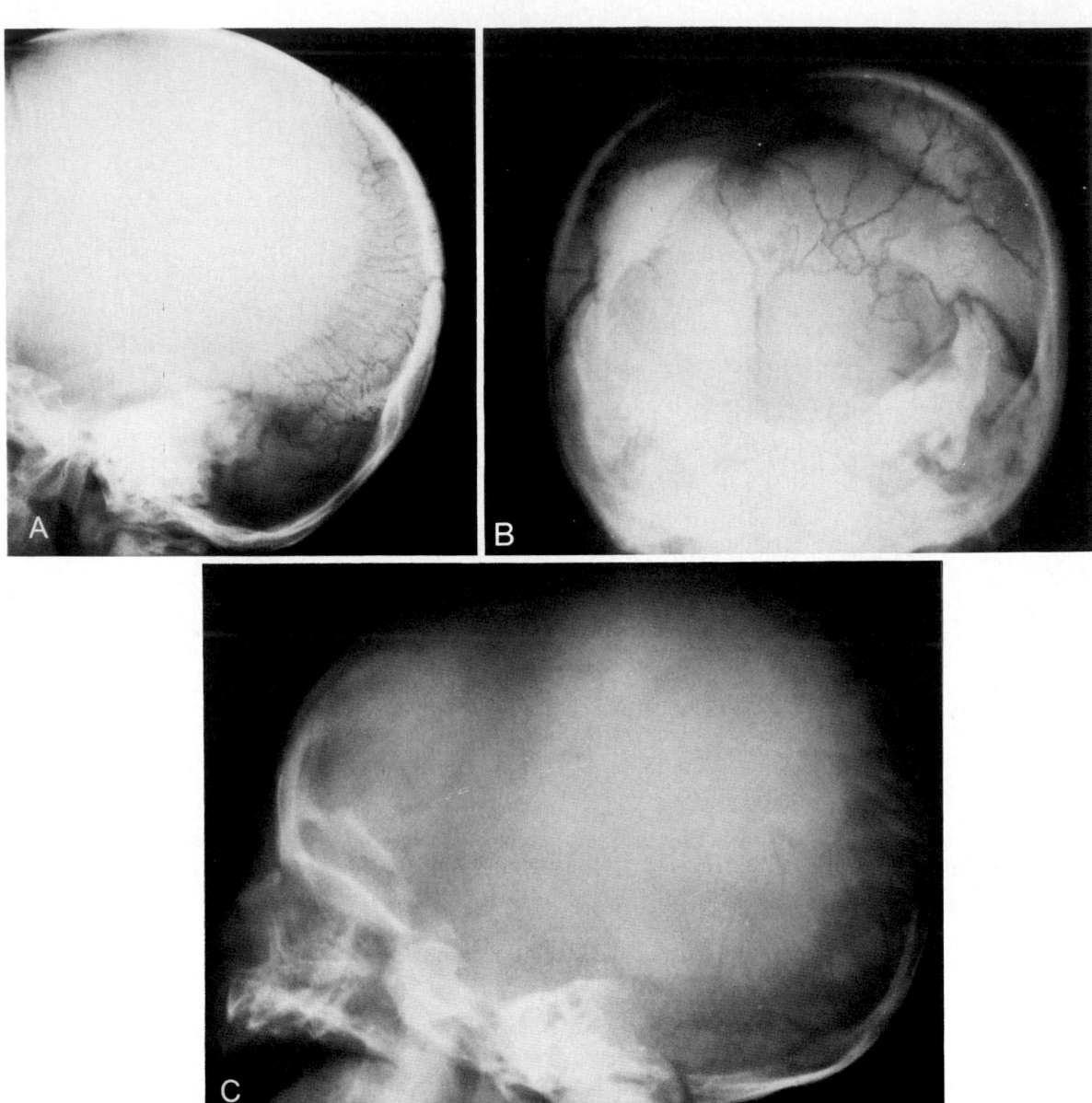

Fig. 5.25. Wormian bones. Note extensive wormian bone formation along the lambdoid suture and posterior parietal regions. Patient with cleidocranial dysostosis. B. Another patient with cleidocranial dysostosis demonstrating more extensive wormian and mosaic bone formation. C. Wormian bone formation, in the posterior parietal region and lambdoid suture areas in osteogenesis imperfecta.

Table 5.12   Wormian Bones

Normal (especially lambdoid) suture)	Commonest
Osteogenesis imperfecta Cleidocranial dysostosis Cretinism Some trisomies Healing rickets	Moderately common
Pycnodysostosis Hypophosphatasia Pachydermoperiostosis Idiopathic acro-osteolysis Hallermann-Streiff syndrome Aminopterin-induced syndrome Kinky hair or Menkes' syndrome Otopalitaldigital syndrome Prader-Willi syndrome Progeria	Relatively rare

BUTTON SEQUESTRUM

A button sequestrum occurs when a round destructive lesion of the calvarium is associated with a small sclerotic piece of sequestrated bone in its center. It is not particularly common in children and, although it can occur in a number of conditions, in childhood it most often is seen with osteomyelitis or eosinophilic granuloma (1–3). However, other causes to be considered include idiopathic, dermoid cysts, healing of a burr hole, fibrous dysplasia, hemangioma, epidermoid cysts, and radiation necrosis. In adults it has been noted with Paget's disease, multiple myeloma, and meningioma, but only the latter condition might be seen in the child.

References

1. Satin R, Usher MS, Goldenberg M: More causes of button sequestrum. *J Can Assoc Radiol* 27:288–289, 1976.
2. Sholkoff SD, Mainzer F: Button sequestrum revisited. *Radiology* 100:649–652, 1971.
3. Wells PO: The button sequestrum of esinophilic granuloma of the skull. *Radiology* 67:746–747, 1956.

CALVARIAL BONE DESTRUCTION

The cause of bone destruction of the calvarium are about the same as those for long bones (see p 311), and in general calvarial destruction may be; (1) mottled and permeative, or (2) discretely lytic (Table 5.13).

Table 5.13 Calvarial Destruction

A. Permeative or mottled	Aneurysmal bone cyst[a] ⎫
Metastatic disease[c] ⎫	Intraosseous hematoma ⎪
Infection[b,d] ⎬ Commonest	Hemangioma of calvarium[b] ⎪
	Calvarial dermoids[b] ⎪
Leukemia-lymphoma[c] ⎱ Moderately common	Congenital syphilis ⎬ Rare
	Primary bone tumor ⎪
Primary bone tumor ⎫	Radiation necrosis ⎪
Hyperparathyroidism ⎬ Relatively rare	Intradiploic ectopic neural tissue[b] ⎪
B. Solitary or multiple, discreetly	Caffey's disease ⎭
lytic lesions	
Histiocytosis X[c] ⎫	C. Large lytic areas
Fibrous dysplasia[d] ⎪	Fibrous dysplasia[b] ⎱ Commonest
Encephaloceles[b] ⎪	Infection[b] ⎰
Normal and accessory fontanelles ⎬ Commonest	
Osteomyelitis[b] ⎪	Histiocytosis X ⎱ Moderately common
Metastatic disease ⎭	Post-op bone flap necrosis ⎰
Venous lakes[b,c] ⎫	Chordoma of clivus ⎫
Healing cephalohematoma[b] ⎪	Meningioma ⎪
Epidermoid inclusion cyst[a] ⎬ Moderately common	Nasopharyngeal tumors and polyps ⎬ Relatively rare
Leukemia-lymphoma[c] ⎭	Neurofibromatosis (sphenoid wing) ⎪
Leptomeningeal cysts[b] ⎫	Radiation necrosis ⎭
Pachyonnian granulations[b] ⎪	
Neurofibromatosis (lambdoid defect) ⎬ Relatively rare	
Scalp tumor or cyst ⎪	
Congenital dermal sinus[b] ⎭	

[a] Markedly sclerotic edge.
[b] Variable but not markedly sclerotic edge.
[c] Frequently multiple.
[d] Occasionally multiple.

Mottled or Permeative Destruction

This type of bone destruction most often is due to infection, metastatic disease, or the leukemia-lymphoma group of diseases. It also occurs with primary bone tumors but, in the calvarium, these are rare. Mottled destruction may be solitary or multiple and, when multiple and peppered, the best possibilities are metastatic disease and the leukemia-lymphoma group of diseases (Fig. 5.26A). Multiple areas of destruction in infection are less common for such destruction usually is solitary (Fig. 5.26B). Diffuse, permeative destruction can be mimicked in hyperparathyroidism, where severe demineralization and osteomalacia are the causes of the appearance (Fig. 5.26C).

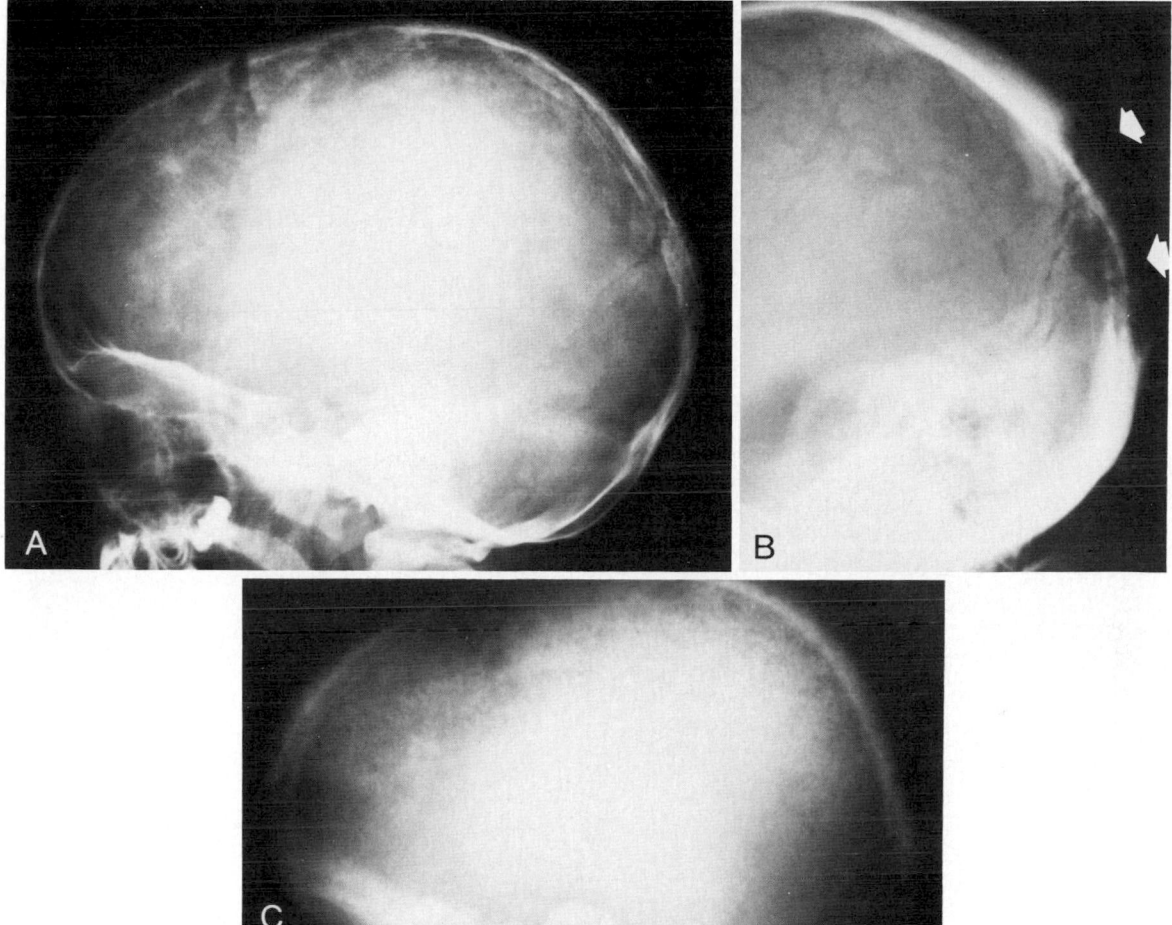

Fig. 5.26. Mottled calvarial destruction. A. Note mottled destruction due to neuroblastoma. B. Permeative destruction due to osteomyelitis-coccidiomycosis (arrow). C. Mottled pseudodestruction secondary to hyperparathyroidism.

Discretely Lytic Destruction

With this type of destruction, the lesions, once again, may be solitary or multiple. For the most part they are characterized by areas of rather homogeneous lysis, rimmed by varying degrees of sclerosis. However, before embarking on a discussion of such lesions of the skull, it should be appreciated that the commonest radiolucent defects in the calvarium are the normal fontanelles. The anterior and posterior fontanelles are no problem, but the so-called third or accessory parietal fontanelle (2), the lateral fontanelles, and the metopic fontanelle can pose difficulties.

The third or accessory fontanelle occurs in the midline, along the sagittal suture, and above the posterior fontanelle (Fig. 5.27, A and B). This is exactly in the same location that normal, persistent parietal foramina occur (Fig. 5.27C). Probably all of these defects are one and the same and usually are quite symmetric and bilateral. They may be very small or very large. The metopic fontanelle is rather rare, but occurs in the midline, below the anterior fontanelle.

The lateral fontanelles occur at the confluence of the posterior fossa sutures, but seldom are they large enough to cause any diagnostic problem. Furthermore, since the posterior fossa sutures join at their site, they readily are identified as normal structures. Other, discretely lytic, nonpathologic, areas of radiolucency in the skull can be seen with intradiploic venous lakes and pachyonian granulations (Fig. 5.27D). Neither one of these are as common as in adults and, clinically, no masses are associated with these lesions.

As far as **pathologic entities** producing solitary or multiple lytic lesions are concerned, they include conditions such as histiocytosis X, congenital epidermoid inclusion cysts (cholesteatoma), dermoids, osteomyelitis, fibrous dysplasia, leptomeningeal cyst, encephalocele, hyperparathyroidism, and metastatic disease (Table 5.13). A wide variety of these lytic lesions is demonstrated in Figures 5.28 through 5.31. Encephaloceles tend to occur in the midline, most often in the occipital region, and then in the frontal area (see Fig.

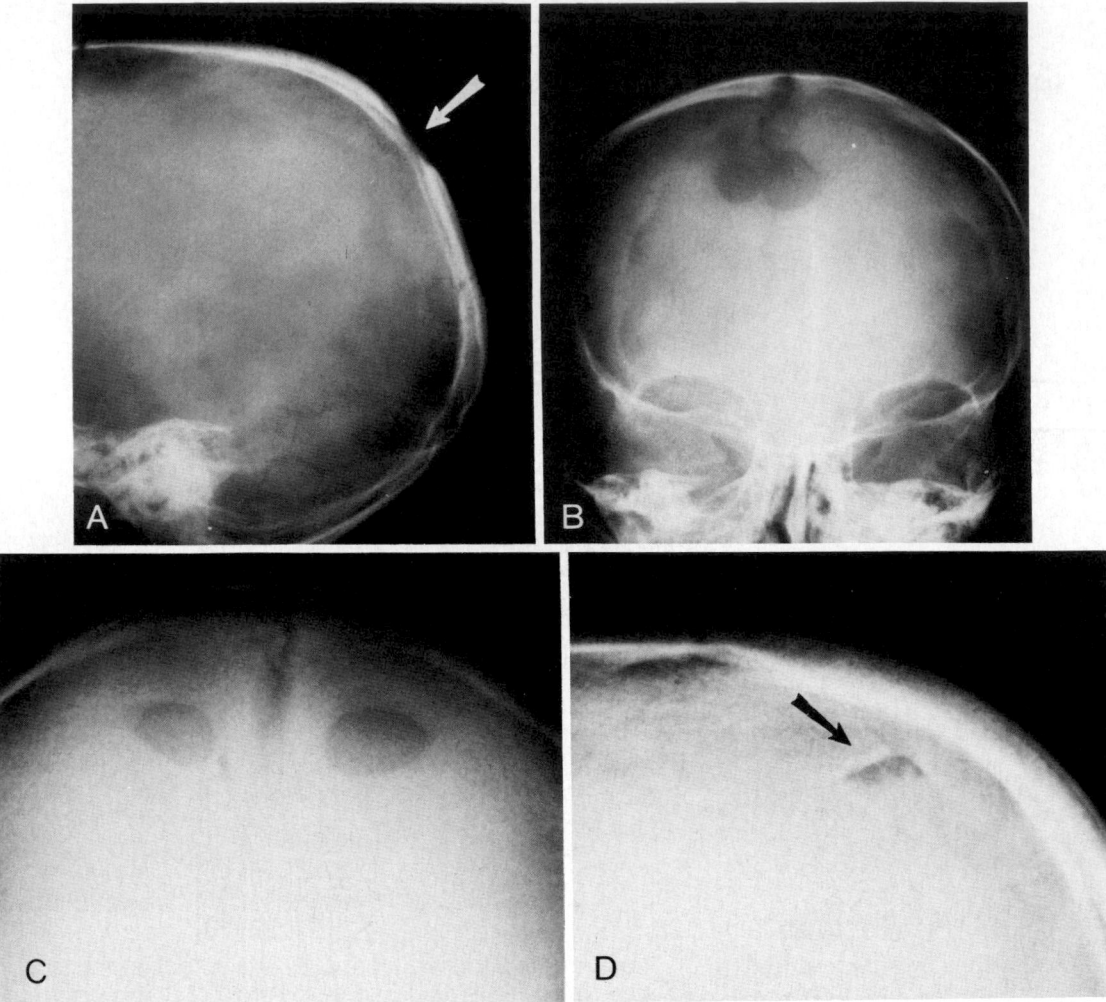

Fig. 5.27.   Solitary calvarial defects. A. Typical location of the so-called accessory or third fontanelle (arrows). B. Frontal view showing same defect. C. Typical posterior parietal foramina. D. Lytic defects in the calvarium due to pachyonian granulation (arrows).

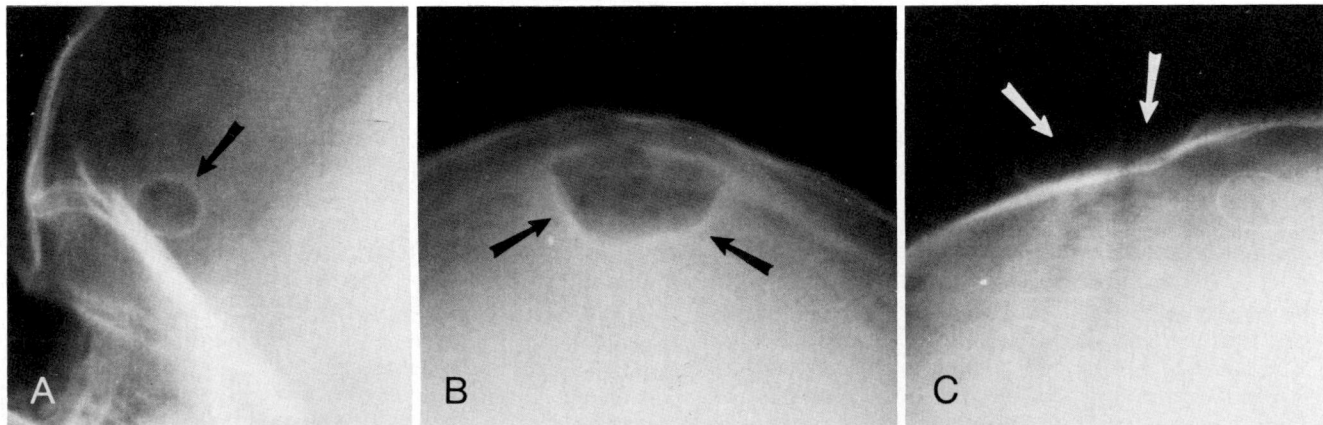

Fig. 5.28.   Solitary lytic lesions of calvarium. A. Typical epidermoid inclusion (congenital cholesteatoma) in frontal bone (arrow). Note sclerosis around its edge. B. Large external table epidermoid (arrows). C. Tangential view showing external table location (arrows).

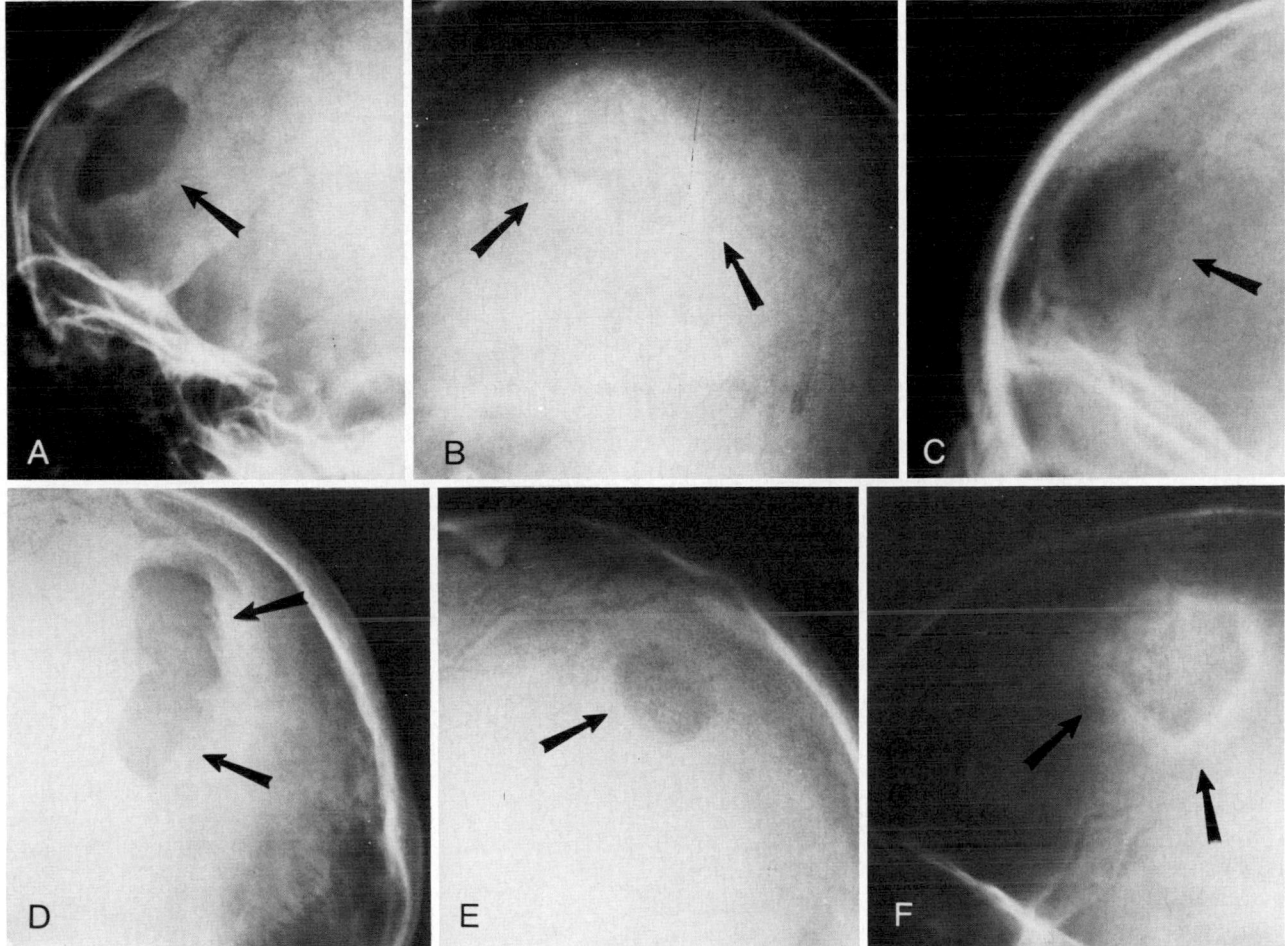

Fig. 5.29. Solitary lytic lesions of calvarium. A. Typical eosinophilic granuloma with no sclerosis around its edges (arrows). B. Vague, lytic area with mild sclerosis in fibrous dysplasia (arrow). C. Solitary lytic area due to metastatic neuroblastoma (arrow). Note absence of sclerosis. D. Typical leptomeningeal cyst (arrows). Note oblong configuration and minimal sclerosis. E. Cranial hemangioma (arrows). In some cases a lattice-work or honeycombed appearance is seen in these lesions. F. Large epidermoid cyst with moderate sclerosis (arrows). This epidermoid was predominantly in the external table.

5.48A). They can, however, occur along the base of the skull and even laterally. Osteomyelitis and metastatic disease can occur anywhere in the skull and so can fibrous dysplasia. Metastatic lesions usually have little sclerosis around their edges (Fig. 5.29C), while sclerosis is variable with fibrous dysplasia (Fig. 5.29B). Some degrees of sclerosis usually is present with osteomyelitis, while the lesions of eosinophylic granuloma and histiocytosis X usually are extremely radiolucent, sharp-edged, and not rimmed by sclerosis (Figs. 5.29A and 5.31A).

Epidermoid inclusion cysts most commonly occur in the frontoparietal region but can be seen almost anywhere. They are characterized by a definite, sclerotic border and can measure anywhere from 1 to 3 cm in diameter (Fig. 5.28). Leptomeningeal cysts occur at the site of old fractures, where associated meningeal tears allow the arachnoid membranes to herniate

through the fractures. With subsequent normal pulsation of the brain, erosion along the margins of the herniation occurs, and chronic widening, with scalloping, of the fracture line is seen. Eventually, a cyst-like calvarial defect is formed. The defect usually is oval or oblong and peripheral sclerosis is absent or minimal (Fig. 5.29D). Minimal brain herniation through the defect can occur.

Rarer causes of solitary lytic lesions of the calvarium include intraosseous hematoma (trauma, headbangers, hemophilia), hemangioma (Fig. 5.29E) (may be honeycombed radiolucency), congenital syphilis, sarcoidosis, neurofibromatosis (idiopathic defect along lambdoid suture) (3) (Fig. 5.30A), primary bone tumor, scalp tumor or cyst causing erosion of the calvarium, leukemia or lymphoma, congenital dermoid sinus (usually midline in the occiput or frontal region), radiation necrosis, intradiploic ectopic neural tissue,

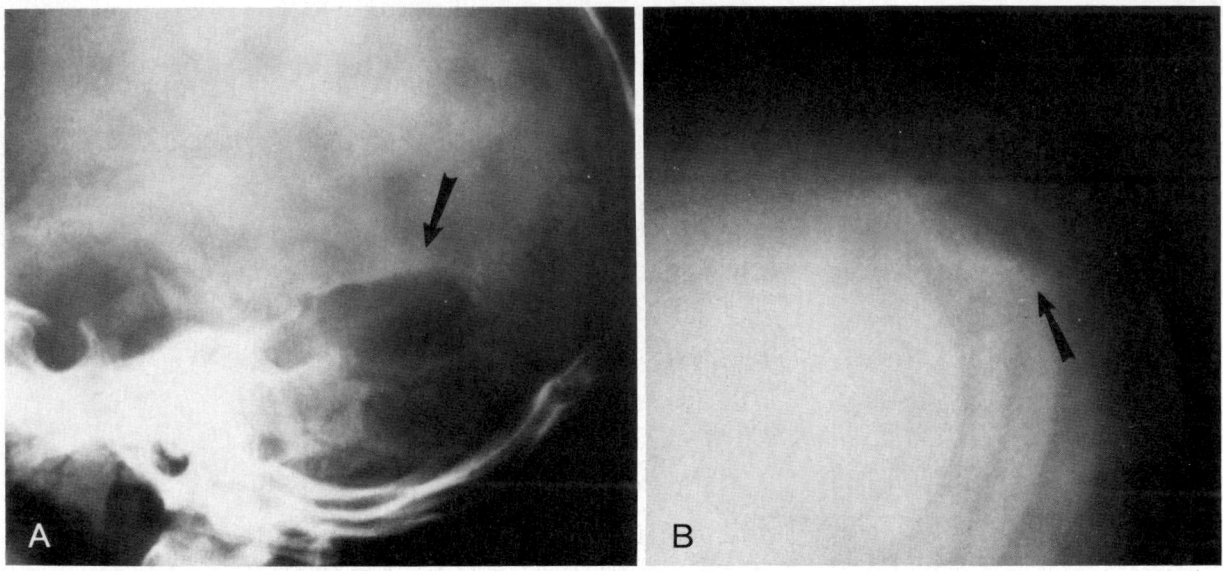

Fig. 5.30. Solitary lytic lesions of calvarium. A. Note characteristic lambdoid defect in neurofibromatosis (arrow). B. Pseudolytic lesion due to healing cephalohamatoma in infant (arrow). In tangential view this lesion can be seen in Fig. 5.10A.

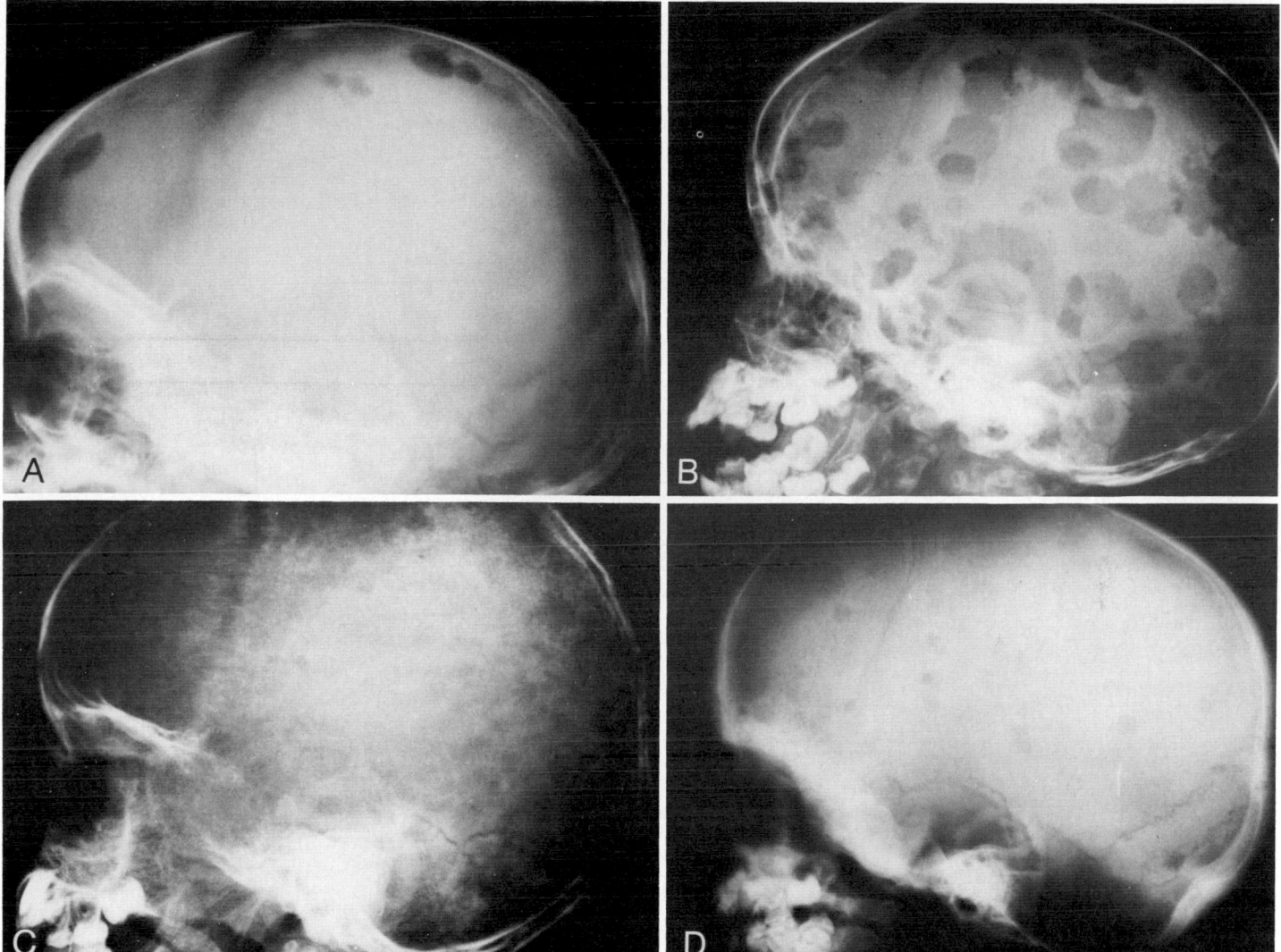

Fig. 5.31. Multiple lytic lesions of calvarium. A. Typical nonsclerotic, punched-out lesions of histiocytosis X. B. More extensive lesions producing geographic skull. Patient with histiocytosis X. C. Multiple areas of moth-eaten destruction in metastatic neuroblastoma. D. Multiple lytic lesions in hyperparathyroidism (renal osteodystrophy). Also note increased density of calvarium. Courtesy Dr. Derek Harwood-Nash, Toronto, Ontario, Canada.

Caffey's disease, and healing cephalohematoma (Fig. 5.30B). Of the foregoing conditions, the most likely to product multiple, discrete lytic lesions are histiocytosis, X, metastatic disease, and leukemia-lymphoma (Fig. 5.31). Rarely, multiple discrete defects occur in hyperparathyroidism (Fig. 5.31D).

References

1. Boyd RDH, Shaw DG, Thomas BM: Infantile cortical hyperostosis with lytic lesions in the skull. *Arch Dis Child* 47:471–472, 1972.
2. Chemke J, Robinson A: Third fontanel. *J Pediatr* 75:617–622, 1969.
3. Handa J, Koyama T, Shimizu Y, Yoneda S: Skull defect involving the lambdoid suture in neurofibromatosis. *Surg Neurol* 3:119–121, 1975.
4. Murphy J, Gooding CA: Evolution of persistently enlarged parietal foramens. *Radiology* 97:391–392, 1970.
5. Neuhauser EBD: Infantile cortical hyperostosis and skull defects. *Postgrad Med* 48:57–59, 1970.
6. Shackelford GD, Shackelford PG, Schwetschenau PR, McAlister, WH: Congenital occipital dermal sinus. *Radiology* 111:161–166, 1974.
7. Swischuk LE: The normal newborn skull. *Semin Roentgenol* 9:101–113, 1974.

INTRACRANIAL CALCIFICATIONS

Intracranial calcifications, much as calcifications anywhere, can be irregular, curvilinear, serpentine, or punctate. In some cases more than one type is seen at the same time, but most often one form prevails. Many times, by utilizing the location and configuration of a calcification, one can determine its most likely etiology (Table 5.14). In this regard, it might be noted that intracranial calcifications now are more easily identified with CT scanning (22) and that many, previously not seen at all on plain films, now commonly are visualized with this modality.

Table 5.14   Intracranial Calcification[a]

Location	Type				
	Irregular	Curvilinear	Linear	Serpentine	Punctate
Pituitary fossa	25, 40	25			
Para and supra sellar	**25**	**25**			
Basal ganglia	2, 13, 20, 41				
Anterior III ventricle	**23, 27**				**37**
Pineal post. III ventricle	11, 27, 38, 39	11?			11?, 38
Convexities	**2–9**	**9**		**18, 19, 22**	
Brain substance (anywhere)	1, 2, 5, 7, 8, 10, 20, 26, 28–32, 34, 36	12		12, 31	12
Periventricular	**1, 2**	**1**			
Entire brain	3, 4?	3			
Falx-tentorium			**14–17, 21**		
Glomi of choroid plex lat vent	39				

[a] 1, Cytomegalic inclusion disease. 2, Toxoplasmosis. 3, Herpes simplex. 4, Rubella. 5, Tuberculosis. 6, Meningitis. 7, Brain infection-abscess. 8, Intracranial bleeding. 9, Subdural hematoma, hygroma. 10, Cerebral infarction. 11, Vein of Galen aneurysm. 12, Other aneurysms. 13, Pseudohypoparathyroidism. 14, Hypervitaminosis D. 15, Hyperparathyroidism. 16, Idiopathic hypercalcemia. 17, Other hypercalcemic states. 18, Folic acid deficiency. 19, Methotrexate therapy. 20, Tuberous sclerosis. 21, Basal cell nevus syndrome. 22, Sturge-Weber disease. 23, Fahr's syndrome. 24, Lissencephaly. 25, Craniopharyngioma. 26, Teratoma. 27, Atypical teratoma (pinealoma). 28, Glioma-astrocytoma. 29, Meningioma. 30, Ependymoma. 31, Hemangioma. 32, Oligodendroglioma. 33, Hemangioblastoma. 34, Metastatic retinoblastoma. 35, Metastatic neuroblastoma. 36, Neuroblastoma (primary). 37, Lipoma corpus callosum. 38, Normal-pineal. 39, Normal-glomi choroid plexus. 40, Pituitary stone. 41, Idiopathic.

Irregular Calcifications

When irregular calcifications are small they may appear punctate, but true punctate calcifications are discussed later. Irregular calcifications most commonly are seen after infection, infarction, or intracranial bleeding, and with intracranial tumors. Less commonly they are seen with metabolic, hypercalcemic states. If irregular calcifications are seen in and around the sella, the most common cause is tumor and most often it is craniopharyngioma (Fig. 5.32A) (2, 17). Occasionally, it can be an atypical teratoma (29) or other tumor, but craniopharyngioma is the most common. With craniopharyngioma, in addition to irregular calcification, curvilinear calcification in the walls of these frequently cystic tumors is common (see Fig. 5.34A).

Irregular calcifications in the basal ganglia can be idiopathic (16), but also are seen with pseudohypoparathyroidism (Fig. 5.32B), tuberous sclerosis (9, 14), cytomegalic inclusion disease (33), toxoplasmosis (21), and radiation therapy. When irregular calcifications are located around the posterior portion of the third ventricle, that is around the pineal gland, almost always they are secondary to atypical teratoma. These tumors also are called ectopic pinealomas, and can coexist with another, similar lesion just anterior and inferior to the third ventricle (29). Physiologic, irregular calcifications of the glomi of the choroid plexuses of the lateral ventricles are not as commonly encountered in children as in adults (Fig. 5.32C) and, rarely, irregular calcifications behind the pineal gland can be seen in a thrombosed vein of Galen aneurysm.

Irregular calcifications, located anywhere in the brain, usually are due to old infection, bleeding, infarction, or brain tumor (Fig. 5.32, D and E). When these calcifications are extremely fine and sand-like, one might consider meningioma, but meningioma is rather rare in children. In addition, meningioma also can calcify in a more irregular pattern (Fig. 5.32E). As far as irregular calcification of other intracranial tumors is concerned, the problem most often is astrocytoma. However, similar calcifications also can be seen in hemangiomas, hemangioblastomas, teratomas (19, 31), intracranial neuroblastoma (13), and along the base of the skull, with chordomas or other cartilaginous tumors of the calvarium. Metastatic disease to the brain seldom calcifies in children, but in infants an exception occurs with retinoblastoma (8).

Irregular calcifications distributed around the walls

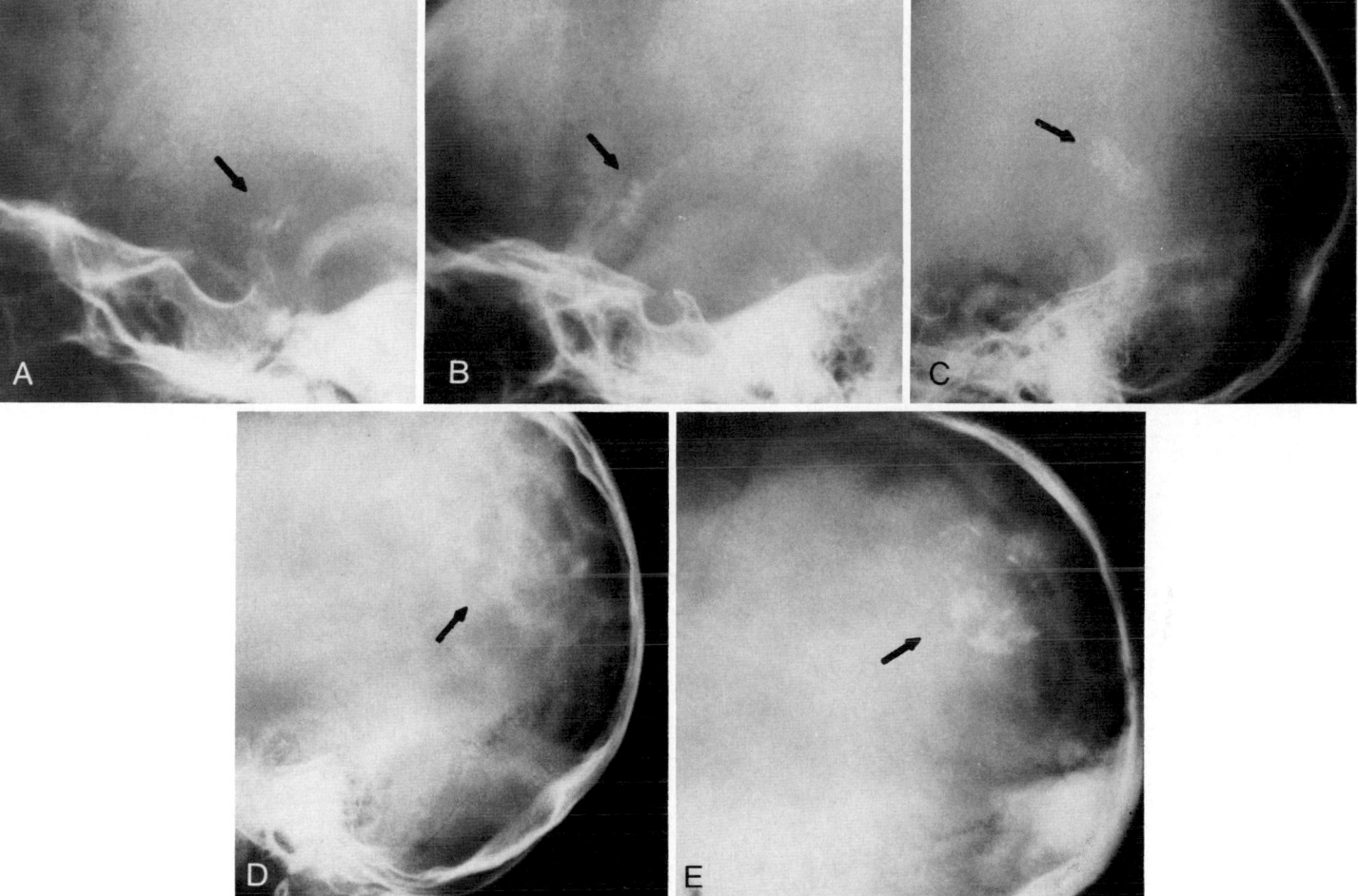

Fig. 5.32. Irregular intracranial calcifications. A. Irregular calcification in craniopharyngioma (arrow). B. Typical irregular calcifications in basal ganglia of patient with pseudohypoparathyroidism (arrow). C. Typical location of normal irregular calcifications in the glomi of the choroid plexus of the lateral ventricles (arrows). These calcifications, on frontal view, are usually bilateral. D. Irregular calcification in old brain infarction (arrow). E. Irregular calcification in parasagittal meningioma.

of the ventricles almost always indicate intrauterine infection, and the commonest cause of this type of calcification is cytomegalic inclusion virus (Fig. 5.33, A and B). Most often, there is associated brain atrophy and a small skull and, although the configuration is not entirely specific for cytomegalic inclusion disease (18), it still should be one's first choice (18, 32). Similar calcifications produced by other intrauterine infections are far less common. Cytomegalic inclusion disease also can cause calcifications elsewhere in the brain substance (33), but the periventricular distribution is most common and characteristic.

In toxoplasmosis, the head may be large or small and, when large, the problem is hydrocephalus. Irregular, flaky calcifications can coexist and can be located almost anywhere (i.e. over the meninges, around the ventricles, in the basal ganglia, along the brain base, etc. (21)—(Fig. 5.33C). Seldom, however, are they as discretely periventricular as in cytomegalic inclusion disease. When very dense calcifications virtually out-

line the external surface of a small, atrophic brain, herpes simplex should be the cause (27). Rubella has been reported to produce a similar configuration (12), but this must be very rare because rubella seldom produces much in the way of intracranial calcification. They have been documented (23, 24), but are rare and focal.

Irregular calcifications over the convexities of the brain, or even along the undersurface of the superior sagittal sinus, most commonly are due to old, subdural hematomas. However, they also can be seen with subdural hygroma, healed meningitis, subdural abscess and, after methotrexate treatment, in leukemia and lymphoma (28). More often, however, the latter calcifications are more serpentine and mimic those of Sturge-Weber disease (6, 20). Ill defined, irregular, calcifications located in the midline, around the anterior third ventricle, have been seen in ferrocalcinosis, or Fahr's disease (3).

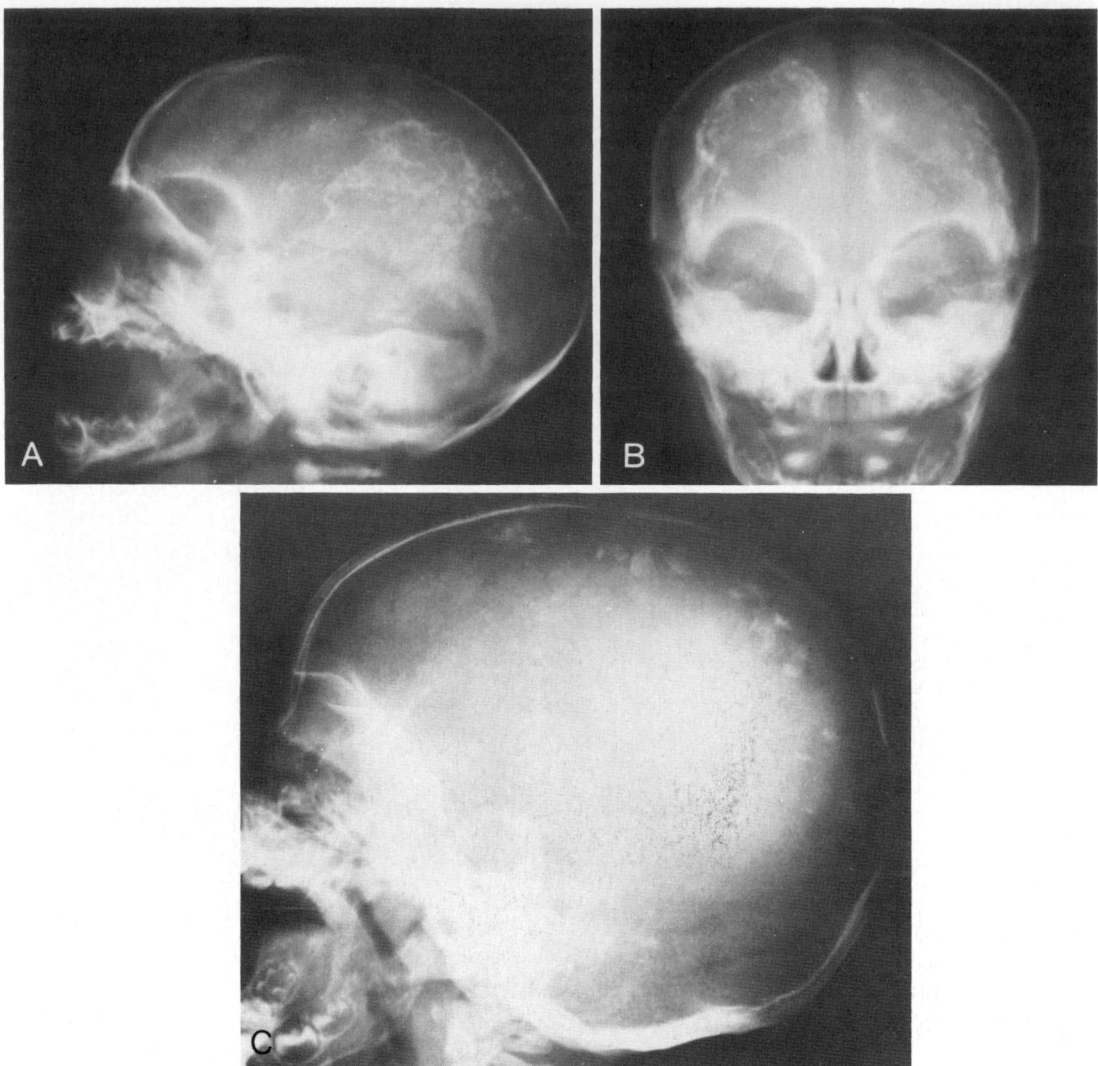

Fig. 5.33. Irregular intracranial calcifications. A. Typical periventricular calcifications of cytomegalic inclusion disease. B. Frontal view demonstrating periventricular configuration. Note that the head is small. C. Typical, scattered, flaky calcifications of toxoplasmosis.

Curvilinear and Linear Calcifications

Curvilinear calcifications almost always occur in a cyst, cystic tumor, or vascular lesion (Fig. 5.34). They are not particularly common in children, except as they occur in cystic craniopharyngioma (Fig. 5.34A). Curvilinear calcifications in aneurysms, either congenital or mycotic, are rare in children (Fig. 5.34B). Similar calcifications over the convexities can be seen with old subdural hematomas, hygromas, or abscesses (Fig. 5.34, C and D).

Purely linear calcifications usually are located in the falx, tentorium, or petroclinoid ligaments, but none are common in children. Indiopathic calcification of the falx, and petroclinoid ligaments is common in adults, but neither is seen very often in children. Indeed, in children, when falx calcification is seen, one could just as easily be dealing with the basal cell nevus syndrome, or a hypercalcemic state such as hypervitaminosis D (Fig. 5.35), hyperparathyroidism, or idiopathic hypercalcemia.

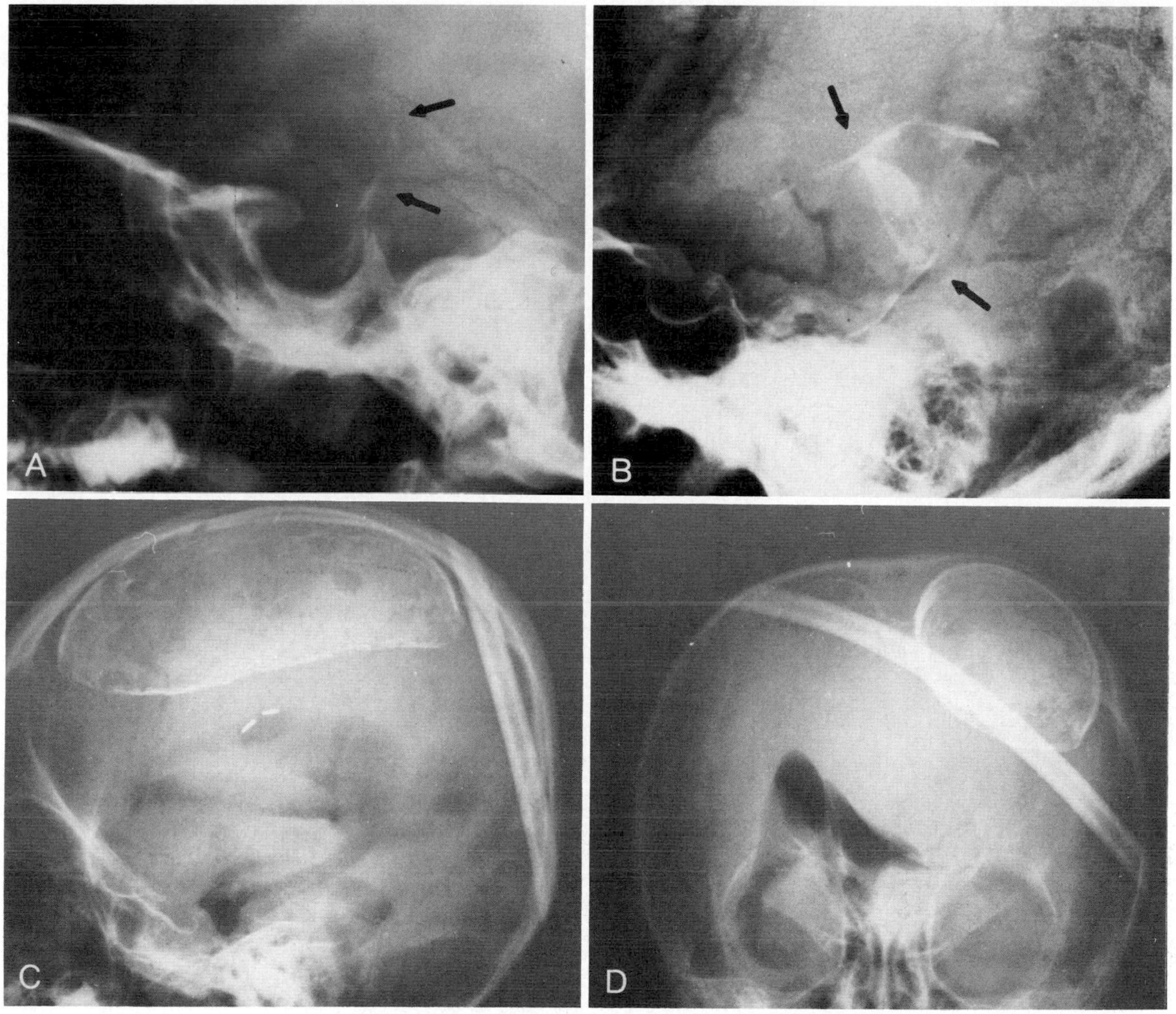

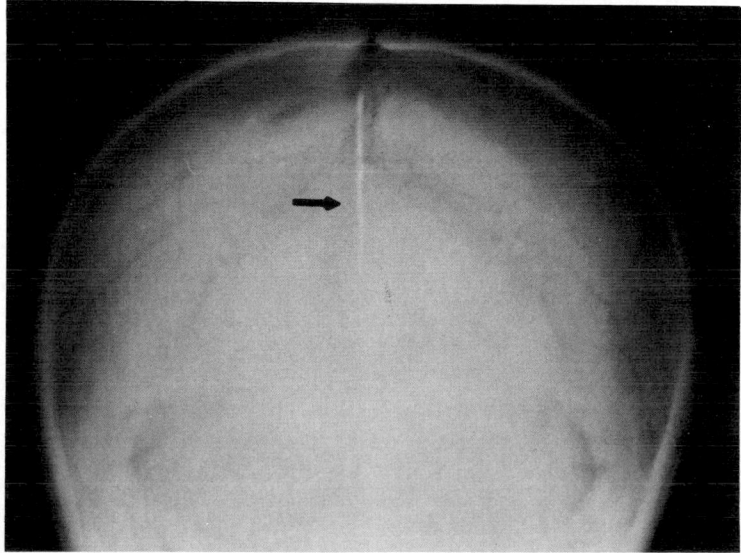

Fig. 5.34. Curvilinear and linear calcifications. A. Typical curvilinear calcification of cystic craniopharyngioma (arrows). B. Calcified congenital aneurysm in young adult (arrows). C. Curvilinear, sheath-like calcification in old subdural hematoma. D. Frontal view of same patient.

Fig. 5.35. Linear intracranial calcification. Calcification of Falx in hypervitaminosis D.

Serpentine Calcifications

These calcifications usually occur within large blood vessels or over the gyri of the brain. Blood vessel calcifications are rare, even in arteriovenous malformations and hemangiomas, and actually when one sees a serpentine calcification in a child, most often the problem is the Sturge-Weber syndrome (7). In this condition, a diffuse subarachnoid angiomatosis leads to pial calcifications over the gyri. Roentgenographi-cally, these calcifications produce double tract serpentine configurations, which are virtually pathogno-monic (Fig. 5.36). Most often they occur in the parietal region. Similar calcifications have been seen in leukemia and lymphoma, after methotrexate therapy (6, 20, 28), and with folic acid deficiency (10). Somewhat serpentine calcifications occasionally are seen in the rare tumor known as oligodendroglioma.

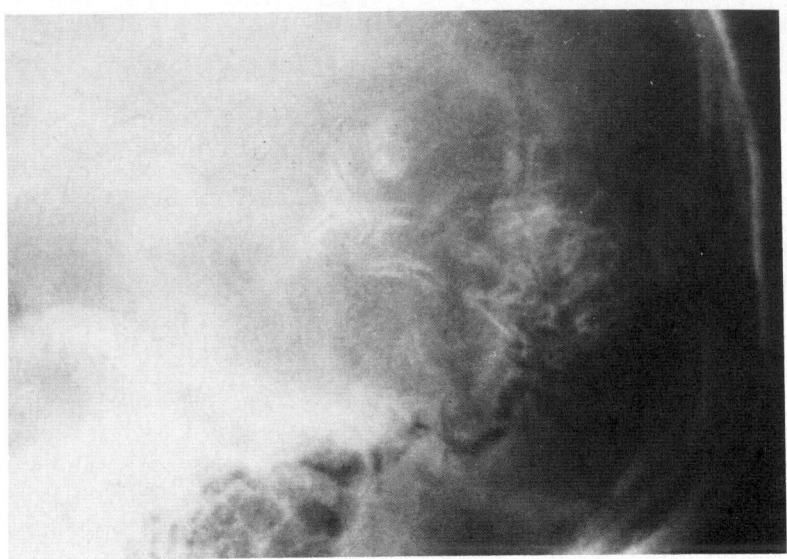

Fig. 5.36. Serpentine calcifications. Typical calcification of Sturge-Weber syndrome.

Punctate Calcifications

The commonest punctate calcification in an adult is the normally calcified pineal gland, but normal pineal gland calcification usually is not encountered in children until after the age of 6 yr (1, 26). Even then it is not particularly common until adolescence (Fig. 5.37A). Larger, similar calcifications in the pineal can be seen with atypical teratoma (Fig. 5.37B), and a small punctate calcification, just anterior to, and above, the pineal gland, occasionally is seen in the calcified splenium of the normal corpus collosum (Fig. 5.37C). Nonspecific punctate calcifications, due to inflammatory disease of the brain, hemorrhage, or infection, are not particularly common (Fig. 5.37D). A small, punctate calcification just anterior to the third ventricle has been documented in congenital lissencephaly (34), a condition characterized by severe mental retardation and lack of normal gyri of the brain. For this reason the condition also is known as congenital agyria. Calcification in the same location occurs with lipoma of the corpus callosum (15) where the presence of an area of fat density surrounding the calcification usually secures the diagnosis. Both these findings can be seen on plain films and with CT scanning.

Small, punctate, or comma-shaped calcifications can be seen with cysticercosis, but the condition, at least in this country, is not common in children. A reverse, small, comma-shaped calcification, seen in the habenular commissure just behind the pineal gland, is not commonly encountered in children. Finally, a small punctate calcification occasionally can be encountered in the pituitary fossa, the so-called pituitary stone (Fig. 5.37E). The finding is of no particular clinical consequence (11).

References

1. Adeloye A, Felson B: Incidence of normal pineal gland calcification in skull roentgenograms of black and white Americans. *Am J Roentgenol* 122:503–507, 1974.
2. Azar-Kia B, Krishnan UR, Schechter MM: Neonatal craniopharyngioma; case report. *J Neurosurg* 42:91–93, 1975.
3. Babbitt DP, Tang T, Dobbs J, Berk E: Idiopathic familial cerebrovascular ferrocalcinosis (Fahr's disease) and review of differential diagnosis of intracranial calcification in children. *Am J Roentgenol* 105:352–358, 1969.
4. Barson AJ, Symonds J: Calcified pituitary concretions in the newborn. *Arch Dis Child* 52:642–645, 1977.
5. Boltshauser E, Wilson J, Hoare RD: Sturge-Weber syndrome with bilateral intracranial calcification. *Radiology*

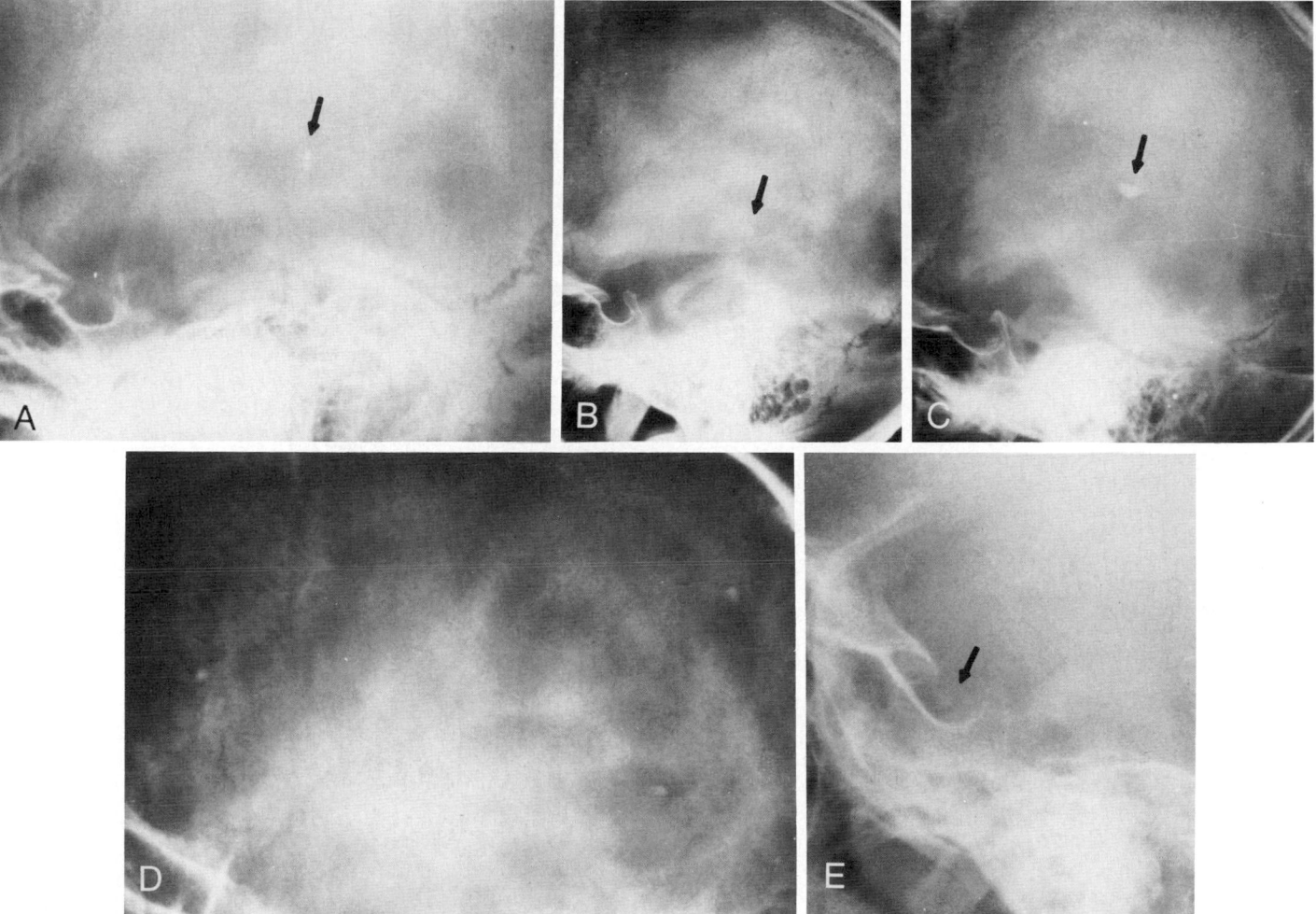

Fig. 5.37. Punctate intracranial calcifications. A. Typical normal pineal calcification in 10-year-old child (arrow). B. Large, pineal calcification in atypical teratoma (ectopic pinealoma). C. Calcification in splenium of normal corpus callosum. D. Punctate calcifications secondary to healed intracranial tuberculosis. E. Punctate calcification in pituitary stone (arrow).

121:767–768, 1976.

6. Borns PF, Rancier LF: Cerebral calcification in childhood leukemia mimicking Sturge-Weber syndrome; report of two cases. *Am J Roentgenol* 122:52–55, 1974.

7. Coulam CM, Brown LR, Reese DF: Sturge-Weber syndrome. *Semin Roentgenol* 11:55–60, 1976.

8. Davis LA, Diamond I: Metastatic retinoblastoma as a cause of diffuse intracranial calcification. *Am J Roentgenol* 78:437–439, 1957.

9. Fitz CR, Harwood-Nash DCF, Thompson JR: Neuroradiology of tuberous sclerosis in children. *Radiology* 110:635–642, 1974.

10. Garwicz S, Mortensson W: Intracranial calcification mimicking the Sturge-Weber syndrome. A consequence of cerebral folic acid deficiency. *Pediatr Radiol* 5:5–9, 1976.

11. Glasser SP, Earll JM: Pituitary "stone." An unusual calcification. *JAMA* 203:367–369, 1968.

12. Harwood-Nash DC, Reilly BJ, Turnbull I: Massive calcification of the brain in a newborn infant. *Am J Roentgenol* 108:528–532, 1970.

13. Horten BC, Rubinstein LJ: Primary cerebral neuroblastoma; a clinicopathological study of 35 cases. *Brain* 99:735–756, 1976.

14. Lagos JD, Holman CB, Gomez MR: Tuberous sclerosis; neuroroentgenologic observations. *Am J Roentgenol* 104:171–176, 1968.

15. List CF, Holt JF, Everett M: Lipoma of the corpus callosum. *Am J Roentgenol* 55:124–134, 1946.

16. Macpherson RI, Hoogstraten J, Tjaden R: Calcification of the basal ganglia in infancy. *J Can Assoc Radiol* 20:159–163, 1969.

17. Majd M, Farkas J, LoPresti JM, Chandra R, Hung W, Lussenhop AJ: A large calcified craniopharyngioma in the newborn. *Radiology* 99:399–400, 1971.

18. Molloy PM, Lowman RM: Lack of specificity of neonatal intracranial paraventricular calcifications. *Radiology* 80:98–102, 1963.

19. Morages A, Vidal MT: Giant congenital intracranial teratoma. *Helv Paediatr Acta* 24:106–110, 1969.

20. Mueller S, Bell W, Seibert J: Cerebral calcifications associated with intrathecal methotrexate therapy in

acute lymphocytic leukemia. *J Pediatr* 88:650–653, 1976.

21. Mussbichler H: Radiologic study of intracranial calcifications in congenital toxoplasmosis. *Acta Radiol Diagn* 7:369–379, 1968.

22. Norman D, Diamond C, Boyd D: Relative detectability of intracranial calcifications on computed tomography and skull radiography. *J Comput Assist Tomogr* 2:61–64, 1978.

23. Peters ER, Davis RL: Cogenital rubella syndrome; cerebral mineralizations and subperiosteal new bone formation as expressions of this disorder. *Clin Pediatr* 5:743–746, 1966.

24. Rowen M, Singer MI, Moran ET: Intracranial calcification in the congenital rubella syndrome. *Am J Roentgenol* 115:86–91, 1972.

25. Sackett GL, Ford MM: Cytomegalic inclusion disease with calcification outlining the cerebral ventricles. *Am J Roentgenol* 76:512–515, 1956.

26. Schey WL: Intracranial calcifications in childhood, frequency of occurrence and significance. *Am J Roentgenol* 122:495–502, 1975.

27. South MA, Tompkins W, Morris R, Rawls WE: Congenital malformation of the central nervous system associated with genital type (type II) herpes virus. *J Pediatr* 75:13–18, 1969.

28. Spehl M, Flament J, Maurus R, Delalieux G, Brihaye J, Cremer N: Diffuse intracranial calcification appearing during the follow-up of acute lymphoblastic leukemia. *Ann Radiol* 17:417–422, 1974.

29. Swischuk LE, Bryan RN: Double midline intracranial atypical teratomas (a recognizable neuroendocrinologic syndrome). *Am J Roentgenol* 122:517–524, 1974.

30. Tabaddor K, Shulman K, Dal Canto MD: Neonatal craniopharyngioma. *Am Dis Child* 128:381–383, 1974.

31. Takaku A, Mita R, Suzuki J: Intracranial teratoma in early infancy. *J Neurosurg* 38:265–268, 1973.

32. Tucker AS: Intracranial calcifications in infants. *Am J Roentgenol* 86:458–461, 1961.

33. Voigt K, Sauer M, Luthardt T: Unusual roentgenological findings in cytomegalic inclusion body disease; large and circumscribed calcereous deposits of the basal ganglia and scattered calcifications of the parieto occipital cortex. *Pediatr Radiol* 3:47–49, 1975.

34. Wesenberg RL, Juhl JH, Daube JR: Radiological findings in lissencephaly (congenital agyria). *Radiology* 87:436–444, 1966.

35. Wilson CB, Roy M: Calcification within congenital aneurysms of the vein of Galen. *Am J Roentgenol* 91:1319–1326, 1964.

INTRACRANIAL RADIOLUCENCIES (AIR AND FAT)

Abnormal intracranial radiolucency is due to either abnormal accumulations of fat or the presence of intracranial gas (1). As far as fat is concerned, almost always, when the finding is seen on plain films, the problem is lipoma of the corpus callosum (3, 5). Characteristically, there is an area of fatty density in the midline, anteriorly (Fig. 5.38), and the lesion is exceptionally well delineated with CT scans. These lipomas can be seen as isolated lesions or in association with other intracranial anomalies. Fat also can be present in dermoids and, now that CT scanning is so popular, previously undetected intracranial epidermoid cysts are being documented more and more (2, 4, 6). Indeed, in some cases fat fluid levels have been demonstrated in these lesions (2, 6).

As far as air in the calvarium is concerned, almost always it is secondary to trauma, either penetrating or with fractures involving the paranasal sinuses or mastoid air cells. The finding is very important to note, especially in trauma cases, and once again is demonstrable both with plain films and CT scanning (Fig. 5.39, A and B). Seldom is intracalvarial gas due to a gas-forming infection. When pneumoencephalography was more popular, iatrogenic intracranial air was a common finding, but iatrogenic gas now is most often postsurgical. Massive air embolus is rare, but can lead to air being seen in the various vessels of the brain.

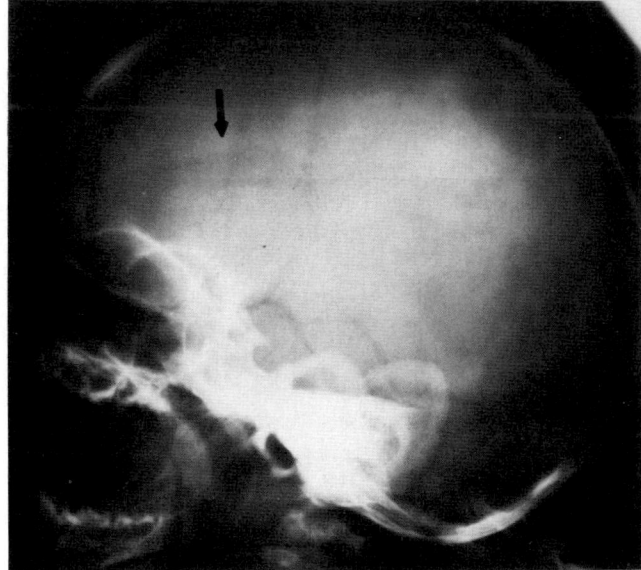

Fig. 5.38. Intracranial radiolucencies. Typical location of fatty density in midline lipoma (arrows).

References

1. Azar-Kia B, Sarwar M, Batnitzky S, Schechter MM: Radiology of the Intracranial Gas. *Am J Roentgenol* 124:315–323, 1975.

2. Cornell SH, Graf CJ, Dolan KD: Fat-fluid level in intracranial epidermoid cyst. *Am J Roentgenol* 128:502–503, 1977.

3. Kushnet MW, Goldman RL: Lipoma of the corpus callosum associated with a frontal bone defect. *Am J Roentgenol* 131:517–518, 1978.

4. Laster DW, Moody DM, Ball MR: Epidermoid tumors with intraventricular and subarachnoid fat: report of two cases. *Am J Roentgenol* 128:504–507, 1977.

5. List CF, Holt JF, Everett M: Lipoma of the corpus callosum. *Am J Roentgenol* 55:124–134, 1946.

6. Maravilla KR: Intraventricular fat-fluid level secondary to rupture of an intracranial dermoid cyst. *Am J Roentgenol* 128:500–501, 1977.

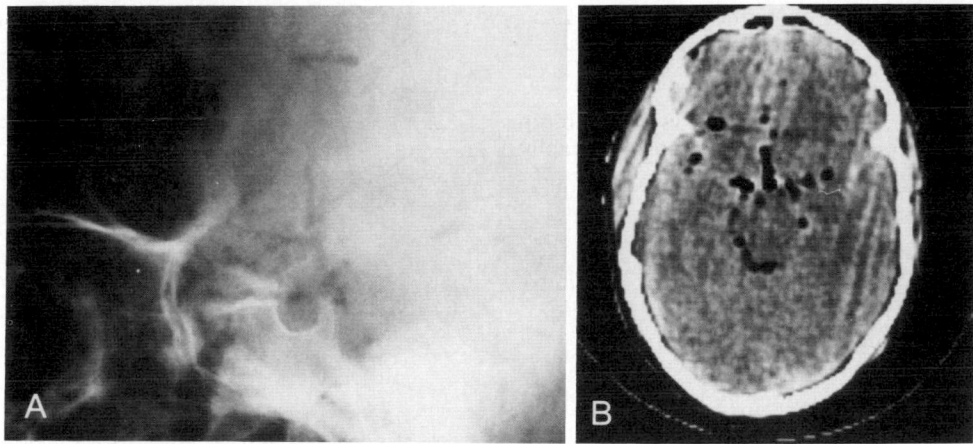

Fig. 5.39. **Intracranial radiolucencies.** A. Scattered radiolucencies due to intracranial air after trauma. B. CT scan demonstrating numerous black areas of intracranial air.

ABNORMALITIES OF THE MASTOID AIR CELLS AND PETROUS BONE

Mastoid Sclerosis and Lysis

The commonest cause of **sclerosis** of the mastoid bone, around the mastoid air cells, is chronic middle ear infection. In such cases, with time, the mastoid air cells can disappear entirely and the bone become very dense and white (Fig. 5.40A). Next most common among the causes of mastoid sclerosis are the various bone dysplasias producing base of the skull thickening (see Table 5.4). Occasionally, one may encounter a sclerotic, primary bone tumor (Fig. 5.40B) and, in addition, sclerosis of the mastoid region can occur after radiation therapy for tumors, and histiocytosis X.

As far as **lysis** or **destruction** of the petrous bone is concerned, the commonest causes are mastoid abscess (Fig. 5.41A) and histiocytosis X (Fig. 5.41B). Abscesses are less common now that antibiotics are so commonplace. Destruction secondary to cholestea-

tomas, with chronic middle ear inflammatory disease is rarely visualized in children (Fig. 5.41C). If the cholesteatomas are large enough, they can be seen on plain films, but usually tomography is required to demonstrate the earliest changes, that is, destruction of the scutum. Indeed, unless performed, many more cholesteatomas will be seen clinically than demonstrated radiographically.

Rarely, a tumor can cause destruction of the petrous bone and, of the primary tumors, the most common in childhood is rhabdomyosarcoma (Fig. 5.41D). Meningioma causing destruction of the petrous bone is rare in childhood and, actually, next most common would be destruction due to leukemia or lymphoma. Metastatic disease always is a possibility, but it is unusual for it to selectively go to the petrous bone.

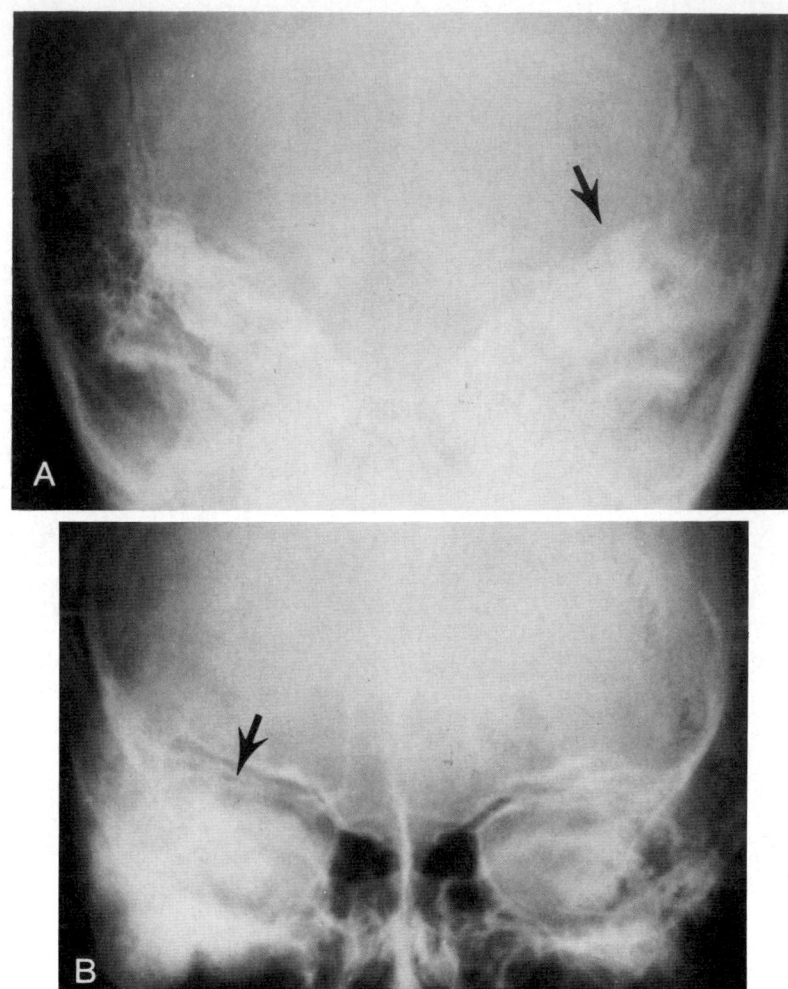

Fig. 5.40.   Mastoid sclerosis. A. Note dense, sclerotic, virtually airless mastoid bone secondary to chronic infection (arrows). B. Marked sclerosis of mastoid bone secondary to primary osteogenic sarcoma (arrows).

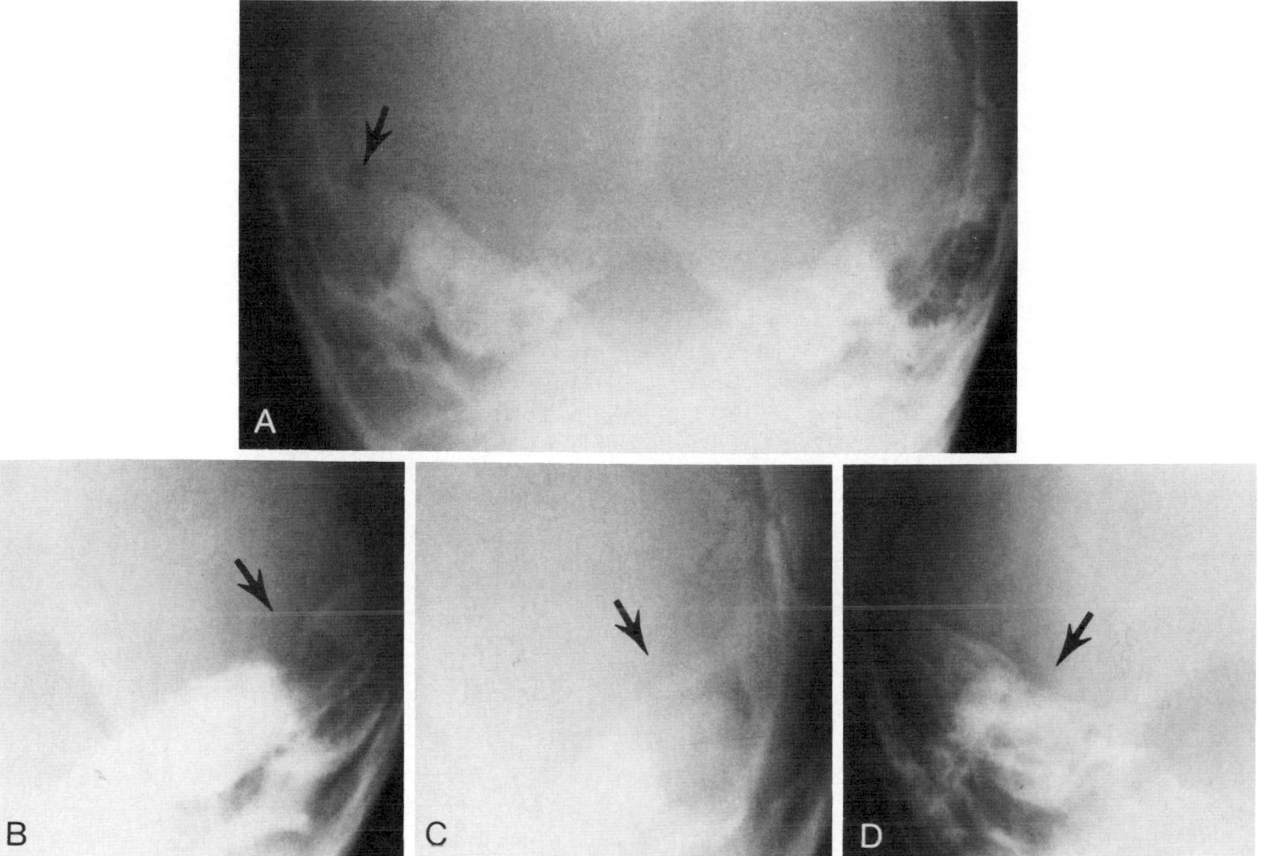

Fig. 5.41. Mastoid destruction. A. Destruction of mastoid bone by mastoid abscess (arrows). B. Mastoid destruction secondary to histiocytosis X (arrow). C. Large cholesteatoma (arrow) producing mastoid destruction. D. Mastoid destruction, somewhat subtle, due to large rhabdomyosarcoma (arrow).

Decreased Aeration of Mastoid Air Cells

The commonest cause of decreased aeration of the mastoid air cells is middle-ear infection. With chronic infection there is inhibition of air cell development and, in long-standing cases, air cells virtually are absent. In such cases the petrous bone also is sclerotic (Fig. 5.42A). However, when the air cells are normally developed, but aeration is decreased, the problem is edema or exudate secondary to acute infection (Fig. 5.42B), or blood associated with a basal skull fracture (Fig. 5.42C). In addition to these causes, any of the conditions producing frank bone destruction, mentioned in the preceding section, can produce associated mastoid air cell underaeration.

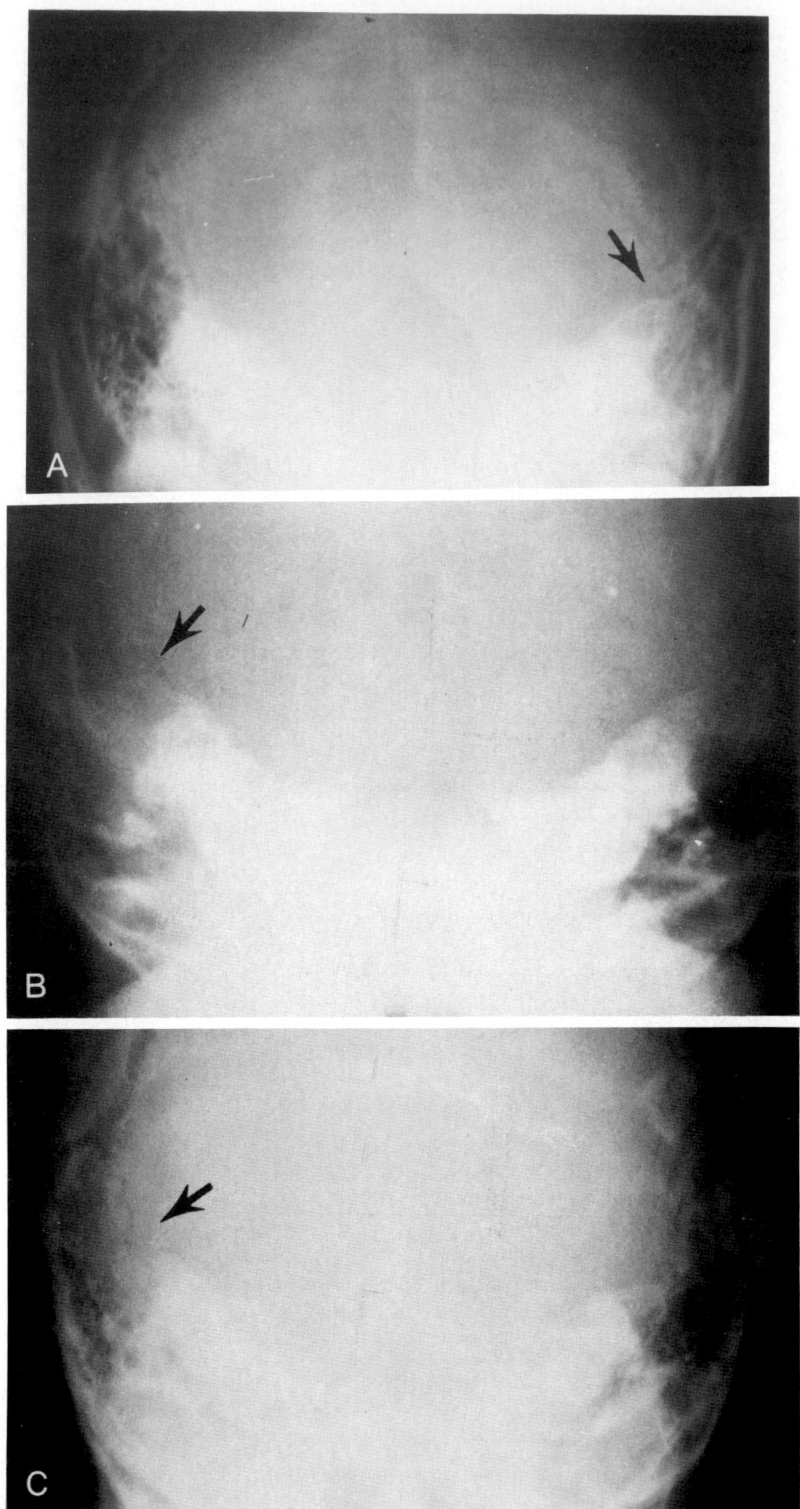

Fig. 5.42. Decrease mastoid air cell aeration. A. Decreased aeration and development of mastoid air cells in chronic middle-ear inflammation (arrow). B. Decreased aeration, on an acute basis, with acute mastoiditis (arrow). C. Markedly decreased aeration of mastoid antrum and air cells (arrow) secondary to bleeding after fracture. Note diastatic lambdoid suture. In some cases the fracture is not visible on standard views.

INTERNAL AUDITORY CANAL ABNORMALITIES

Basically, abnormalities of the internal auditory canals deal with size and contour changes. Smallness of the canals can occur on a congenital basis and with any condition leading to hyperostosis or thickening of the base of the skull (see Table 5.4). Contour changes usually consist of canal enlargement and are seen with intracanalicular tumors or neurofibromatosis. In adults, acoustic neuromas account for most cases of internal auditory canal enlargement, but this tumor is not particularly common in children. Meningiomas also are uncommon in children and, actually, in children, if the canals appear wider than normal, one should first consider normal variation. An unusual cause of enlargement is dural ectasia as seen in neurofibromatosis (1, 2). In such cases, no tumor is present but rather dural ectasia, as part of the generalized mesenchymal abnormality in neurofibromatosis, leads to widening of the canals (Fig. 5.43). Actually, the problem is similar to that seen with posterior scalloping and spinal canal widening in neurofibromatosis (see Fig. 6.12B).

References

1. Hill MD, Oh KS, Hodges FH: Internal auditory canal enlargement in neurofibromatosis without acoustic neuroma. *Radiology* 122:730, 1977.
2. Sarwar M, Swischuk LE: Bilateral internal auditory canal enlargement due to dural ectasia in neurofibromatosis. *Am J Roentgenol* 129:935–936, 1977.

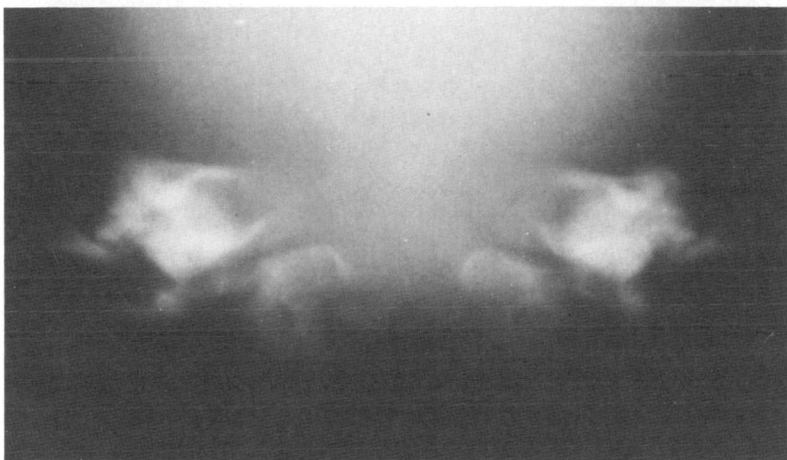

Fig. 5.43.   Enlarged internal auditory canals. Bilateral internal auditory canal enlargement due to dural ectasia in neurofibromatosis.

ABNORMALITIES OF THE ORBIT

Orbital Calcifications

The commonest intraorbital calcification is that seen with retinoblastoma. However, it is not always easy to detect (Fig. 5.44A) and, currently, is more readily demonstrable with CT scanning (1). This is important to note because calcification is said to occur in up to 75% of cases of retinoblastoma (3). Usually, the calcification is granular and irregular. Irregular intraorbital calcifications also occur in ocular dermoids, retrolental fibroplasia (usually in and around the limbus of the lens), infection, trauma, with foreign bodies, and in hypercalcemic states such as hypervitaminosis D, hyperparathyroidism, and idiopathic hypercalcemia (2, 4). In retrolental fibroplasia, the lens itself can be outlined with calcification (Fig. 5.44B).

Finally, it might be noted that, in some patients, with just certain degrees of steepness of the Water's view, the lenses appear denser than the soft tissues. In such cases one should not erroneously believe that calcium is present (Fig. 5.44C).

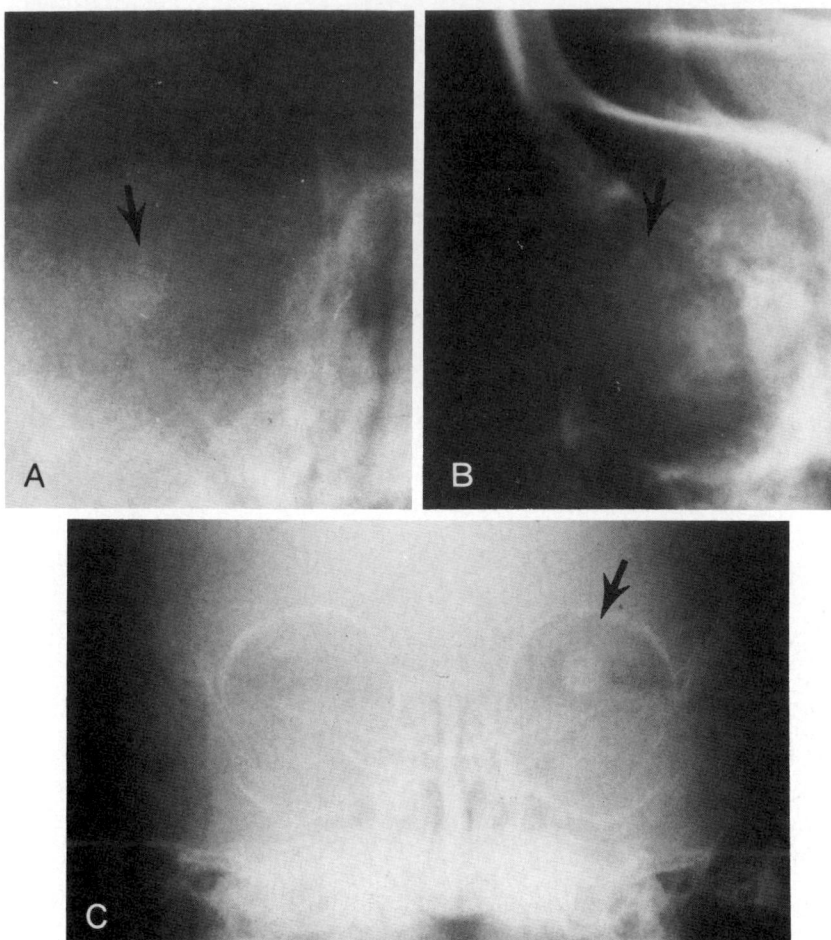

Fig. 5.44. Orbital calcifications. A. Poorly visualized orbital calcification of retinoblastoma (arrow). B. Lens calcification in retrolental fibroplasia (arrow). C. Pseudocalcification of lens on Water's view (arrow). This is an artifact and no calcification is present in such cases.

References

1. Danziger A, Price HI: CT findings in retinoblastoma. *Am J Roentgenol* 133:695–697, 1979.
2. Fleischner FG, Shalek SR: Conjunctival and corneal calcification in hypercalcemia; roentgenologic findings.

N Engl J Med 241:863–865, 1949.
3. Fulton H: A roentgenographic aid in the diagnosis of retinoblastoma. *Am J Roentgenol* 64:735–739, 1950.
4. Taybi H: Ocular calcification and retrolental fibroplasia. *Am J Roentgenol* 76:583–593, 1956.

Orbital Size Abnormalities

The orbit can be too large or too small, but seldom are both orbits enlarged. In terms of unilateral enlargement, the commonest cause is a growing orbital tumor in a young infant (Fig. 4.45A). Thereafter, one should consider orbital enlargement as part of the skeletal dysplasia of neurofibromatosis (Fig. 4.45B). Occasionally, destructive lesions of the orbit can cause slight orbital enlargement, and this can occur with histiocytosis X (Fig. 5.45C).

A unilateral small orbit most commonly is due to congenital underdevelopment of the globe (Fig. 5.46A), and the face usually also is underdeveloped on the same side. However, a small orbit also can be seen after enucleation of the eye (Fig. 5.46B) and in cases where hyperostosis of the calvarium causes smallness of the orbit. This can occur with fibrous dysplasia (Fig. 5.46C), osteopetrosis, Cooley's anemia, etc. Bilaterally small orbits are seen with many of the forebrain hypoplasia syndromes causing hypotelorism (see Fig. 5.47).

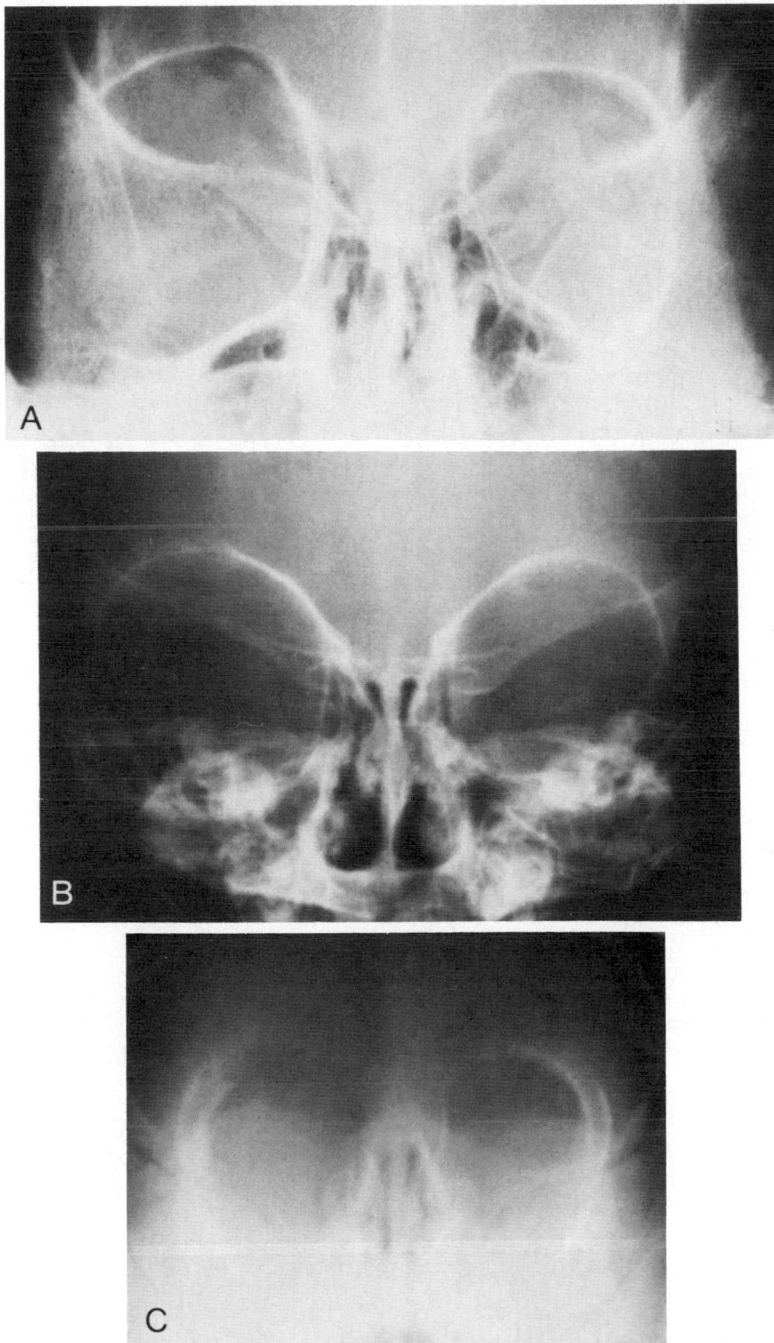

Fig. 5.45. Large orbits. Orbital enlargement on the right secondary to intraorbital hemangioma. B. Orbital enlargement on the right due to skeletal dysplasia of neurofibromatosis. C. Slight orbital enlargement on the right due to bone destruction in histiocytes X.

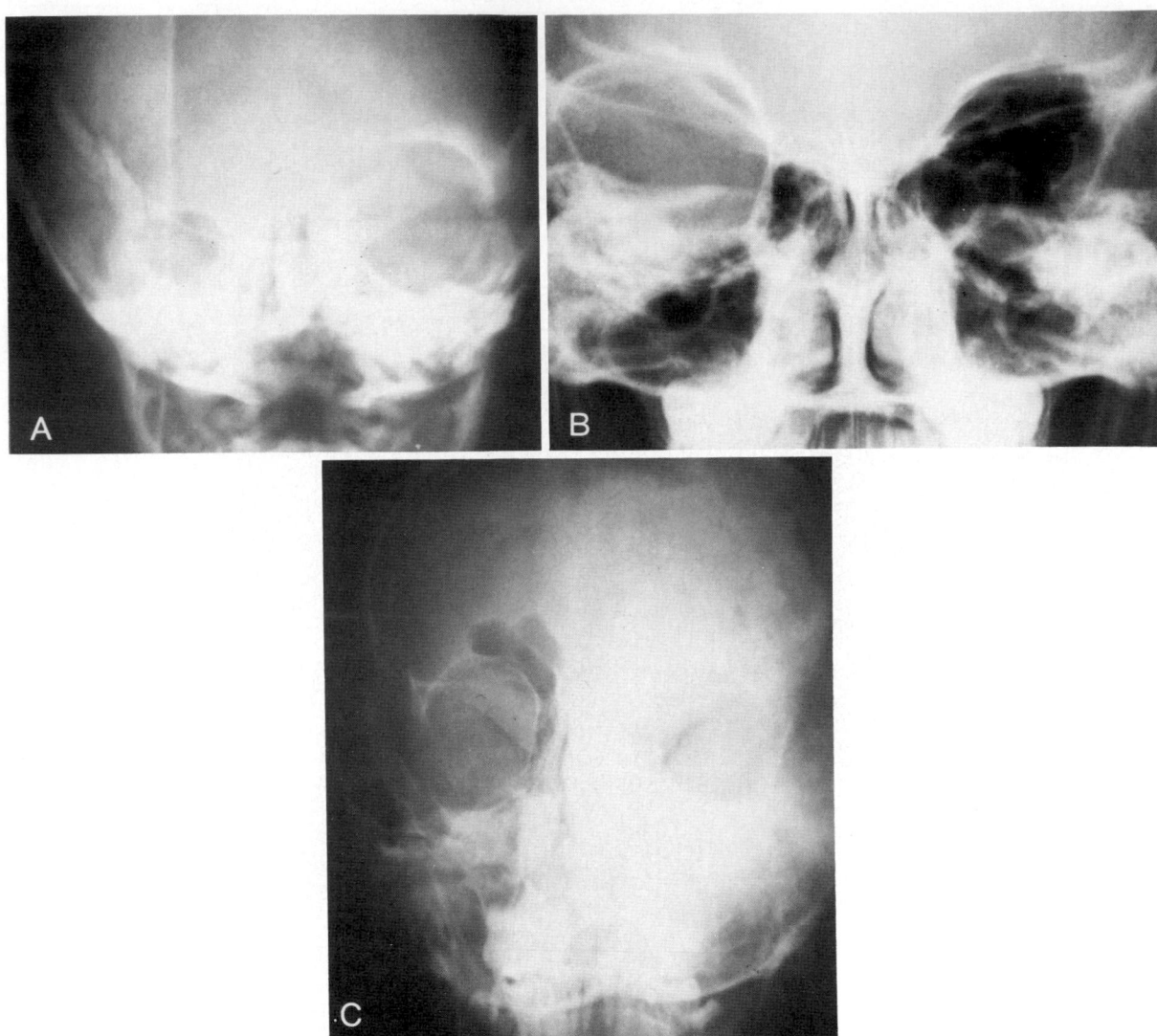

Fig. 5.46.   Small orbits. A. Congenital underdevelopment of the face and orbit on the right. B. Small orbit on the left after enucleation of the eye. C. Small orbit due to hyperostosis, in fibrous dysplasia.

Hypotelorism

Hypotelorism, in its severest form, is seen with arrhinencephally (1), cebocephaly, and the cyclops deformity (Fig. 5.47, A and B). In all of the these conditions, the forebrain is poorly developed and, in addition, the orbits usually are small and round. Hypotelorism also occurs with simple trigoencephaly secondary to premature closure of the metopic suture. In such cases, the close set orbits also have a slanted, worried appearance (Fig. 5.47C). Mild degrees of hypotelorism are seen with sagittal craniosynostosis and in syndromes such as Down's syndrome and the Trisomy 13 syndrome.

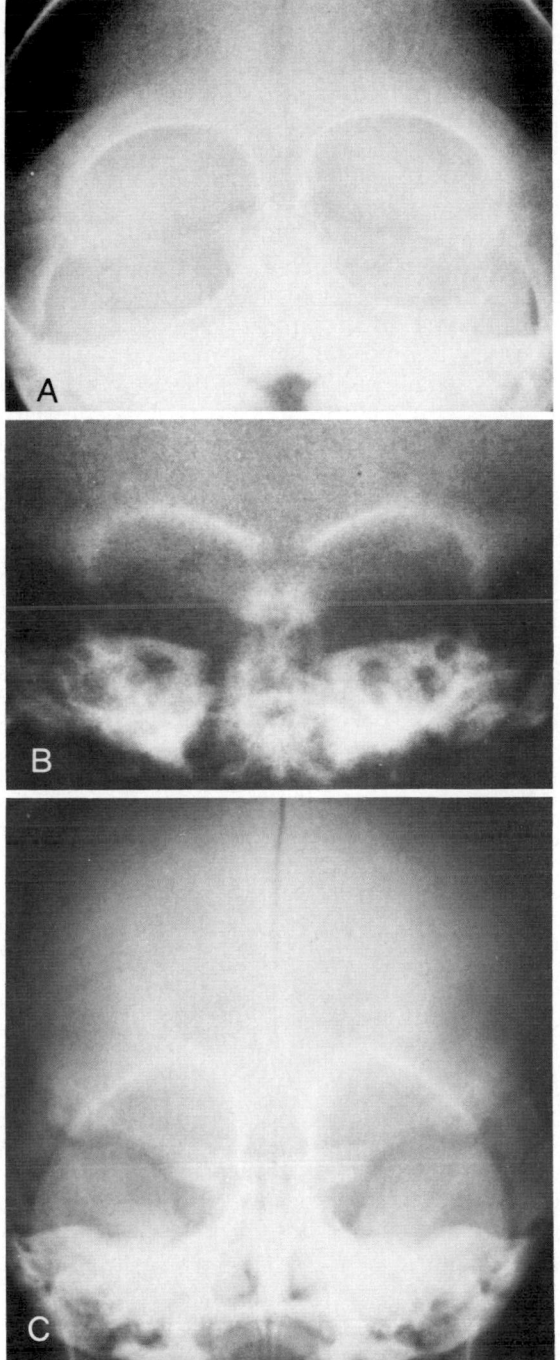

Fig. 5.47. Hypotelorism. A. Severe hypotelorism in arrhinencephaly syndrome. B. More severe hypotelorism, almost a cyclops deformity in another patient with arrhinencephaly. C. Hypotelorism in metopic suture synostosis. Note characteristic slanted appearance of superior orbital margins.

Hypertelorism

Hypertelorism occurs as a normal familial variant in some infants. In such cases, it usually is mild and probably not true hypertelorism. The eyes may appear to be set apart more than usual but, when the bony margins of the orbit are measured, intraorbital distance still is normal. It is the clinical appearance of some of these patients that suggests hypertelorism. True hypertelorism probably is confined to conditions such as frontal encephalocele (Fig. 5.48A), and the median cleft face or Greig's syndrome (3, 4) (Fig. 5.48B), and bony dysplasias such as cleidocranial dysostosis, Crouzon's craniofacial dysostosis, and bilateral coronal premature synostosis. Indeed, mild hyperterlorism occurs in so many syndromes that it is of questionable diagnostic value. Most of these conditions are listed in various syndrome books available today. In the median cleft face syndrome, some patients demonstrate a peculiar bony spicule in the frontal portion of the skull (Fig. 5.48B). Final causes of hypotelorism are nasal tumors, such as fibromas and gliomas, and chronic nasal polyps as seen in cystic fibrosis.

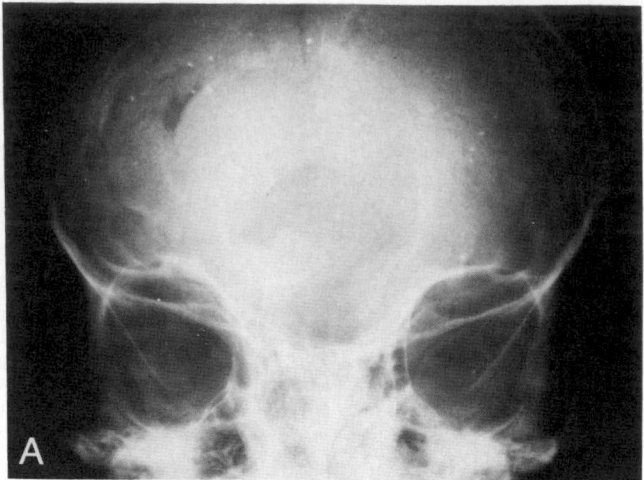

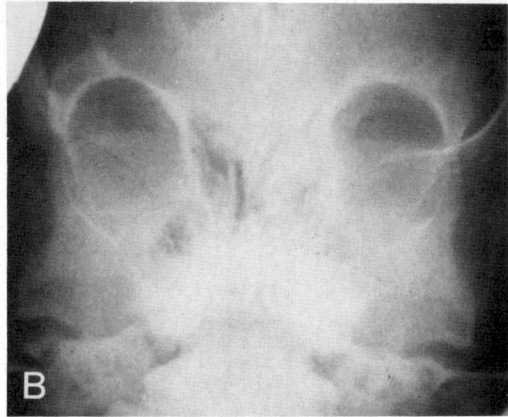

Fig. 5.48. **Hypertelorism.** Hypertelorism in frontal encephalocele. Note bony defect. B. Grieg's syndrome with hypertelorism.

Abnormal Orbital Shapes

Small and large orbits have been discussed previously, and the slanted orbital roof of metopic synostosis has been alluded to in a previous section (see Fig. 5.47C). Irregular deformity of the orbital margins occurs after trauma and after extensive surgery, and exceptionally round orbits occur in the forebrain hypoplasia, arrhinencephaly syndromes (see Fig. 5.47A), and in more advanced cases of cerebral atrophy and mental retardation (Fig. 5.49).

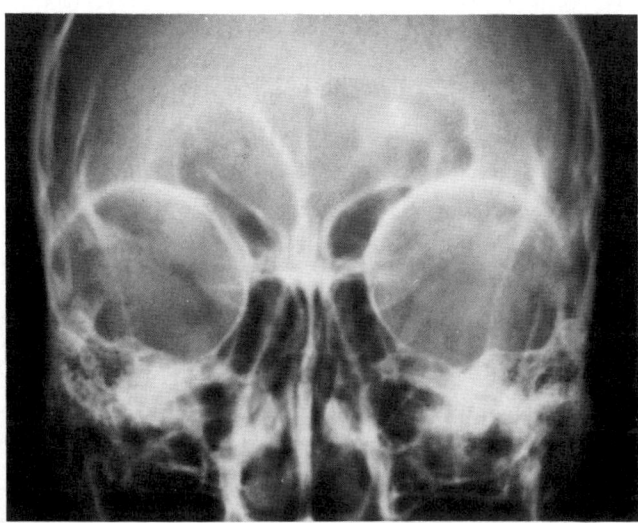

Fig. 5.49. **Round orbits.** Overly round orbits in patient with severe brain atrophy and mental retardation.

Optic Canal Size Abnormalities

Enlargement of the optic canal is almost always secondary to an intracanalicular tumor such as an optic glioma, neurofibroma, or meningioma. In children, optic glioma is most common (Fig. 5.50A), and the finding now is most easily demonstrable with CT scanning. A small optic canal can be seen with optic nerve atrophy (Fig. 5.50B), either congenital or after enucleation of the eye. As with the orbit, lesions leading to hyperostosis of the calvarium also cause smallness of the optic canal (i.e., Cooley's anemia, hypercalcemia, fibrous dysplasia, osteopetrosis, etc.).

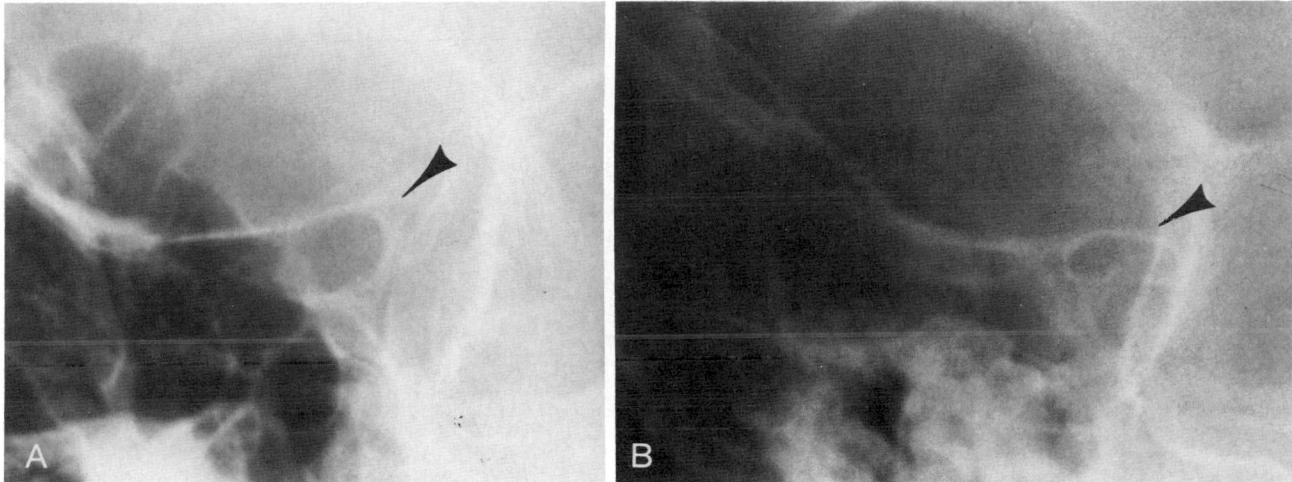

Fig. 5.50. Optic canal size abnormalities. A. Enlarged optic canal (arrow), in patient with optic glioma. B. Small optic canal (arrow) secondary to optic nerve atrophy.

Proptosis

Proptosis can occur with intraorbital tumors, intraorbital inflammations secondary to sinusitis, nonspecific intraorbital soft tissue inflammations, Caffey's disease (inflammatory hyperostosis of the bone), hyperthyroidism, bony tumors of the retro-orbital bones, fibrous dysplasia of the bones, and with hyperostosing abnormalities such as osteopetrosis, Cooley's anemia, etc. Proptosis also can occur with retrobulbar, intraorbital infarcts in sickle cell disease. A peculiar form of proptosis is that which occurs with thinning of the sphenoid bone due to the skeletal dysplasia of neurofibromatosis. Because the bone is absent, exophthalmus often is pulsating in these cases. It might also be noted that proptosis and its causes now are most readily demonstrable with CT scanning.

Intraorbital Air

Intraorbital air almost always is secondary to penetrating trauma (Fig. 5.51A). However, occasionally such air can be mimicked by air outlining the normal palpebral fissures (Fig. 5.51B) or in patients with sunken eyes and prominent supraorbital ridges (Fig. 5.51C).

References

1. Currarino G, Silverman FN: Orbital hypotelorism arhinencephaly and trigonencephaly. *Radiology* 74:206–217, 1960.
2. Keats TE: Ocular hypertelorism (Grieg's syndrome) associated with Springel's deformity. *Am J Roentgenol* 110:119–122, 1970.
3. Kurlander GJ, DeMyer W, Campbell JA: Roentgen of the median cleft face syndrome. *Radiology* 88:473–478, 1967.

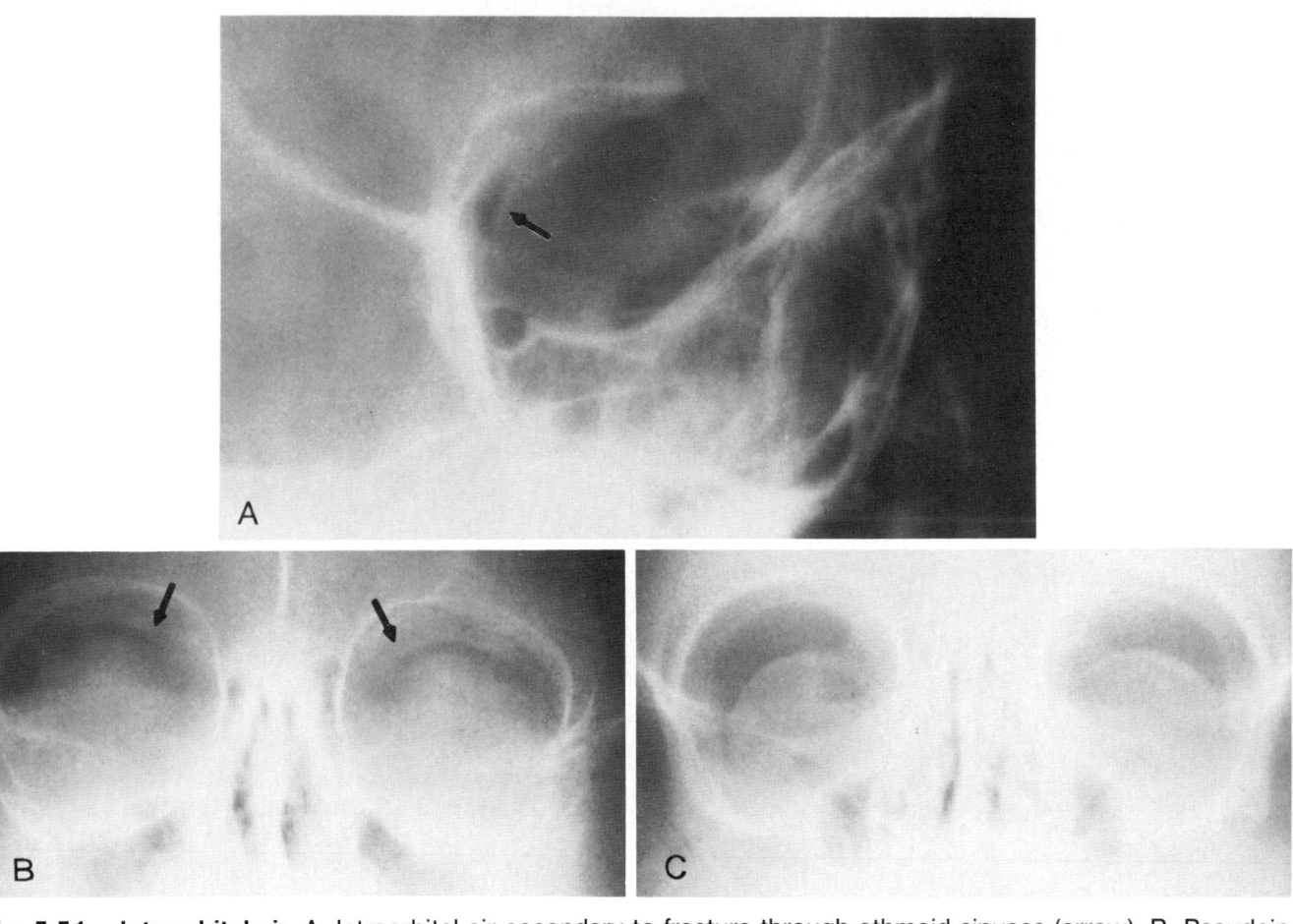

Fig. 5.51.   Intraorbital air. A. Intraorbital air secondary to fracture through ethmoid sinuses (arrow). B. Pseudointraorbital air due to air outlining palpebral fissure (arrow). C. Pseudointraorbital air due to deep set globes and prominent orbital ridges (arrows) in patient with Cockayne's syndrome.

Chapter 6

THE SPINE

ABNORMALITIES OF MINERALIZATION

Generalized Abnormalities

Abnormalities of mineralization consist of (*a*) demineralization (osteomalacia and osteoporosis), (*b*) increased density or osteosclerosis, and (*c*) the **bone in bone vertebra.** As far as causes of generalized demineralization and osteosclerosis are concerned, they are the same as those encountered for other parts of the skeleton. For a list of these conditions, see Tables 4.1 and 4.2. The **bone in bone** appearance of

the vertebral bodies most commonly is seen as a physiologic phenomenon in the newborn (often premature) infant (Table 6.1). In such cases, with the stresses of the perinatal period, enchondral bone formation is temporarily impaired, and a ring of radiolucency develops. However, the ring is not appreciated until normal growth resumes, and a white line of healthy bone is deposited around it (Fig. 6.1A). The finding is comparable to that which occurs with trophic (growth arrest) lines in the long bones and is entirely nonspecific. Occasionally these growth arrest lines can be seen in older children (Fig. 6.1B).

Otherwise, when a bone in bone appearance is encountered, one should consider conditions such as osteopetrosis (Fig. 6.1C), chronic lead poisoning, healing renal osteodystrophy, and occasionally, hypercalcemia. In these conditions, rather than a ring encircling the entire vertebral body, one usually sees two horizontal white lines, at the top and bottom of the body. For this reason the terms **"sandwich vertebra"** and **"Rugger jersey spine"** are utilized.

Table 6.1   Bone-in-Bone and Sandwich Vertebra

Physiologic in premature infant	}	Commonest
Healing renal osteodystrophy[a]	}	Moderately common
Osteopetrosis[a] Chronic lead poisoning[a] Hypercalcemia Chronic illness-trophic lines[a]	}	Relatively rare

[a] Usually sandwich vertebra.

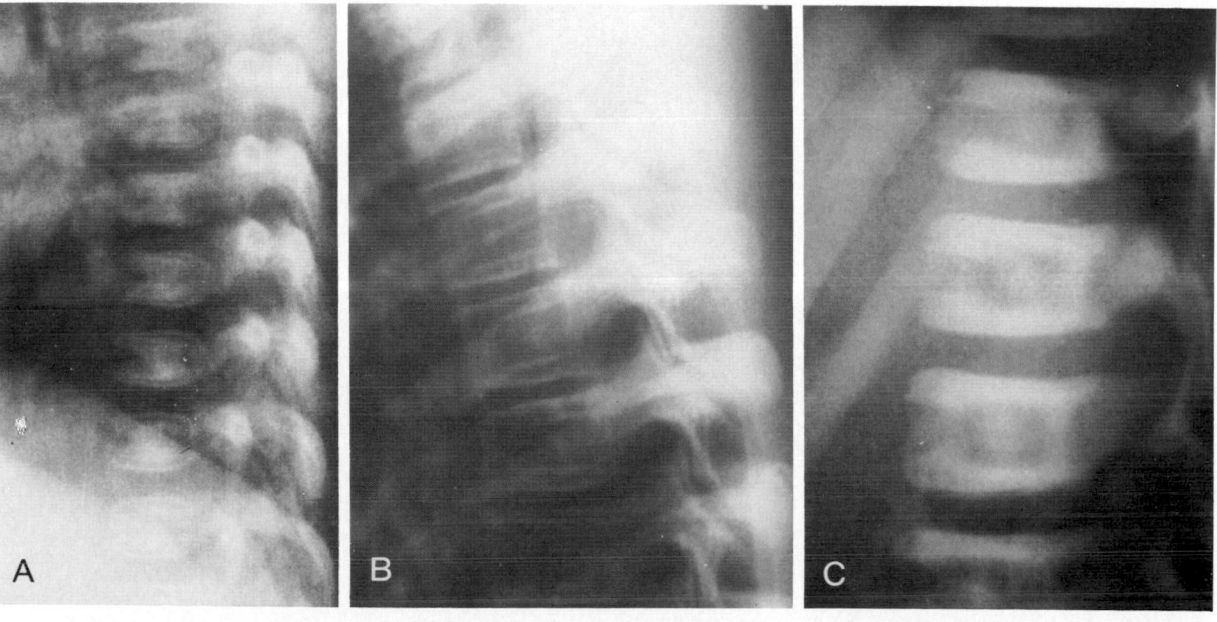

Fig. 6.1   Bone in bone vertebra. A. Typical bone in bone vertebra in newborn infant. B. Bone in bone vertebra due to growth arrest lines in patient with asthma. C. Bone in bone appearance in osteopetrosis.

Focal Sclerosis

Focal sclerosis of a vertebral body, or its posterior elements is not common in children (Table 6.2). Bone islands and osteoblastic metastases are virtually unheard of, and about the only primary malignant bone tumors producing focal sclerosis in the spine are osteogenic sarcoma, Hodgkins disease-lymphoma (3), and Ewing's sarcoma (4) (Fig. 6.2A). The so-called "solitary sclerotic pedicle" (5) also is rare in children and when seen should be due to an osteoid osteoma. Actually, osteoid osteoma, even though relatively rare,

probably is the commonest cause of focal sclerosis in the pediatric spine (Fig. 6.2B). It may be a cause of occult pain or undiagnosed scoliosis (1, 2) and, until sclerosis around the abberant nidus of osteoid tissue becomes apparent, the lesion may elude even the most experienced observer. For this reason tomography, CT scanning, and isotope scans usually are employed. Large osteoid osteomas are termed "giant osteoblastomas" and are more lytic than blastic.

Focal sclerosis of the apophyseal joints, extending into the pedicles, can be seen with congenital abnormalities of joint alignment and articulation. Most often this occurs in a lumbosacral region. Other causes of focal sclerosis include healed osteomyelitis, healed histiocytosis X, healed trauma, and tuberous sclerosis.

Table 6.2 Focal Sclerosis of Vertebra

Osteoid osteoma Sclerosis with apophyseal joint malalignment	Commonest
Bone islands Osteoblastic metastases Ewing's sarcoma Osteogenic sarcoma Solitary sclerotic pedicle Lymphoma Tuberous sclerosis Healed trauma, infection	Rare

References

1. Caldicott WJH: Diagnosis of spinal osteoid osteoma. *Radiology* 92:1192–1195, 1969.
2. Keim H, Reina E: Osteoid Osteoma as a cause of scoliosis. *J Bone Joint Surg* 57-A:159–163, 1975.
3. Mandell GA: Resolution of Hodgkin's induced ivory vertebrae. *Pediatr Radiol* 7:178–179, 1978.
4. Whitehouse GH, Griffiths GJ: Roentgenologic aspects of spinal involvement by primary and metastatic Ewing's tumor. *J Can Assoc Radiol* 27:290–297, 1976.
5. Wilkinson RA, Hall JE: The sclerotic pedicle: tumor or pseudotumor? *Radiology* 111:683–688, 1974.

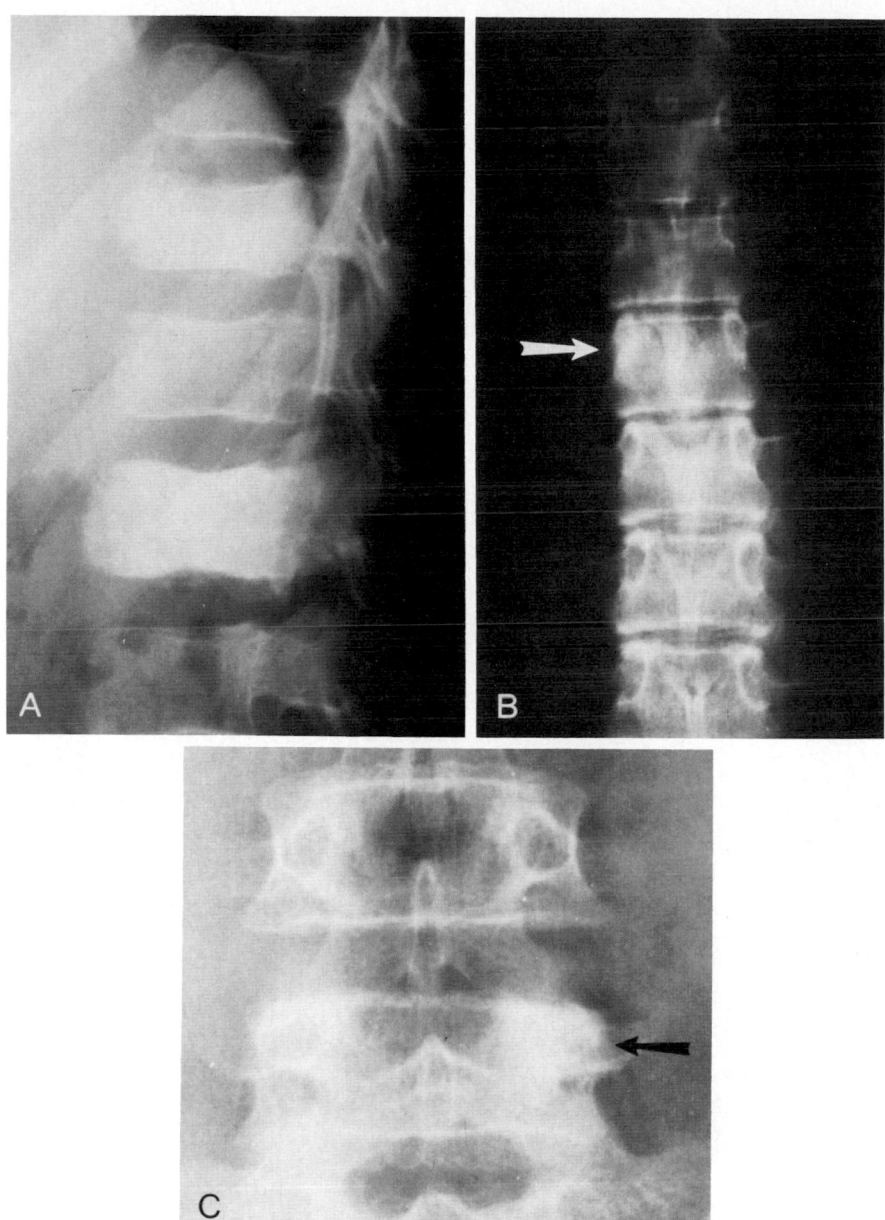

Fig. 6.2. Focal sclerosis of vertebra. A. Multiple sclerotic vertebra in healed metastatic Ewing's sarcoma. B. Slightly sclerotic pedicle (arrow), due to osteoid osteoma. C. Ideopathic, normal, sclerotic pedicle (arrow).

ABNORMALITIES OF THE PEDICLES

Abnormalities of the pedicles consist of (*a*) abnormal sizes and shapes, (*b*) absence or destruction, and (*c*) sclerosis.

Abnormal Shapes

Abnormal shapes of the pedicle include flattened and dysplastic pedicles (Table 6.3), and dysplastic pedicles occur with congenital anomalies such as meningomyelocele, diastematomyelia, Klippel-Feil syndrome, and neurofibromatosis (7). Flattened pedicles occur with intraspinal expanding lesions (i.e., tumor, cyst). In such cases the pedicles are flattened and somewhat concave along their inner aspects (Fig. 6.3A). The deformity may be more pronounced on one side than the other and should be differentiated from normal flattening of the pedicles, most commonly occurring in the upper lumbar region (Fig. 6.3B). Normal pedicles, although flattened, are not eroded or concave along their inner aspects (2) and, overall, comprise the commonest cause of flattened or oval pedicles in childhood.

Table 6.3   Abnormal Pedicle Shapes

A.	Flattened pedicles		
	Normal (lumbar region)	}	Commonest
	Intraspinal expanding tumor	}	Moderately common
	Intraspinal expanding cyst	}	Relatively rare
B.	Dysplastic pedicle		
	Part of other spinal anomaly	}	Commonest
	Neurofibromatosis	}	Moderately common

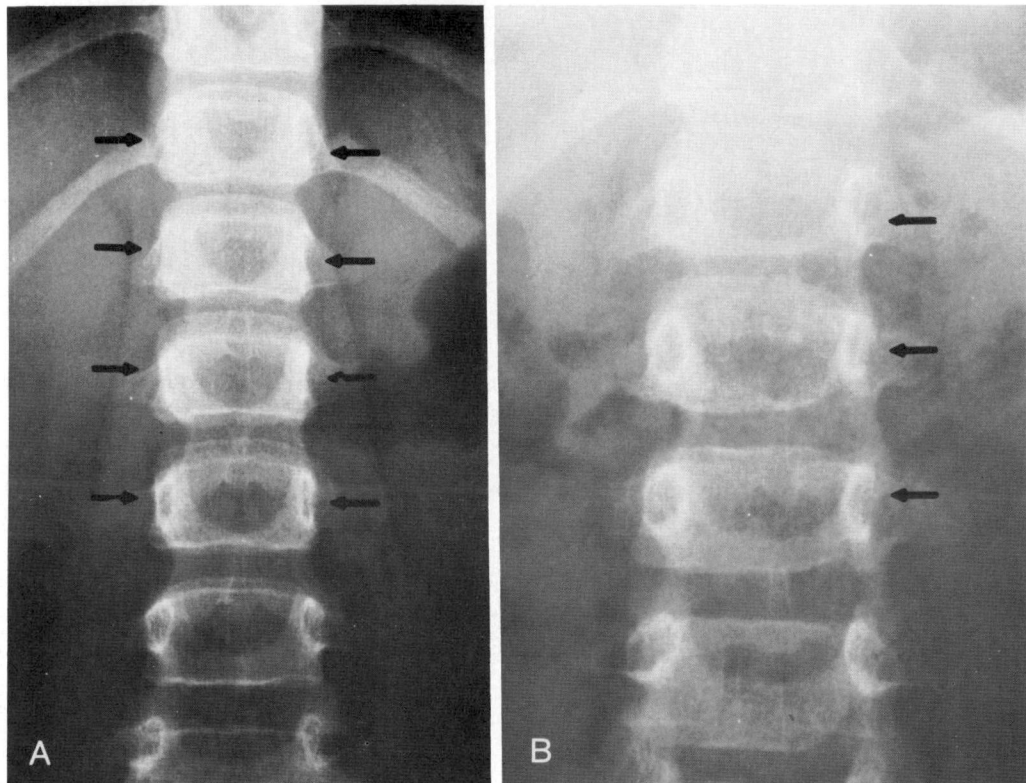

Fig. 6.3.   Flattened pedicles. A. Flat pedicles due to intraspinal tumor (arrows). B. Normal flat pedicles in upper lumbar spine (arrows). Note that they do not have a concave inner aspect. Very often these normal flat pedicles are bilateral.

Abnormal Size

Pedicles can be too small or too large (Table 6.4), but neither deformity is particularly common in children. Small pedicles most often are congenital in origin (1, 8) (see Fig. 6.26B), but can result from hypoplasia secondary to previous radiation therapy of lesions such as Wilm's tumor. Enlarged pedicles can occur on an isolated basis with contralateral arch deficiency and are believed to result from compensatory hypertrophy (6). Enlargement of a number of pedicles on one side, in the absence of arch deficiency, also has been described (4), but the adjacent ribs also appeared expanded and dysplastic, and the problem may have been a disease such as fibrous dysplasia or neurofibromatosis. Pedicles also can enlarge when they are involved by bony tumors such as osteoid osteoma, giant osteoblastoma, hemangioma, lymphangioma, osteochondroma, etc.

Table 6.4 Abnormal Pedicle Size

A. Enlarged pedicle
   Osteoblastoma
   Hemangioma
   Lymphangioma
   Other tumor
   Isolated contralateral arch deficiency
	Relatively rare

B. Small pedicle Congenital with other anomaly	Commonest
Postradiation therapy	Moderately common
Congenital absence or hypoplasia	Relatively rare

Destruction or Absence of a Pedicle

Isolated destruction of a pedicle can occur with metastatic disease, leukemia, lymphoma, and primary bone tumor (Table 6.5). Congenital absence is rare in children (3, 5, 9), and the cervical spine seems to be the most common location for this abnormality. However, it can be seen elsewhere (Fig. 6.4), but in the cervical spine it may be associated with symptoms.

Table 6.5 Destroyed, Absent and Sclerotic Pedicles

Destroyed or absent pedicles Destruction with metastatic disease	Commonest
Destruction with leukemia, lymphoma	Moderately common

Primary bone tumor
   Histiocytosis X
   Congenitally absent pedicle (cervical spine usually)
	Relatively rare

Sclerotic pedicle Osteoid osteoma	Commonest
Stress with abnormal apophyseal joint alignment	Moderately common

Ewing's sarcoma
   Hodgkin's lymphoma
   Osteogenic sarcoma
	Rare

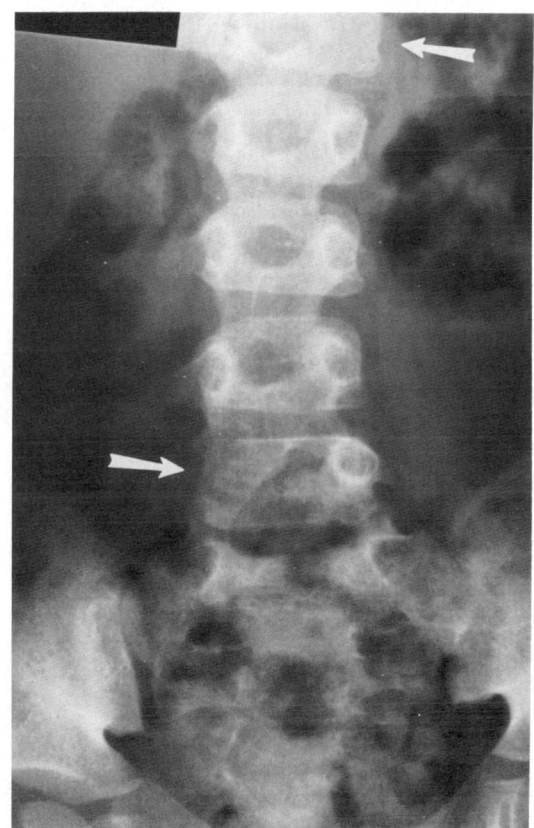

Fig. 6.4. Absent pedicle. Two absent pedicles (arrows) in patient with trisomy 21.

Sclerotic Pedicle

A sclerotic pedicle is not particularly common in the pediatric age group but it does occur (Table 6.5). The commonest cause is osteoid osteoma (see Fig. 6.2B), and the next most common is stress-induced sclerosis secondary to abnormal alignment of apophyseal joints or frank spondylolisthesis. Rarely one can see a sclerotic pedicle with Ewing's sarcoma, Hodgkin's lymphoma, or osteogenic sarcoma.

References

1. Bardsley JL, Hanelin LG: The unilateral hypoplastic lumbar pedicle. *Radiology* 101:315–317, 1971.
2. Benzian SR, Mainzer F, Gooding CA: Pediculate thinning; a normal variant at the thoracolumbar junction. *Br J Radiol* 44:936–939, 1971.
3. Danziger J, Jackson H, Block S: Congenital absence of a pedicle in a cervical vertebra. *Clin Radiol* 26:53–56, 1975.
4. Hart KZ, Brower AC: Unilateral hypertrophy of multiple pedicles. *Am J Roentgenol* 129:739–740, 1977.
5. Kaufman RA, Poznanski AK, Hensinger RN: Congenitally absent thoracic pedicle in a child with rhabdomyosarcoma. *Pediatric Radiol* 9:173–174, 1980.
6. Maldaque BE, Malghem JJ: Unilateral arch hypertrophy with spinous process tilt: A sign of arch deficiency. *Radiology* 121:567–574, 1976.
7. Mandell GA: The pedicle in neurofibromatosis. *Am J Roentgenol* 130:675–678, 1978.
8. Morin ME, Palacios E: The aplastic hypoplastic lumbar pedicle. *Am J Roentgenol* 122:639–642, 1974.
9. Oestreich AE, Young LW: The absent cervical pedicle syndrome: A case in childhood. *Am J Roentgenol Radium Ther Nucl Med* 107:505–510, 1969.

DEFECTS AND ABSENCE OF THE POSTERIOR ARCHES

The commonest defect of the posterior vertebral arches is that due to the various normal synchondroses, which are especially well visualized on oblique views of the cervical spine (Fig. 6.5). Other defects are relatively uncommon but can be congenital or acquired (Table 6.6). Congenital defects occurring in association with anomalies such as meningocele, meningomyelocele, sacral dimple, diastomatomyelia, etc., are straightforward. However, when isolated, they always are a problem in differentiation from fractures. In this regard, the most common such defect is that which occurs in the posterior arch of C$_1$ (6, 9), and the resulting configurations are endless and bizarre (Fig. 6.6, A and B). However, the smooth pointed, or triangular, appearance of the fragments, and wide gap between them should suggest a congenital etiology.

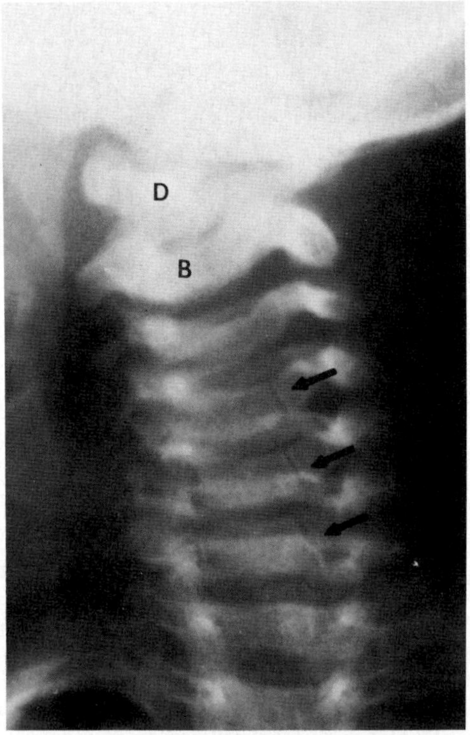

Fractures through the posterior arch of C$_1$ usually produce narrow defects, without sclerotic edges, and are due to hyperextension injuries (Fig. 6.6C). Differentiating the rare congenital defect of C$_2$ from the more common hangman's fracture (4) is more difficult. However, once again congenital defects usually have smooth, somewhat sclerotic edges, an appearance quite different from that seen with fractures (Fig. 6.7, A and B). Furthermore, with flexion and extension, the congenital defect is stable, while the fracture is not.

The defect of spondylolysis (Fig. 6.8A), and subsequent spondylolisthesis, usually seen in the lower lum-

Fig. 6.5. Normal posterior arch synchondroses. Note the normal synchondroses in the posterior arches of the cervical vertebra (arrows). Also note the synchondrosis between the dens (D) and body (B) of C$_2$.

Table 6.6 Posterior Arch Defects or Underdevelopment

Congenital defects C$_1$ Spondylolysis-spondylolisthesis (lower lumbar spine) Normal synchondroses between the body and arches	Commonest
Fractures with hyperextension injury (hangman's fracture C$_2$, other areas) Congenital defects with myelomeningocele, etc.	Moderately common
Congenital defects other than C$_1$ Defects acquired after infection, tumor, etc.	Rare

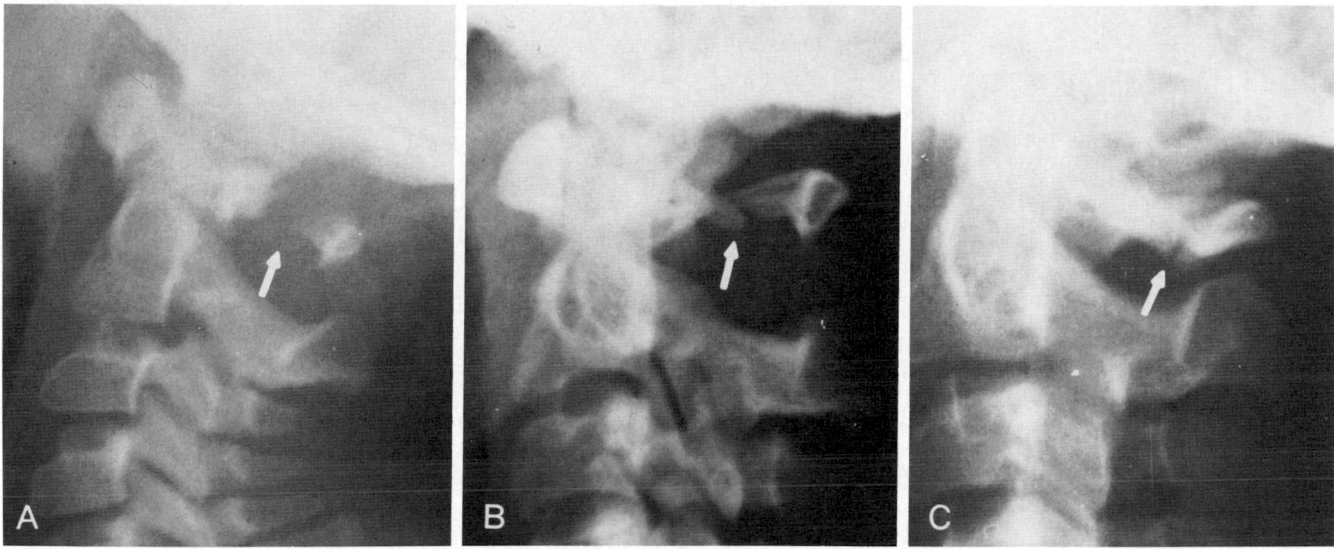

Fig. 6.6 Posterior arch defects of C₁. A. Large congenital defect of C₁ (arrow). B. Smaller defect (arrow), associated with peculiarly shaped bony remnants. C. Thin, discrete defect due to fracture (arrow) secondary to hyperextension injury of C₁.

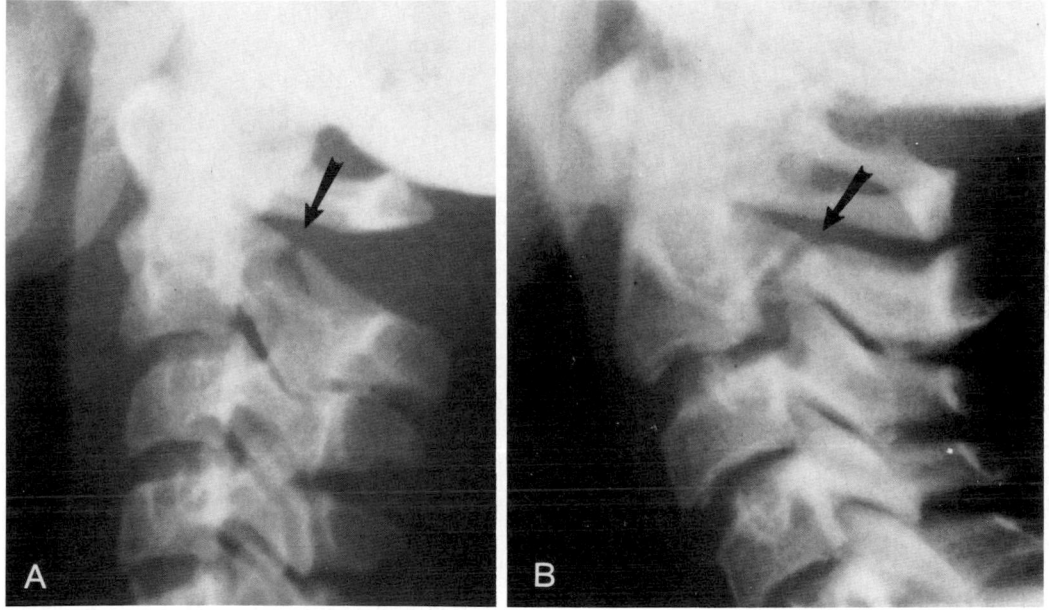

Fig. 6.7. Posterior arch defects of C₂. A. Typical Hangman's fracture (arrow). Note indistinct margins of defect. B. Rare congenital defect (arrow). Note sclerotic margins. On flexion and extension this defect did not change its configuration.

bar spine, generally is considered acquired (2, 7). It is likely that the subclinical stress leads to fracturing, a phenomenon which may be more apt to occur in a neural arch which is congenitally hypoplastic. Spondylolysis at other levels is much less common (1, 3, 5, 8). Overt fractures resulting in the same problem are less common, except at the C₂ level where the classic hangman's fracture occurs. Arch defects secondary to infections, histiocytosis X, tumors, etc., are rare. Ex-

tensive congenital defects of the neural arches can be associated with considerable instability of the neck (Fig. 6.8B).

References

1 Azouz EM, Chan JD, Woo R: Spondylolysis of the cervical vertebrae: report of three cases, with a review of the English and French literature. *Radiology* 111:315–318, 1974.

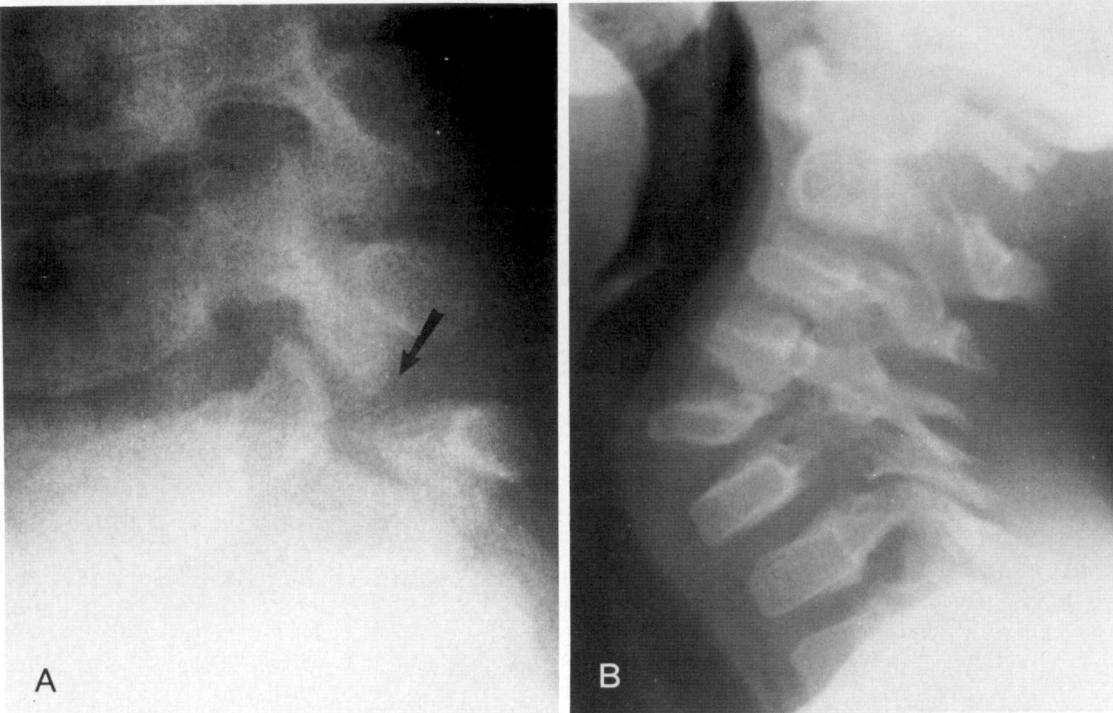

Fig. 6.8. Posterior arch defects. A. Spondylolysis (arrow) of L₅. Extensive congenital defects of neural arches in cervical spine, leading to marked instability and, eventually, cord compression.

2. Beeler JW: Further evidence on the acquired nature of spondylolysis and spondylolisthesis. *Am J Roentgenol* 108:796–798, 1970.
3. Charlton OP, Gehweiler JA Jr, Morgan CL, Martinez S, Daffner RH: Spondylolysis and spondylolisthesis of the cervical spine. *Skeletal Radiol* 3:79–84, 1978.
4. Elliott JM Jr, Rogers LF, Wissinger JP, Lee JF: The hangman's fracture. Fractures of the neural arch of the axis. *Radiology* 104:303–307, 1972.
5. Gehweiler JA Jr, Martinez S, Clark WM, Miller MD, Stewart GC Jr: Spondylolisthesis of the axis vertebra. *Am J Roentgenol* 128:682–684, 1977.
6. Logan WW, Stuard ID: Absent posterior arch of the atlas. *Am J Roentgenol* 118:431–434, 1973.
7. McKee BW, Alexander WJ, Dunbar JS: Spondylosis and spondylolisthesis in children. *J Can Assoc Radiol* 22:100–109, 1971.
8. Moseley I: Neural arch dysplasia of the sixth cervical vertebra, "congenital cervical spondylolisthesis." Case report. *Br J Radiol* 49:81–83, 1976.
9. Sauvegrain J, Mareschal JL: Cranio-cervical malformations in childhood. About 35 cases. *Ann Radiol* 15:263–277, 1972.
10. Swischuk LE, Hayden CK Jr, Sarwar M: The dens-arch synchondrosis versus the hangman's fracture. *Pediatr Radiol* 8:100–112, 1979.

VERTICAL DEFECTS OF VERTEBRAL BODIES

The commonest vertical defect of the vertebral bodies is that due to congenital sagittal cleft vertebra (Table 6.7). On frontal view these defects occur in the midsagittal plane and result in a variety of clefting abnormalities ranging from a simple cleft to a typical butterfly vertebra (Fig. 6.9A). Most often seen on an isolated, sporadic basis, they also are common in many syndromes and, in some rare chondrodystrophies may involve all the vertebral bodies (5). Congenital coronal defects are less common, and of these the commonest are those seen in neonates in the lower thoracic and upper lumbar regions (Fig. 6.9B). These clefts tend to occur more in males than in females and are a common feature of the trisomy 13 syndrome (1, 2, 4, 6). They are believed, by some, to result from notochordal remnants (5), but most likely are just congenital ossification defects.

Acquired vertical defects of the vertebral bodies, for

Table 6.7 Vertical Defects of Vertebral Bodies

Pseudo defect—posterior arch synchondrosis Sagittal cleft vertebra	Commonest
Compression fractures	Moderately common
Coronal cleft vertebra	Relatively rare

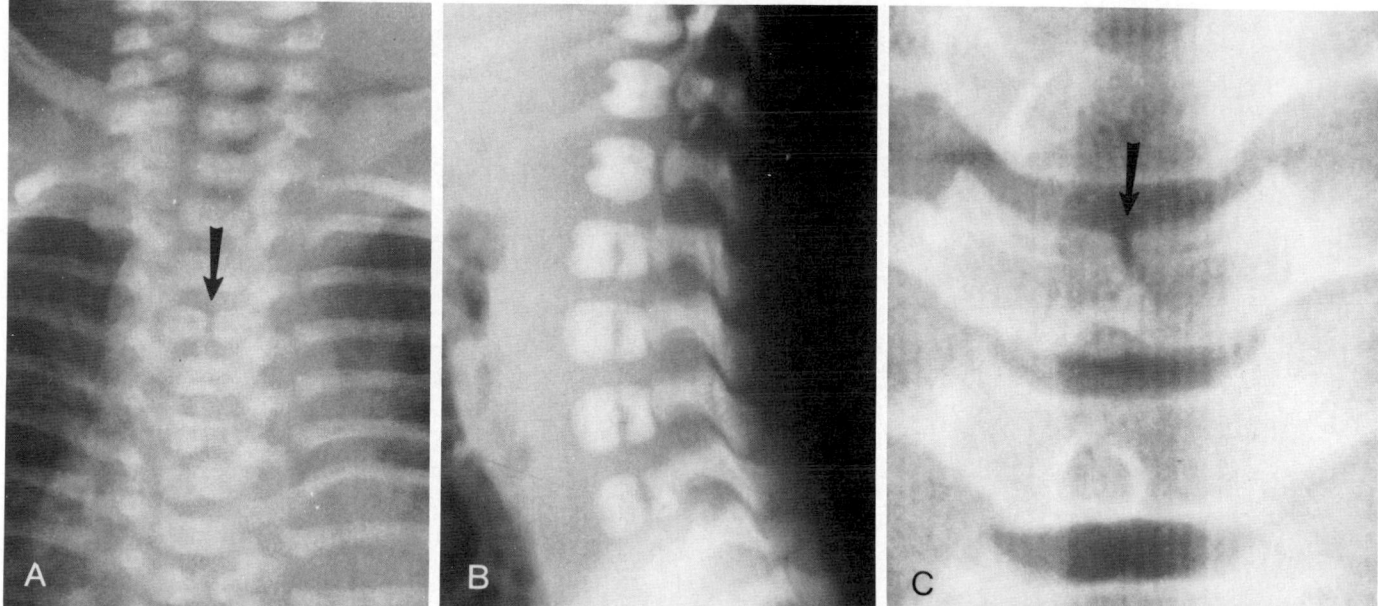

Fig. 6.9. Vertical defects of vertebral bodies. A. Typical defect of sagittal cleft (butterfly) vertebra (arrow). B. Coronal cleft vertebrae in lumbar region (arrow). C. Vertical cleft due to flexion compression fracture (arrow).

the most part, occur with compression fractures resulting from anterior flexion or combined anterior flexion-axial compression injuries (3). In such cases, a vertical, body fracture occurs and is most clearly demonstrable with ordinary or computerized tomography (Fig. 6.9C). In infants, a similar, pseudodefect is produced with superimposition of the posterior, midsagittal synchrondroses over the vertebral bodies.

References

1. Cohen J, Currarino G, Neuhauser EBD: Significant variant in the ossification centers of the vertebral bodies. *Am J Roentgenol* 76:469–475, 1956.
2. Fielden P, Russell JGB: Coronally cleft vertebra. *Clin Radiol* 21:327–328, 1970.
3. Richman S, Friedman RL: Vertical fracture of cervical vertebral bodies. *Radiology* 62:536, 1954.
4. Rowley KA: Coronal cleft vertebra. *J Fac Radiol* 6:267–274, 1955.
5. Swischuk LE: *Radiology of the Newborn and Young Infant*, ed 2. Baltimore, Williams & Wilkins, 1980, p 839.
6. Wollin DG, Elliott GB: Coronal cleft vertebrae and persistent notochordal derivitives of infancy. *J Can Assoc Radiol* 12:781–80, 1961.

PROMINENT CENTRAL VEIN GROOVES

Normally in infants, the anterior central vein groove is readily visible, and in some infants the posterior groove also is seen (3). This is an entirely normal finding (Fig. 6.10A), and even can be seen in some young children. The groove does, however, become more prominent, and persists longer, in the immature spine of hypothyroidism (see Fig. 6.18C). It also is more prominent in osteopetrosis (Fig. 6.10B), and also has been noted to be more prominent in marrow packing disorders such as thalassemia major, sickle cell anemia, Gaucher's disease, leukemia, lymphoma, and metastatic neuroblastoma (1). The relative incidence of these conditions is noted in Table 6.8.

References

1. Mandell GA, Kricun ME: Exaggerated anterior vertebral notching. *Radiology* 131:367–369, 1979.
2. Riggs W Jr, Rockett JF: Roentgen chest findings in childhood sickle cell anemia. A new vertebral body finding. *Am J Roentgenol* 104:838–845, 1968.
3. Wagoner G, Pendergrass EP: The anterior and posterior "notch" shadows seen in lateral roentgenograms of the vertebrae of infants. *Am J Roentgenol* 42:663–670, 1939.

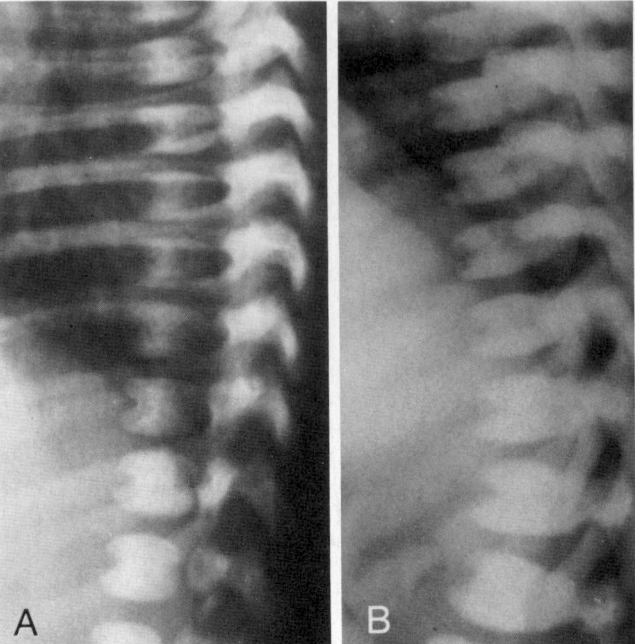

Fig. 6.10. Central vein grooves. A. Note prominent, normal anterior central vein grooves in vertebrae of an infant. The posterior grooves are less visible in the thoracic region. B. Prominent central vein grooves in young child with osteopetrosis.

Table 6.8 Prominent Central Vein Grooves

Normal—infants	}	Commonest
Hypothyroidism	}	Moderately common
Osteopetrosis		
Thalassemia major		
Sickle cell disease		
Gaucher's disease	}	Relatively rare
Leukemia		
Lymphoma		
Metastatic neuroblastoma		

VERTEBRAL DESTRUCTION

Destruction of the vertebra occurs for the same reasons as does bone destruction in general. However, with vertebral body destruction it is important to note whether there is associated disk destruction. Disk destruction is manifest primarily by disk space narrowing and is the hallmark of infection (Fig. 6.11A). With destruction secondary to tumor, primary or secondary, or histiocytosis X, the disk usually is preserved (Fig. 6.11, B and C). It is only with fungal infections such as coccidiomycosis, aspergillosis, and actinomycosis, that destruction of a vertebral body secondary to infection is associated with preservation of the disk space (Fig. 6.11D).

The commonest cause of vertebral destruction is infection, but destruction secondary to metastatic tumor and histiocytosis X is not uncommon. With histiocytosis X, especially marked degrees of vertebral compression and flattening often are seen, and the end result is a plate-like, classic **vertebra plana** (see Fig. 6.14B). Vertebral destruction secondary to primary bone tumors and aneurysmal bone cysts is uncommon. With the latter, often there is preceding bubbly expansion of the compressed vertebral body (see Fig. 6.19).

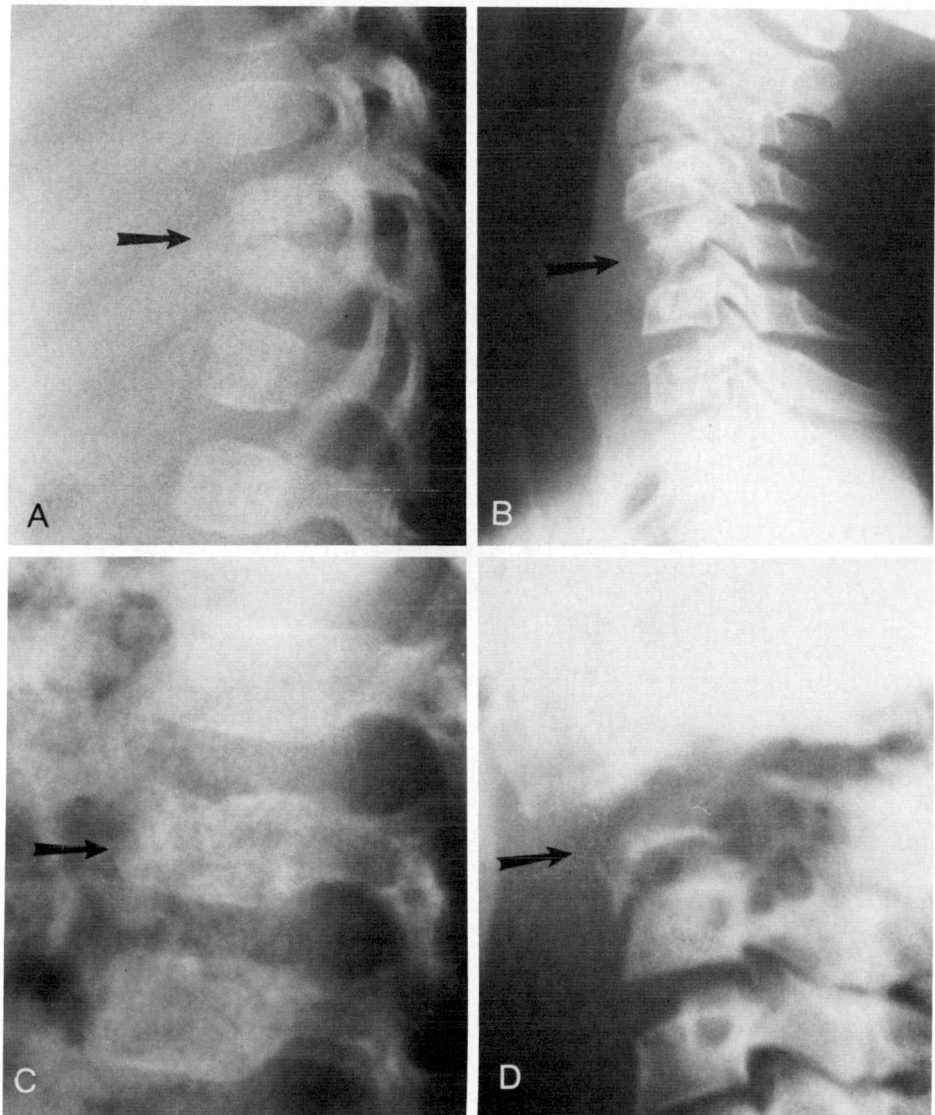

Fig. 6.11. Vertebral destruction. A. Note destruction of two vertebral bodies, and intervening disk space (arrow) due to osteomyelitis. B. Nearly complete destruction of cervical vertebra with relative, if not absolute, preservation of the disk spaces above and below the collapsed vertebral body (arrow). Histiocytosis X. C. Slightly compressed, destroyed vertebral body secondary to metastatic disease (arrow). Note that the disk spaces are preserved. D. Complete destruction of C_2 by actinomycosis (arrow). Note preservation of disk space below.

VERTEBRAL SCALLOPING

The commonest cause of vertebral scalloping is that due to the normal variation (Table 6.9) and most often this occurs along the posterior aspect of the vertebral bodies in the lumbar region (Fig. 6.12A). Less commonly, but certainly not rarely, normal anterior scalloping is seen, in approximately the same area (Fig. 6.12B). However, as opposed to posterior scalloping, which rarely, if ever, extends into the thoracic region, normal anterior scalloping commonly extends into the lower thoracic spine. It does not, however, involve the upper thoracic or cervical spine to any degree.

As far as pathologic scalloping is concerned, most often it is seen posteriorly and is due to some expand-

ing intraspinal lesion (Fig. 6.12C). The lesion may be neoplasm, cyst, syringomyelia, hydromyelia, uncontrolled communicating hydrocephalus (2), or dural ectasia. The most common condition to produce the latter problem is neurofibromatosis (Fig. 6.12C). In these cases it is not an intraspinal tumor which produces the finding, but rather a defect in mesenchymal development leading to dural ectasia and expansion of the spinal canal. In addition to neurofibromatosis, the problem is seen in Marfan's syndrome, Ehlers-Danlos syndrome, and idiopathically (1).

Increased posterior scalloping also occurs with the chondrodystrophies, mainly achondroplasia and its related conditions (Fig. 6.12C). In most of these cases, the spinal canal also is narrower than normal, and it is crowding of the normally growing spinal cord which causes pronounced scalloping of the vertebral bodies. The phenomenon also is seen in diastrophic dwarfism, thanatophoric dwarfism, etc., and in later life, because the spinal canal is narrowed, patients with achondroplasia suffer from early and severe disk compression of the cord and roots.

As far as pathologic anterior scalloping is concerned, the causes are relatively few. It can be seen with adjacent, eroding tumors, destruction of the vertebra by lymphoma or metastatic disease, but most often is seen as an inherent mesenchymal deformity in neurofibromatosis (Fig. 6.13E). Erosions secondary to adjacent aortic aneurysms are uncommon in children.

When both exaggerated posterior and anterior scalloping occur together, a spindle or spool-shaped vertebra results. To a mild degree this can be seen in the chondrodystrophies and storage diseases, and even on a normal basis. In more pronounced form, however, it is seen in trisomy 21, some of the other trisomies, Melnick-Needles osteodysplasia, and neurofibromatosis (see Fig. 6.24).

References

1. Katz SG, Grunebaum M, Strand RD: Thoracic and lumbar dural ectasia in a two year old boy. *Pediatr Radiol* 6:238–240, 1978.
2. Mitchell GE, Lourie H, Berne AS: The various causes of scalloped vertebrae with notes on their pathogenesis. *Radiology* 89:67–74, 1967.

Table 6.9   Vertebral Scalloping

A. Posterior	
Normal; lumbar	Commonest

Intraspinal tumor, cyst
    Neurofibromatosis (dural ectasia)
    Achondroplasia, other chondrodystrophies (small canal)
    Storage diseases
	Moderately common

Ehler-Danlos syndrome (dural ectasia)
    Marfan's syndrome (dural ectasia)
    Hydromyelia, syringomyelia
    Uncontrolled communicating hydrocephalus
	Rare

B. Anterior	
Normal; lower thoracic and upper lumbar	Commonest

Neurofibromatosis (dysplastic vertebra)
    Leukemia, lymphoma (destruction)
    Metastatic disease (destruction)
	Moderately common

Adjacent intra-abdominal tumors, cysts (erosion)	Rare

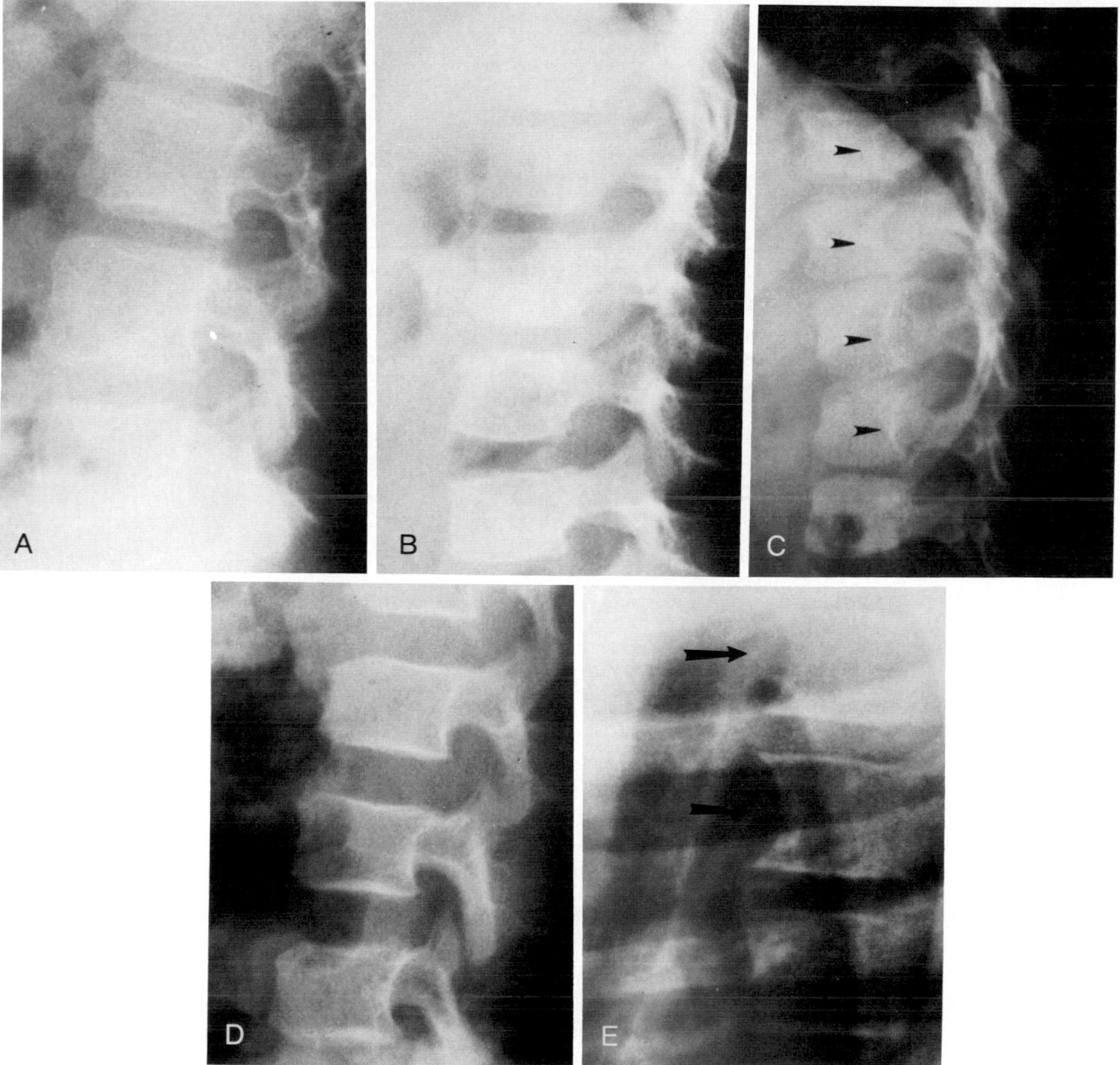

Fig. 6.12. Vertebral scalloping. A. Normal posterior lumbar vertebral scalloping. B. Normal anterior lumbar and lower thoracic vertebral scalloping. C. Pathologic scalloping due to dural ectasia in neurofibromatosis (arrows). D. Pathologic posterior scalloping in achondroplasia. E. Pathologic anterior scalloping of thoracic vertebra in neurofibromatosis (arrows).

VERTEBRAL BODY SHAPE ABNORMALITIES

Vertebral shape abnormalities include (a) flat vertebrae (platyspondyly), (b) cuboid vertebrae, (c) biconcave vertebrae, (d) tall vertebrae, (e) round or oval vertebrae, (f) expanded vertebrae, (g) wedged vertebrae, (h) hooked or beaked vertebrae, (i) spool-shaped vertebrae.

Flat Vertebrae

Flat vertebrae usually result from compression fractures or developmental abnormalities (Table 6.10).

Occasionally, especially in the thoracic spine, a little flattening of the vertebrae can be seen in normal

Table 6.10 Flat Vertebrae

A. Single or multiple but not all
vertebral bodies

Fracture Eosinophilic granuloma, his- tiocytosis X	Commonest
Metastatic disease Congenital variation Osteogenesis imperfecta Osteomalacia-osteoporosis Leukemia-lymphoma	Moderately common

B. All vertebral bodies

Severe osteoporosis-osteo- malacia[a,c] Sickle-cell disease[c]	Commonest
Severe osteogenesis imper- fecta[a,c] Other anemias[a,c] Leukemia, lymphoma[a,c] Spondyloepiphyseal dyspla- sia[a,b]	Moderately common
Thanatophoric dwarfism[a] Metatrophic dwarfism[a] Morquio's disease[b]	Relatively rare
Achondrogenesis Kniest's syndrome[a] Dyggve-Melchoir-Clausen syndrome[b]	Rare

[a] Uniformly flat.
[b] Pear-shaped.
[c] Biconcave.

children and, indeed, some may demonstrate slight anterior wedging. In terms of pathologic vertebral flattening, it is important to note whether the phenomenon is isolated to one or two vertebral bodies or generalized throughout the spine. If all of the vertebral bodies are flattened, a bony dysplasia (Fig. 6.13, A and B), or severe osteoporosis or osteomalacia (Fig. 6.13C) should be considered (1, 2). If only one or two vertebral bodies are flattened, one should consider either an ordinary or pathologic fracture.

Conditions leading to universal platyspondyly include spondyloepiphyseal dysplasia, Morquio's disease (storage disease which resembles spondyloepiphyseal dysplasia), achondrogenesis, thanatophoric dwarfism, metatrophic dwarfism, Kniest's syndrome, and the Dyggve-Melchior-Clausen syndrome (findings resemble Morquio's disease or spondyloepiphyseal dysplasia). In spondyloepiphyseal dysplasia, Morquio's disease, and Dygvve-Melchior-Clausen syndrome, the vertebral bodies often also are **pear-shaped** (Fig. 6.13D). When universal platyspondyly is seen in osteogenesis imperfecta, the problem is multiple com-

pression fracturing and a mixture of flat and biconcave vertebrae can result.

As noted earlier, when only one or two vertebral bodies are flattened, and especially if they are **anteriorly wedged**, one should consider compression fracture. Such fractures, regular or pathologic, commonly occur with hyperflexion or axial compression injuries (Fig. 6.14A). When a vertebra is flattened entirely, the term **vertebra plana** is utilized, and most often is seen in histiocytosis X. Indeed, in some cases the vertebral body becomes wafer thin (Fig. 6.14B). Other conditions leading to single or multiple, but not universal, vertebral body compression include metastases, leukemia, osteogenesis imperfecta, and any cause of osteomalacia or osteoporosis.

References

1. Kozlowski K: Platyspondyly in childhood. *Pediatr Radiol* 81–88, 1974.
2. Schorr S, Legum C: Radiological aspects of the vertebral components of osteochondrocysplasias. *Br J Radiol* 50:302–311, 1977.

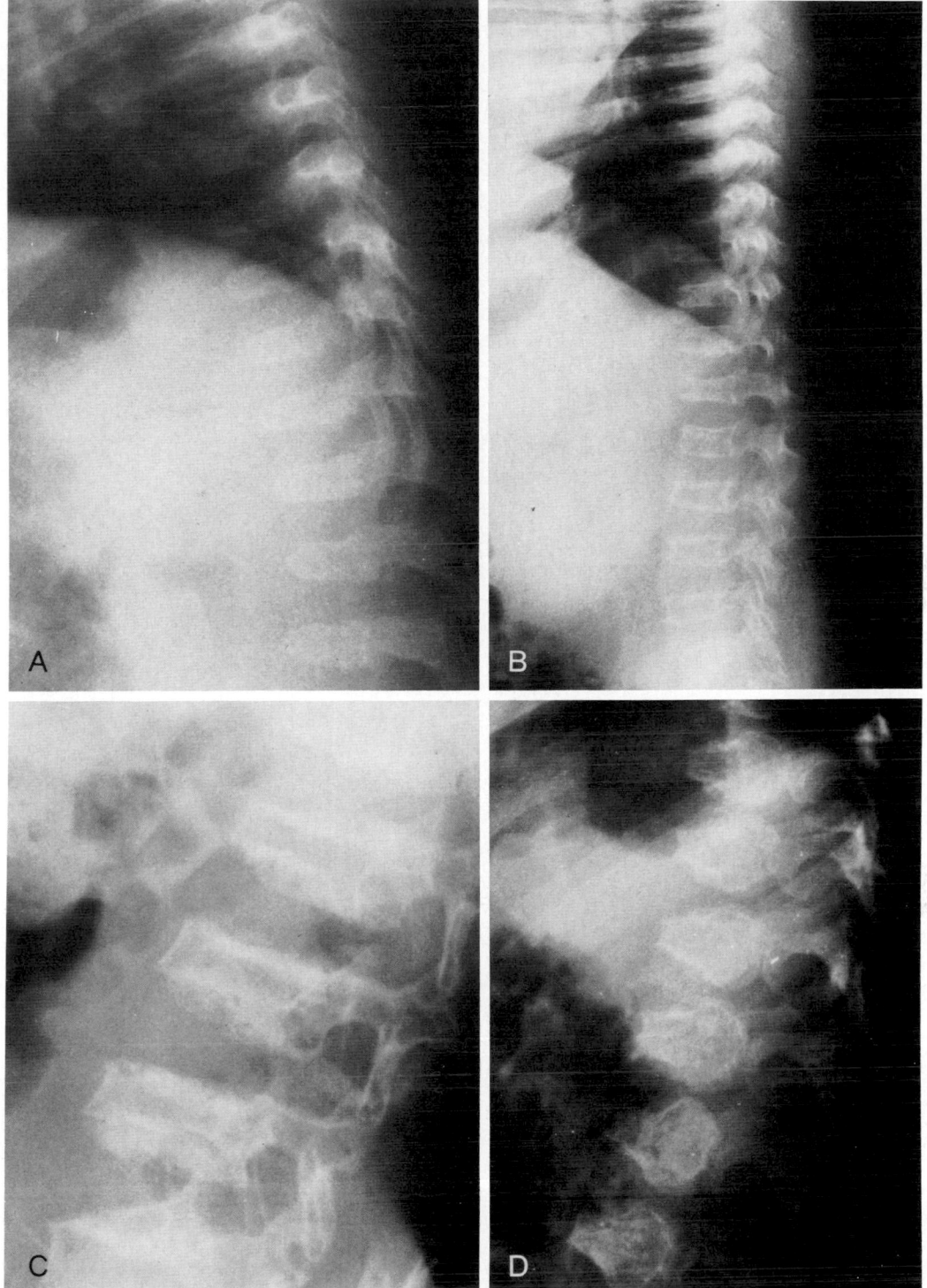

Fig. 6.13. Flat vertebra. A. Flat vertebra in Morquio's disease. B. Flat vertebra in spondyloepiphyseal dysplasia. C. Flat vertebra due to severe osteoporosis in Cushing's syndrome. D. Flat, pear-shaped vertebra in spondyloepiphyseal dysplasia.

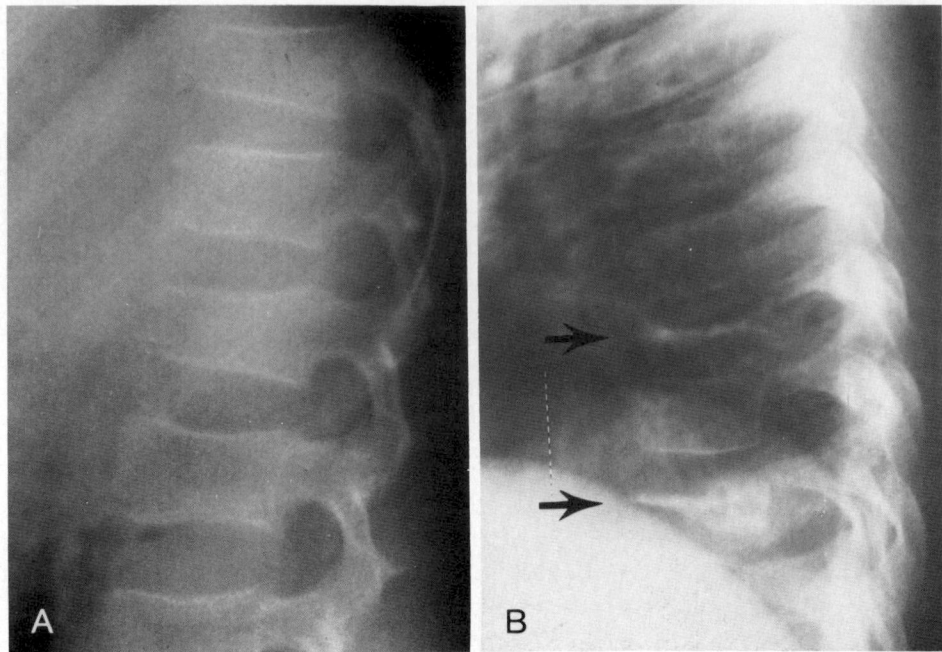

Fig. 6.14. Flat vertebral bodies. A. Anteriorly wedged, flat body due to compression fracture in patient with lymphoma. B. Typical vertebra plana, wafer thin, compressed vertebra in histiocytosis X (arrows).

Cuboid Vertebrae (Table 6.11)

Cuboid vertebrae can be encountered in the cervical spine or lower thoracolumbar region on a normal basis. When abnormal, they are seen throughout the spine and, for the most part, occur in chondrodystrophies such as achondroplasia (Fig. 6.15A), thanatophoric dwarfism, diastrophic dwarfism, hypochondroplasia, and the short-limbed polydactyly syndromes of Saldino-Noonan and Majewski. In these latter conditions, the vertebra also are quite hypoplastic and, in some cases, even more round than cuboid. Somewhat cuboid vertebra also occur in the storage diseases (Fig. 6.15B).

Table 6.11 Cuboid Vertebrae

Normal (cervical and T–L spine) Achondroplasia	Commonest
Hypochondroplasia Other chondrodystrophies Storage diseases	Moderately common
Short-limbed polydactyly dwarfs	Rare

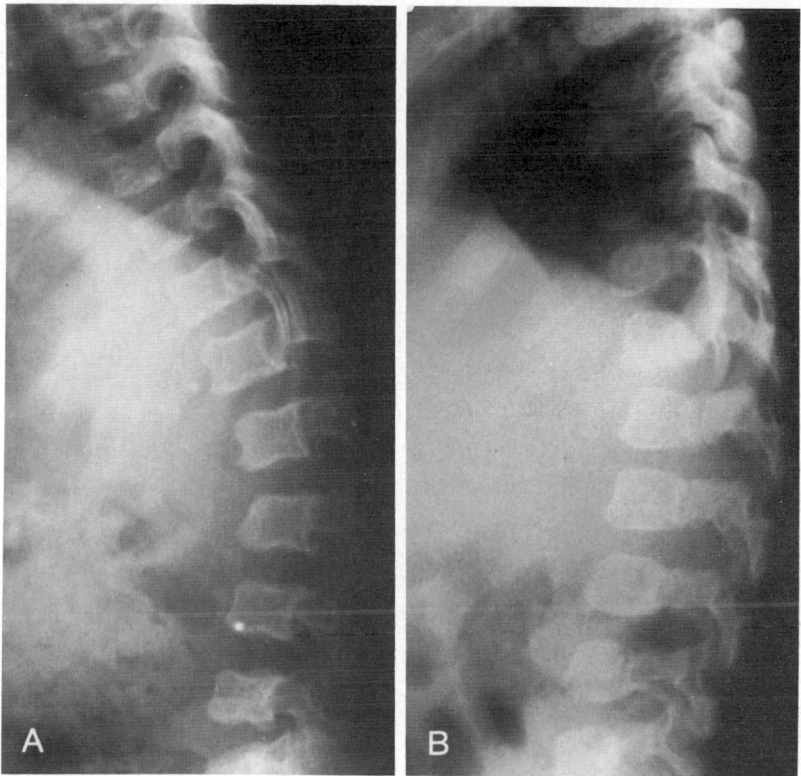

Fig. 6.15. Cuboid vertebrae. A. Cuboid vertebrae in achondroplasia. B. Mucopolysaccharidosis with cuboid vertebrae.

Biconcave Vertebrae (Table 6.12)

The best known, and one of the most common, biconcave or fish vertebra occurs with sickle cell disease (1, 2). In these cases it is believed that end plate infarction causes bone necrosis and subsequent expansion of the intervening disks into the vertebrae. Because of the infarction, a typical square cornered, **step-like appearance** to the depression is seen (Fig. 6.16A). However, the step-like configuration does not occur in all cases, and furthermore, similar step-like deformities have been noted with renal osteodystrophy, thalassemia, homocystinuria, and Gaucher's disease (3–7). Biconcave vertebrae, without step-like compression, usually occur when there is extreme softening of the vertebral bodies. In such cases, the disks expand and bulge into the vertebral bodies (Fig. 6.16B), and some of the more common conditions in which this occurs are outlined in Table 6.10. Basically, however, they include the more severe forms of osteomalacia and osteoporosis (i.e., osteogenesis imperfecta, rickets, hypophosphatasia, steroid therapy, hyperparathyroidism, Cushing's syndrome, severe malnutrition, and marrow packing disorders such as sickle cell disease, Cooley's anemia, lymphoma, and metastases). A complete list of conditions leading to osteomalacia or osteoporosis is available in Tables 4.1 and 4.2. A mild degree of biconcaving of the vertebra is seen in some normal individuals and is due to the normally prominent nucleus pulposus of the intervertebral disks (Fig. 6.16C).

References

1. Hansen GC, Gold RH: Central depression of multiple vertebral end-plates: A "pathognomonic" sign of sickle hemoglobinopathy in Gaucher's disease. *Am J Roentgenol* 129:343–344, 1977.
2. Riggs W, Rockett JF: Roentgen chest findings in childhood sickle cell anemia: a new vertebral body finding. *Am J Roentgenol Radium Ther Nucl Med* 104:838–845, 1968.
3. Rohlfing BM: Vertebral end-plate depression: report of

Table 6.12   Biconcave Vertebrae (also Table 6.10)

Sickle-cell disease[a] Osteoporosis-osteomalacia	Commonest
Osteogenesis imperfecta Renal osteodystrophy Normal Schmorl's nodes	Moderately common
Thalassemia[b] Gaucher's disease[b] Homocystinuria[b]	Relatively rare

[a] Often step-like depression.
[b] Occasionally step-like depression.

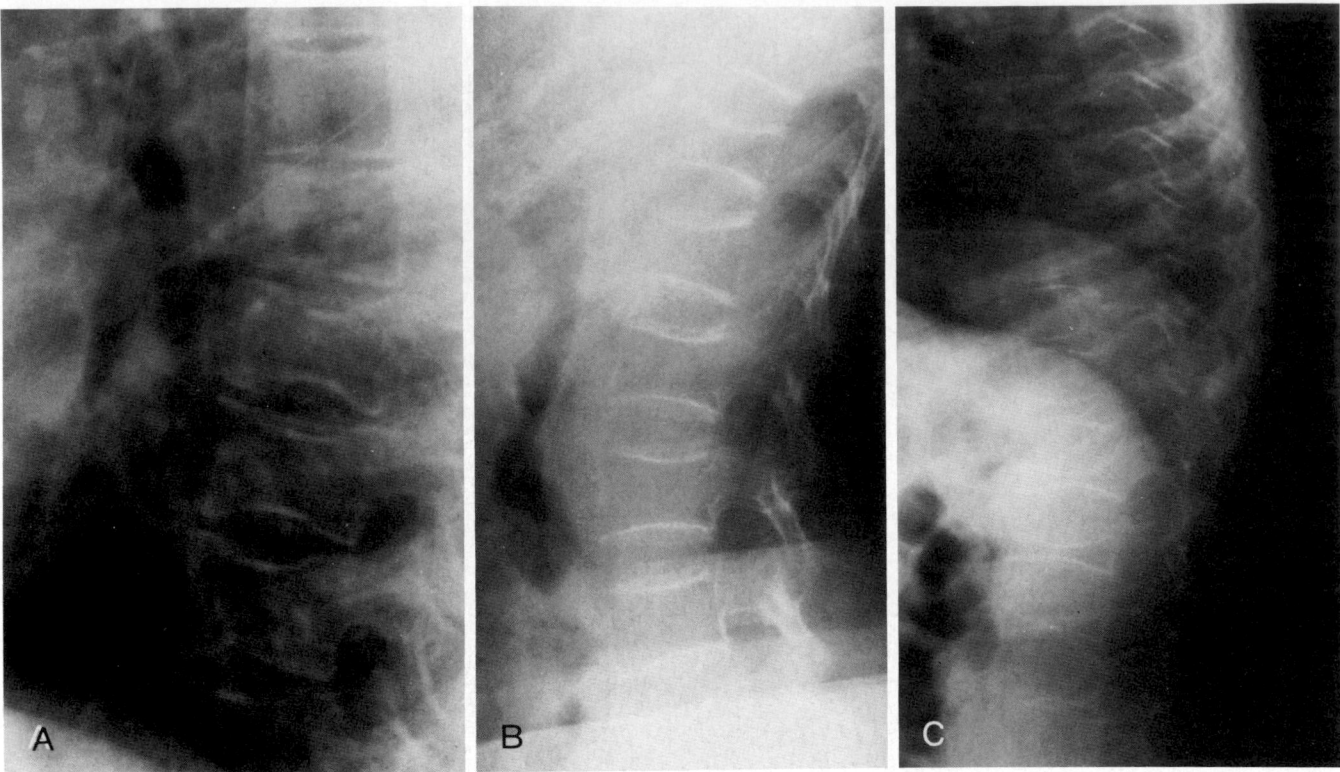

Fig. 6.16. Biconcave vertebrae. A. Biconcave vertebrae with step-like central depressions in sickle cell disease. B. Biconcave vertebrae, associated with grossly expanded disks in patient with leukemic and steroid induced osteoporosis. C. Mild biconcave vertebrae due to normally prominent nucleus pulposus.

two patients without hemoglobinopathy. *Am J Roentgenol* 128:599–600, 1977.

4. Schwartz AM, Homer MJ, McCauley RGK: Step-off vertebral body: Gaucher's disease versus sickle cell hemoglobinopathy. *Am J Roentgenol* 132:81–85, 1979.

5. The "typical" spine changes of sickle-cell anemia in a patient with thalassemia major (Cooley's anemia). *Radiology* 89:1065.

6. Westerman MP, Greenfield GB, Wong PWK: "Fish vertebrae", homocystinuria, and sickle cell anemia. *JAMA* 230:261–262, 1974.

7. Ziter FMH Jr: Central vertebral end-plate depression in chronic renal disease: Report of two cases. *Am J Roentgenol* 132:809–811, 1979.

Tall Vertebrae (Table 6.13)

Tall vertebrae, for the most part, are seen in hypotonic infants and children. Absence of vertical stresses cause the vertebrae to become tall (1) and canine in shape. The configuration can be seen in a variety of syndromes where hypotonia exists and, thus, with many underlying neurologic or neuromuscular disorders (Fig. 6.17).

Table 6.13   Tall Vertebrae

Trisomy 21	}	Commonest
Rubella syndrome		
Other causes of hypotonia	}	Moderately common

Reference

1. Gooding CA, Neuhauser EBD: Growth and development of the vertebral bodies in the presence and absence of normal stress. *Am J Roentgenol* 93:388–393, 1965.

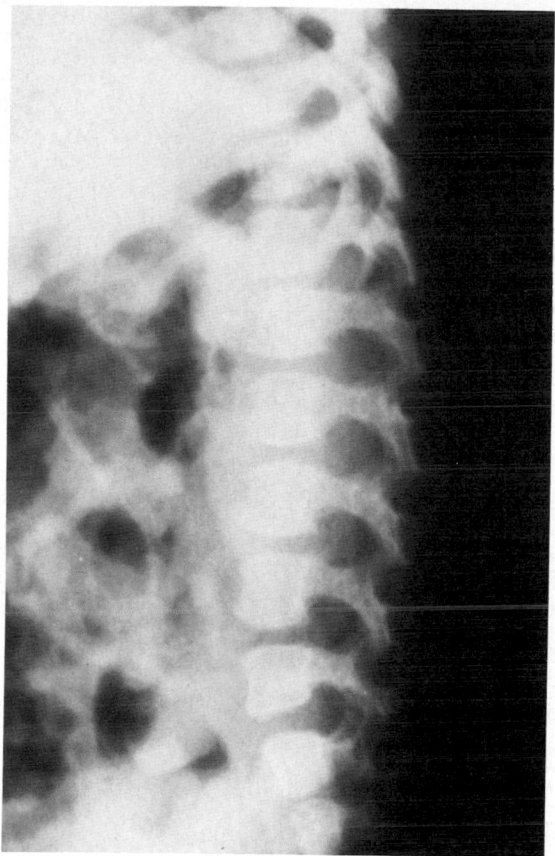

Fig. 6.17.   Tall vertebrae. Typical tall vertebrae in retarded patient. Note slight spool-shaped appearance of the vertebrae, not an uncommon associated finding.

Round Vertebrae (Table 6.14)

Normal, round vertebral bodies commonly are seen in the neonatal period, in the thoracolumbar junction (Fig. 6.18A). As the infant grows older, the vertebrae become more rectangular in shape and, eventually, as the ring epiphyses develop, their corners become quite square. In some children, under normal circumstances, the ringed epiphyses may be late in appearing, and then a rounded to oval vertebral body configuration temporarily persists (Fig. 6.18B). The same problem occurs with certain pathologic conditions and, basically, these include (*a*) vertebral body underdevelopment in association with anomalies such as meningomyelocele, and (*b*) retarded bone maturation as seen in untreated hypothyroidism (Fig. 6.18C). Round, actually more oval, vertebrae due to underdevelopment are seen in the pear-shaped platyspondylic vertebrae occurring in certain bony dysplasias (see Fig. 6.13D).

Table 6.14 Round and Expanded Vertebrae

Round vertebrae		
Normal neonate (especially T–L junction) Meningocele	}	Commonest
Hypothyroidism	}	Moderately common
Short-limbed polydactyly syndromes Bone dysplasias with pear-shaped vertebrae (see Table 6.10)	}	Rare
Expanded vertebrae		
Compression fracture with lateral expansion	}	Commonest
Aneurysmal bone cyst Hemangioma-lymphangioma	}	Relatively rare
Osteoblastoma Ewing's sarcoma (sclerotic-treated)	}	Rare

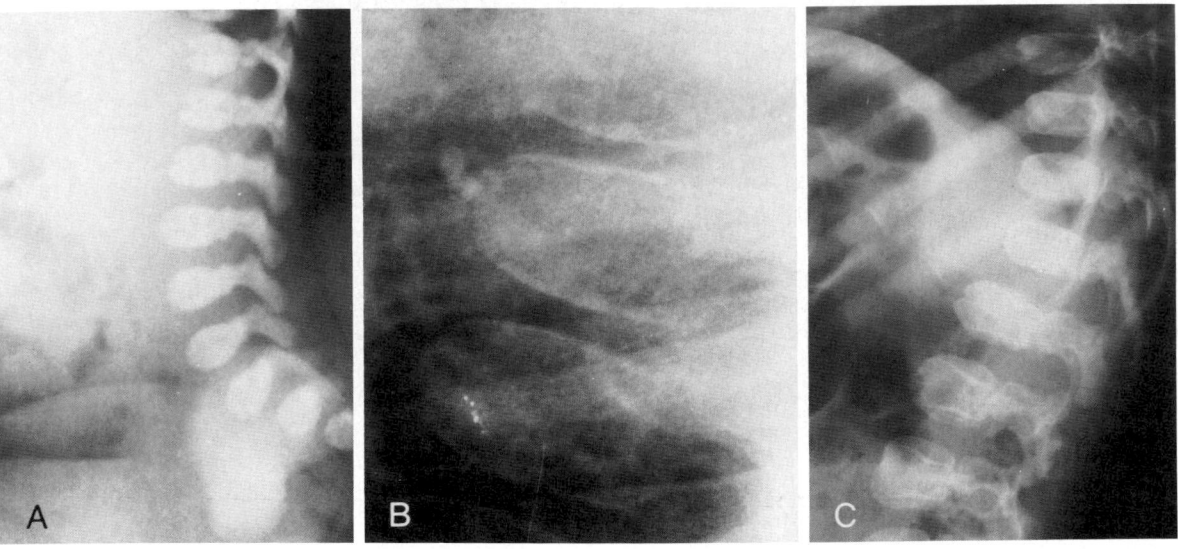

Fig. 6.18. Round vertebrae. A. Normal, round vertebrae in noeonate. B. Oval to round vertebrae in normal child with delayed appearance of ringed epiphyses. C. Round to oval vertebrae in child with untreated hypothyroidism. Also note persistent prominence of the central vein grooves.

Expanded Vertebrae (Table 6.14)

Isolated, expanded vertebrae are seen with bone cysts and tumors, and the most common bone cyst in the spine is the usually bubbly appearing aneurysmal bone cyst (Fig. 6.19A). These lesions also can extend into the posterior elements, and a similar configuration can be seen with giant cell tumors. The latter, however, are uncommon in children. Cystic, somewhat honeycombed expansion also occurs with hemangiomas and lymphangiomas (Fig. 6.19B), and sclerotic, expanded vertebrae can be seen with treated Ewing's sarcoma (see Fig. 6.2A). Expanded vertebrae also occur with giant osteoid osteoma (osteoblastoma), and the vertebrae can expand laterally with severe compression fractures.

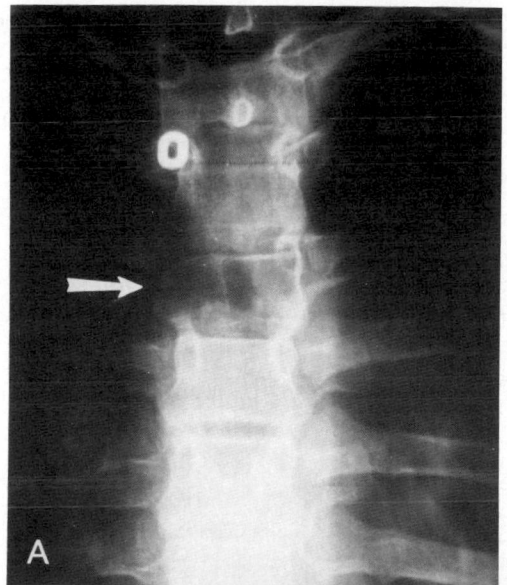

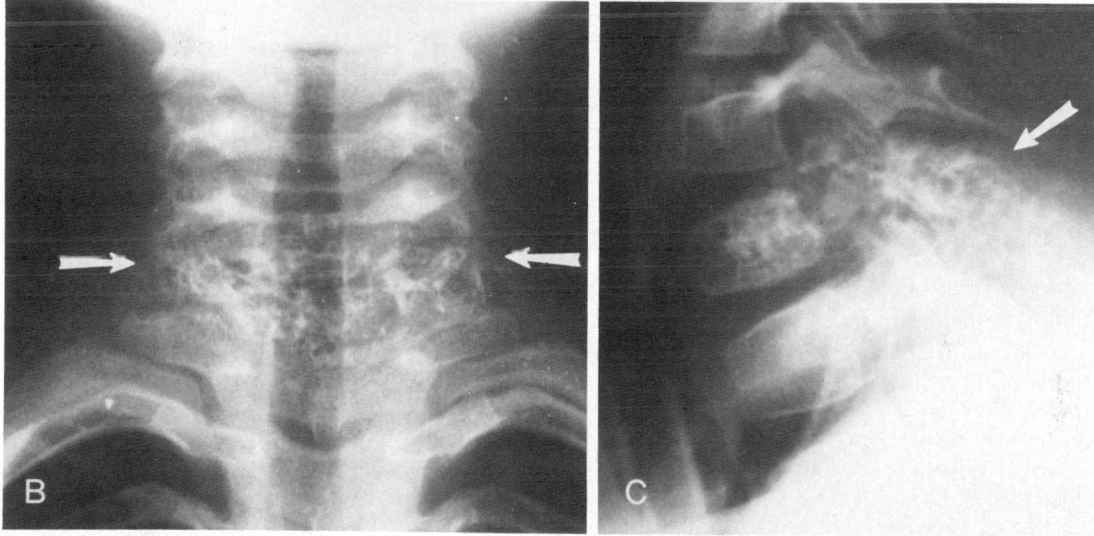

Fig. 6.19. **Expanded vertebrae.** A. Slightly expanded, radiolucent, bubbly appearing aneurysmal bone cyst (arrow). B. Markedly expanded, bubbly appearing vertebra secondary to hemangioma (arrows). C. Lateral view showing extension into posterior elements (arrow).

Wedged Vertebrae (Table 6.15)

Wedging of the vertebrae can occur anteriorally or laterally, but anterior wedging is more common. Occasionally, mild anterior wedging, especially in the thoracic region, can be seen in normal individuals, but otherwise, wedging should be considered abnormal and usually is due to acute trauma (more common) or chonic flexion-compression (Fig. 6.20). On a chronic basis, anterior wedging occurs with Scheuermann's disease, with the so-called gibbus spine, in the thoracolumbar junction (see Fig. 6.40) and, indeed, any time there is chronic hyperflexion of the spine (Fig. 6.20B). Lateral wedging occurs with trauma and also with scoliosis.

Table 6.15 Wedged Vertebrae

Anterior compression fracture Rotoscoliosis (lateral wedging)	Commonest
Kyphosis (various causes) Scheuermann's disease Normal (thoracic spine minimal) Hemivertebrae-sagittal (lateral wedging)	Moderately common
Hemivertebrae-coronal (gibbus) Gibbus—other causes (see p 430)	Relatively rare

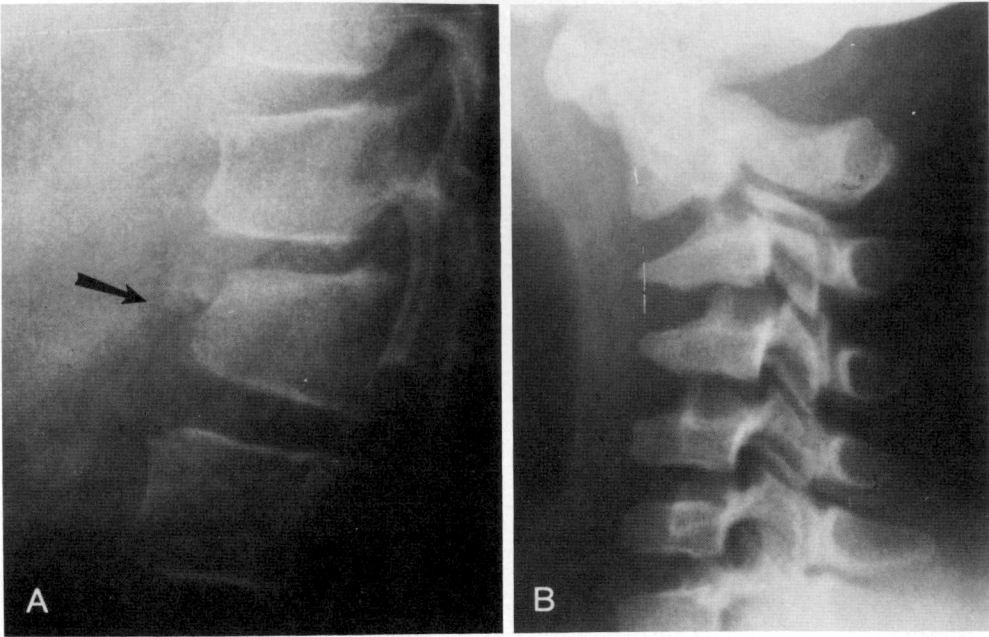

Fig. 6.20. Wedged vertebrae. A. Typical wedged vertebra due to flexion-type fracture (arrow). The verteba above also is slightly wedged and a small corner fracture is present. B. Severe anterior wedging due to chronic hyperflexion of cervical spine. The exact etiology of this patient's prolonged hyperflexion deformity was never determined, but he was hypotonic and did have pseudohypoparathyroidism.

Hooked or Beaked Vertebrae (Table 6.16)

The hooked or beaked vertebra can show a smooth or irregular hook, but in either case, results from acute or chronic hyperflexion (4). There may or may not be associated disk material extrusion (1, 3), but when extrusion occurs there is associated narrowing of the disk space. For the most part, irregular hooking or beaking is seen with overt hyperflexion injuries, either acute or chronic (Fig. 6.21, A and B). The latter occur with Scheuermann's disease and any time prolonged hypotonia leading to chronic bending of the spine is present. Acute trauma, causing notching, most often is seen on a legitimate basis, but also can be seen in the battered child syndrome (5).

When a smooth, hooked, or beaked vertebra is seen,

the problem still is hyperflexion, but in these cases hyperflexion is prolonged and irregular fragmentation of the vertebral corners does not occur. Rather, there is a smooth notching deformity (Fig. 6.22). Smooth notching most commonly is seen in normal infants, at the thoracolumbar junction (Fig. 6.22A). The deformity usually is rather mild and entirely reversible. It results because of exaggerated thoracolumbar kyphosis, secondary to hypotonia which is normal in infancy. The problem is exaggerated when the infant is placed in a sitting position. On a pathologic basis, hypotonia also is the basic underlying problem, but in addition there may be abnormality of bone maturation. Most commonly this is seen in the various stor-

Table 6.16   Hooked or Beaked Vertebrae

Normal in infants (thoracolumbar junction)	Commonest
Storage diseases Hypothyroidism Acute and chronic trauma Scheuermann's disease Neurogenic or neuromuscular disease with hypotonia	Moderately common
Achondroplasia Bone dysplasia in neurofibromatosis	Relatively rare

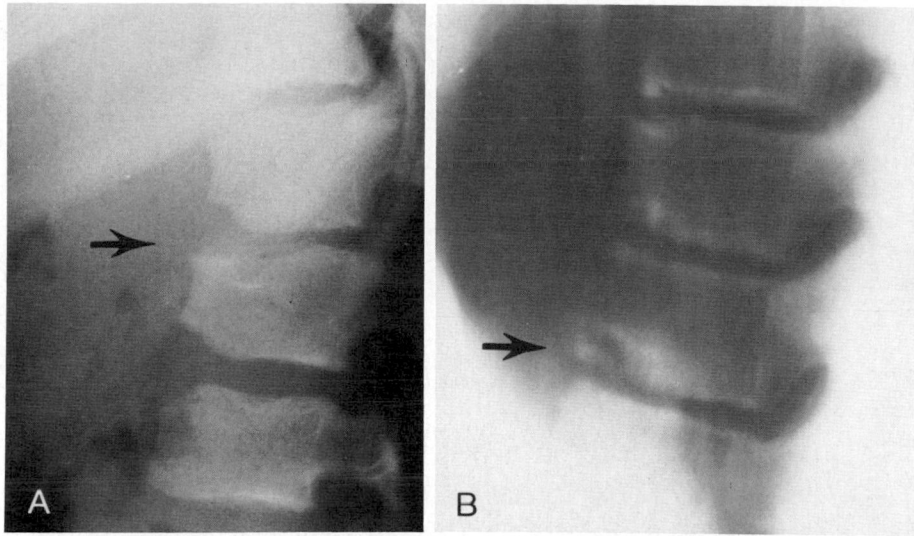

Fig. 6.21. Hooked or beaked vertebrae; irregular hooking or beaking. A. Note irregular notching due to acute flexion injury (arrow). Note associated disk space narrowing. B. Similar finding in Scheuermann's disease (arrow).

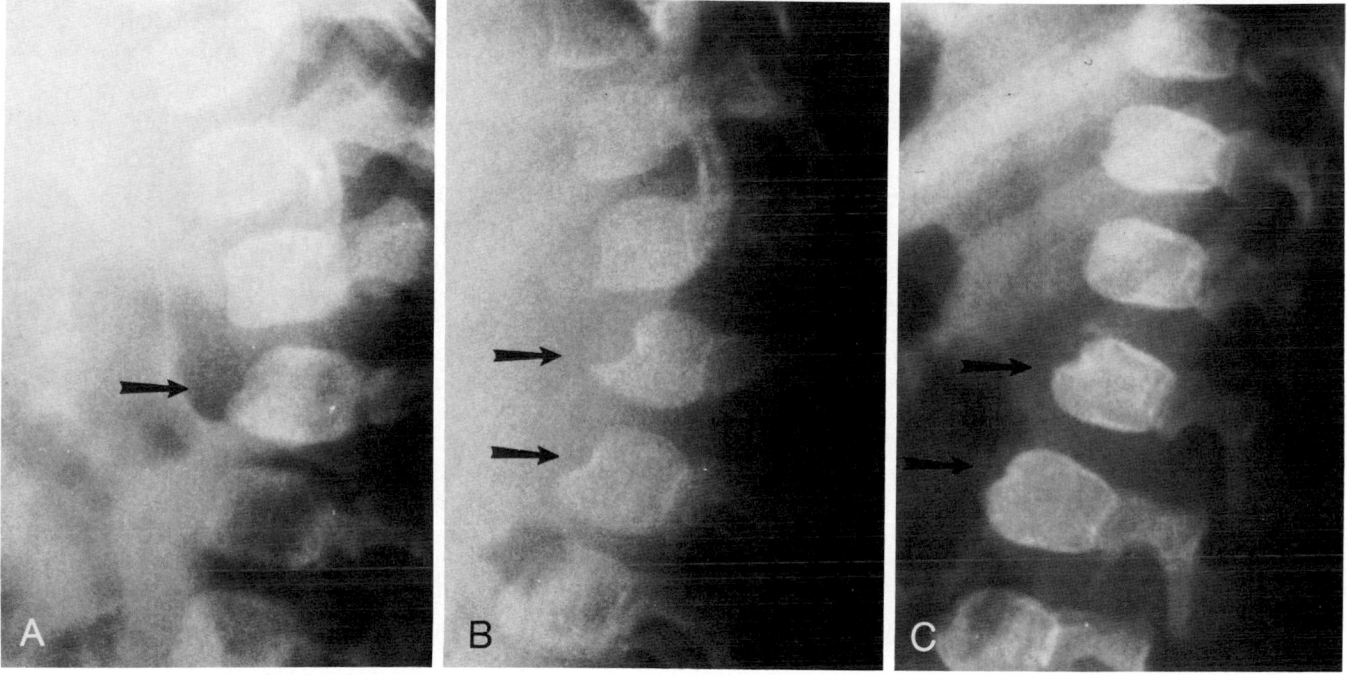

Fig. 6.22. Smooth notching or beaking. A. Normal notching in infant (arrow). B. Severe notching in Hurler's disease (arrows). C. Similar notching in hypothyroidism (arrow).

age diseases (Fig. 6.22B), but also in hypothyroidism (Fig. 6.22C). Occasionally, it also is seen in some case of achondroplasia, the hypotonic trisomies (4) and, indeed, in any condition where neuromuscular hypotonia exists. In any of these cases, if hypotonia is reversed, regression of the deformity occurs (Fig. 6.23).

References

1. Begg AC: Nuclear herniation of the intervertebral disc; their radiological manisfestations and significance. *J Bone Joint Surg* 36B:180–193, 1954.
2. Evans PR: Deformity of vertebral bodies in cretinism. *J Pediatr* 41:706–712, 1952.
3. Rabinowitz JG, Sacher M: Gangliosidosis (GM₁): a re-evaluation of the vertebral deformity. *Am J Roentgenol* 121:155–158, 1974.
4. Swischuk LE: The beaked, notched, or hooked vertebra; its significance in infants and young children. *Radiology* 95:661–664, 1970.
5. Swischuk LE: Spine and spinal cord trauma in the battered child syndrome. *Radiology* 92:733–738, 1969.

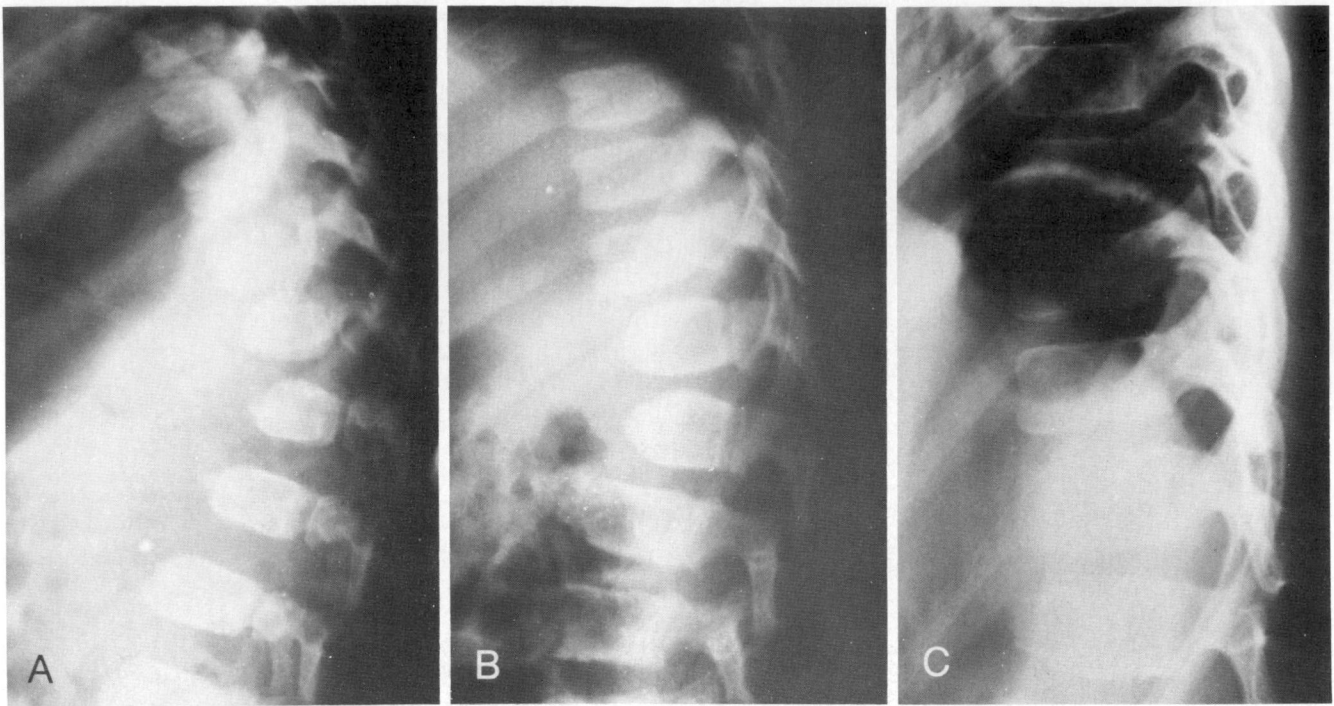

Fig. 6.23. Smooth notching with regression. A. Severe notching in hypothyroidism. B. Somewhat later, after therapy was initiated, changes were less pronounced. C. Patient is now an adolescent and only minimal deformity remains.

Spool-Shaped Vertebrae

Spool-shaped vertebrae are not particularly common. In the normal lumbar spine, where mild degrees of anterior and posterior scalloping are common, a mild spool-shaped deformity can be seen. In exaggerated form, however, spool-shaped vertebrae are seen with the tall vertebrae of hypotonia (see Fig. 6.17) and with bony dysplasias such as the Melnick-Needles osteodysplasia syndrome, neurofibromatosis (Fig. 6.24), trisomy 21, some other trisomies, and some chondrodystrophies and storage diseases.

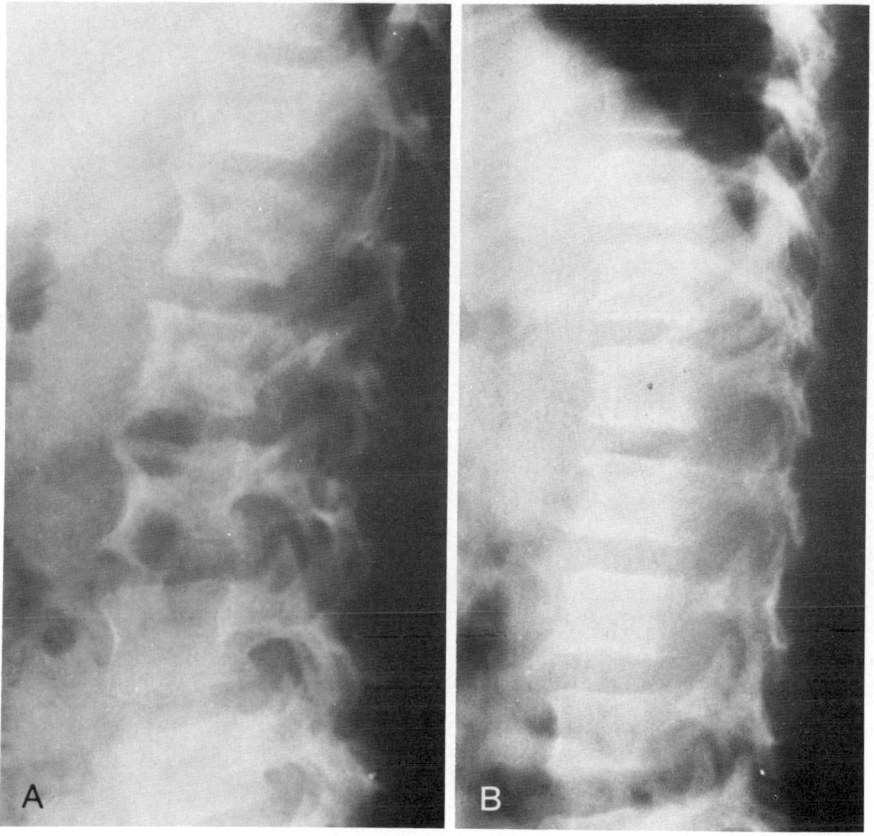

Fig. 6.24. Spool-shaped vertebrae. A. Spool-shaped vertebrae in neurofibromatosis. B. Melnick-Needles osteodysplasia with spool-shaped vertebrae.

Absent Vertebral Bodies

Occasionally, on a congenital basis, an entire vertebral body is absent and spondylolisthesis results. However, most often only a part of the vertebral body is absent and then either a sagittal or coronal cleft hemivertebra is seen.

Blocked Vertebrae (Table 6.17)

Blocked vertebrae are associated with an extremely narrow or totally obliterated disk. The commonest cause of such blocking or fusion is congenital and very often is seen at the C_2–C_3 area (Fig. 6.25A). Such blocking can be seen in isolated form or in association with the Klippel-Feil syndrome (1–7). In this latter condition, numerous, bizarre fusion segmentation anomalies of the cervical spine exist (Fig. 6.25B). The result is a short neck and varying degrees of torticollis. In spite of the severe bony abnormality, neurologic deficit is uncommon. Sprengel's deformity of the scapula (elevated, rotated scapula) is commonly associated (8), and some of these patients may have renal agenesis and/or congenital deafness. Blocked vertebrae are less common elsewhere and, in fact, when seen, usually are not totally blocked but associated with a very narrow disk (see Fig. 6.34A).

Acquired blocked vertebrae result when intervening disks are destroyed and subsequent healing occurs. Very often a kyphotic, or frank Gibbus, deformity results (see Fig. 6.40A). Most often the problem is infection, but occasionally it is severe discovertebral trauma. On a chronic basis, this latter phenomenon occurs in Scheuermann's disease. Ankylosing spondylitis also can lead to acquired blocked vertebrae, but the condition is rare in children.

Table 6.17 Blocked Vertebrae

Congenital; with spinal dysraphism }	Commonest
Congenital; isolated Acquired; after infection Congenital; Klippel-Feil syndrome }	Moderately common
Acquired; after trauma Scheuermann's disease }	Relatively rare

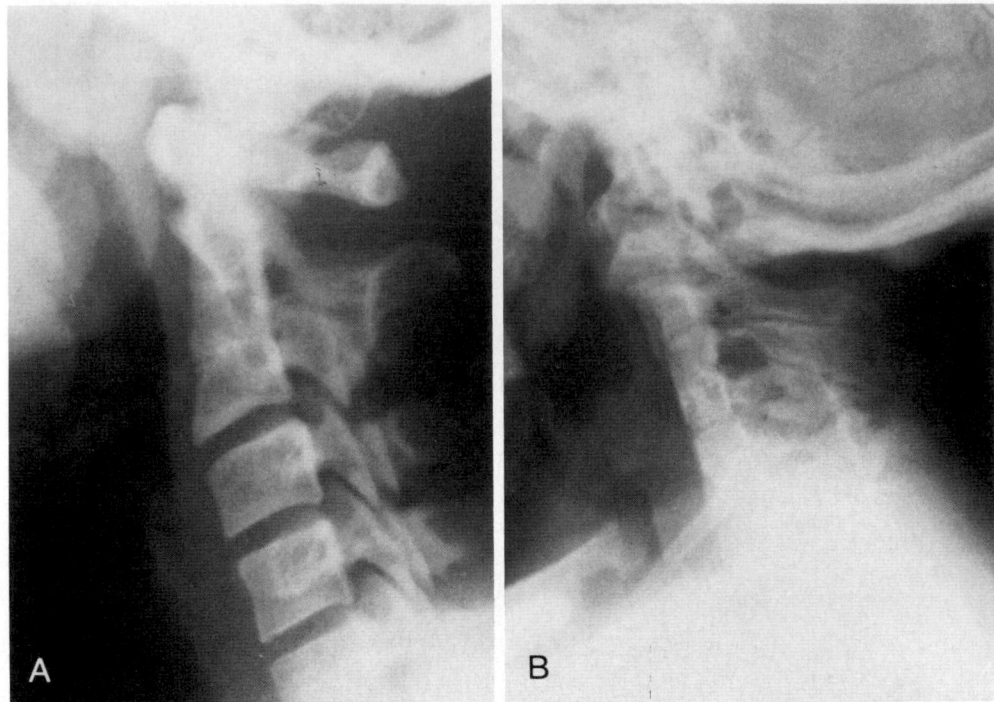

Fig. 6.25. Blocked vertebrae. A. Typical blocking of C_2–C_3. Note that fusion extends into the posterior elements and apophyseal joints. B. Typical, bizarre appearance of fusion segmentation anomalies in the Klippel-Feil syndrome.

References

1. Hensinger R, Lang J, MacEwen G: Klippel-Feil syndrome: constellation of associated anomalies. *J Bone Joint Surg* 56-A:1246–1253, 1974.
2. Moore W, Matthews TJ, Rabinowitz R: Genitourinary anomalies associated with the Klippel-Feil syndrome. *J Bone Joint Surg* 57-A:355–357, 1975.
3. Palant DI, Carter, BL: Klippel-Feil syndrome and deafness. A study with polytomography. *Am J Dis Child* 123:218–221, 1972.
4. Ramsey J, Bliznak J: Klippel-Feil syndrome with renal agenesis and other anomalies. *Am J Roentgenol* 113:460–463, 1971.
5. Sherk HH, Shut L, Chung S: Iniencephalic deformity of the cervical spine with Klippel-Feil anomalies and congenital elevation of the scapula: Report of three cases. *J Bone Joint Surg* 56:1254–1259, 1974.
6. Shoul ML, Ritvo M: Clinical and roentgenographic manifestations of the Klippel-Feil syndrome. *Am J Roentgenol* 68:369–385, 1952.
7. Stark EW, Borton TE: Hearing loss and the Klippel-Feil syndrome. *Am J Dis Child* 123:233–235, 1972.
8. Wilson MG, Mikity VG, Shinno NW: Dominant inheritance of Sprengel's deformity. *J Pediatr* 79:818–821, 1971.

SPINAL CANAL DIAMETER ABNORMALITIES

The abnormal spinal canal can be too wide or too narrow (Table 6.18), but before considering canal diameter abnormalities it should be remembered that the normal spinal canal, on frontal view, usually appears wide in the cervicothoracic and lumbosacral region of infants (Fig. 6.26A). As far as pathologic widening is concerned, the commonest cause is a congenital anomaly such as a meningocele or meningomyelocele. Less commonly, other dysraphic problems such as diastematomyelia (Fig. 6.26B), congenital dermal sinus, and a variety of intraspinal tumors or cysts can be encountered (Fig. 6.26C). Another rare cause of spinal canal enlargement, in the cervical region, is hydrosyringomyelia (Fig. 6.26D). Meningomyeloceles most often are seen in the lumbosacral region and

Table 6.18   Spinal Canal Diameter Abnormalities

A. Enlarged	
Normal, cervical and lumbosacral	
Meningocele-meningomyelocele	Commonest
Intraspinal tumor, cyst	Moderately common
Syringomyelia, hydromyelia	Relatively rare
B. Narrowed	
Chondrodystrophies (achondroplasia, etc.)	Commonest
Congenital narrowing (other)	Rare

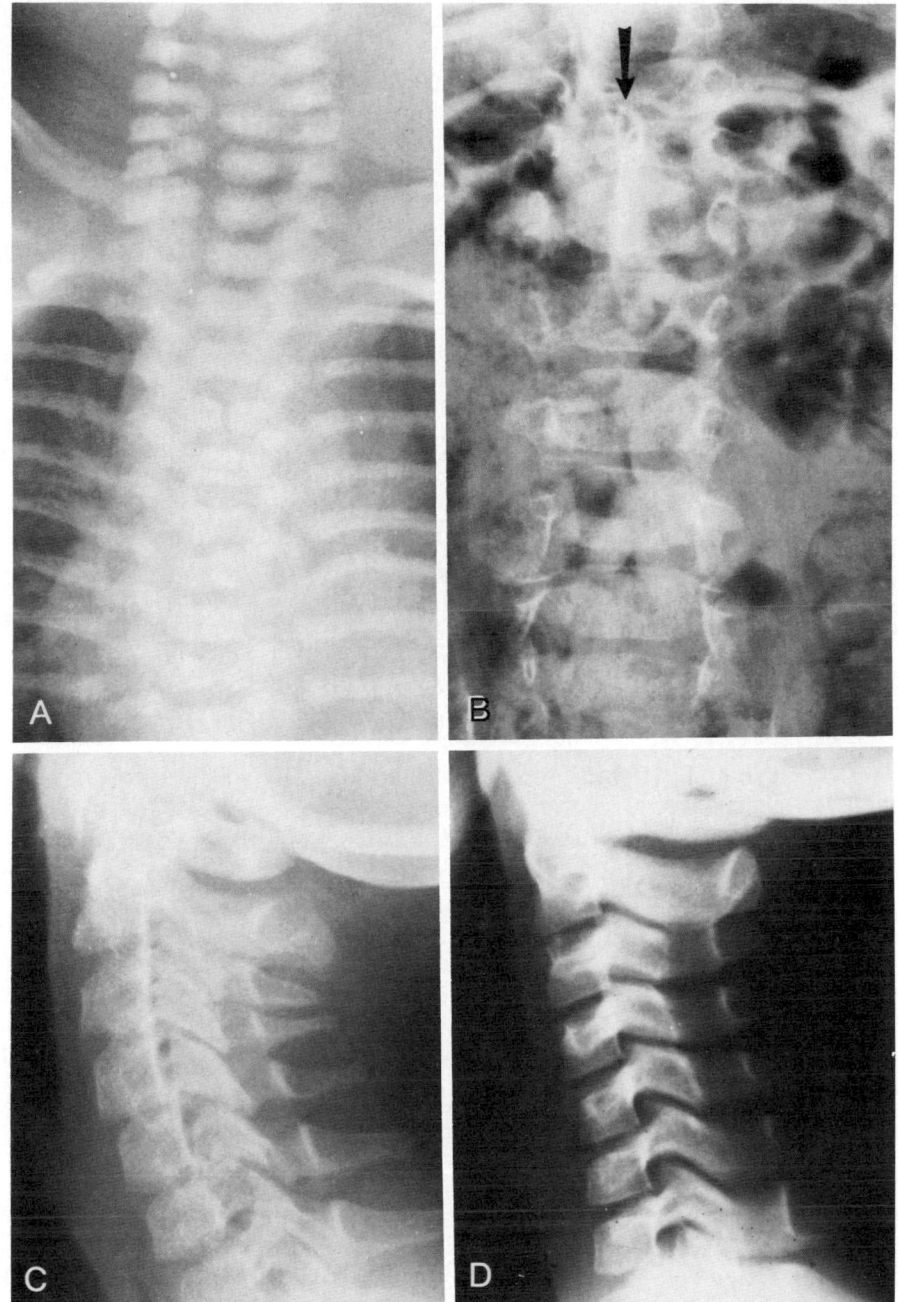

Fig. 6.26. **Enlarged spinal canal.** A. Normal, pseudowidened, cervical spinal canal in infant. Such erroneous impression of widening is common in infants. B. Widened spinal canal due to diastematomyelia. Note bony spicule (arrow). C. Widening of the canal in the cervical region due to an intraspinal tumor. D. Spinal canal widening due to syringomyelia.

then at the cervicothoracic junction. Diastematomyelia most common occurs at the thoracolumbar junction and, if the transfixing bony spicule is visualized, the diagnosis is assured (Fig. 6.26B). However, many times the spicule is fibrous or cartilaginous and then CT myelography is required for final definition (3). As the spicule transfixes the spinal cord, it prevents its normal ascent, causes it to stretch, and induces neurologic symptoms.

Narrowing of the spinal canal, as opposed to expansion, most often is generalized and almost always due to impaired enchondral bone formation seen with an underlying bony dysplasia. Of these, the chondrodystrophies are most common, and the best example is achondroplasia (Fig. 6.27). Similar narrowing, however, is seen with achondrogenesis, thanatophoric dwarfism, metatrophic dwarfism, diastrophic dwarfism, the Kniest syndrome, and some of the storage

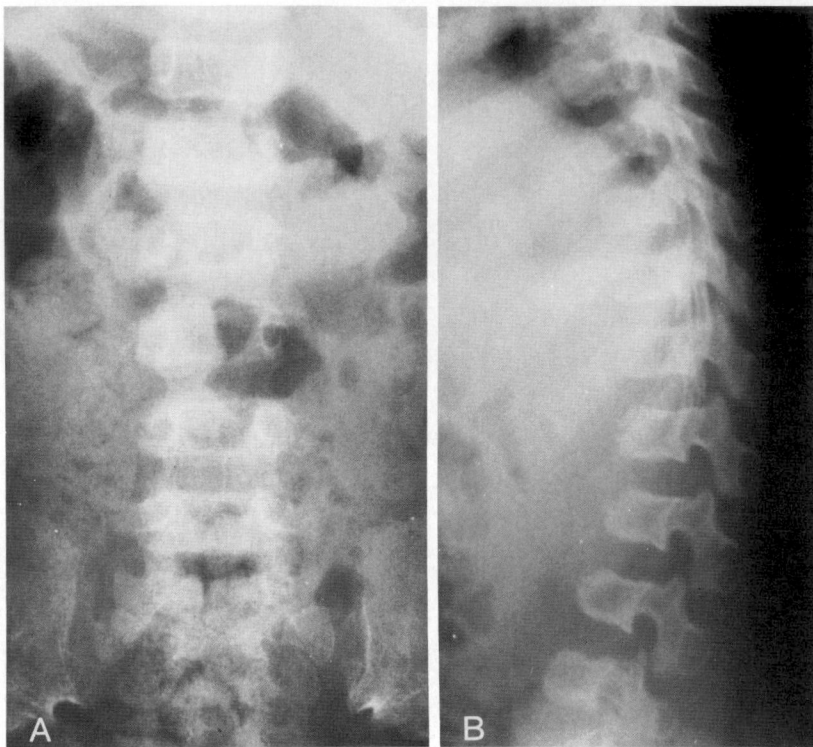

Fig. 6.27. Narrow spinal canal. A. Note generalized narrowing of spinal canal, manifest by rather uniform interpedicular distance. Normally, the canal should be wider in the thoracolumbar junction and lower cervical regions. This patient was an achondroplast. B. Lateral view showing generalized narrowing of the spinal canal, and some exaggerated posterior scalloping.

diseases. A congenitally small spinal canal, under other circumstances, is uncommon in childhood.

References

1. Hilal S, Marton D, Pollack E: Diastematomyelia in children; radiographic study of 34 cases. *Radiology* 112:609–621, 1974.
2. Neuahuser EBD, Wittenborg MH, Dehlinger K: Diastematomyelia. *Radiology* 54:659–664, 1950.
3. Weinstein MA, Rothner AD, Duchesneau P, Dohn DF: Computed tomography in diastematomyelia. *Radiology* 117:609–611, 1975.

INTERVERTEBRAL FORAMEN ABNORMALITIES

The intervertebral foramina can be larger or smaller than normal (Table 6.19). The latter is quite uncommon and almost always is secondary to congenital maldevelopment as seen with other congenital abnormalities such as the Klippel-Feil syndrome, fused vertebra, unilateral bar leading to scoliosis, diastematomyelia, and meningomyelocele (Fig. 6.28A). Small intervertebral formana, secondary to posttraumatic and/or degenerative arthritis are rare in children.

Large intervertebral foramina are more common and can be seen with absence or hypoplasia of a neural arch or an expanding intracanalicular tumor. In regards to the latter, one should think first of an intra-extraspinal dumbbell type lesion (Fig. 6.28B). In children, however, such tumors of the nerve roots (i.e., neurofibroma, etc.) are uncommon and, actually, in younger children a dumbbell tumor is more apt to be a neuroblastoma or ganglioneuroma (2, 4, 5). Rarely,

a paraspinal sarcoma can produce such a dumbbell configuration.

Other causes of large intervertebral foramina include the bony dysplasia and associated dural ectasia seen in neurofibromatosis, lateral meningoceles, posttraumatic nerve root avulsion diverticula, and hypertrophic interstitial polyneuritis (6). None are particularly common in children. Occasionally, dural ectasia also can be seen with the Marfan's and Ehler-Danlos syndromes, and on an idiopathic basis (1, 3).

References

1. Binet EF, Lustgarten MD: Enlarged neural foramen in a child. *N Y State J Med* 7:449–452, 1971.
2. Fagan CJ, Swischuk LE: Dumbbell neuroblastoma or ganglioneuroma of the spinal canal. *Am J Roentgenol* 120:453–640, 1974.

Table 6.19   Intervertebral Foramen Size Abnormalities

A. Small	
Congenital with other anomalies ⎫	Commonest
Posttraumatic ⎫	Relatively rare
B. Enlarged	
Congenital with dysraphism anomalies ⎫	Commonest
Dumbbell tumor (usually neuroblastoma–ganglioneuroma) ⎫	Moderately common
Neurofibromatosis (bony dysplasia-dural ectasia) ⎭	
Intraspinal tumor (other)	
Posttraumatic nerve root diverticulum	
Congenital absence or hypoplasic pedicle ⎬	Rare
Lateral meningocele	
Interstitial polyneuritis	
Dural ectasia, idiopathic	

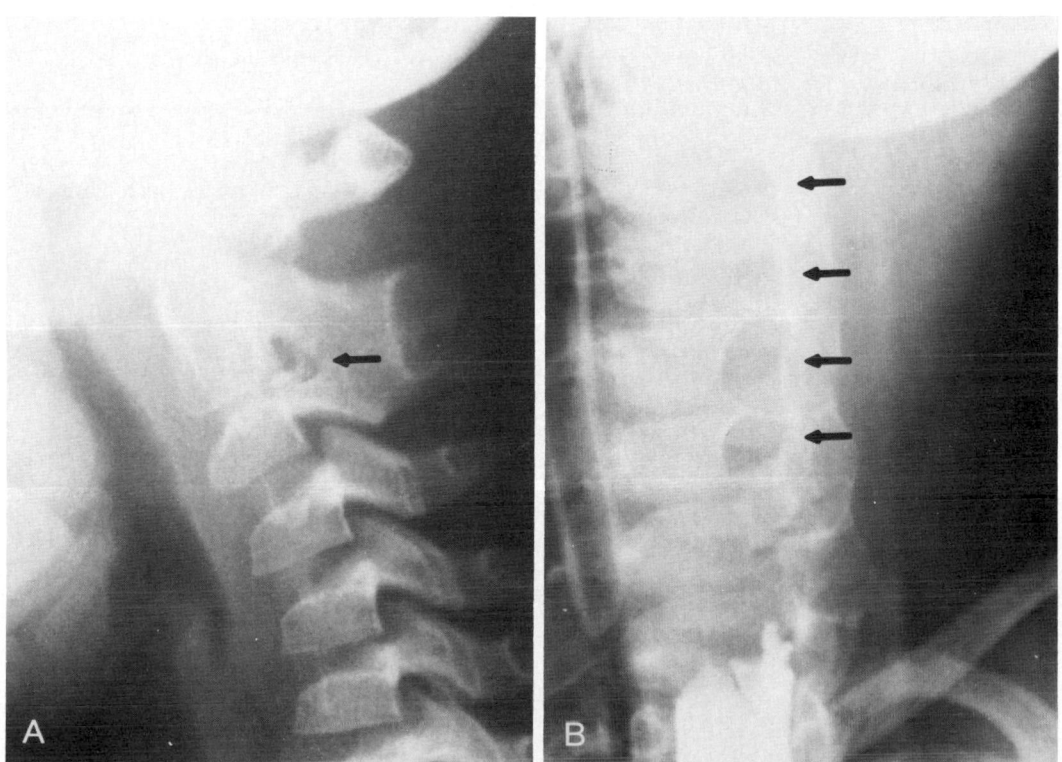

Fig. 6.28.   Intervertebral foramen size abnormalities. A. Small intervertebral foramen secondary to fusion of posterior elements of C_2–C_3 (arrow). B. Large intervertebral foramina due to dumbbell neurofibroma (arrows). Note complete block on this myelogram.

3. Katz SG, Grunebaum M, Strand RD: Thoracic and lumbar dural ectasia in a two-year old boy. *Pediatr Radiol* 6:238–240, 1978.
4. King, D, Goodman J, Hawk T, Boles ET, Sayers MP: Dumbbell neuroblastomas in children. *Arch Surg* 110:888–891, 1975.
5. Kirks DR, Berger PE, Fritz CR, Harwood-Nash DC: Myelography in the evaluation of paravertebral mass lesions in infants and children. *Radiology* 119:603–608, 1976.
6. Patel DV, Ferguson L, Schey WL: Enlargement of the intervertebral foramina: an unusual cause. *Am J Roentgenol* 131:911–913, 1978.

DISLOCATED VERTEBRAL BODIES

Vertebral body dislocation usually results from trauma, but also can be seen with disk, or vertebral body, infection, and severe congenital defects of the vertebral bodies and neural arches. However, physiologic, anterior dislocation in the upper cervical spine is the commonest cause of vertebral body dislocation in childhood (Table 6.20). Almost always such dislocation occurs anteriorly on flexion (Fig. 6.29A), but it also can occur posteriorly on extension (Fig. 6.29B). When such dislocations occur at multiple levels, as illustrated in Figure 6.29, A and B, accepting them as physiologic is not difficult, but when the phenomenon is isolated to one level, solving the problem can be more difficult. Most often such isolated dislocation occurs anteriorly at the C_2–C_3 level of the cervical spine (Fig. 6.30A). Indeed, so disturbing is the finding that one's first consideration usually is that of pathologic dislocation. Pathologic dislocation does occur at this level, with a hangman's fracture (Fig. 6.30C), and to facilitate differentiating of the two conditions, one can utilize the posterior cervical line (1). This line, applied from the anterior cortex of the spinous process of C_1 to the anterior cortex of the spinous process of C_3, should not pass more than 1 to 1.5 mm anterior to

the cortex of the spinous process of C_2 (1). If it does, a fracture should be suspected (6.30C), and contrarily, if it falls within normal range, no matter how serious the problem appears, physiologic dislocation only is present (Fig. 6.30B).

As far as true, traumatic dislocations of the vertebral bodies are concerned, most often these occur anteriorly, in the cervical spine, and are the result of flexion–rotation, or whiplash injuries (Fig. 6.31A). In any of these cases, disruption of the disk space and its surrounding ligaments is the cause of dislocation. Lateral dislocation also occurs with trauma, but is less

Table 6.20 Vertebral Body Dislocation

Physiologic—cervical spine	}	Commonest
Traumatic dislocation Lumbar spondylolysis—spondylolisthesis	}	Moderately common
Dislocation with infection Dislocation with congenital anomalies	}	Relatively rare

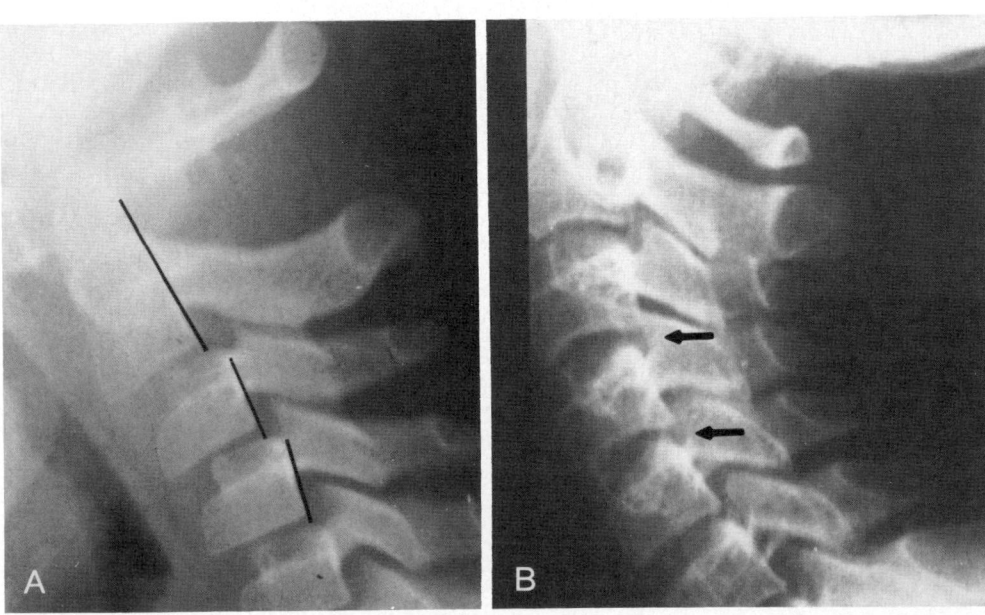

Fig. 6.29. Dislocated vertebral bodies. A. Physiologic anterior dislocation of cervical spine at multiple levels. B. Physiologic posterior dislocation of the cervical spine at two levels (arrows). Posterior dislocation rarely occurs beyond this degree.

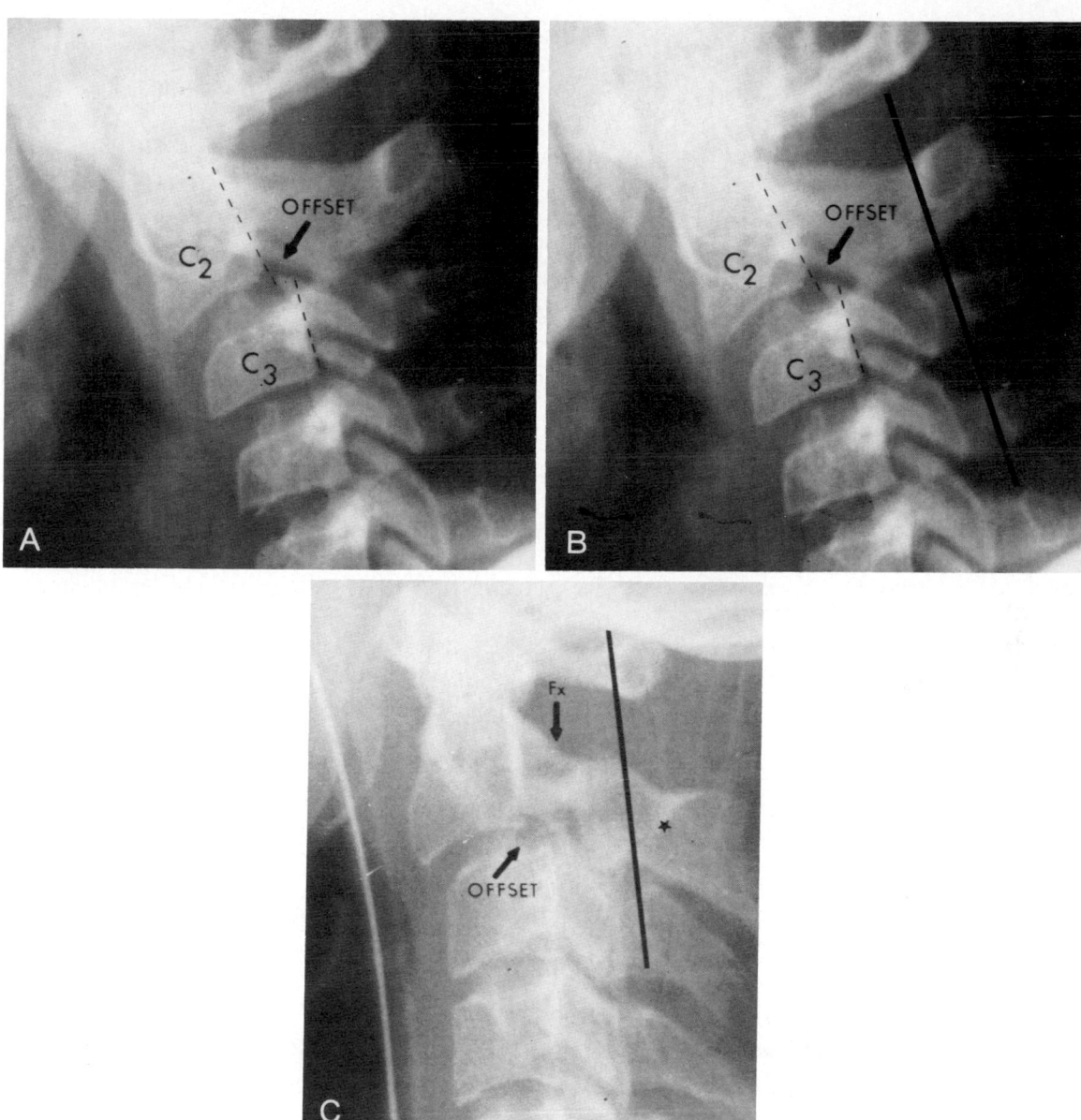

Fig. 6.30. Physiologic versus pathologic dislocation C₂–C₃. A. Note dislocation or offsetting of C₂ on C₃. Spine is flexed. B. Posterior cervical line touches the cortex of C₂ because the posterior elements of C₂ have moved forward with the body. No true dislocation is present. C. Hangman's fracture (Fx) with anterior displacement of C₂. Because of the fracture, the posterior elements of C₂ remain posterior, and the distance between the posterior cervical line and spinus process of C₂ now is increased beyond 2 mm. This signifies pathologic dislocation.

common and usually is due to severe, combined rotation-flexion or extension injuries. Dislocations associated with disk or apophyseal joint infection are relatively uncommon and so are congenital dislocations due to absence, or large defects, of the vertebral bodies and neural arches (Fig. 6.31, B and C).

References

1. Swischuk LE: Anterior displacement of C₂ in children: Physiologic or pathologic? A helpful differentiation. *Radiology* 122:759–763, 1977.

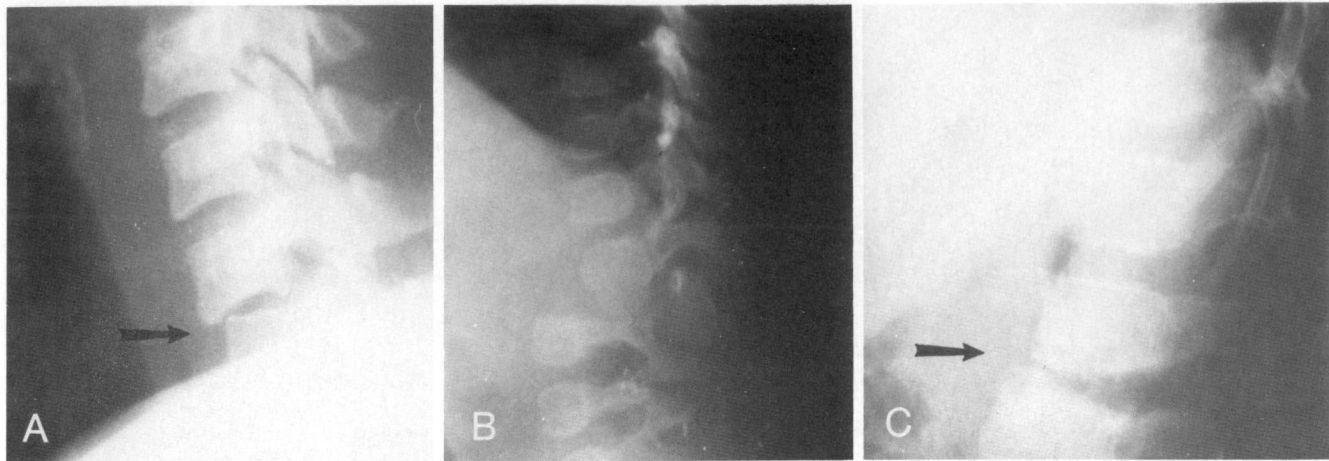

Fig. 6.31. Vertebral body dislocation. A. Anterior dislocation of C_6 on C_7 (arrow), due to unilateral locked facet. Also note that the disk space is narrow. This occurs with this type of injury. B. Gross dislocation due to congenital absence of vertebral body and partial absence of posterior elements. C. Dislocation secondary to diskitis (arrow).

SPINOUS TIP MALALIGNMENT

Midline malalignment of the spinous tips occurs with rotatory injuries resulting in unilateral locked or perched facets. In such cases the spinous tips above and below the level of rotation are offset, one on the other. In other words, they do not follow a straight line down the midsagittal plane. A note of caution is offered here, as one should be aware that congenital anomalies of the spinous tips may make the tips appear displaced.

Increased vertical intraspinous distance is seen with hyperflexion injuries causing rupture of the posterior ligaments, and also with Chance fractures (1–3), of the thoracolumbar spine. This type of spinous mala-lignment also can be mimicked by anomalous maldevelopment of the posterior elements. In children, the distance between C_1 and C_2, on flexion normally is quite wide.

References

1. Chance GQ: Note on type of flexion fracture of spine. *Br J Radiol* 21:452–453, 1948.
2. Smith WE, Kaufer H: Patterns and mechanisms of lumbar injuries associated with lap-seat belts. *J Bone Joint Surg* 51-A:239, 1969.
3. Steckler RM, Epstein JA, Epstein BS: Seat Belt trauma to lumbar spine: unusual manifestation of seat belt syndrome. *J Trauma* 9:508–513, 1969.

ABNORMALITIES OF THE APOPHYSEAL JOINTS

Deformity of the apophyseal joints associated with congenital anomalies of the spine are straightforward. Apart from this, apophyseal joint abnormalities are rather uncommon in children, but basically consist of joints being too wide, too narrow, or dislocated (Fig. 6.32). Joints which are too wide result from injuries associated with ligamentous tears, and widening often is accentuated with traction (Fig. 6.32A). Many times these injuries are the result of flexion-rotation forces and then, the apophyseal joints may become dislocated in the so-called locked, or perched, facet position (6.32C).

Congenital narrowing of the apophyseal joints does occur and, actually, most often takes the form of fusion (Fig. 6.32B). However, narrowing of the apophyseal joints also occurs with rheumatoid arthritis (Fig. 6.33). Many times these changes lag behind clinical symptoms, and most often joint involvement first is noted at the C_2–C_3 area, or in the lower cervical spine. In the most severe form of rheumatoid arthritis, that is Still's disease, one occasionally can have obliteration of all of the apophyseal joints, and ankylosis to the point of bamboo spine formation (Fig. 6.33). Narrowing of the apophyseal joints also can occur with traumatic dislocation, and with pyogenic infection causing destruction.

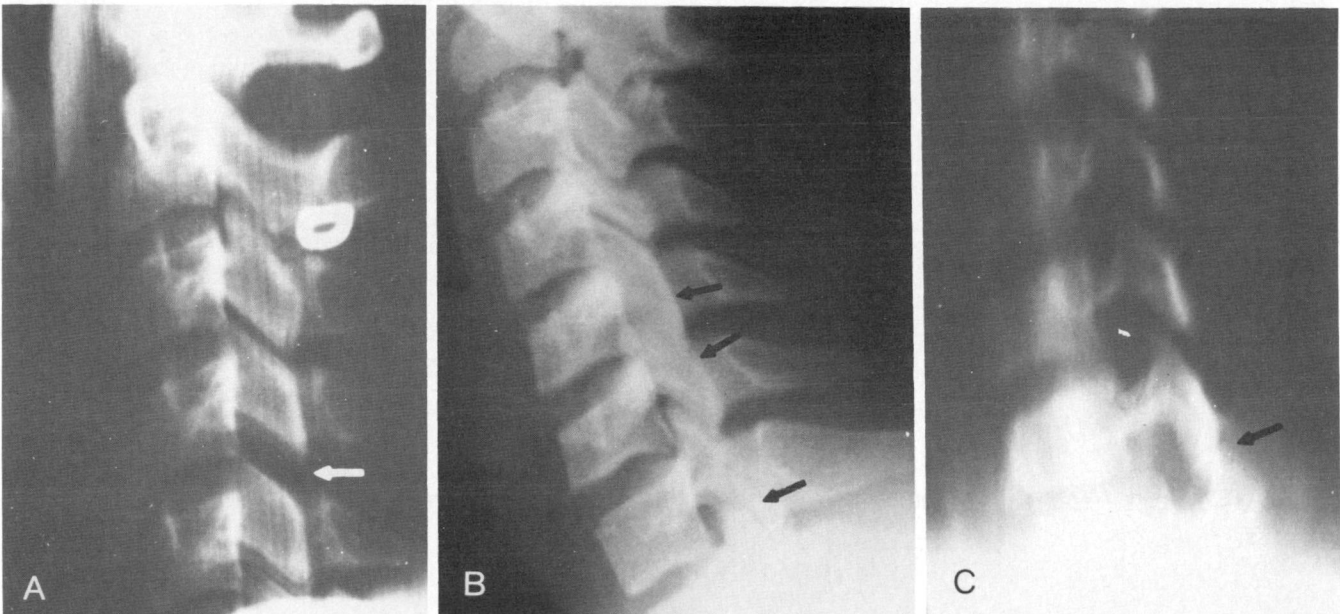

Fig. 6.32.   Apophyseal joint abnormalities. A. Widening of the apophyseal joint after traumatic dislocation (arrow). Patient is in traction. The initial injury was locked facet. B. Congenital narrowing of the lower cervical and upper thoracic apophyseal joints (arrows). Also note associated rudimentary disk at the C_7–T_1 level. The apophyseal joints in the midcervical spine are completely ankylosed on a congenital basis. C. Dislocated, locked, or jumped facet (arrow) visualized on oblique view.

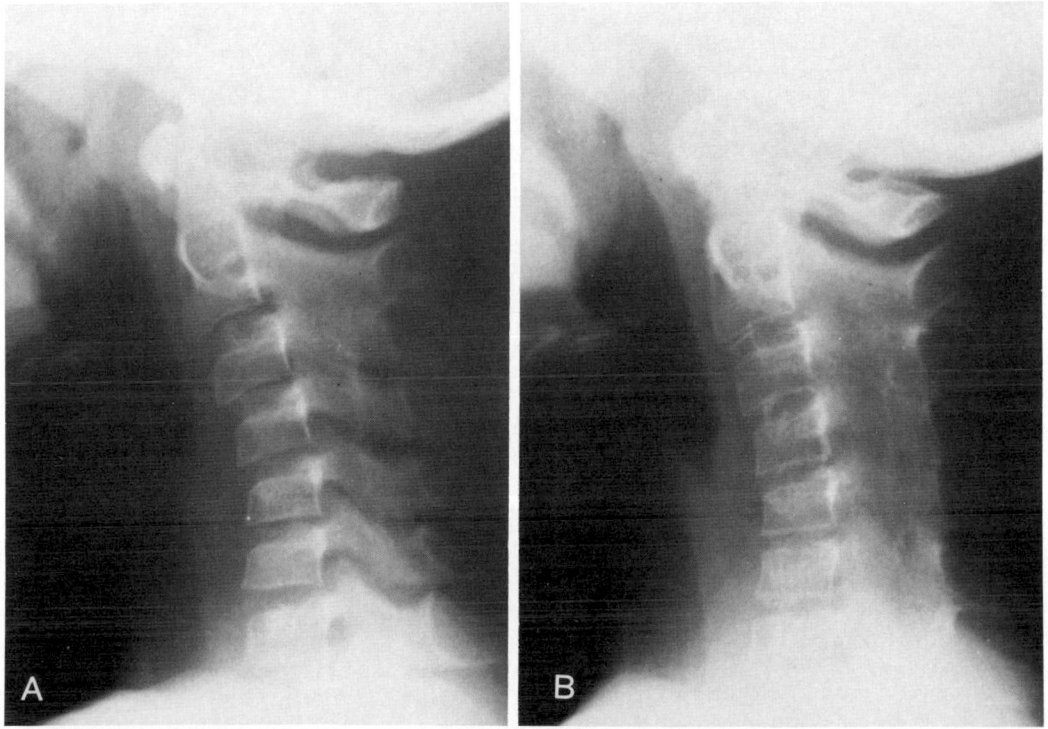

Fig. 6.33.   Apophyseal joint fusion in rheumatoid arthritis. A. Note early fusion of apophyseal joints. B. Later on, complete fusion and a bamboo spine result. This usually occurs in Still's disease.

DISK ABNORMALITIES

The intravertebral disks can be (a) narrower than normal, (b) thicker than normal, or (c) calcified (Table 6.21). When narrow they may be smooth or irregular but when thick they usually are smooth and biconvex.

Table 6.21 Disk Abnormalities

Narrowed disks	
Infection (diskitis, spondyloarthritis, osteomyelitis)	Commonest
Scheuermann's disease Congenital narrowing (blocked vertebra)	Moderately common
Acute trauma (flexion-rotation) Spondyloepiphyseal dysplasia Morquio's disease	Relatively rare
Cockayne's syndrome Ruvalcaba syndrome Ankylosing spondylitis Kniest's syndrome	Rare
Widened disks	
Osteoporosis, osteomalacia End plate infarction (sickle cell, Gaucher's)	Commonest
Trauma (hyperextension)	Moderately common
Disk calcification	
Idiopathic (cervical)	Commonest
Idiopathic (thoracolumbar) Ochronosis Hemochromatosis Hyperparathyroidism Hypervitaminosis D Pseudogout Ankylosing spondylitis	Rare

Disk Narrowing

Disk narrowing can be due to congenital underdevelopment of a disk (i.e., blocked vertebra), disk and adjacent vertebral infection or inflammation, and discovertebral trauma. Congenitally narrowed disks can occur anywhere and may be single (Fig. 6.34A) or multiple. Usually there is some underdevelopment of the adjacent vertebral bodies but the vertebral bodies themselves are rather smooth and otherwise, intact. With disk infection or inflammation, disk space narrowing eventually is associated with adjacent vertebral body destruction, but this may not be overtly apparent in the early stages (Fig. 6.34, B and C). Such infection can occur anywhere in the spine, but most often it is seen in the upper lumbar region (1, 3, 4, 9, 14, 18–20). When seen in the thoracic spine, tuberculosis should be considered first (8), but in other areas, nontuberculous, pyogenic infection is more likely.

When disk narrowing, associated with adjacent vertebral body destruction, occurs in the lumbar spine, often it is referred to as childhood diskitis or spondyloarthritis. There is difference in opinion as to whether the problem always is secondary to infection. However, most favor this etiology, even though organisms cannot be cultured from all patients. Most often symptoms consist of back pain and an inability to bend over. In addition, there may be a limp or actual refusal to walk. The degree and rate of vertebral destruction in the adjacent vertebral bodies is variable and some cases apparently are self-limiting, even without antibotic therapy. This is one of the reasons why those who favor a traumatic etiology (i.e., subclinical trauma) support the trauma concept. Whatever the cause, the roentgenographic findings are rather characteristic. In the early stages, when plain films are inconclusive, isotope bone scans are in order (7, 15).

Disk destruction, secondary to infection, also can be seen after spinal puncture (12), and also has been reported in sarcoidosis (19). It might be noted at this point that, with infections such as coccidioidomycosis and aspergillosis (16), even though vertebral body destruction may be extensive, the intervening disks usually remain intact. Disk space narrowing, as it

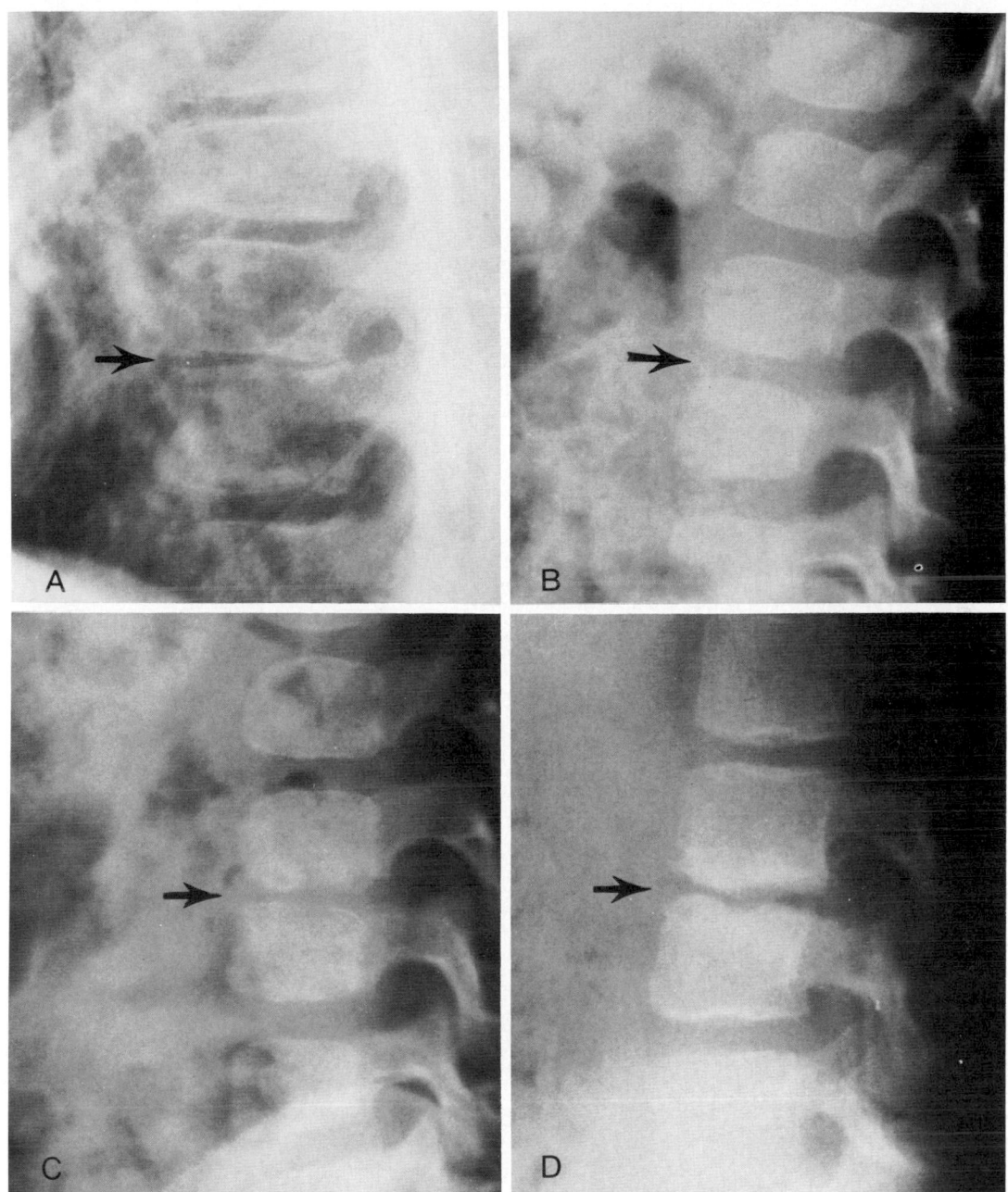

Fig. 6.34. Disk narrowing. A. Congenitally narrowed intravertebral disk (arrows). B. Early disk narrowing in diskitis (arrow). C. Two weeks later, disk narrowing is more pronounced (arrow). Early vertebral destruction also is seen. D. Another patient in later stages, showing persistent narrowing (arrow) and irregularity of the end plates.

occurs in ankylosing spondylitis in adults (4, 6), is not common in children, mostly because the disease is not common in children (10, 11).

Spine trauma leading to disk disruption almost always is due to flexion or flexion-rotation forces (Fig. 6.35A). Contrarily with extension injuries, there is tendency for the disk space to become wider than normal (Fig. 6.35A). In Scheuermann's disease the problem also probably is trauma, but trauma is sub-

clinical (15). In these patients, kyphosis of the thoracic spine, pain in many instances, and irregular disk space narrowing constitute the findings (Fig. 6.35B).

Herniation of disk material into the end plates is common and if it occurs anteriorly, notched or beaked vertebrae result (see Fig. 6.21). Disk irregularities similar to those seen in Scheuermann's disease have been noted in the Ruvalcaba syndrome (17), Cockayne's syndrome, spondyloepiphyseal dysplasia, Mor-

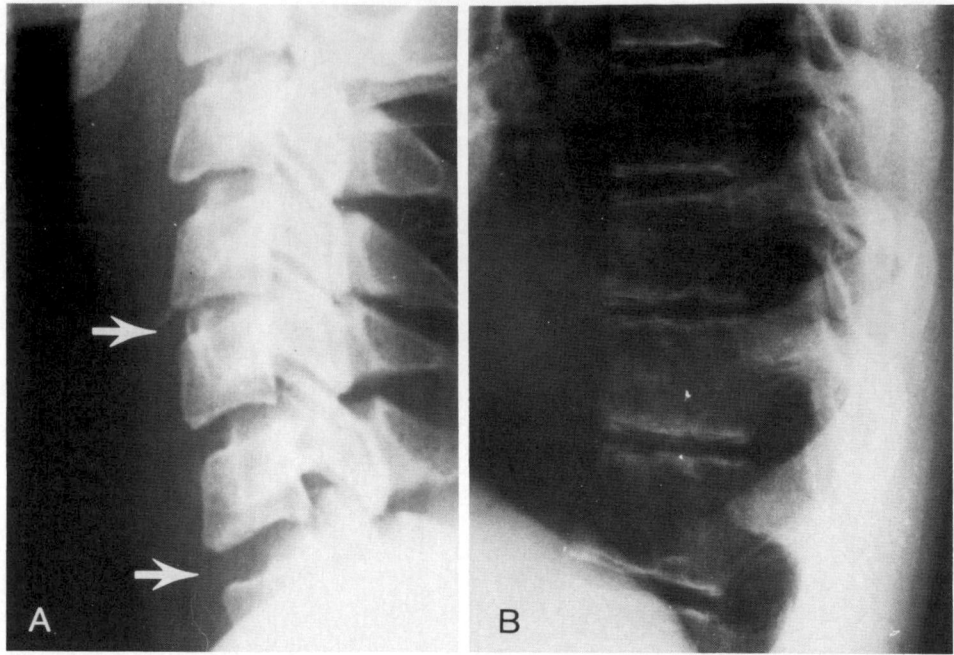

Fig. 6.35. Disk narrowing and widening. A. Note disk narrowing due to flexion injury (upper arrow). Also note associated avulsion fracture. Disk widening (lower arrow) is present and is due to an extension injury. This patient had both extension and flexion injuries. B. Uniformly thin, irregular disks in Scheuermann's disease.

quio's disease, and Kniest's syndrome. Acute disk herniation leading to narrowed disk spaces is uncommon in children.

References

1. Alexander CJ: The aetiology of juvenile spondylarthritis (discitis). *Clin Radiol* 21:178–187, 1970.
2. Bolivar R, Kohl S, Pickering LK: Vertebral osteomyelitis in children: report of four cases. *Pediatrics* 62:549–553, 1978.
3. Childe AE, Tucker FR: Spondyloarthritis in infants and children. *J Can Assoc Radiol* 12:47–51, 1961.
4. Dihlmann W, Delling G: Disco-vertebral destructive lesions (so-called Andersson lesions) associated with ankylosing spondylitis. *Skeletal Radiol* 3:10–16, 1978.
5. Fischer GW, Popich GA, Sullivan DE, Mayfield G, Mazat BA, Patterson PH: Discitis: a prospective diagnosis analysis. *Pediatrics* 62:543–548, 1978.
6. Frank P, Gleeson J: Destructive vertebral lesions in ankylosing spondylitis. *Br J Radiol* 48:755–758, 1975.
7. Gates GF: Scintigraphy of discitis. *Clin Nucl Med* 2:20–25, 1977.
8. Goldblatt M, Cremin BJ: Osteoarticular tuberculosis: its presentation in colored races. *Clin Radiol* 29:669–677, 1978.
9. Jamison RC, Heimlich EM, Miethke JC, O'Loughlin, BJ: Nonspecific spondylitis of infants and children. *Radiology* 77:355–367, 1961.
10. Kleinman P, Rivelis M, Schneider R, Kaye JJ: Juvenile ankylosing spondylitis. *Radiology* 125:775–780, 1977.
11. Ladd JR, Cassidy JT, Martel W: Juvenile ankylosing spondylitis. *Arthritis Rheum* 14:579–590, 1971.
12. Lintermans JP, Seyhnaeve V: Spondylotic deformity of the lumbar spine and previous lumbar punctures. *Pediat Radiol* 5:181–182, 1977.
13. Martel W: Pathogenesis of cervical discovertebral destruction in rheumatoid arthritis. *Arthritis Rheum* 20:1217–1225, 1977.
14. Moes CAF: Spondylarthritis in children. *Am J Roentgenol* 91:578–587, 1964.
15. Norris S, Ehrilich MG, Keim DE, Guitermann H, McKusick KA: Early diagnosis of disc-space infection using Gallium-67. *J Nucl Med* 19:384–386, 1978.
16. Rassa M: Vertebral aspergillosis with perservation of the disc. *Br J Radiol* 50:918–920, 1977.
17. Ruvalcaba RHA, Reichert A, Smith DW: A new familial syndrome with osseous dysplasia and mental deficiency. *J Pediatr* 79:450–455, 1971.
18. Spiegel PG, Kengla KW, Isaacson AS, Wilson JC Jr: Intervertebral disc-space inflammation in children. *J Bone Joint Surg* 54A:284–296, 1972.
19. Stump D, Spock A, Grossman H: Vertebral sarcoidosis in adolescents. *Radiology* 121:153–155, 1976.
20. Wenger DR, Bobechko WP, Gilday DL: The spectrum of intervertebral disc-space infection in children. *J Bone Joint Surg* 60:100–108, 1978.

Thickened Disks

Disks do not thicken per se, but rather they become thick because (a) they expand into softened vertebral bodies or (b) ligament injury allows adjacent vertebral bodies to be separated, causing the disk to expand. The latter occurs, for the most part, with extension injuries of the spine (Fig. 6.35A). Universally thickened disks usually are associated with biconcave vertebral bodies, and very often the problem is extensive osteoporosis or osteomalacia of the spine (see Fig. 6.16B). The disks also become a little widened with end plate infarction as seen in sickle cell disease and Gaucher's disease. Indeed, the disk spaces appear wider than normal with any cause of biconcave vertebral bodies.

Schmorl's Nodes

Schmorl's nodes are herniations of the nucleus pulposis into the adjacent vertebral bodies. When they occur in the center, they produce characteristic bulges and are most often seen in normal individuals (see Fig. 6.16C). If they occur around the periphery of the vertebral body, vertebral notching results (see Fig. 6.21).

Disk Calcification

Disk calcification is uncommon in children, except as it occurs on an idiopathic basis in the cervical spine (1, 3, 4, 6). The etiology of such calcification is unknown, but subclinical trauma or viral infection have been suggested. Most often these patients have neck pain, a wry neck deformity, and considerable spasm of the paraspinal muscles. The calcified disks, often slightly expanded, are characteristic (Fig. 6.36A). The condition is self limiting and the calcifications tend to disappear with time. In the interval, however, there may be anterior or posterior herniation of the calcifications, but this does not seem to lead to neurologic sequelae (2, 5). Less frequently, these calcifications can be seen in the thoracic or even, upper lumbar spine (Fig. 6.36B).

Other causes of disk calcification, such as ochronosis, ankylosing spondylitis, gout, hemochromatosis, hyperparathyroidism, hypervitaminosis D, degenerative disease, and pseudogout are very rare in children.

References

1. Henry MJ, Grimes HA, Lane JW: Intervertebral disk calcification in childhood. *Radiology* 89:81–84, 1967.
2. Mainzer F: Herniation of the nucleus pulposus. A rare complication of intervertebral disk calcification in children. *Radiology* 107:167–170, 1973.
3. Melnick JC, Silverman FN: Intervertebral disk calcifications in childhood. *Radiology* 80:399–408, 1963.
4. Mikity VG, Isenbarger J: Intervertebral disk calcification in children. *Am J Roentgenol* 95:200–202, 1965.
5. Sutton TJ, Turcotte B: Posterior herniation of calcified intervertebral disks in children. *J Can Assoc Radiol* 24:131–136, 1973.
6. Swick H: Calcification of intervertebral disks in childhood. *J Pediatr* 86:364–369, 1975.

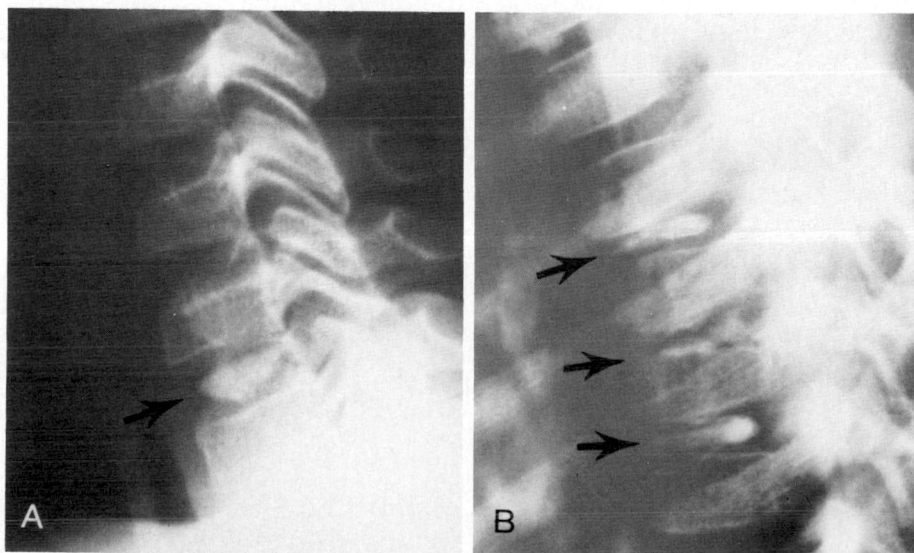

Fig. 6.36. Disk calcification. A. Note typical cervical disk calcification (arrow). B. Another patient with similar calcifications in the thoracic spine (arrows).

ABNORMAL SPINAL CURVATURES

Abnormal curvatures of the spine consists of scoliosis, kyphosis, and lordosis (Tables 6.22–6.23). In some patients, kyphosis and scoliosis are combined, but lordosis usually is an isolated problem.

Table 6.22   Scoliosis

Paraspinal muscle spasm Idiopathic rotoscoliosis	Commonest
Rotoscoliosis with muscle hypotonia Scoliosis with vertebral anomalies Congenital heart disease	Moderately common
Radiation therapy Scoliosis with intraspinal and spinal tumors Scoliosis with neurofibromatosis Scoliosis with unilateral bar	Relatively rare

Table 6.23   Kyphosis

Normal-thoracolumbar in infants Cervical spine angulation, C_2–C_3-normal	Commonest
Compression fractures (regular-pathologic) Infection with vertebral destruction Congenital spine anomalies Storage diseases Chondrodystrophies and Scheuermann's disease	Moderately common
Absent vertebral body Spine and spinal cord tumors Radiation therapy Underlying spinal cord disease (other than tumor)	Relatively rare

Scoliosis

The commonest cause of scoliosis is paraspinal muscle spasm secondary to some spinal, paraspinal, intraabdominal or intrathoracic inflammatory or traumatic lesion. After muscle spasm, scoliosis usually is idiopathic in nature. This form of scoliosis is most common in females and suspected to be due to inherent muscle imbalance (3, 5, 9, 11, 12, 17). Scoliosis of this type is termed rotoscoliosis because, together with a

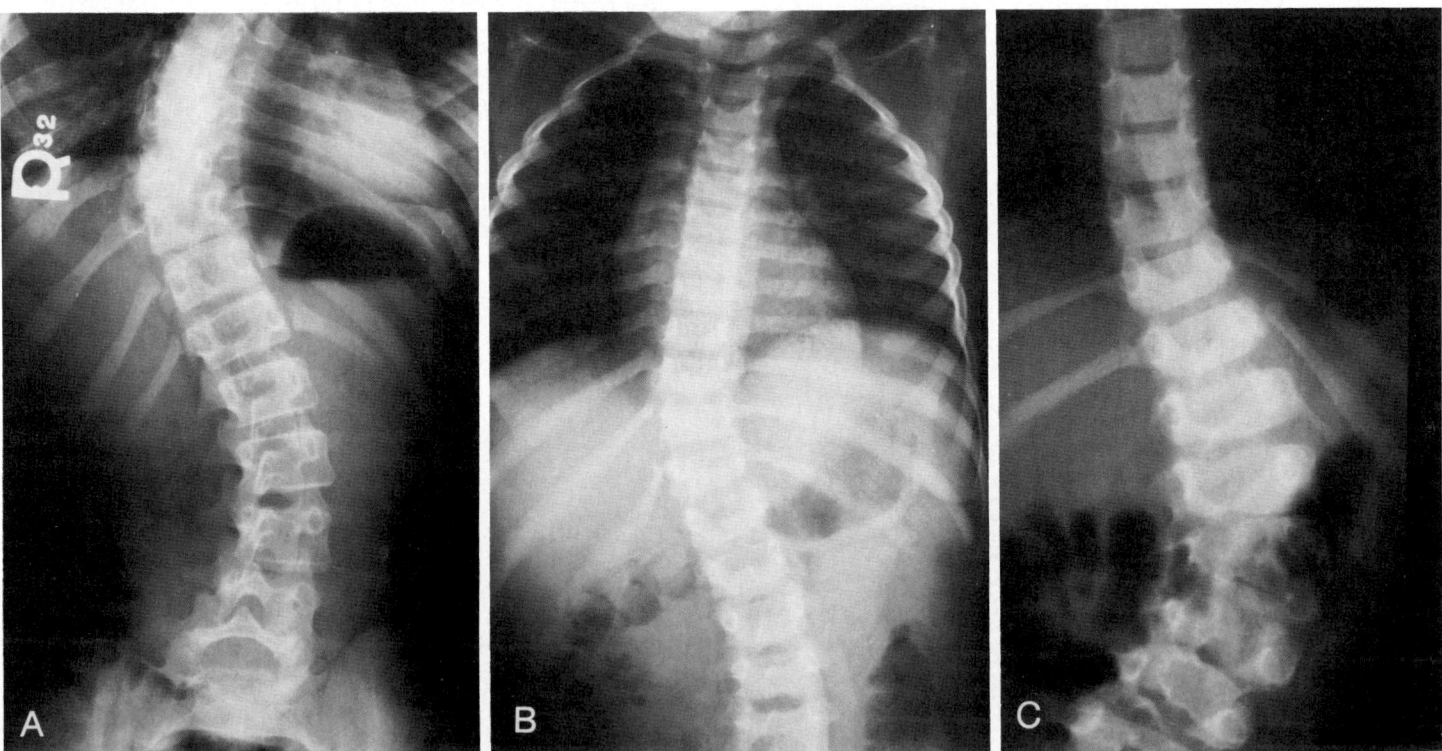

Fig. 6.37.   Scoliosis. A. Typical rotatory scoliosis. B. Angular scoliosis in neurofibromatosis. C. Angular scoliosis due to unilateral bar on the right.

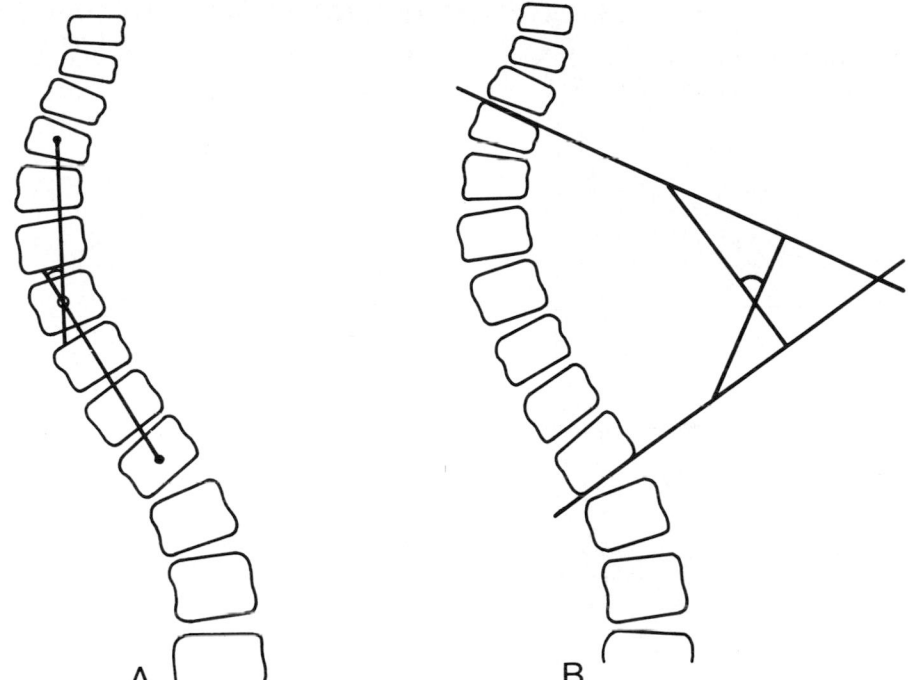

Fig. 6.38.   Scoliosis measurement. A. Ferguson method of scoliosis measurement. B. Lippman-Cobb method of scoliosis measurement. Redrawn after McAlister et al. (10).

compensatory upper curve, a rotatory arrangement of the vertebral bodies is present. The rotatory component is best assessed by noticing the position of the spinus processes and pedicles (Fig. 6.37A). In mild cases, the rotatory component is barely perceptible, while in advanced cases, associated kyphosis may be seen. This type of scoliosis also is seen in cerebral palsy and other neuromuscular conditions with muscular imbalance or hypotonia.

When scoliosis is due to some underlying spine or spinal cord problem, (i.e., tumor, infection, neurofibromatosis, etc), or to an anomaly such as a sagittal hemivertebra or a unilateral bar, often it is more angular than rotatory (Fig. 6.37, B and C). It is important to appreciate this configuration, for slight degrees of angular scoliosis may provide the first clue to the presence of a significant abnormality of the spine or spinal cord. Congenital anomalies of the spine leading to such scolioses are rather straightforward, except for the so-called unilateral bar, which may require laminography for adequate delineation. In this condition there is fusion, in a bar-like fashion, of the vertebra on one side, and this inhibits growth to the point of causing scoliosis (Fig. 6.37C).

There are numerous methods of measuring scoliosis, but the two used most often are the methods of Lippman and Cobb, and Ferguson (10). Both are illustrated in Figure 6.38.

Kyphosis

The commonest cause of kyphosis is normal, physiologic bending of the thoracolumbar spine in infants (Table 6.23). Because of natural hypotonia, especially in the sitting position, kyphosis of the thoracolumbar junction occurs, and can be associated with vertebral notching (see Fig. 6.22A). As these normal infants grow older, muscle tone increases, and the kyphosis and notching disappear (15). If, however, hypotonia is pathologic, for any number of causes, kyphosis and notching persist (15). For the most part this occurs in many of the storage diseases, achondroplasia and other chondrodystrophies, hypothyroidism, and any neurologic or neuromuscular condition leading to hypotonia.

Another time when kyphosis may appear dramatic, and yet be normal, is when it occurs at the C_2–C_3 level. Because of muscle spasm or voluntary flexion, a child's head becomes cocked forward. The resulting angulation of C_2 on C_3 may at first erroneously suggest pathologic dislocation (Fig. 6.39). However, when it is noted that C_2 is not anteriorly displaced in C_3, but merely angulated, one can discount thoughts of dislocation. When actual displacement of C_2 on C_3 occurs, differentiation from a hangman's fracture becomes important (see Fig. 6.30).

Localized kyphosis, at any level, is seen with anterior compression fractures of the vertebral bodies (see Fig. 6.20), and with vertebral and disk infections. In addition, such localized kyphosis can be seen secondary to congenital defects of the vertebral bodies, hy-

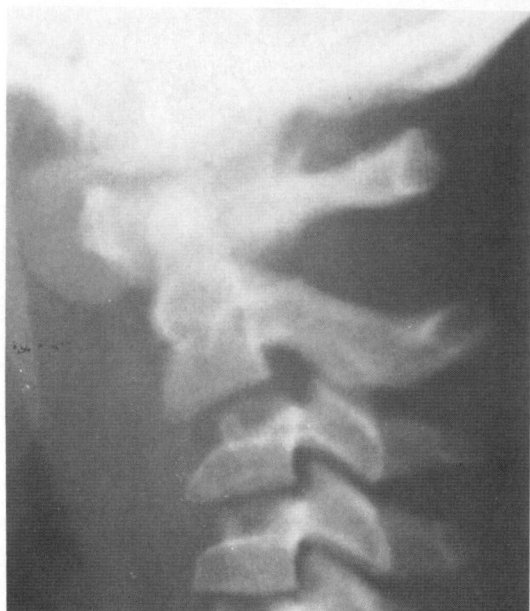

Fig. 6.39. Kyphosis. Normal angulation of C₂ on C₃, causing kyphosis, often erroneously suggesting pathologic dislocation.

poplasia of the vertebral bodies due to radiation therapy, deformity in neurofibromatosis, and with spine and spinal cord tumors. In long standing infection with healing, especially tuberculosis, the spine may fuse in a typical **gibbus deformity** (Fig. 6.40A). In some of the other conditions producing focal kyphosis, chronic anterior flexion produces underdevelopment of the vertebral bodies, and a similar gibbus deformity, without vertebral body fusion, can be seen (Fig. 6.40, B and C).

Generalized kypohosis also occurs in Scheuermann's disease (1, 4), an affliction of teenagers often associated with back pain. Its precise etiology is not known, but it is believed to represent a problem of subclinical trauma to the vertebral end plates. In essence, it is a traumatic osteochondritis (1) but, in addition, there is some feeling that there may be a genetic predisposition to the problem. The roentgenographic findings are rather typical, with irregular disk space narrowing, anterior wedging of the involved vertebral bodies, and varying degrees of kyphosis (see Fig. 6.34D). In more advanced cases, fusion of the vertebral bodies with a gibbus deformity can result (Fig. 6.40D).

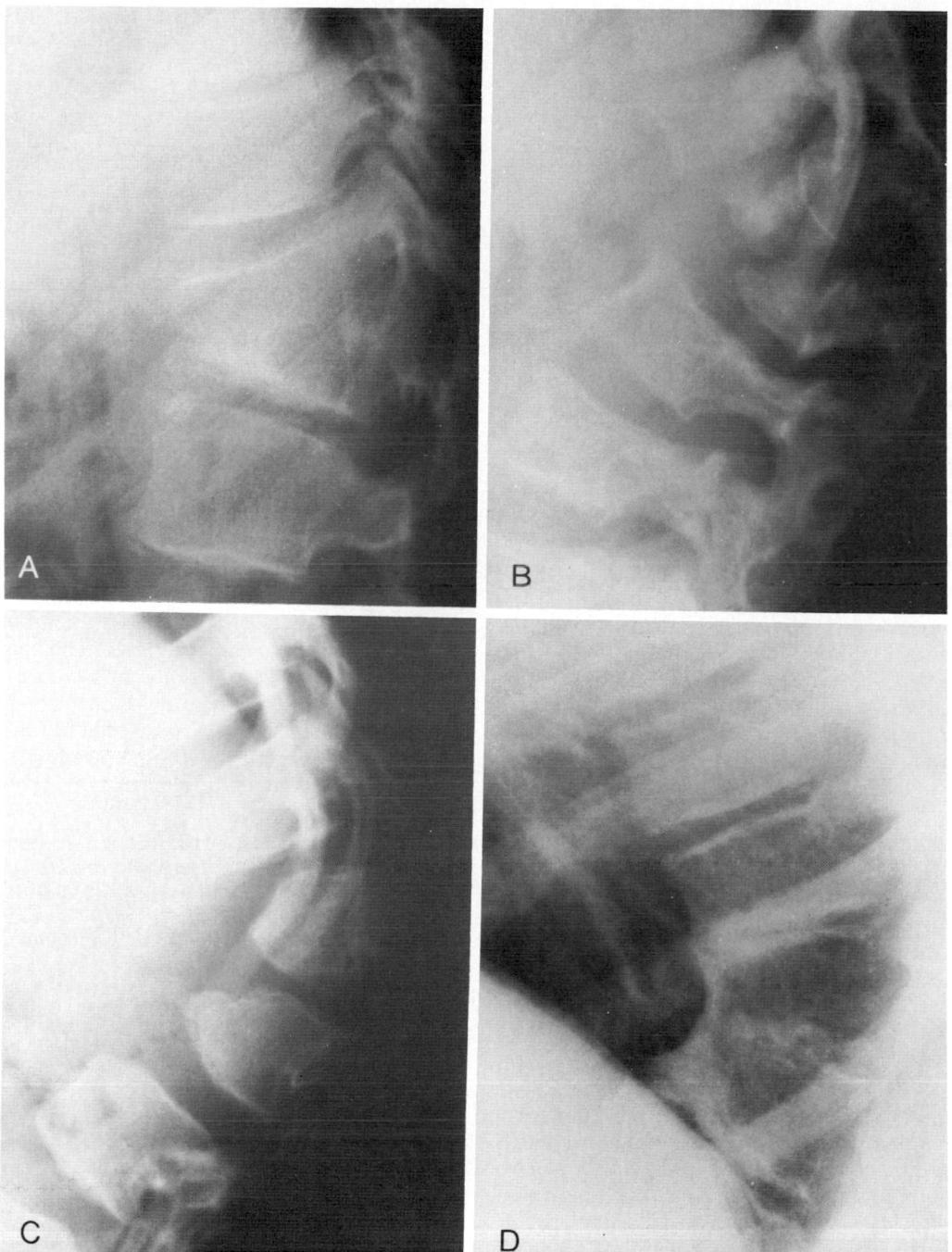

Fig. 6.40. Kyphosis-Gibbus deformity. A. Typical Gibbus deformity due to destroyed, fused vertebra in tuberculosis. B. Gibbus deformity in neurofibromatosis. C. Gibbus deformity in achondroplasia. D. Gibbus deformity secondary to kyphosis and fusion in Scheuermann's disease.

Lordosis

The commonest cause of lordosis is normal development of the spine in the lumbar region. However, exaggerated lordosis in the thoracolumbar region occurs with many chondrodystrophies, especially achondroplasia (see Fig. 6.27B). Lordosis also occurs with lumbar spondylolisthesis. Such defects currently are believed secondary to overt or subclinical trauma.

Severe degrees of lordosis also can be seen with extensive, contiguous posterior element defects.

References

1. Alexander CJ: Scheuermann's disease: a traumatic spondylodystrophy? *Skeletal Radiol* 1:209–221, 1977.
2. Fellows KE Jr, Rosenthal A: Extracardiac roentgeno-

graphic abnormalities in cyanotic congenital heart disease. *Am J Roentgenol Radium Ther Nucl Med* 114:371–379, 1972.

3. Gore DR, Passehl R, Sepic S, Dalton A: Scoliosis screening: results of a community project. *Pediatrics* 67:196–200, 1981.
4. Halal F, Gledhill RB, Fraser FC: Dominant inheritance of Scheuermann's Juvenile kyphosis. *Am J Dis Child* 132:1105–1107, 1978.
5. Jeffries BF, Tarlton M, De Smet AA, Dwyer SF II, Brower AC: Computerized measurement and analysis of scoliosis: a more accurate representation of the shape of the curve. *Radiology* 134:381–385, 1980.
6. Jordan CE, White RI Jr, Fischer KC, Neill C, Dorst JP: The scoliosis of congenital heart disease. *Am Heart J* 84:463–469, 1972.
7. Luke MJ, McDonnel EJ: Congenital heart disease and scoliosis. *J Pediatr* 73:725–733, 1968.
8. MacEwen GD, Conway JJ, Miller WT: Congenital scoliosis with a unilateral bar. *Radiology* 90:711–715, 1968.
9. McAlister WH, Schackelford GD: Classification of spinal curvatures. *Radiol Clin N Am* 13:93, 1975.
10. McAlister WH, Schackelford GD: Measurement of spinal curvatures. *Radiol Clin N Am* 13:113–121, 1975.
11. Nachemson AJ, Sahlstrandt T: Etiologic factors in adolescent idiopathic scoliosis, spine. *J Bone Joint Surg* 59A:176–184, 1977.
12. Newest views on scoliosis. *Clin Orth* 93:1–238, 1973.
13. Rickles LN, Peterson HA, Bianco AJ, Weidman WH: The association of scoliosis and congenital heart defects. *J Bone Joint Surg* 57:449–455, 1975.
14. Rothner AD, Keim H, Chutorian AM: Occult neuromuscular disease in 100 consecutive patients with scoliosis. *J Pediatr* 86:748–750, 1975.
15. Swischuk LE: The beaked, notched, or hooked vertebra: its significance in infants and young children. *Radiology* 95:661–664, 1970.
16. Wright WD, Niebauer JJ: Congenital heart disease and scoliosis. *J Bone Joint* 38A:1131–1136, 1956.
17. Young LW, Oestreich AE, Goldstein LA: Roentgenology in scoliosis: contribution to evaluation and management. *Am J Roentgenol* 108:778–795, 1970.

WRY NECK OR TORTICOLLIS

The commonest cause of wry neck or torticollis is muscle spasm, either idiopathic, or secondary to inflammation or trauma (2, 3, 5) (Table 6.24). Congenital torticollis can be seen with a shortened sternocleidomastoid muscle. As far as idiopathic torticollis is concerned, its etiology is unknown but it may represent a mild rotatory subluxation of C_1 on C_2. With true rotatory dislocation of C_1 on C_2, the C_1-dens distance is increased, while with idiopathic torticollis it is not.

Wry neck or torticollis also can be a presenting symptom of upper cervical spine or posterior fossa tumors and it is also seen in Sandifer's syndrome (1, 4). In Sandifer's syndrome, gastroesophageal reflux leads to peculiar posturing of the neck and apparent torticollis. Just why this occurs is not known but when the reflux is corrected, the abnormal posture disappears.

On frontal view, with torticollis, the spinus tip of C_2 lies on the same side of a line drawn through the dens, as the tip of the mandible (Fig. 6.41). This does not occur with simple rotation of the spine because, with simple rotation, the spinus tip of C_2 lies on the other side of the line. On lateral view, the upper cervical spine may appear very disorganized, but it is still important to note the distance between the anterior arch of C_1 and the dens. The reason for this is that idiopathic torticollis is associated with a normal distance while, in rotatory dislocation, it is increased (see Fig. 6.42C). These rotational abnormalities of C_1–C_2 currently are best demonstrated with CT scanning.

References

1. Bray PF, Herbst JJ, Johnson DG, Book LS, Ziter FA, Condon VR: Childhood gastroesophageal reflux: neurological and psychiatric syndromes mimicked. *JAMA* 237:1342–1345, 1977.
2. Clark RN: Diagnosis and management of torticollis. *Pediatr Ann* 5:43–57, 1976.

Table 6.24 Torticollis or Wry Neck

Idiopathic Trauma-spasm	Commonest
Congenital short muscle Upper cervical or posterior fossa tumor	Moderately common
Sandifer's syndrome—gastroesophageal reflux	Rare

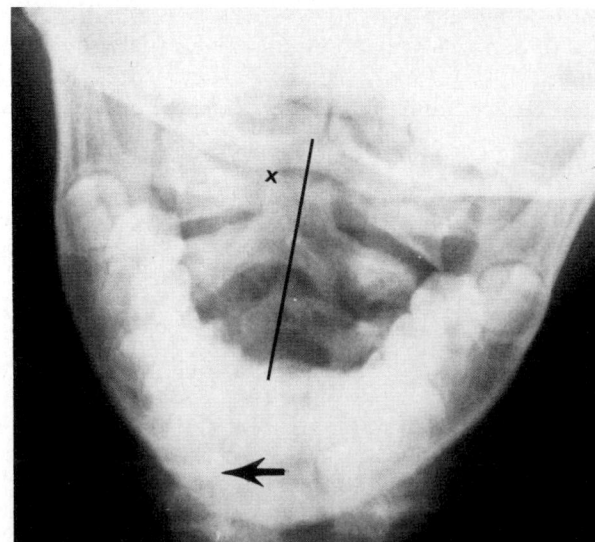

Fig. 6.41. Torticollis. Note that the spinus tip of C_2 (X) lies on the same side of a line drawn through the dens as the tip of the mandible (arrow).

3. Donaldson JS: Acquired torticollis in children and young adults. *JAMA* 160:458–461, 1956.
4. Murphy WJ Jr, Gellis SS: Torticollis with hiatus hernia in infancy. *Am J Dis Child* 131:564–565, 1977.

5. Shapiro R, Youngberg AS, Rothman SLG: The differential diagnosis of traumatic lesions of the occipito-atlanto-axial segment. *Radiol Clin N Am* 11:505–526, 1973.

UPPER CERVICAL SPINE ABNORMALITIES

Hypoplastic or Absent Dens

The commonest cause of hypoplasia or absence of the dens is congenital anomaly (1, 2, 5, 6) (Table 6.25). In such patients there often is an associated problem of C_1–C_2 instability because, along with underdevelopment of the dens, there is generalized underdevelopment of C_1–C_2 and the stabilizing ligaments (see Fig. 6.42B). In addition, the os terminale, the normal ossification center at the tip of the dens, becomes larger and more bizarre in shape, in many cases of dens hypoplasia. When this occurs, it is termed the "os odontoideum" (see Fig. 6.43C). Hypoplasia of the dens also can be acquired and usually is secondary to cervical spine injury in infancy (3, 4). In these cases, blood supply is disrupted and resorption of the dens occurs. Problems with instability also can occur in these patients. Congenital hypoplasia of the dens can occur in normal individuals but does have an increased incidence in achondroplasia, trisomy 21, Morquio's disease, other storage diseases, and punctate epiphyseal dysplasia.

Table 6.25 Hypoplastic or Absent Dens

Congenital anomaly (with certain syndromes—see text) }	Commonest
Congenital anomaly (isolated) }	Moderately common
Resorption after trauma }	Relatively rare

References

1. Garber JN: Abnormalities of the atlas and axis vertebrae—congenital and traumatic. *J Bone Joint Surg* 46A:1782, 1964.
2. Gwinn John L, Smith JL: Acquired and congenital absence of the odontoid process. *Am J Roentgenol* 88:424–431, 1962.
3. Hawkins RJ, Fielding JW, Thompson WJ: Os odontoideum—congenital or acquired: A case report. *J Bone Joint Surg* 58A:413–414, 1976.
4. Ricciardi JE, Kaufer H, Louis DS: Acquired Os odontoideum following acute ligament injury: report of a case. *J Bone Joint Surg* 58A:410–412, 1976.
5. Shapiro R, Youngberg AS, Rothman SLG: The differential diagnosis of traumatic lesions of the occipitoatlanto-axial segment. *Radiol Clin N Am* 11:505–526, 1973.
6. Von Torklus D, Gehle W: *The Upper Cervical Spine.* New York, Grune and Stratton, 1972.

Increased C₁-Dens Distance

The C_1-dens distance normally is wider in children than in adults and, indeed, this is the commonest cause of widening in children (Table 6.26). A distance of 2 to 3 mm is very common and, actually, measurements up to 4 to 5 mm in 2 to 3% of normals can be seen (3, 7). Nonetheless, pathologic widening still occurs and, just because a normal measurement can be in the realm of 4 to 5 mm, this should not be taken to infer that all such measurements are normal. On the other hand, it does indicate the need for a certain degree of caution in interpreting C_1-dens distance in children (Fig. 6.42A). In addition, it should be noted that the C_1-dens distance can open up to 2 mm with flexion and still be normal.

With pathologic widening of the C_1-dens distance, one should first consider congenital laxity of the ligaments and associated hypoplasia of the dens and C_1 (Fig. 6.42B). This can occur on an isolated basis, but more often is seen in syndromes such as trisomy 21, Morquio's disease, the storage diseases, and punctate epiphyseal dysplasia (1, 2, 5). In some of these cases, the degree of dislocation is rather profound and neurologic sequelae result (4).

The next most common cause of C_1-dens distance increase is trauma and, for the most part, such trauma consists of simple anterior dislocation of C_1 on C_2 or rotatory dislocation of C_1 on C_2 (Fig. 6.42C). After trauma, one might consider laxity of the ligaments predisposing to C_1–C_2 dislocation as is seen in rheumatoid arthritis (6) and purportedly, retropharyngeal abscess. With rheumatoid arthritis, laxity of the ligaments leads to the dislocation, but it is debatable whether retropharyngeal abscess causes any pathological widening.

Table 6.26 Increased C₁–Dens Distance

Normal }	Commonest
Congenital hypoplasia of the dens and C_1 (isolated or with syndromes—see text) }	Moderately common
Rotatory dislocation C_1–C_2 Dislocation of C_1–C_2 }	Relatively rare
Rheumatoid arthritis Morquio's disease Other storage diseases }	Rare

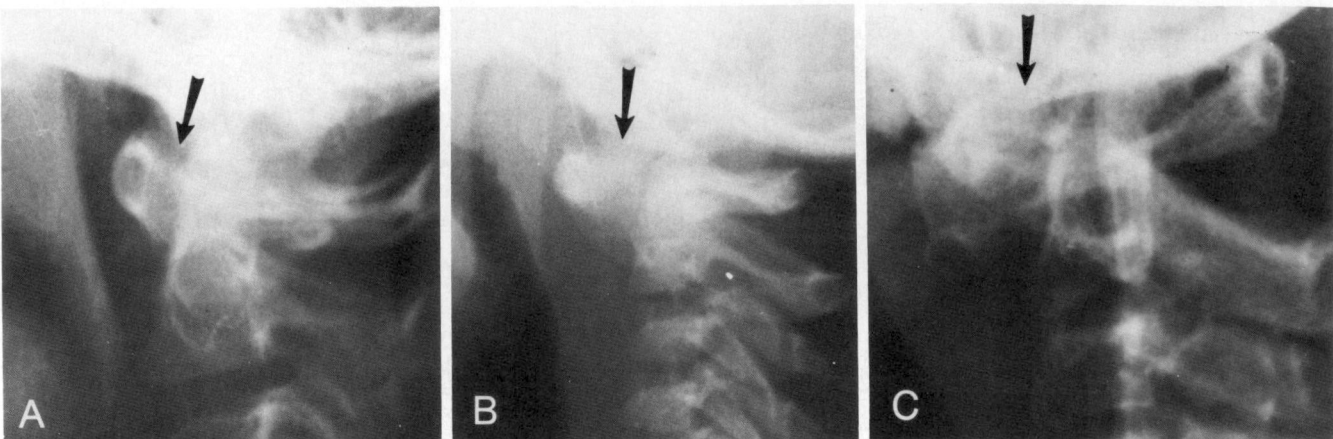

Fig. 6.42. Increased C_1-dens distance. A. Normal, generous C_1-dens distance in child. B. Hypoplastic dens and anterior dislocation of C_1 on C_2. C_1-dens distance is markedly increased. C. Increased C_1-dens distance secondary to rotatory dislocation of C_1 and C_2.

References

1. Afshani E, Girdany BR: Atlanto-axial dislocation in chondrocysplasia punctata: report of the findings in 2 brothers. *Radiology* 102:399–401, 1972.
2. Brill CB, Rose JS, Godmilow L, Sklower S, Hirschhorn K: Spastic quadriparesis due to C_1–C_2 subluxation in Hurler syndrome. *J Pediatr* 92:441–443, 1978.
3. Locke GR, Gardner JI, Van Epps EF: Atlas-dens interval (ADI) in children: a survey based on 200 normal cervical spines. *Am J Roentgenol* 97:135–140, 1966.
4. Ochiai Y, Yamamoto M, Takeshita K, Arima M: Myelopathy in infancy complicating congenital atlantoaxial dislocation. *Am J Dis Child* 130:1270–1271, 1976.
5. Pueschel SM, Scola FH, Perry CD, Pezzullo JD: Atlanto-axial instability in children with Down syndrome. *Pediatr Radiol* 10:129–132, 1981.
6. Reid GD, Hill RH: Atlantoaxial subluxation in juvenile ankylosing spondylitis. *J Pediatr* 93:531–532, 1978.
7. Swischuk LE: *Emergency Radiology of the Acutely Ill or Injured Child.* Baltimore, Williams & Wilkins, 1979, p 442.

Cervical-Occipital Ossicles

A number of ossicles normally occur at the cervical-ossicle junction because the embryologic development of this area is rather complex. Basically, however, ossicles are identified around the lip of the foramen magnum, around the anterior arch of C_1, and over the tip of the dens. The latter is completely normal and is the ossification center for the tip of the dens; the os terminale (Fig. 6.43, A and B). The os terminale can overgrow and become quite large with congenital or acquired hypoplasia of the dens. It is then termed the os odontoideum (Fig. 6.43C). The most important point about all the remaining ossicles around the cervical occipital junction is not to misinterpret them for avulsion fractures. Usually, they are quite smooth and often, totally incidental findings. Seldom are they seen in infants and young children, and it is only in adults and teenagers that one encounters them with any regularity. In the adult, however, they are quite common.

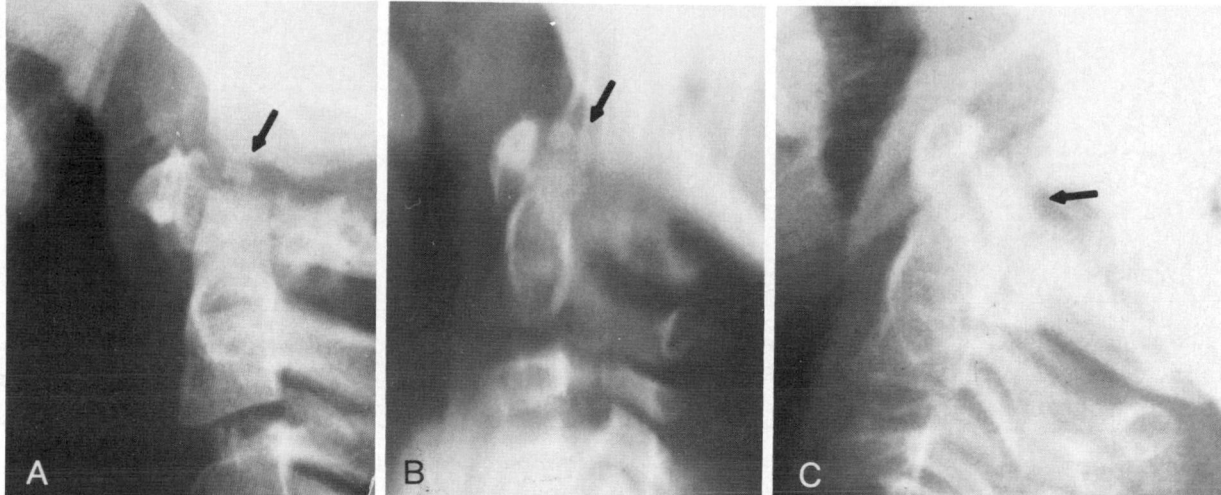

Fig. 6.43. Os terminale. A. Normal os terminale (arrow). B. Multiple, slightly larger os terminale (arrow). C. Hypoplastic dens and overgrown os terminale, resulting in os odontoideum (arrow).

SACRAL ABNORMALITIES

The sacrum can be destroyed, much as the spine in general. However, destructive lesions such as metastatic tumor, histiocytosis X, infection, etc., occur much less commonly in the sacrum than in the remainder of the spine. In the sacrum, erosion or even frank destruction can be seen with presacral tumors (12), including teratoma, sarcoma, and the rare sacral chordoma. Some of these tumors, and a variety of presacral cysts can, in some cases merely deviate the sacrum.

A curved, or sickle deformity of the sacrum (Fig. 6.44A), usually signifies some associated sacral anomaly. This can take the form of an anterior, lateral, or intrasacral meningocele, or the condition known as tether cord (Fig. 6.44B). In the latter condition, the cord is bound to the abnormal area of sacral development and, with growth, unable to rise to its normal position. Consequently, there is stretching of the cord and neurologic symptoms develop. Very frequently, an intra or, indeed, intra-extra spinal lipoma is present. Similar curving deformities and other anomalies also are seen with imperforate anus. Finally, somewhat similar sacral deformities can be seen in association with presacral teratoma and imperforate anus (1, 2, 7).

Absence of the sacrum (4, 8, 14) results in significant neurologic deficit and a characteristic appearance of the sacrum and pelvis (Fig. 6.44C). In extreme form, the condition is referred to as the caudal regression or mermaid deformity syndrome (3, 5, 9, 13). Sacral hypoplasia or agenesis is believed to result from a vascular insult to the lower spine in fetal life and is more common in infants of diabetic mothers (3, 13). Sacral agenesis also has been noted in association with presacral teratoma (1, 2, 7).

References

1. Ashcraft KW, Holder TM: Congenital anal stenosis with presacral teratoma. *Ann Surg* 162:1091–1095, 1956.
2. Ashcraft KW, Holder TM: Hereditary presacral teratoma. *J Pediatr Surg* 9:691–697, 1974.
3. Assemany SR, Muzzo S, Gardner LI: Syndrome of phocomelic diabetic embryopathy (caudal dysplasia). *Am J Dis Child* 123:489–491, 1972.
4. Banta JV, Nichols O: Sacral agenesis. *J Bone Joint Surg* 51:693–703, 1969.
5. Becker MH, Szatkowski JA, Brant EE: Case report 75, diagnosis; caudal regression syndrome. *Skeletal Radiol* 3:191–192, 1978.
6. Cohn J, Bay-Nielsen E: Hereditary defect of sacrum and coccyx with anterior sacral miningocele. *Acta Paediatr Scand* 58:268–272, 1969.
7. Currarino G, Coin D, Votteler T: Triad of Anorectal, sacral, and presacral anomalies. *Am J Roentgenol* 137:395–398, 1981.
8. Dassel PM: Agenesis of the sacrum and coccyx. *Am J Roentgenol* 85:697–700, 1961.
9. Duhamel B: From mermaid to anal imperforation syndrome of caudal regression. *Arch Dis Child* 36:152–155, 1961.
10. Grand M, Eichenfeld S, Jacobson HG: Sacral aplasia (agenesis). *Radiology* 74:611–617, 1960.
11. Kenefick JS: Hereditary sacral agenesis associated with presacral tumors. *Br J Surg* 60:271–274, 1973.
12. Macpherson RI, Young F: Sacrococcygeal tumors. *J Can Assoc Radiol* 21:132–142, 1970.
13. Passarge E, Lenz W: Syndrome of caudal regression in infants of diabetic mothers; observations of further cases. *Pediatrics* 37:672–675, 1966.
14. Thompson IM, Kirk RM, Dale M: Sacral agenesis. *Pediatrics* 54:236–238, 1974.

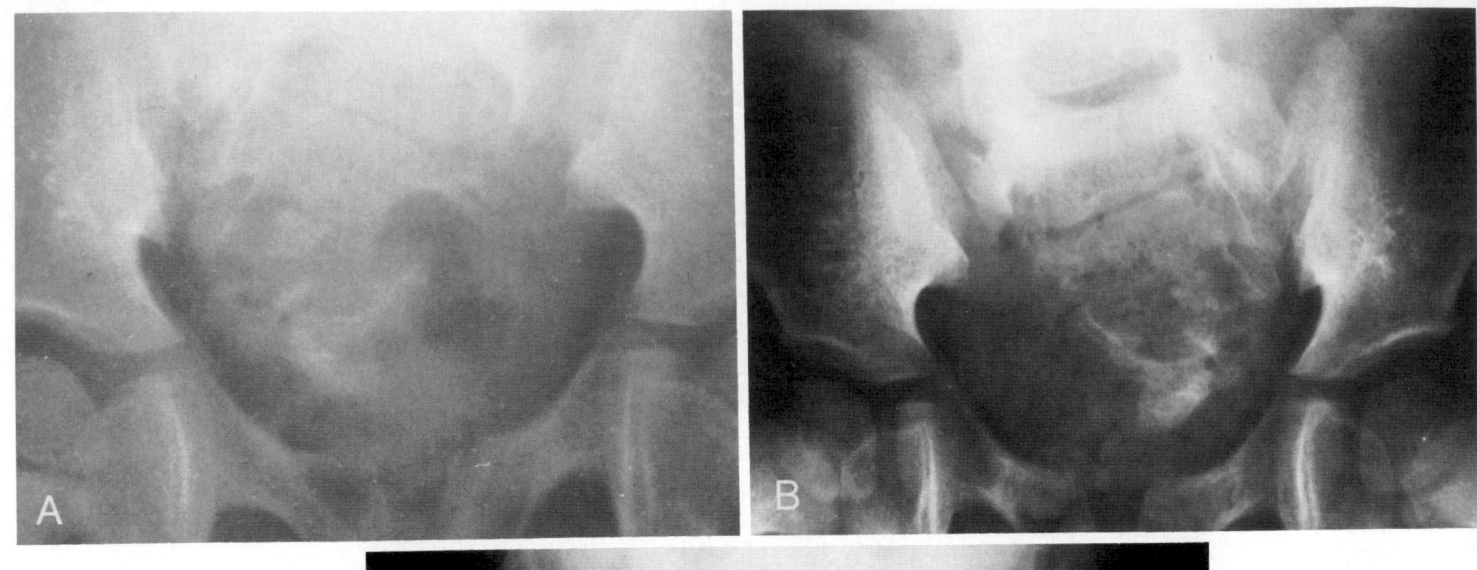

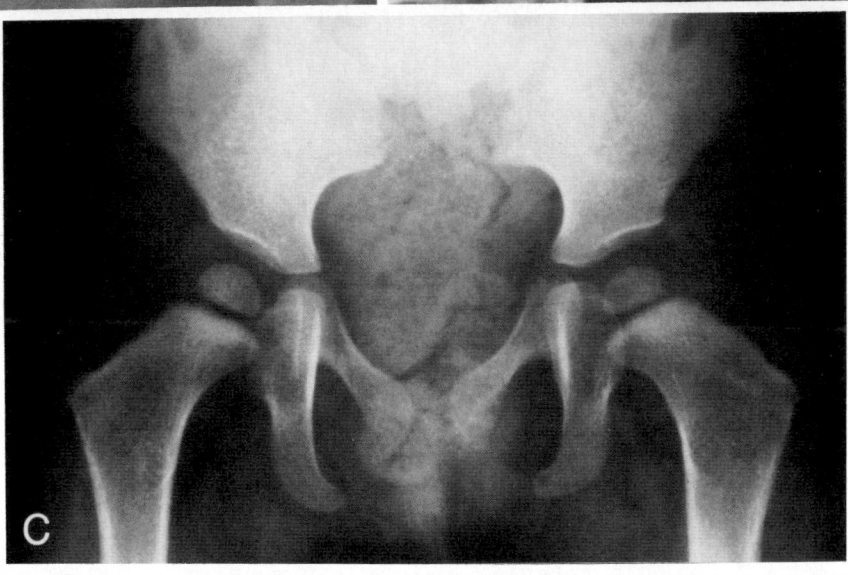

Fig. 6.44. Sacral abnormalities. A. Curved or sickle-shaped sacrum in patient with lateral meningocele. B. Curved, deformed sacrum with tethered cord. C. Absent sacrum. Note close positioning of the iliac wings.

SACROILIAC JOINT ABNORMALITIES

Widening of the sacroiliac joints can occur with traumatic separation, infection, or inflammation. All of these problems have been discussed at an earlier point (see p 277).